FLUID-ELECTROLYTE;
Acid-Base Metabolism
and Disorders

FLUID-ELECTROLYTE;

Acid-Base Metabolism and Disorders

A Clinical Emphasis Related to Physiology and Molecular Mechanisms

MICHAEL KINGSTON

Library of Congress Control Number:		2011961061
ISBN:	Hardcover	978-1-4653-0179-6
	Softcover	978-1-4653-0178-9
	Ebook	978-1-4653-0587-9

To order additional copies of this book, contact:
Xlibris Corporation
1-800-618-969
www.xlibris.com.au
Orders@xlibris.com.au
501054

CONTENTS

Rationale of Manuscript

This book may be of interest to: General Physicians, Nephrologists, Intensivists, Anaesthetists, Endocrinologists, Emergency Department Physicians, Researchers, Physiologists and Advanced Trainees. - to cover the field of Fluid-Electrolyte disorders .

This book is unique because:

- It is written by one rather then several authors as is usual in most texts on this subject. This imparts a consistent approach and style.

- It is written by a General Physician with 50 years medical experience with an academic background who has also worked as an Intensivist, Paediatrician, Surgeon and Anaesthetist and has a lifetime interest, including a MD degree in the field. There is therefore a broader focus compared to subspecialists who author most texts.

- It has a focus on Clinical aspects of Fluid-Electrolyte Disorders but relates this to current physiology and molecular mechanisms.

- It contains applied disorders which other texts often do not. For example: Chapters on Shock; Diuretics and Genetic Disorders of Tubular Transport; Interpretation of Urine Electrolytes; Approach to Oliguria, Renal Failure and Hyponatremia and Low Cardiac Output; Gastrointestinal Disorders and Electrolytes; Starvation, Diabetic Ketoacidosis and Hyperosmolar States.

- It contains challenges to traditional beliefs in several areas based on the author's experience, observations combined with critical appraisal of the literature.

- It contains the most comprehensive account of treatment of both hyperkalaemia and hypokalemia in the chapter on Potassium based on personal observations, including work successfully submitted for the MD (thesis) degree, and critical appraisal of the literature.

- It contains up to date and personal observation in the chapters on Magnesium and Phosphorous. It explains and discusses the traditional and newer Stewart-Fencl approach to Acid-base balance and Disorders and reconciles the two.

INTRODUCTION

It is not necessarily the strongest of the species that survives, nor the most intelligent; It is the one most adaptable to change. Charles Darwin.

Matter is made up of elements. Each element has identical particles called atoms and electrons.

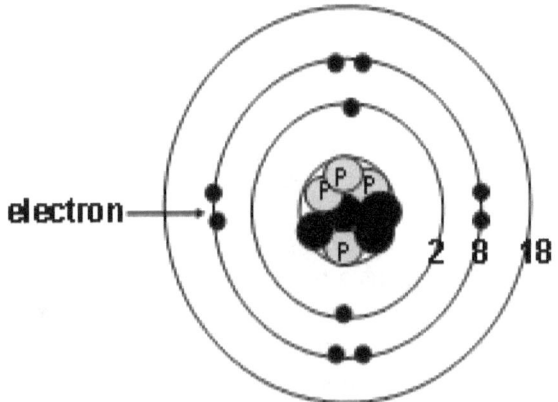

Figure 1. Model of an atom.
(P =proton; larger black circle =neutron; smaller black circle = electron)

The nucleus contains positively charged protons, neutrons of similar mass, but no charge. Electrons have minimal mass and a negative charge of similar magnitude to protons and orbit the nucleus in shells. The inner shell has 2 electrons, the next 8, the next 18 and the next (not shown) a maximum of 32 electrons.

Atoms are made up of:

- a nucleus, containing protons with a positive charge, and neutrons of similar mass but no charge.
- electrons with negative charge, equal to the charge on protons, which orbit the nucleus but have approximately 2000 times less mass

Atoms are divisible into smaller particles. To satisfy <u>electro-neutrality</u> electrons (-) must equal the number of protons (+). Atoms, which have an extra electron (negative charge), unmatched by a proton, are highly unstable, reactive and destructive and are called free radicals. For example, an extra electron added to the molecule O_2, is highly unstable. Elements are classified in the Periodic table based on the number of protons -called the atomic number. This also equals the number of electrons. Isotopes differ only in the number of neutrons in the nucleus. The simplest element hydrogen(H) contains one proton and one electron.

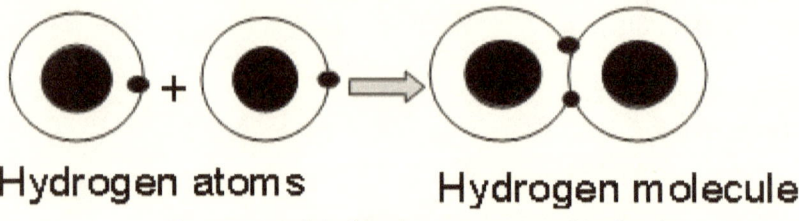

Hydrogen atoms   Hydrogen molecule

Figure 2. Model of Hydrogen atom and molecule

Electrons orbit around the nucleus at specific distances from it—called shells. Each shell only contains a maximum number of electrons specific for that shell. Shells further away from the nucleus contain more electrons. The first shell has a maximum complement of 2 electrons, the second 8, the third 18 and then 32. When a shell has a full complement of electrons additional electrons orbit around the next shell. The attraction between nucleus and electrons decreases with distance from their shells. The outer shell has the greatest tendency to react with electrons from other atoms.

Most atoms do not exist in a free state but combine to achieve stability by sharing or exchanging electrons to fill their outer shell. The number of electrons which exchange to achieve this is their valence. Exchange of electrons may occur with the same element or with different elements. For example hydrogen (H) shares an electron with another H forming the molecule hydrogen gas (H_2). (figure 2).

3 major types of bonds form between elements:

- **Ionic:** electrons are donated or accepted
- **Covalent:** electrons are shared
- **Hydrogen bonds.**

IONIC.

Sodium has a single electron and chlorine 7 electrons in their outer shells. Both are unstable because their outer shells are incomplete. When they react sodium donates its single outer shell electron to chlorine: the unstable metal sodium combines with the corrosive gas chlorine to form stable common salt (NaCl). Loss of an electron leaves sodium with a positive charge and gain of an electron leaves chloride with a negative charge. (Figure 3). In solution electrolytes conduct electricity, essential for muscle and nerve function, exert osmotic pressure, and influence acid base balance.

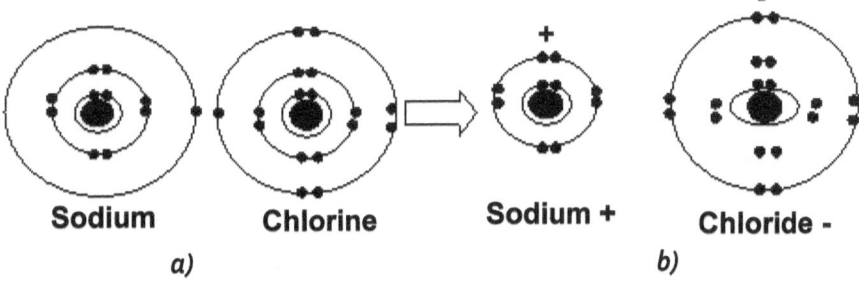

Sodium   Chlorine   Sodium +   Chloride -

a)   b)

Figure 3. Unstable sodium and chlorine react to form stable sodium chloride-common salt. Sodium donates an electron in its outer shell to chlorine which results in a completed outer shell in each case. Note that in b) sodium and chloride now have complete outer shells of 8 electrons which results in stability.

COVALENT BONDS.

One, two (double bond) or three electrons (triple bond) **are shared rather than donated between two atoms** or uncommonly one atom may provide both electrons to form covalent bonds. For example carbon (C), with 4 electrons in its outer shell, can share electrons with 4 hydrogen atoms which complete the outer shells of both C and H to form methane (CH$_4$). The valence of Carbon is 4 because it shares 4 electrons. Compounds which contain carbon are called organic.

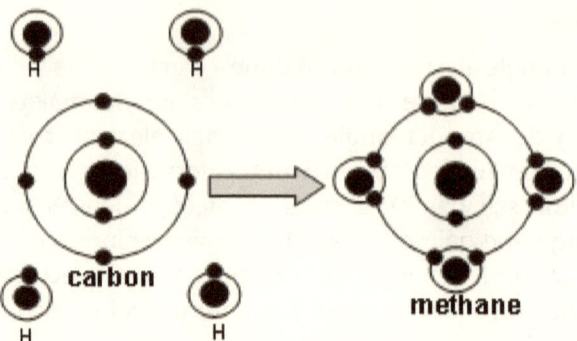

Figure 4. Model showing covalent bond formed by carbon and hydrogen to form methane. Carbon has 4 electrons in its outer shell. This achieves its full complement of 8 electrons by sharing electrons with 4 hydrogen atoms.

POLAR COVALENT BONDS.

Molecules with covalent bonds but in which sharing of electrons is slightly unequal. Electrons orbiting closer to one atom of a molecule for more than 50% of the time impart a weak negative charge, called δ^-; electrons orbiting further away from an atom results in a weak positive charge, called δ^+. Polar molecules are able to form weak bonds with other polar molecules. The best example is the hydrogen bond.

HYDROGEN BONDS.

These are polar covalent bonds involving hydrogen and either an oxygen or nitrogen atom. Water (H_2O) is formed by oxygen sharing two electrons with hydrogen. However there is an important difference compared to carbon. The positive nucleus of the oxygen atom exerts a stronger attraction for electrons of hydrogen atoms than does the hydrogen nucleus for its own electron. This skews the orbiting electrons of H toward the oxygen atom creating a small negative charge (delta -) at the oxygen end and positive charge (delta+) at the H end of the water molecule (figure 5.)

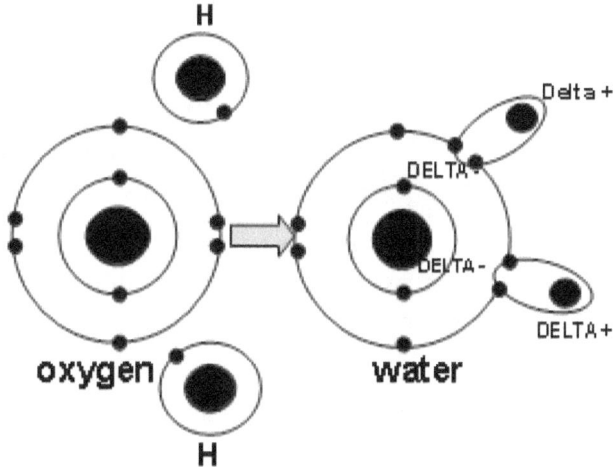

Figure 5. Model showing combination of oxygen with 2 hydrogen atoms to form water. Note that the electron of H atoms in water are nearer to the nucleus of the oxygen atom than the nucleus of the H atom.

This imparts unique properties to water called polarity which gives water its stability, solvent properties, surface tension, cohesiveness and facilitates ionisation of molecules with ionic bonds such as Na^+ Cl^-. When NaCl is placed in water the slight electronegativity of oxygen atoms in water attracts Na^+ and slightly electropositive H^+ ions in water attract Cl^- ions: ionic bonds are separated as individual ions interact with positive or negative ends of polar water molecules. A hydration shell forms around each ion.

Water also dissociates, although to a very small extent, to OH^- and H^+ ions (more accurately H_3O^+ and OH^- ions). This influences hydrogen ion concentration $[H^+]$ (pH) of body fluids: when H^+ increases to exceed OH^- more associate to form water (H_2O) which limits change in $[H^+]$. This is crucial because H^+, although of low concentration, binds and alters the properties and structure of other molecules. At 25°C H_2O dissociates into 0.0000001 mol H^+ (10^{-7}) and 0.0000001 mol OH^- (10^{-7}). The solution is neutral. An acid solution is one in which $H^+ > OH^-$ and an alkaline solution one in which $OH^- > H^+$.

95% of body weight is composed of 4 elements: carbon, oxygen, hydrogen and nitrogen. Elements which are important in electrolyte fluid physiology are shown in table1.

- <u>Atomic number</u> is the number of protons in an atom (which also equals the number of electrons).
- <u>Atomic mass</u> is the number of protons plus neutrons. Mass may not be double the atomic number, and may not be a whole number, because of a variable number of neutrons in the element. (Called isotopes).
- <u>Valence</u> is the number of <u>unpaired</u> electrons—the number required to complete the outer shell
- Charges result from elements which ionise: by donating electrons (left with + charges) or accepting electrons (left with negative charges). The number of charges is the same as the valence.

	Symbol	Atomic Number	Mass	Valence
Hydrogen	H	1	1	1
Carbon	C	6	12	4
Nitrogen	N	7	14	3
Oxygen	O	8	16	2
Sodium	Na	11	23	1
Magnesium	Mg	12	24	2
Phosphorus	P	15	31	3
Sulphur	S	16	32	2
Chlorine	Cl	17	35.5	1
Potassium	K	19	39	1
Calcium	Ca	20	40	2

Table 1. Elements important in electrolyte –fluid physiology

POLYATOMIC IONS

Atoms which interact as a <u>group</u> rather than as individual atoms and have negative or positive charges; commonly HCO_3^-, NH_4^+ and SO_4^{2-} and phosphate(PO_4^{3-}).

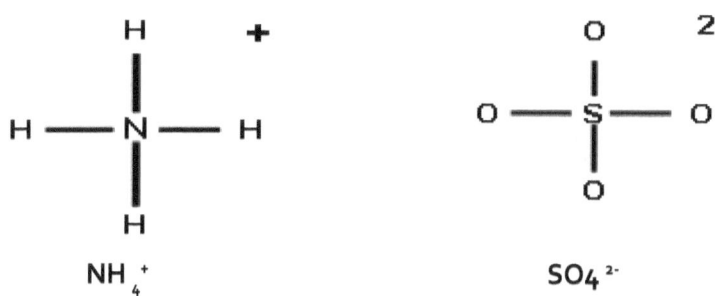

Figure 6. Polyatomic ions Ammonium and Sulphate. These react as a group.

Elements react in proportion to their atomic mass. Thus 23g of Na^+ (AW 23) reacts with 35.5g Cl^- (AW35.5) to form 58.5g or 1 mole of NaCl.

Molecular weight and Equivalents.

Molecules are 2 or more atoms held together by bonds. The molecular weight (MW) is the sum of atomic weights which compose a molecule. For example the MW of NaCl (AW Na 23, Cl 35.5) is 23 + 35.5 = 58.5. The measure of molecular weight is the mole which is the mass of a molecule divided by its MW. For example 58.5g NaCl is 1 mole (58.5 ÷ 58.5(MW)). The unit of measurement, the mole is used in physiology and medicine because molecules react in relation to their molar concentration but not their mass; and their dissociation in water is related to their molar concentration.

Valence.

The valence of an atom in ionic compounds is the number of electrons which must be gained or lost in order to complete the outer electron shell.

Equivalent is the mole x valence: it is a measure of the number of charges which molecules give rise to when they dissociate: Thus 1 mole of NaCl gives rise to one positive and one negative charge- Na^+ and Cl^-.

1Mol of Calcium Chloride ($CaCl_2$) MW (40 + 35.5 +35.5 = 111) dissociates in water to form Ca^{2+} + $2Cl^-$ which is 1 mol Ca^{2+} and 2 mol Cl^- but 2 equivalents of calcium (2 positive charges) and 2 equivalents of chloride (2 single negative charges).

The mole and equivalent are inconveniently large and are usually converted to more manageable numbers shown below.

Mole	mol	1	Equivalent
Millimole,	mmol	10^{-3}	mEq
Micromole	μmol	10^{-6}	μEq
Nanomole	nmol	10^{-9}	nEq
Picomole	pmol	10^{-12}	picoEq

L is the symbol for litre. Serum Na^+ is usually measured in mmol/L; H^+ in nmol/L and some hormones in pmol/L.

Isomers: molecules of the same formula but different shape.

Solutes are substances which <u>dissolve</u> in water. They may be charged eg Na^+Cl^- or without charge, for example, glucose and urea. Substances which dissolve in water (solvent) exert an osmotic pressure.

Osmoles. Osmosis is an important concept. Osmotic pressure is related to the total number of particles in solution. If an impermeable solute is added to water on one side of a semipermeable membrane, permeable to water but not to solute, water will move to equalise the osmotic pressure generated by the difference in concentration of solute across the membrane. Water will move until the increase in pressure exerted by additional water counteracts the further transfer of water. A solute which is freely permeable across membranes, such as urea, does not exert an osmotic force but increases the total number of particles and thus osmolality.

Figure 7. Result of adding solute to one side of a container of water, separated by a semipermeable membrane, permeable to water but impermeable to solute. Water passes into the side with the higher solute concentration until pressure exerted by additional water counteracts the force exerted by the higher solute concentration.

Unionised substances, which do not dissociate in solution, contribute 1 particle to osmolality whereas ionised substances contribute according to the number of particles to which they dissociate.

$$Glucose \rightarrow Glucose \qquad\qquad = 1\ particle$$

$$Na\ Cl \rightarrow Na^+ + Cl^- \qquad\qquad = 2\ particles$$

$$CaCl_2 \rightarrow Ca^+ + Cl^- + Cl^- \qquad\qquad = 3\ particles$$

The molecular weight (MW) in grams of a solute gives rise to the same number of particles. For example 58.5g NaCl (AW Na^+ 23, AW Cl^- 35.5) gives rise to 1 Osmol of Na^+ and 1 Osmol Cl^-.

Tissues are composed of cells surrounded by interstitial fluid. On average cells contain approximately 70% water.

The cellular cytoplasm is a viscous proteinaceous fluid which is interspersed by a network of filaments and tubular structures, the cytoskeleton, which connects various parts of the cell to membranes. It supports, maintains cellular shape, and contains microtubules for transport. The cell contains a nucleus, organelles, endoplasmic reticulum, ribosomes, Golgi apparatus and mitochondria. Cells are separated from each other and the interstitial fluid by semi permeable membranes.

Intracellular water is the total water contained in all cells in the body.

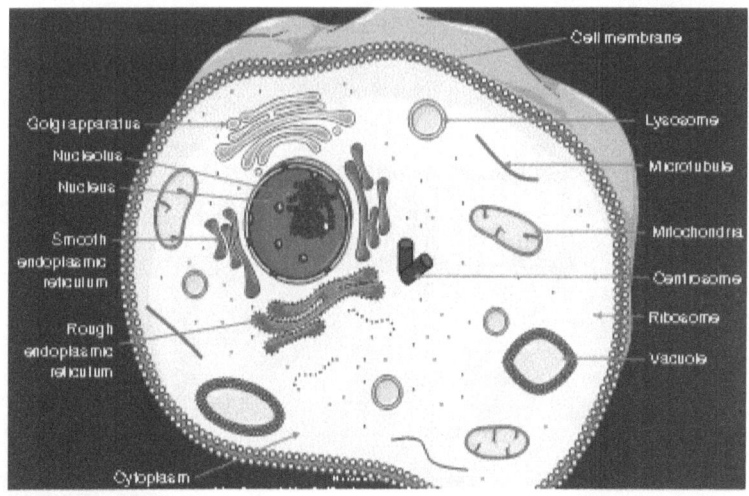

Figure 8. Model of cell. (Produced by using Servier medical art)

Interstitial Fluid.

Cells are surrounded by interstitial fluid which enables delivery and exchange of CO_2, O2, nutrients and waste products. Interstitial fluid is composed of small proteoglycan fibrils and fluid in the form of a gel. The gel decreases free flow of fluids and enables even distribution of fluid to cells. Collagen and smaller amounts of elastic fibres provide a supportive framework. A small amount of free water does form and increases considerably when oedema is present. This is carried to the thoracic duct by a lymphatic network.

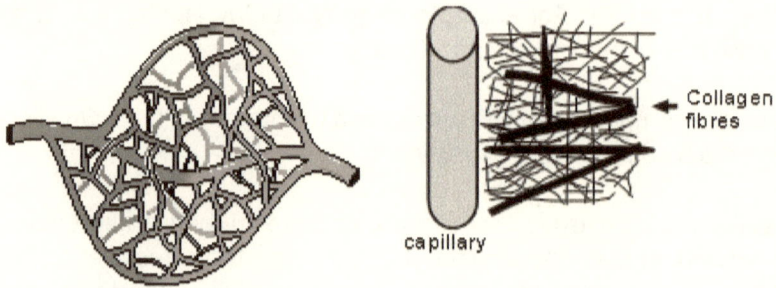

Capillary network

Figure 9. Model showing capillary network proteoglycan fibrils and collagen fibres. The fibrils and interstitial fluid form a gel. (Produced using Servier medical art)

The membrane is a phospholipid bi-layer in which the heads facing outwards are polar—can interact with water (hydrophilic-literally love of water)) while the tails composed of fatty acids face inwards and are hydrophobic. (Water hating).

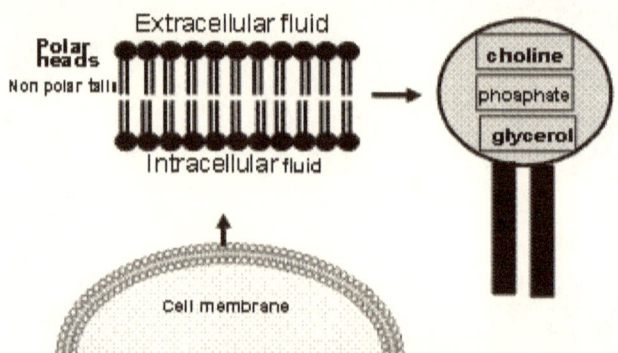

Figure 10. Model of cell membrane at different magnifications.

The polar heads face the interstitial fluid and intracellular fluid in the cell and can interact with water (hydrophilic). The hydrophobic fatty acid tails face inwards. (produced using Servier medical art)

The plasma membrane is impermeable to large molecules such as proteins. Lipid soluble substances such as carbon dioxide (CO_2) and oxygen (O_2) rapidly diffuse through membranes. Water, which is polar, diffuses slowly and ions are impermeable. However the membrane is embedded with proteins which serve 2 main functions:

- Act as receptors for signals (from ligands)
- Transport ions, water, nutrients and waste products, which are relatively impermeable, into and out of cells.

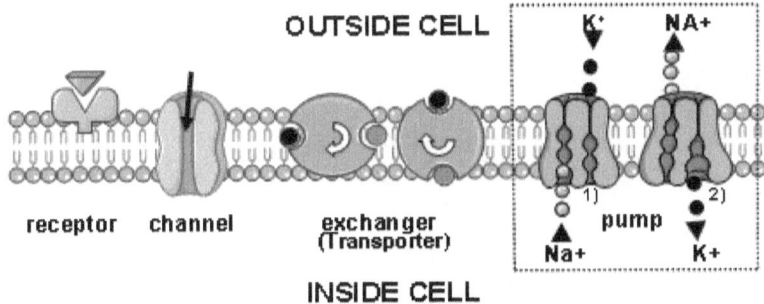

Figure 11. Model of the cellular membrane with transport proteins (produced using Servier medical art).

Transport through the membrane is provided by:

Pumps.

Pumps move ions against electrical or chemical gradients using hydrolysis of ATP as a source of energy. For example, Na^+: K^+ ATPase pumps.

Transporters.

Transporters use concentration or electrical gradients, produced by pumps, to transport one or more ions or solutes. These move 2 or more solutes in the same direction (called symporters) or in the opposite direction (called antiporters or exchangers). For example: glucose coupled with Na^+ uses the gradient favouring Na^+ reabsorption, generated by Na^+ K^+ ATPase pumps; the Na^+ K^+ $2Cl^-$ co-transporters use the Na^+ gradient, generated by Na^+:K^+ pumps, to reabsorb Na^+, K^+ and $2Cl^-$ from the renal tubular lumen;

$Na^+:H$ (NHE) exchangers(antiports) mediate 1:1 exchange of Na^+ for H^+. Stoichiometry is the ratio of solutes involved in transport. For example, the Na^+ glucose symport has a stoichiometry of 1:1: one Na^+ is transported with one glucose molecule.

Channels.

Channels, located in membranes of cells, transport ions or water in response to ionic or osmotic gradients without requiring energy to function. They may be open most of the time or gated- closed but open in response to chemical, electrical signals or osmotic gradients. Disturbances may involve their structure or the retrieval process: channels are moved to the membrane, where they are active, or to the cytosol, where they are inactive, by cytoskeletal proteins.

Receptors

Receptors are the receptor components of the signal transduction pathway of cells. Stimulation of receptors by a ligand usually results in large numbers of intermediate steps which amplify the signal before it has an effect. Thus the effect of 1 molecule of a ligand is multiplied by up to a million times. An example of this process is as follows:

Ligand binds to receptor

Activates membrane bound enzyme (eg adenyl cyclase

Produces cAMP from ATP

Activates protein kinase

Phosphorylates an enzyme

Produces a specific action

Cell membrane electric potential

The cell membrane has an electrical potential, which is important in electrolyte—fluid physiology. The main cations in cells are potassium (K^+) and Magnesium (Mg^{2+}); the main anions are phosphorous (P) and protein which have negative charges. The main cation in the interstitial fluid outside the cell is sodium (Na^+) and main anion chloride (Cl^-).

Electric charges separate on each side of the membrane as shown in figure 12.

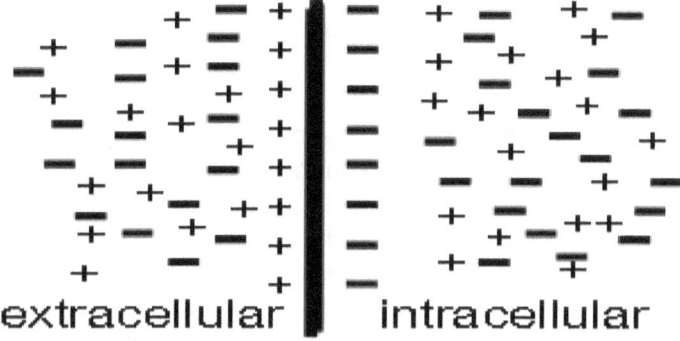

Figure 12.Model of separation of charges on each side of the plasma membrane. Note that opposite charges only line up adjacent to the membrane. The charges in the remainder of the intracellular and extracellular fluid are scattered randomly.

The membrane potential is crucial for muscle and nerve function. Ions gradually leak from membranes through ionic channels. The leak of K^+ is 50 -70 times greater than leak of Na^+. Ions would eventually equalise on each side of membranes in response to concentration gradients. This would dissipate the transmembrane electrical charge. Na^+: K^+ pumps, present in all cells, pump Na^+ of cells and potassium into cells using hydrolysis of ATP as a source of energy.

The electromotive force (EMF) is generated as follows

K^+ leaks out of cells through potassium channels due to the large concentration gradient across cell membranes. Na^+ is much less permeable and lesser amounts diffuse into cells. Net movement of positive potassium ions out of the cell increases net negative charges on protein and phosphate because they are impermeable and remain within cells

The electrical force attracting K^+ back into the cell increases as the cell interior becomes increasingly negative. Potassium efflux (movement out of the cell) ceases when the force due to the concentration gradient is balanced by the increase in negative potential in the cell. By convention when a cation leaves the cell the intracellular potential is called negative).

At the balance point the EMF for K^+ is given by the NERNST equation:

EMF =   -61 log (K (i) / (K o) (i = inside o = outside of cell)
   =   ~ -61 log 150/5.0
   =   -61 x log 30 (log30=1.48)
   =   <u>~ 90 mV</u>

However other ions which move into or out of cells also exert an EMF. The transmembrane potential depends on their:

- Concentration difference across the membrane.
- Permeability across the membrane.
- Polarity. For example Na^+, which enters rather than leaves cells, exerts a positive rather than negative EMF. Although the transcellular concentration gradient of Na^+ is approximately $150_{(o)}/10(i)$ its contribution to EMF is much lower than $K^{+ (o)}$ because its permeability is much lower.

The approximate net EMF of most cells is:

K^+ leak	-90mV
Na^+ leak	+ 6mV
Na^+K^+ ATPase pump	- 6mV
Net EMF	-90mV

Na^+: K^+ ATPase pumps exert a negative potential because 3 Na^+ ions are transported out of the cell in exchange for 2K^+ transported into the cell. (Stoichiometry 3:2)

The leak of K^+ and Na^+ would eventually lead to equilibrium where the concentration of Na^+ and K^+ are equal inside and outside the cell. This would dissipate the cellular negative potential. An energy requiring pump, utilising adenosine triphosphate (ATP), pumps 3 Na⁺ out of the cell in exchange for 2 K⁺ ions into cells and thus maintain normal ionic concentrations.

The combination of leak and rectifying Na⁺K⁺ ATPase pumps maintain the transmembrane voltage. The leak contributes 95% and pumps 5%.

Depolarisation is the process of rapid dissipation of negative potential in cells.

Sodium channels have voltage gates which open in response to decrease in voltage in nerve and muscle. When a specific lower voltage is reached, spontaneously or due to a stimulus, Na⁺ moves rapidly into cells and decreases intracellular negative potential—called depolarisation. The sudden conformational change in Na⁺ channels, which leads to marked increase in sodium permeability, occurs when voltage decrease to approximately -50 to -70mV.

Pumps and other cellular functions require energy to function. Adenosine triphosphate, ATP, is the source of energy used by cells to carry out biological work. ATP contains high energy phosphate bonds which release large amounts of energy when phosphate ($\approx$P), called high energy phosphate, is split off.

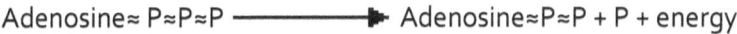

Adenosine$\approx$ P$\approx$P$\approx$P ⟶ Adenosine$\approx$P$\approx$P + P + energy

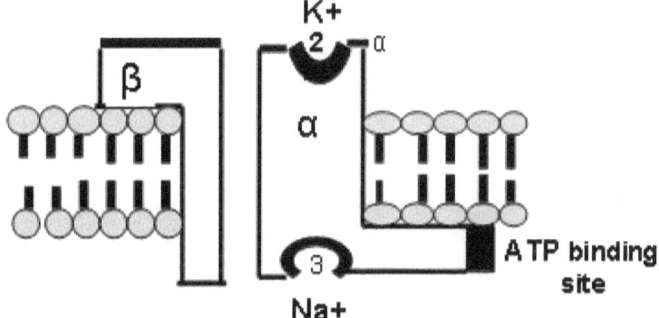

Figure 13. Simplified model of the Na: K⁺ ATPase pump located in the cell membrane. α =alpha subunit; β = beta subunit. Magnesium is a cofactor required for action of ATPase. The work of the pump in transferring K⁺ into the cell and Na⁺ out is fuelled by the breakdown of ATP to ADP.

ATP is resynthesised from ADP using energy released from oxidation of carbohydrate, fat and to a lesser extent protein; shown in figure 14. Carbohydrates and fat are broken down to provide energy in 4 main stages provided oxygen is available.

1. Breakdown to the 2 carbon molecule acetyl coenzyme A (AcCoA).
2. Metabolism of AcCoA in Krebs cycle in mitochondria to carbon and hydrogen (H) atoms. Carbon combines with oxygen to form CO_2.
3. Pairs of H atoms are split into hydrogen ions (H^+) and electrons (e^-) catalysed by dehydrogenases in mitochondria.

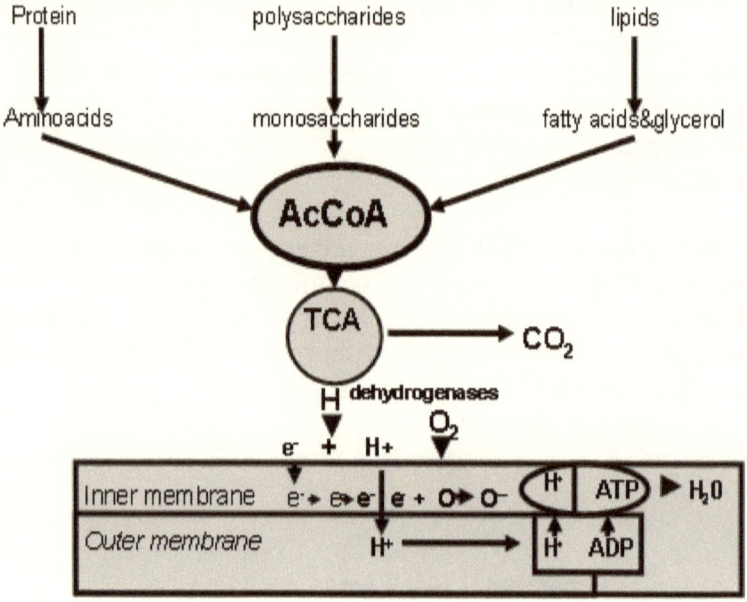

Figure 14: Model of the synthesis of ATP from food.(see text)

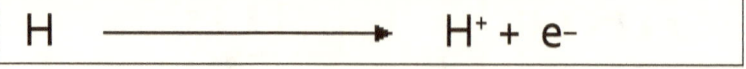

4   H, H^+ and e^-, in combination with dehydrogenases, are transferred to the electron chain on inner mitochondrial membranes. The most common of several dehydrogenase involved is NAD^+ (nicotinic adenine dinucleotide)

The net result of a more complex process is that H^+ and e- are presented to the electron chain on the inner mitochondrial membrane. NAD^+ is reformed when H^+ and e^- are transferred to the electron chain. Electrons enter the electron transport chain and energy is released at each stage of transfer to different electron acceptors. The energy is used to transport H^+ (remaining from splitting of H to H^+ and e^-.) through the inner mitochondrial membrane to the space between the inner and outer membranes. As a result this develops a high electrical (proton) potential difference.

This provides the force to move H^+ through the outer mitochondrial space back into the inner mitochondrial space through ATPase protein molecules embedded in the membrane. The energy enables ADP to combine with $\approx$P to form ATP.

The final electron acceptor, molecular oxygen (O), combines with 2 electrons to form $O^{..}$. This is highly unstable and combines with $2H^+$, which has passed into the inner from outer mitochondrial membranes, to form water.

$$O^{..} + 2H^+ \longrightarrow H_2O$$

In conclusion the main source of energy is breakdown of food in stages to hydrogen which is split into H, H^+ ions (protons) and electrons (e^-). At each stage of the electron chain energy released is used to move (H^+) through membranes. This results in a high proton (H^+) EMF in the outer mitochondrial compartment. Movement of H^+ through the ATPase molecule back through the membrane into the inner compartment, in response to this force, causes a high energy phosphate bond to attach to ADP.

Despite the complexities of glycolysis and Krebs cycle only a small amount of ATP is formed by these processes. Over 90% of energy is produced by oxidation of hydrogen atoms: 3 ATP molecules are synthesised for each 2 electrons (produced by the ionisation of 2 H atoms) passing down the electron chain.

Glycolysis and the oxidation of H atoms are controlled by the cells need for ATP. In general **re**duction- **ox**idation reactions (**redox**) involve loss of electrons from one chemical, which is oxidised, and its gain by another chemical which is reduced. The flow of electrons is responsible for all work by living organisms. Cells contain several other molecular energy transducers which convert the energy of electron flow to useful work.

The source of electrons and H is reduction of compounds in food (with higher electron affinities). The energy used originated from photosynthetic bacteria and plants which captured sunlight in synthesis of more complex molecules, such as carbohydrate, from CO_2 and H_2O.

ATOMS, ELEMENTS AND MOLECULES

1. Marshall W J. Clinical chemistry, 4th edition 2000 Edinburgh Mosby.
2. Waugh A, Grant A. Introduction to the Chemistry of Life p18-28. in Ross and Wilson's Anatomy and Physiology in Health and Illness.9th edition 2002. Churchill Livingston.
3. Martini p31-37 in Fundamentals of Anatomy and Physiology. 4th edition 1996. Williams and Wilkins.
4. Tortara GJ, Derrickson B. How matter is organised; p 29-41 in Principles of Anatomy and Physiology. 11th edition 2003 John Wiley and Sons.
5. Marieb EN. P 26-29. in Essentials of Human Anatomy and Physiology. 8th edition. 2006. Pearson-Benjamin Cummings.

CELLS, CELL MEMBRANE AND CELL ELECTRICAL POTENTIAL

6. Porth, Carol M: Cell and tissue characteristics p 3-31 in Pathophysiology—Concepts of Altered Health States. 5th edition. 1998 Lippincott
7. Banasik JL. Chapter 3.Cell structure and Function. In Pathophysiology, Biology and Behavioural Aspects. 2nd edition. Eds Copstead. 2000 WB Saunders

8. Boron WF, Boulpaep EL. Physiology of cells and molecules p9-114 in Medical Physiology, updated edition.2005 Elsevier Saunders.

9. Banasik.C. Cell Structure and Function.Ch.3 in Pathophysiology, Biological and Behavioural Aspects. 2nd edition. Eds Copstead. 2000 WB Saunders

10. Sherwood, L: p 49-87 Ch3: The Plasma Membrane and Membrane Potential. Human Physiology (From Cells to Systems).2001 Brooks/Cole

11. Guyton, A.C. and Hall, J.E, Membrane potentials and action potentials. P. 57-71 and the cell and its function p 11-26 in Textbook of Medial Physiology, 11th edition 2006, Elsevier Saunders: Philadelphia.

12. Guyton, A.C and Hall JE, The microcirculation and lymphatic System: Capillary Fluid exchange, Interstitial Fluid, and Lymph flow. P181-203 in Textbook of medical physiology, 7. A.C. Guyton and J.E. Hall Editors. 2006, Elsevier Saunders: Philadelphia. P. 57-71.

13. Cellular mechanisms: excitation, contraction and secretion in Pharmacology.Eds Rang H P, Dali MM, Ritter JM, Moore P K. 5th edition.2004. Churchill Livingstone.

ENERGY METABOLISM

14. Ganong WF. Energy balance, Metabolism and Nutrition p 4-50. Review of Medical Physiology. 20th Edition 2001.McGraw-Hill

15. McArdle WD, Katch FI, Katch VL. Exercise Physiology 4th edition. 1996 Williams and Wilkins.

16. Champe PC, Harvey RA. Lippincotts Illustrated Review: Biochemistry. 2nd edition 1994. J B Lippincott Company.

17. Marieb E N. Concepts of Matter and energy in Essentials of Human Anatomy and Physiology. 8th edition. 2006. Pearson-Benjamin Cummings.

Anatomy and Function of Body Fluid Compartments. [1-4]

'The stability of the milieu interiur is the primary freedom and independence of existence; the mechanism which allows of this is that which ensures in the milieu interiur the maintenance of all the conditions necessary to the life of the elements'. Claude Bernard.

Approximately 50% of body weight of a young adult female is water. Young males have 55-60% water as body weight and neonates 70%. The differences are due to the relative amounts of skin, muscle, internal organs, which contain 70-80% water; bone 22% water; and adipose tissue only 10% water. Ageing results in loss of muscle and relative increase in adipose tissue. Thus total body water (TBW), as a percent of body weight, declines with ageing. After adjusting for total body fat or fat free mass there is no difference with ageing in males and very small differences in females [5]. The total body water (TBW) at different age groups in both males and females is shown in table 1. [5]

Age groups (Years)		20-29	30-39	40-49	50-59	60+
Total body water.	M. (n=292)	56%	53%	52%	51%	46%
	F. (n=274)	47%	46%	44%	43%	43%

Table 1. Total Body water by age as a % of body weight. [5] n=number measured M= male; F = female.

The figure of 50% for total body water in females is both easy to remember and useful in calculations. Unfortunately recent increases in adiposity in developed countries have resulted in a decrease of body water as a percent of weight. Recent, compared to past estimates, show males aged 20-29yrs have a TBW of 56% of body weight which declines to 46% at age 60; females aged 20-29yrs have a TBW of 47% body weight which decreases to 43% at about 60yrs of age. [5, 6]

Water, distributed among trillions of cells in the body, is considered collectively as intracellular water. The cells are surrounded by interstitial fluid which has a composition similar to primeval seas. This provides an optimum supportive environment that allows exchange of O_2, CO_2, ions, removal of waste products and transfer of hormones.

Extracellular fluid is composed of interstitial fluid, inaccessible water in bone, cartilage and dense connective tissue and transcellular fluid. Transcellular water is the small amount of fluid in specialised compartments such as the cerebrospinal, intraocular fluid and gastrointestinal tract. A substantial volume of interstitial fluid in bone, cartilage and transcellular fluid exchanges slowly. Measurement of extracellular volume (ECV) is much more difficult than TBW and there are marked differences reported in textbooks and publications.

These differences are due to variations in methods of measurement- especially whether tracers enter cells and whether exchange occurs with slowly exchanging components of interstitial fluid; and measurement reported in subjects with differences in body weight, height and age.

Silva et al [7] measured and established reference values for extracellular water (ECW) in 1538 healthy subjects of different races, gender, age, height and weight. Average ECW was 0.25 L/kg in females and 0.26 L/kg in males. ECW varied according to weight and height and in males with age; and there was considerable interindividual variation even when these variables were taken into account.

Given this; variations in methodology; variation between healthy subjects and those with disease; and the marked differences reported; the assignment of values for ECW are very approximate and difficult to individualise.

The volume of extracellular fluid that exchanges rapidly is commonly reported as slightly more than half intracellular water or one third (20%), of the total body water. The ratio of intracellular to extracellular water is approximately 2:1

The structure and composition of interstitium differs considerably depending on the tissues and organ it surrounds. All interstitium is viewed collectively for body fluid purposes. The majority of interstitial fluid is combined with mucopolysaccharides (proteoglycans) as a gel and water adsorbed onto collagen fibres. This acts like a sponge to trap interstitial fluid leaving small amounts of free water. The interstitium has traditionally been considered to play a passive role in fluid balance: changes in interstitial hydrostatic and colloid osmotic pressure counteract changes in capillary filtration-a form of autoregulation. However interstitial matrix is dynamic: connective tissue cells can contract collagen gel by influencing the tension of the fibre networks. [8]

Interstitial fluid and cells are supplied by a large network of capillaries linked to larger blood vessels and heart. The vascular system contains approximately 5% of body water as plasma. The blood volume, approximately 7 % of body weight, (79mL/kg) contains approximately 60% plasma and 40% red cells. Red cell mass is related to the mass of body cells to which it supplies oxygen.

Plasma volume is approximately one quarter of extracellular volume which gives a ratio of plasma volume to interstitial fluid of approximately 1:3. This is important because 500 mL colloid is equivalent to 1500 mL saline and not 1L as is often recommended in trials of fluid infusion in those in shock.

A second important function of interstitial fluid is to buffer blood volume losses by transfer of saline into the vascular compartment. Distribution of total body water (TBW) is shown in figure 1. Interstitial fluid is separated by capillary pores on one side and from cells by a semipermeable membrane on the other.

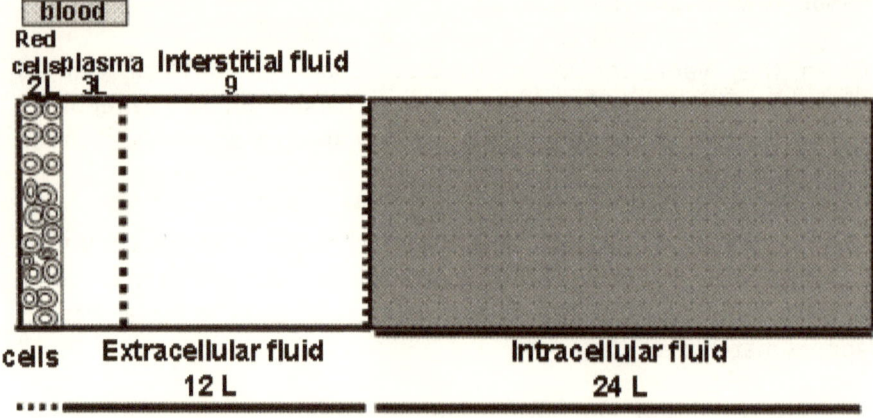

Figure 1: Body fluid compartments assuming Total body water = 36L. Interstitial water is separated from cellular water by a semipermeable membrane and plasma by capillary pores.

The ratios of intracellular to extracellular water is ~ 2:1

The ratio of interstitial to plasma water is ~ 3:1

Body water contains solutes: electrolytes which dissociate in water to form ions with an electric charge and non electrolytes such as urea and glucose which do not dissociate and have no electric charge. Positive charges on cations must equal negative charges on anions to satisfy electroneutrality. The solute composition of the plasma, cellular and interstitial water is shown in figure 2.

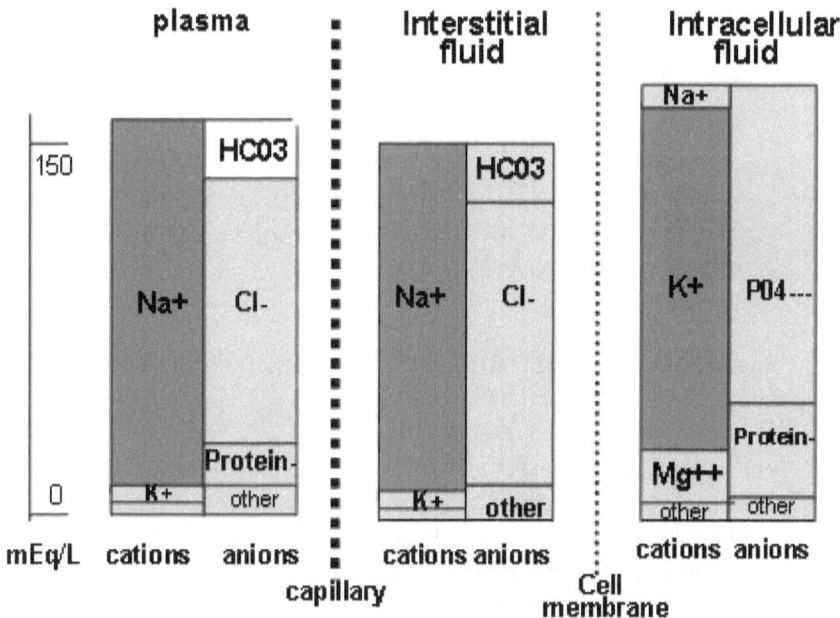

Figure 2 Composition of plasma, interstitial fluid and intracellular fluid. Values are in mEq/L of water.

The main cation in interstitial fluid and plasma is Na+ and anions- Cl- and HCO3-.

Donnan effect

The concentration of protein, mainly albumin, is higher in plasma than interstitial fluid. Albumin has net negative charges which attract sodium. Thus plasma contains a higher Na+ concentration and interstitial fluid lower Na+ but higher Cl- concentration. The main cations in cells are Potassium (K+) and magnesium (Mg^{++}) and main anions protein—and phosphate. The K$^+$ concentration in cell water is approximately 150 mEq/L and similar to the Na+ concentration, 150 mEq/L, in interstitial water.

Electrolytes are commonly measured in plasma rather than plasma water. Plasma contains 93% water and 7% solids. The concentration of electrolytes in mmol/L is higher in 1L of plasma water than in 1L of plasma because non-electrolytes contribute volume but not electrolytes to plasma. (Figure 3)

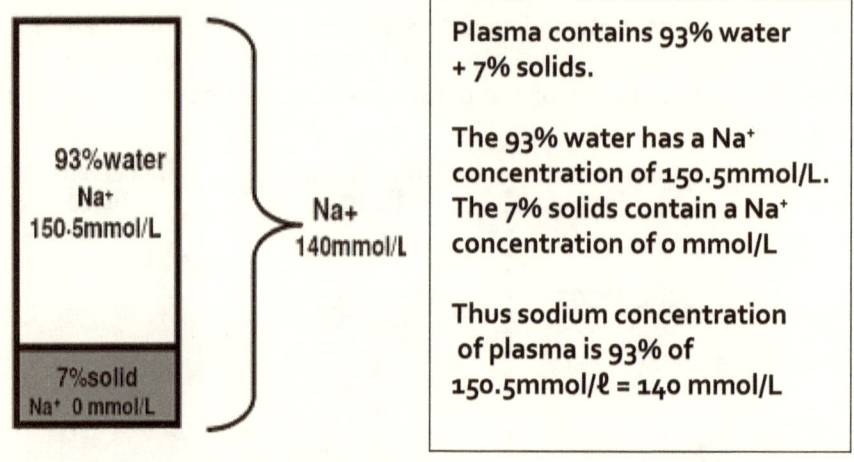

Figure 3. Sodium concentration in the water and solid component of plasma.

Thus an increase in the percent of solids decreases concentration of Na^+ in plasma but not in the water component of plasma. An increase in solids from hyperlipidaemia or hyperproteinaemia lowers plasma Na+, but not tonicity, which is a function of solutes dissolved in water.If plasma Na+ of 140mmol/L in the above example is measured by atomic spectrometry, which measures sodium in the water component of plasma alone, the concentration is 150 mmol/L.

Water is freely permeable between membranes. Thus addition or loss of water without electrolytes (free water) distributes between cells and extracellular water in the ratio of their volumes so that osmolality remains equal in all body compartments.

Osmosis is net diffusion of water across a selectively permeable membrane from a region of high water concentration to one of lower concentration. [3] The osmotic pressure relates to the number of particles in solution. If an impermeable solute is added to water on one side of a semipermeable membrane, permeable to water but not solute, water moves to the compartment containing additional solute to equalise osmotic pressure.

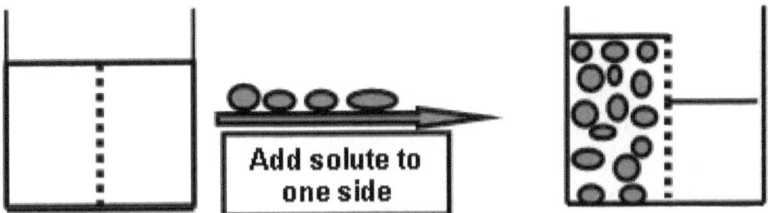

Figure 4. The effects of addition of a solute, which is impermeable, to one side of a semipermeable membrane, but permeable to water.

Water moves until the increased pressure exerted by additional water, in response to the osmolal gradient, counteracts further transfer of water.

Unionised solutes, which do not dissociate in solution, contribute 1 particle whereas ionised substances contribute according to the number of particles to which they dissociate.

Glucose Glucose   = 1 particle.

$NaCl \longrightarrow Na+ + Cl-$ = 2 particles.

$CaCl_2 \longrightarrow Ca+ + Cl- + Cl-$ = 3 particles.

Osmolality of a solution is a function of the total number of particles dissolved in solvent—usually water. Osmolality of extracellular and intracellular fluid are the same because a change is osmolality (number of particles) in one compartment causes water, which is freely permeable, to pass through semipermeable membranes in order to equalise osmolality.

Extracellular solutes only exert an osmotic effect if they are unable to pass through membranes into cells. Solutes such as urea, which diffuse rapidly into cells, do not exert an osmotic effect: no net movement of water occurs and cells do not increase in volume because urea increases osmolality of both extracellular and intracellular water equally. Therefore urea increases plasma osmolality, but not tonicity. It is an ineffective osmole.

Symptoms develop from swelling or shrinking of cells and not from osmolality per se. This is called tonicity or 'effective osmolality'. The signalling process which turns ADH on or off is responsive to tonicity not osmolality.

Osmolality of Body Fluids

The osmolality of ECF and ICF are equal and approximately 290mOsm/kg water. Plasma has a slightly higher osmolality than interstitial fluid because it contains plasma proteins. The plasma osmolality is less than the theoretical sum of particles because dissociation of some ions, such as NaCl, is not 100%.

The total body osmolality is mainly due to Na^+, the main extracellular cation, and K^+ the main intracellular cation, and their accompanying anions.

Total Body Osmolality = approximately 2 x (Na^+ + K^+) / TBW

Na^+ + K^+ are doubled to account for accompanying anions.

Blood enters the microcirculation at the arteriole and leaves at the venule.

Precapillary sphincters, composed of muscle surrounding the arteriolar end of capillaries, control blood flow to the capillary network. Some channels have no sphincter, bypass the capillary network and link directly to the venule.

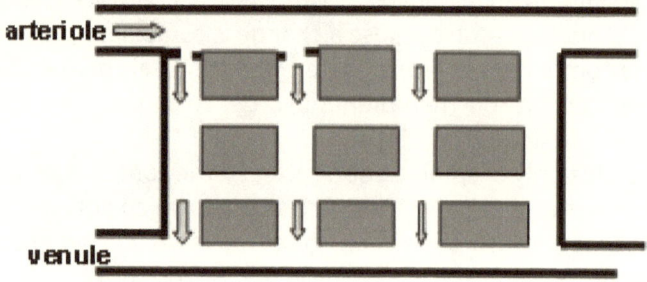

Figure 5. Model of capillary flow

The interstitial fluid is separated from blood in the microcirculation by capillary pores. Capillary pores are permeable to water and electrolytes, but not to plasma proteins or red cells. Water either passes between cells (paracellular) or through cells (transcellular) through Aquaporin channels.

Figure 6 shows net forces moving fluid into the interstitial space at the arteriolar end of the capillary and net forces attracting fluid back at the venular end.

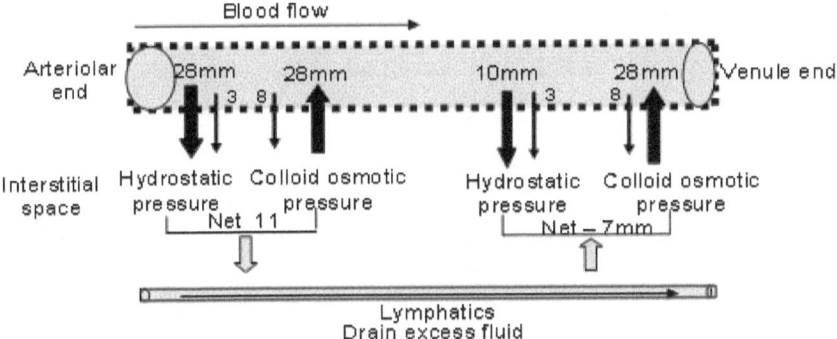

Figure 6. Forces moving fluid into interstitial space at the arterial end of the capillary and net forces attracting fluid back at the venular end. The negative interstitial pressure (approximately 3mm Hg) and the interstitial colloid osmotic pressure (approximately 8 mm Hg) are shown by small arrows.

Forces moving fluid out of and into capillaries are summarised Table (1).

	Outward forces	
Arteriolar end (mm Hg)		**Venous end (mm Hg)**
Outward cap pressure	28	10
Interstitial neg pressure	3	-3
Interstitial colloid OP	8	-8
	Inward forces	
Plasma colloid OP	28	28
Net pressure	11	7

Table 1. Forces at the arteriolar and venous end of the capillary which determine net fluid flow. cap =capillary; OP = osmotic pressure; neg = negative. Out ward forces are from capillary to the interstitial space.

Net capillary filtration is also determined by the capillary coefficient.

The capillary coefficient (Kf) is a product of the capillary surface area and the endothelial permeability. It varies in different tissues.

> Filtration= Kf x net filtration pressure

> Net filtration is approximately 3-4 L /day.

A small amount of protein leaks. This and fluid filtered in excess of that reabsorbed is taken up by lymphatics which drain into the thoracic duct and enter the venous circulation.

If blood volume decreases lower pressure at the arteriolar side of the microcirculation increases movement of interstitial fluid into the circulation. Losses of blood or plasma are thus buffered by interstitial fluid.

Approximately 65% of the blood volume is contained within veins and only approximately 13 % - 0.7l in the arterial system. Veins have a high compliance due to their large volume and distensibility and serve an important reservoir function to buffer changes in blood volume.

Extracellular volume (ECV) is determined by the amount of sodium in the body because sodium is mainly confined to the extracellular space. The term saline deficiency or excess is used to include water accompanying sodium in the same ratio as plasma (eg 140mmol Na with 1L water represents 1L saline if the serum Na is 140mmol/L).

Initially sodium losses are isotonic or hypotonic and accompanied by water loss in the same or greater ratio as occurs in plasma. If water is ingested in excess of saline loss it is initially excreted by the kidney to maintain normal plasma tonicity.

Free water retention in excess of saline represents an additional (free) water excess. Free water depletion, in addition to saline loss, (net water loss greater than the ratio of 1L water to 140 mmol/L sodium), causes hypernatraemia. In practice thirst usually results in water ingestion so that hypernatraemia is uncommon.

For example the loss of 140 mmol sodium and 1L water in a subject with serum Na^+ of 140 mmol/L is conceptualised as having 1L saline loss alone; the loss of 140 mmol sodium and 2 L water is conceptualised as the loss of 1L saline and 1L of free water; and the net loss of 280 mmol sodium and 1L net water loss as 2L saline loss with 1L free water excess.

It is essential to understand the differences between saline depletion and (free) water depletion. Figure 7

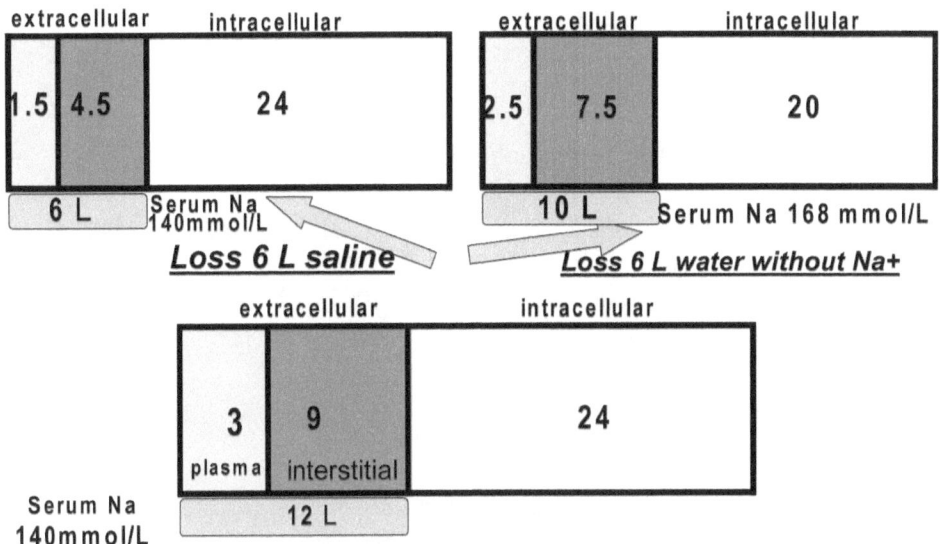

Figure 7. Model showing fluid compartments of a normal subject with TBW of 36 L and the response to loss of 6L saline contrasted with 6L of free water. (See text)

In the model shown in the diagram loss of 6L saline (at 140mmol/L) is borne entirely by the extracellular compartment leading to decrease of 4.5 L in interstitial fluid and 1.5 L in plasma volume (if the ratio of 3:1between interstitial and plasma compartment remain the same). The decrease of 1.5L in plasma volume of 3L represents 50% deficit (1.5 L ÷ 3L) and a 30% decrease in blood volume (1.5L ÷ 5). Plasma Na$^+$ or osmolality does not change.

Loss of 6L (free) water (without Na$^+$) is shared between extracellular water and intracellular water in the ratio of their volumes: This leads to loss of 4L of intracellular and 2L of extracellular water. Loss of 2 L of ECW decreases interstitial water by 1.5 L and plasma volume by 0.5 L.The ratio of interstitial fluid to plasma is 3-1.Therefore plasma volume decreases by 17% (0.5/3) and blood volume by only 10 %. (0.5/5) However plasma Na$^+$ increases to 168 mmol/l and plasma osmolality to approximately 336 mOsm/kg H$_2$O. The increase in plasma Na$^+$ is due to the same amount of sodium contained in a lesser extracellular volume.

Initial plasma Na$^+$ =140 mmol/L and ECW =12 L.

Extracellular body Na$^+$ = 140 x 12 = 1680 mmoL

Following loss of 6l free water 2 L is lost from the extracellular and 4 L from the intracellular compartment. Total Na^+ is now contained in 10 L extracellular water:

Plasma Na = 1680 ÷ 10 = 168 mmol/l.

<u>Thus loss of saline leads to severe plasma fluid loss (hypovolaemia) whereas (free) water depletion has a trivial effect on blood volume, but a major effect on plasma Na^+.</u> Increase in tonicity causes cells to shrink.

<u>In conclusion:</u>

<u>In saline loss without free water loss plasma Na^+ is normal.</u>

<u>A raised plasma Na^+ indicates (free) water deficiency is present.</u>

<u>Low plasma Na^+ (if it reflects low tonicity) indicates that relative excess of free water is present.</u>

Plasma Na^+ may be low, normal or high when hypovolemia (low vascular volume) or saline depletion is present depending on whether there is associated (free) water deficit or excess. Plasma Na^+ is low when there is saline loss plus (free) water excess and high in saline loss plus free water deficiency.

<u>A low plasma Na^+, by itself, does not indicate that saline (sodium) deficiency is present: hyponatraemia may occur in association with hypovolaemia, euvolaemia or hypervolemia.</u>

<u>Indiscriminate use of the term dehydration causes confusion and therapeutic errors:</u> [9] <u>the terms hypovolaemia or saline depletion and free water depletion are preferable.</u>

The account given is in keeping with the traditional view that ions in body compartments are in an osmotically active form. Thus extracellular accumulation of 140 mmol Na is accompanied by 1 L of water. Recent data suggest that Na^+ can accumulate without equivalent water retention in interstitial fluid.

The polyanionic structure of glucosaminoglcans may allow Na^+ to be stored in interstitial fluid in skin in an osmotically inactive form and serve as a reservoir for sodium. [10] This may have been an important buffer in

Paleolithic times when salt was scarce but vital to survival following trauma, childbirth and diarrhoea in children. [11] Plasma volume, but not <u>extracellular volume,</u> increases by as much as 10% in those taking high sodium containing "Western" diets compared to those taking low sodium or Paleolithic diets. [12, 13] More importantly sodium retention is much greater than can be accounted for by increase in plasma volume or gain in weight. On a high sodium diet osmotically inactive sodium may be sequestered in the interstitial space [10, 12, 13] and bone. [14, 15] This may be important in salt sensitive hypertension. [15] Transcription factors, such as tonicity enhancer binding protein (Ton EBP), which activate osmoprotection genes, may protect cells exposed to a hypertonic hostile microenvironment. The interstitium may be a separately regulated space rather than merely a passive reservoir to support plasma volume. [10]

A salt –sensing system-salt appetite, has evolved to ensure optimum salt intake to fill the extracellular space. In mice EnaC-the sodium channel has been proposed as the sodium taste receptor. [16]

References.

1. Gamble JL. Chemical Anatomy, Physiology and Pathology of Extracellular Fluid. Harvard University Press. 6th edition 1964.

2. University of Washington Teaching Syllabus for the course on Fluid and Electrolyte Balance. Edited by BH Scribner. 1953. University of Washington School of Medicine.

3. Guyton, A.C. and Hall, J.E., The Body Fluid Compartments. p 291-306 in Textbook of Medical Physiology, 11th edition 2006., Elsevier Saunders: Philadelphia.

4. Kleeman CR. Body fluid compartment.p 233 in Massry & Glassock's Textbook of Nephrology. 4th edition. 2001. Eds Massry SG, Glassock RJ.

5. Chumlea WC, Guo SS, Zeller CM et al. Total body water reference values and prediction equations for adults. Kidney International **59** 2250-2258 2001.

6. Chumlea WC, Guo SS, Zeller CM et al. Total body water data for white adults 18-64 years of age: The Fels Longitudinal Study. Kidney International: **56**:244-252.1997.

7. Silva AM, Wang J, Pierson RN et al.Extracellular water across the adult life span: reference values for adults.Physiol Meas **28**:489-502 2007.

8. Wilg H, Rubin K, Reed RK.New and active role of the interstitium in control of interstitial fluid pressure: potential therapeutic consequences. Acta Anaesthesiol Scand. **47:** 111-121.2003.

9. Mange K, Matsuura D, Cizman B et al.Language Guiding Therapy: The Case of Dehydration versus Volume Depletion. Annals Intern Med. **127:** 848-852.1997.

10. Titze J, Machnik A. Sodium sensing in the interstitium and relationship to hypertension. Current opinion in Nephrol Hypertens.**19:** 385-392.2010.

11. Hollenberg NK: Set point for Sodium Homeostasis: Surfeit, deficit and their implication. *Kidney Int.* **17**:423-429, 1980 . . .

12. Humphreys MH: Salt intake and body fluid volumes: Have we learned all there is to know? *Amer. J. Kidney Dis.* **37**:648-652, 2001.

13. Heer M, Baisch F, Kropp J. et al: High dietary sodium chloride consumption may not induce body fluid retention in humans. *Amer. J. Physiol. Renal Physiol.* **278**:F585-595, 2000.

14. Palacios C, Wigertz K, Martin BR et al.Sodium Retention in Black and white Female Adolescents in Response to Salt Intake. Clin Endocrinol Metabolism. **89:** 1858-1863.2004.

15. Kanbay M, Chen Y, Solak Y, Sanders PW. Mechanisms and consequences of salt sensitivity and dietary salt intake. Current Opinion in Nephrology and Hypertension.**20**:37-43.2011.

16. Chandrasekhar et al The cellular and molecular components of sodium taste. Nature **464**: 297-301.2010.

RENAL FUNCTION [2-13]

What is man but an ingenious machine designed to turn, with 'infinite artfulness, the red wine of Shiraz into urine'. Story Teller, Seven Gothic Tales, Bak Dinesens. [1]

Life began in primordial seas similar in composition to extracellular fluid. Cells evolved to contain 70-80% water; potassium as the main cation; protein and phosphate as the main anions; enclosed by a semi permeable membrane. The need for oxygen, elimination of CO_2 and waste products occurred by simple diffusion through the membrane to the outside sea. A slow leak of sodium and potassium from cells was counteracted by Na^+: K^+ pumps using Adenosine Triphosphate (ATP) as a source of energy. The pump and the leak of ions through channels in membranes generated a negative intracellular membrane potential essential for cardiac, neuromuscular and cellular function.

At a later stage in evolution mitochondria, derived from bacteria, were incorporated to become the power house of the cell. When our ancestors moved from sea to fresh water a glomerulus and tubule evolved to eliminate excess water and retain sodium. On moving to land the kidney evolved further to:

* Concentrate urine and eliminate waste products, hydrogen ions and potassium in low volume.
* Conserve sodium, of low concentration in most foods, but excrete large potassium loads in the diet.
* Conserve water on land by developing a hypertonic medulla generated by a counter current multiplier system. This was enhanced by using the waste product urea for urinary concentration, recycling it to the medulla and by preventing wash out by low medullary blood flow.
* Reabsorb large amounts of filtered calcium and phosphate, important for skeletal structure, while maintaining low cellular ionic concentration of Ca^{2+} (~100 nmol/L); preventing the harmful renal effects of Ca^{2+}; and excreting phosphate efficiently to prevent calcification in blood vessels and tissues.
* Reabsorb large amounts of solutes filtered as a result of the high glomerular filtration rate (GFR) required to excrete waste products generated by metabolism.

It is important to emphasise the importance of sodium and chloride reabsorption given the present widespread availability of common salt. Food without added salt, often the case in the past, provided a daily intake of only 7-30 mmol of sodium in Paleolithic times [14]. The neonate receives only approximately 3 mmol/day from breast milk. (5.0mmol/L).

Moreover salt was crucial to survival given its role in buffering blood losses during birth or trauma and high losses from gastrointestinal disease or sweating. Indeed salt was highly prized, the subject of wars, taxes, protected salt routes and the payment of salary in salt (sal=salt) to Roman soldiers rather than money. Status was determined by proximity to the salt container in the middle Ages (worth his salt)—often a highly ornate and valuable centrepiece. [15]

Potassium has always been plentiful in the diet—in both plants and protein foods and in starvation available from tissue catabolism.

Starvation, alternating with gorging, was common in many animals including man. Gorging could result in intake of ~ 300mmol K^+ in one meal, which is rapidly absorbed and enters an extracellular space containing only 50-60mmol of potassium at a concentration of 4.0 mmol/L. The membrane potential is due to the ratio of intracellular to extracellular K^+. Increase in extracellular potassium concentration has a potentially dangerous effect on cellular and neuromuscular function. Moreover, 25,000mmol sodium is filtered daily compared to only ~ 700mmol of K^+.

Thus the kidney has evolved to efficiently reabsorb Na^+, but to excrete potassium loads. The main actor in this process is the Na^+: K^+ pump, the main source of renal energy consumption, located in basolateral membranes of cells adjacent to capillaries.

The pumping of Na^+ out of cells in exchange for K^+ provides both an electrical and concentration gradient for luminal absorption of sodium; co-transport of glucose and amino acids; chloride absorption to maintain electroneutrality; H^+ secretion by exchange with Na^+; and water reabsorption secondary to the osmotic gradient produced by NaCl absorption.

The main functions of the kidney are summarised in Table 1:These are achieved by filtration, followed by tubular reabsorption and secretion.

- Elimination of waste products and poisons, especially from protein breakdown. This results in urea ~ 300-600mmol/day; ammonium(NH_4^+), sulphate (SO_4^{2-}), phosphate (PO_4^{3-}), H^+, uric acid and creatinine which require excretion.
- Maintenance of Na^+, Cl^- and K^+ balance with emphasis on <u>conservation of Na$^+$</u>—important in defence of vascular volume, but <u>excretion of potassium</u>.
- Concentration and dilution to maintain water balance and tonicity.
- Maintenance of acid-base balance: excretion of H^+ or HCO_3^- ions derived from the diet and reclamation or excretion of filtered HCO_3^-; or in the Stewart-Fencl model the excretion or retention of chloride.
- Maintenance of divalent cations (Mg^{2+}, Ca^{2+}) and phosphate homeostasis.
- Endocrine functions: production of erythropoietin,1,25 $(OH)_2$ D_3, renin and other hormones.

Table. *Main functions of the kidney.*

Each kidney has approximately 1 million nephrons. (Figure 1.)The renal artery divides into 5 segmental arteries at the hilus which then subdivide into lobar arteries which in turn give rise to interlobular arteries at the cortico-medullary junction. These form arcuate arteries which arch across pyramids. Smaller arteries radiate from these to supply the cortex. (figure 2) The majority of blood flow supplies the cortex and only 10% supplies the medulla. The afferent arterioles divide into a meshwork of capillaries which coalesce to form efferent arterioles.

These branch into a network of capillaries, surrounding the tubule, and drain into the interlobular and then renal vein. Compared to the glomerular capillaries, which have a higher hydrostatic pressure than other capillaries, the peri tubular network is a low pressure system which promotes reabsorption.

The glomerulus consists of a tuft of capillaries containing 3 layers:

- Endothelium.
- basement membrane.
- epithelial cells.

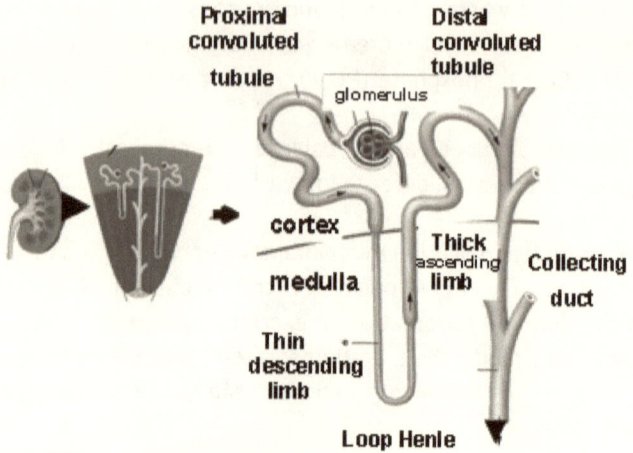

Figure 1. Model showing Kidney, pyramid and individual nephron.
(Produced using Servier medical art.)

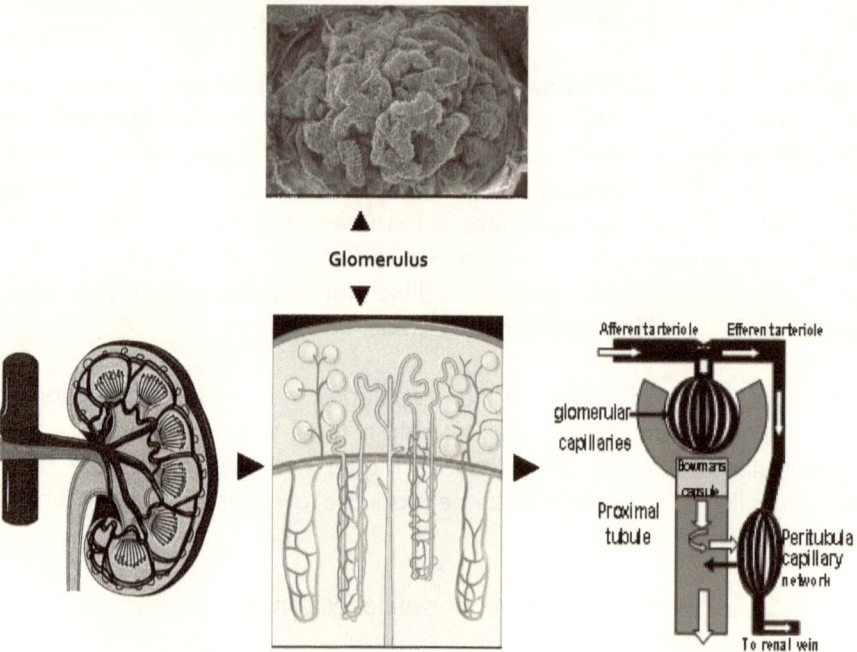

Figure 2. Model of renal blood supply: *The renal afferent arteriole divides into the glomerular tuft and gives rise to the efferent arteriole. This divides into a peritubular network which surrounds tubules.*
(Produced using Servier medical art.)

Endothelium contains numerous pores. Basement membrane, which surrounds endothelium, is composed of a mesh work of collagen and proteoglycans, which are negatively charged, and large spaces which permit passage of water and solute. The negative charge, rather than capillary pores, decrease filtration of negatively charged albumin.

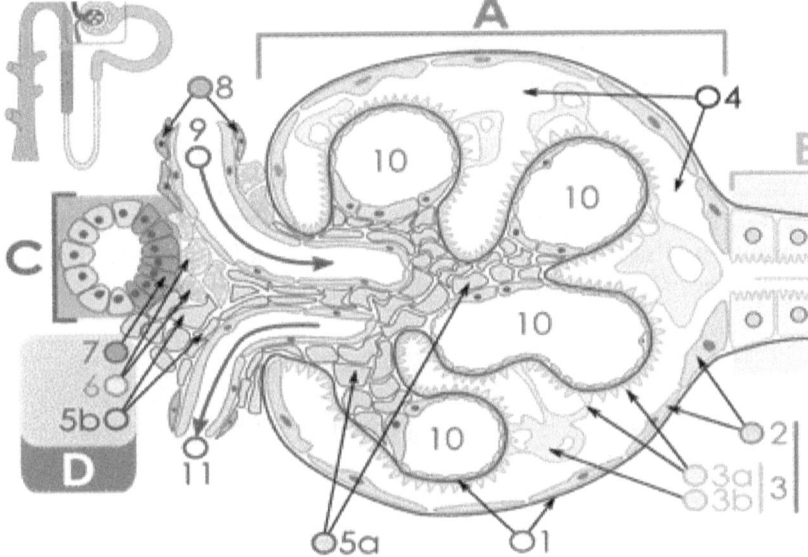

Figure 3A. Renal corpuscle. (Permission Michal Komorniczak, Medical illustrations, Poland)

A-renal corpuscle; B-proximal tubule C-distal convoluted tubule; D-juxtaglomerular aooaratus; 1-basement membrane;2-Bowmans capsule parietal layer 3a-Pedicels(foot processes from podocytes) 3b-podocyte;4-bowmans space; 5a Mesangium 5b- Mesangium (extraglomerular) 6-juxtaglomerular cells;7-macula densa; 9-afferent arteriole; 10-glomerular capillaries; 11-Efferent arterioles.

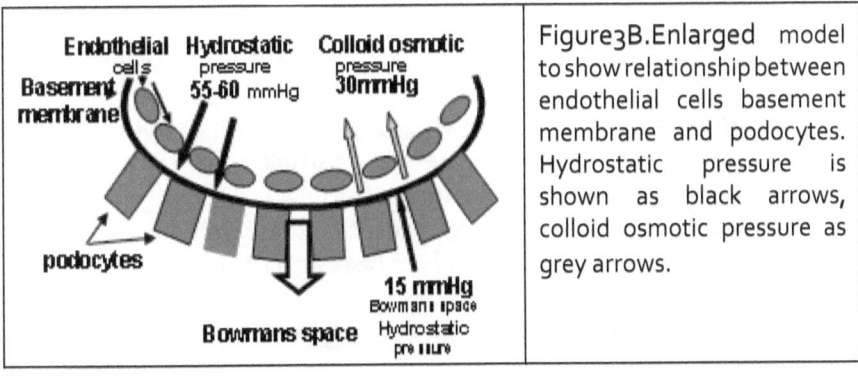

Figure3B.Enlarged model to show relationship between endothelial cells basement membrane and podocytes. Hydrostatic pressure is shown as black arrows, colloid osmotic pressure as grey arrows.

Figure 3B. Model of the glomerulus.

Epithelial cells, covering the glomerulus, are continuous with cells lining Bowman's space. They extend long foot processes called podocytes, which make contact with basement membranes, but contain slits, through which glomerular filtrate passes. Mesangial cells are located in the triangular space between afferent and efferent arterioles and extend into the glomerulus to provide a supporting and contractile function.

Approximately 20-25% of cardiac output (CO) (~ 1L) supplies the kidney. Twenty percent of protein free fluid flows from capillaries of glomerular tufts into Bowmans capsule while 80% emerges from efferent arterioles to enter a peritubular network. The renal plasma flow in a woman with haematocrit of 0.45 and renal blood flow of 950mL is:

$$0.55 \times 950 = 500\text{mL/minute.}$$

If the filtration fraction is 20% the glomerular filtration rate (GFR) =0.2x 500. = 100mL/minute.

Blood in peritubular capillaries, which surround proximal tubules, has a higher oncotic pressure than plasma at 36mm because 20% of protein free fluid has been filtered off. (Figure 3) The higher oncotic pressure and low peritubular capillary pressure promote tubular reabsorption. GFR is determined by the:

* Net filtration pressure.
* Capillary filtration coefficient (Kf), a measure of the surface area and conductivity of capillaries and basement membranes.

The net filtration pressure is the difference between:

1. Capillary hydrostatic pressure (55-60mmHg), which is higher than in other capillaries.
2. Hydrostatic pressure in Bowmans space into which fluid is filtered (~15mmHg). Papillary or ureteral obstruction to flow increases hydrostatic pressure in Bowmans capsule.
3. Colloid osmotic pressure (oncotic pressure) in capillaries, (~30mmHg), which attracts fluid back into the capillary.

Net Filtration pressure= 55 -15 -30 = 10mmHg.

Glomerular filtration rate is net filtration pressure x capillary filtration coefficient (Kf).

GFR = Kf x net filtration pressure.

Capillary filtration coefficient (Kf) is decreased in diabetes, hypertension and capillary inflammation, which increase the thickness and decreases conductance of capillaries and basement membranes. Decrease in basement membrane negative charge, which normally repels negatively charged albumin, may also cause albuminuria.

GFR is regulated by constriction and relaxation of afferent and efferent arterioles. Constriction of efferent arterioles increases glomerular pressure and filtration, while afferent arteriolar constriction decreases pressure and filtration. Shock, afferent arteriolar constriction, by the sympathetic nervous system, angiotensin II, n-adrenaline and endothelin, produced both systemically and locally in the kidney, cause afferent arteriolar constriction. This decreases glomerular filtration.

Prostaglandins partly counteract afferent arteriolar vasoconstriction in order to maintain a critical level of blood flow. The predominant prostaglandins, E2, PGE2 and prostacyclin are important in maintaining renal blood flow and GFR ; inhibiting tubular sodium reabsorption ; antagonising the action of ADH and renin secretion during low cardiac output. [16, 17]

Cycloxygenase (COX) 1 and 2 inhibitors, which decrease synthesis of PGE2 and prostacyclin, decrease renal blood flow, increase sodium retention and may rarely cause hyperkalaemia. Renal failure is especially likely to occur during hypovolaemia if COX inhibitors are administered because modulation of vasoconstriction is inhibited.

Tubular Glomerular Feedback and autoregulation of blood flow.

GFR is kept constant over a wide range of blood pressure and is matched to flow down tubules in individual nephrons, called tubuloglomerular feedback, by several mechanisms.

- Decrease in afferent arteriolar pressure leads to vaso-dilatation, by direct myogenic relaxation, and change in sympathetic and hormonal action. Natriuretic peptides relax mesangial cells and increase capillary surface area available for filtration. Increase in afferent arteriolar pressure results in opposite changes.

- Microvilli of brush borders of proximal tubules are flow sensors and modulate sodium reabsorption by acting on NHE3 exchangers and H^+ ATPase pumps. [18]
- Increase in GFR increases flow of NaCl in thick ascending limbs loops of Henle (TALH) which could exceed their capacity for Na^+ and Cl^- reabsorption. Increased flow is sensed by macula densa cells of the TAL in contact with afferent arterioles (figure 4). Nitric oxide (NO) release is inhibited causing afferent arteriolar constriction and decrease in GFR. The opposite sequence of events occurs if GFR falls below normal. Thus flow of NaCl down nephrons is regulated by changes in GFR.

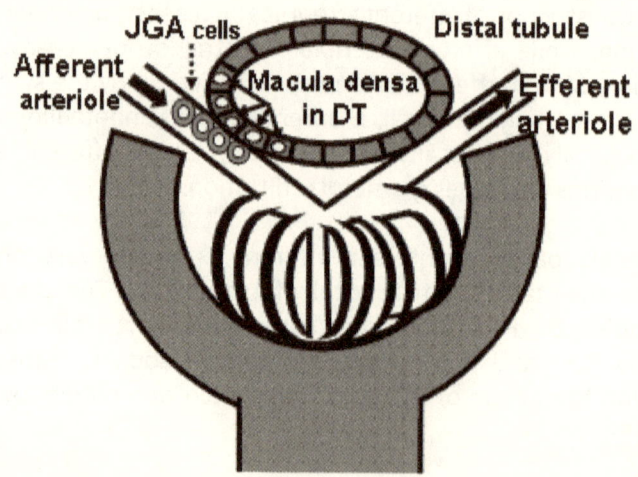

Figure 4. Relation of macula densa cells in distal tubule to afferent arteriole.

One fifth of nephrons are juxtaglomerular: glomeruli near the cortico-medullary junction. These extend long loops of Henle which reach into the inner medulla and are accompanied by long arterioles (vasa recta). They are important for maximum urine concentration.

The following diagram shows different segments of the nephron. The proximal tubule, 2-3mm long, comprises a convoluted and straight section, the pars recta, which enter the Loop of Henle at the outer medulla.

Loops of Henle, which descends into the medulla, consists of thin descending limbs, short thin ascending and long thick ascending limbs (TALH). These ascend to the cortex, where they bend to form distal convoluted tubules.

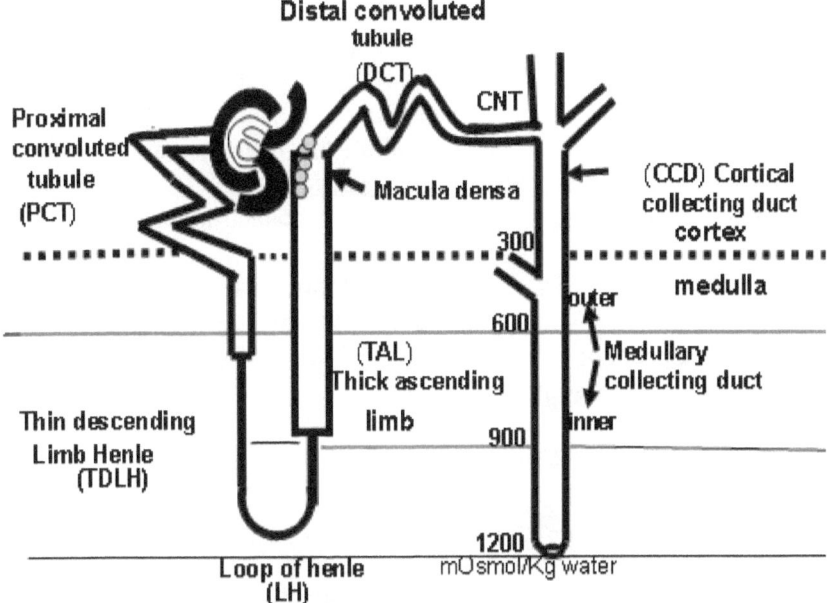

Figure 5. Nephron and osmolal gradients from cortex to medulla. *Horizontal lines are osmolality in mOsmol/kg H$_2$O. CNT=connecting tubule.*

The kidney filters and reabsorbs an enormous amount of water and solute. The following are approximately filtered and excreted in a subject with a GFR of 100mL/min. (table 2).

	Filtered	Excreted
Water	14,400mls	1000-1500ml/L
Na$^+$	20,160mmol	1 00-mmol
K$^+$	576mmol	100-mmol
Cl	14,400mmol	100-mmol
HCO$_3^-$	3,600mmol	0 -mmol
Urea	720mmol	~ -400 mmol
Glucose	720mmol	0-mmol
Ca^{2+}	172mmol	5.0 mmol
Mg^{2+}	115mmol	~10.0mmol

Table 2: Approximate substances filtered per day in a subject with GFR of 100mL/ min on a usual diet. Substances filtered = 100(mL/min) x 60(min) x 24(hours) x mmol of solute in 100mL

Thick ascending limbs establishes contact with the arteriole of its glomerulus at the bend (figure 4 and 5) and give rise to specialised cells—the Macula densa. This senses flow of Cl^- and Na^+ in tubular fluid. At this point the ascending loops of Henle become distal convoluted tubules (DCT). This becomes the connecting tubule (CNT) and joins with adjacent tubules of other nephrons to form cortical collecting ducts. These descend into the medulla as outer and inner medullary collecting ducts.

The high glomerular filtration of solutes and water require a highly efficient system for reabsorption. During sodium deficiency the kidney can reabsorb all except 1-2mmol of the 20,000mmol sodium filtered daily and all except for 300-400mL water

MAIN PROCESSES OF REABSORPTION.

- Proximal tubules reabsorb most filtrate, including water, sodium, HCO_3^-, Cl^-, P anions, aminoacids and glucose.
- Distal tubules reabsorb Na^+, H_2O, K^+, Ca^{2+}, Mg^{2+}, H^+/Cl^- to determine final urine composition.

Sodium Reabsorption

The force for sodium reabsorption is generated by action of Na^+:K^+ pumps which export three Na^+ out of cells in exchange for importing $2K^+$ into cells. This provides a high concentration gradient for Na^+ and negative intracellular potential. This promotes Na^+ reabsorption into cells. Sodium reabsorption provides the mechanism for:

1) Anion reabsorption (Cl^-, HCo_3^- and PO_4^-) to maintain electroneutrality.
2) Water reabsorption to maintain isotonicity in proximal tubules.
3) Aminoacid, glucose and organic compound reabsorption in proximal tubules, in co-transport with Na^+, using energy provided by the Na^+ gradient generated from activity of Na^+:K^+ pumps.
4) Divalent cations—Ca^{2+}, Mg^{2+} absorption in proximal tubules, in response to an increase in their concentration, secondary to sodium, anion and water reabsorption.

Sodium reabsorption takes place in all parts of the tubule except descending limbs, loops of Henle (Table 3).Following reabsorption into cells Na^+ exits via Na^+:K^+ pumps on basolateral membranes.

Tubular Site		Transport Mechanism	Mechanism
Proximal tubule	60-70%	NHE	Na$^+$ H$^+$ exchange
		Paracellular	Na$^+$ reabsorption between cells
		cotransport	NaCl reabsorption with glucose and aminoacids.
Ascending limbs loops of Henle	25-30%	NKCC2	Na$^+$ K$^+$ 2Cl$^-$ co-transport.
Distal convoluted tubule	5-10%	NCC	Na$^+$ Cl$^-$ cotransport.
Collecting tubule	3%	ENaC	Na$^+$ channels.

Table 3: Na$^+$ absorption in different parts of tubule [4, 5, 8, 11, 12, 9,20].

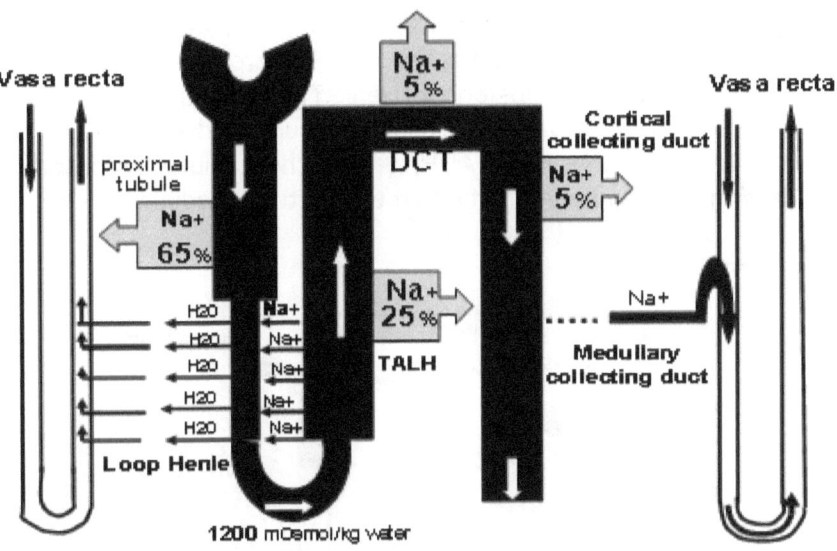

Figure 6: Model of reabsorption of sodium and its recycling into the descending limb loop of Henle and descending vasa recta. In the vasa recta Na$^+$ moves in the direction of the medulla while water moves away from the medulla to the cortex. This promotes high medullary but low cortical sodium concentration. TALH=thick ascending limb loop of Henle; DCT =distal convoluted tubule.

Anion Reabsorption

Cl^-, HCo_3^- and phosphate anions are linked to Na^+ reabsorption in proximal tubules to maintain electroneutrality. 99% of bicarbonate is reabsorbed (reclamation) as a result of Na^+ reabsorption in exchange for H^+ by NHE transporters. Chloride is reabsorbed into cells by Cl^--anion exchangers in luminal membranes or through the gaps between cells—paracellular reabsorption. The extent of each is uncertain. Chloride-formate exchangers, which work in parallel with apical Na^+:H^+ exchangers, may be the most important.[21] Phosphate is reabsorbed by Na^+ phosphate cotransporters (NPT2a) which move from the interior of the cell, where they are inactive, to the luminal (apical) membrane. This occurs in response to low dietary phosphate, 1, $25(OH)_2 D_3$ and hypophosphataemia, while PTH and FGF 23 move transporters from the membrane to cytosol, to promote phosphate excretion.

Water reabsorption.

Water is reabsorbed passively in proximal tubules in response to the osmotic gradient created by sodium anion reabsorption. Water is reabsorbed without sodium in descending thin loops of Henle (DTLH) which concentrates tubular fluid as the bend is approached. The opposite occurs in thick ascending limbs loops of Henle, (TALH): sodium and chloride are reabsorbed without water thus diluting tubular fluid as TALH ascends to the cortex. In the presence of ADH, water without solute, is reabsorbed in collecting ducts by movement into the hypertonic medulla.

Potassium [22-24]

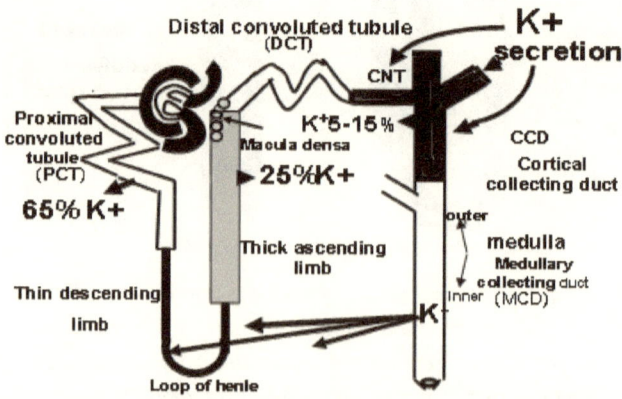

Figure 7. Model showing K^+ reabsorption and secretion in tubule. Secretion is shown as blacked out area. Potassium is recycled into the descending loops of Henle.

Over 90% of filtered potassium is reabsorbed: 65-80% in proximal tubules through the paracellular route; 10-25% in the TALH through cells; and the remainder in medullary collecting ducts. Thus nearly all K^+ is reabsorbed proximal to the DCT. Nearly all urine K^+ results from secretion by principal cells of collecting ducts and CNT in exchange for Na^+. (Shown in black in figure7)

Maximum K^+ secretion, in response to a concentration gradient, requires that tubular fluid K^+ concentration is kept low by sufficiently high flow rates in collecting ducts.—is flow rate dependent.

During K^+ excess cortical collecting ducts and proximal medullary collecting ducts secrete K^+. During deficiency or low potassium diet potassium is reabsorbed by K^+: H^+ exchange in α intercalated cells of collecting ducts. Potassium is recycled from collecting ducts to medulla and into descending thin limbs loop of Henle (DTLH) [25].

Divalent Cations (Ca^{2+} Mg^{2+})

- The proximal tubule reabsorbs 20% Mg^{2+} and 60% Ca^{2+} between cells due to increase in their concentration as Na^+- anion and water are reabsorbed.
- Most remaining Ca^{2+} and Mg^{2+} are reabsorbed in TALH by the paracellular route secondary to the positive lumen potential created by recycling of K^+ into the lumen: the positive lumen potential drives positive divalent ions through tight junctions between adjacent cells. Proteins in tight junctions, called claudins, are selectively permeable to these ions.
- Approximately 10% of Mg^{2+} and Ca^{2+} are reabsorbed in distal convoluted tubules (DCT) through cells (transcellular route): Ca^{2+} by TRPV5 (transient receptor protein vanilloid 5) channels and Mg^{2+} by TRPM6 (transient receptor protein melastin 6) channels. This is where fine tuning of Ca^+ and Mg^+ occur.

Acid base balance [5, 7, 8, 11-13] is achieved by:

* Reclamation of filtered HCO_3^- in proximal tubules utilising Na^+: H^+ exchangers.
* Excretion of filtered HCO_3^- in excess of normal extracellular HCO_3^- (~24mmol/L).
* NH_4Cl and $H_2PO_4^{2-}$ (converted from HPO_4^-) excretion in distal tubules, in response to acidosis or high acid containing diets.

It is important to appreciate that for each Cl^- excreted, without an accompanying cation, a HCo_3^- ion must be reabsorbed and vice versa to maintain electroneutrality. The most important function in acid-base balance is <u>excretion or retention of Cl^- without an accompanying cation:</u> this is achieved by synthesis and excretion of NH_4^+ to accompany Cl^-.

Water Balance. [2-6, 26-30]

Water is isotonic at the end of proximal tubules. Production of an isotonic cortex but hypertonic medulla, in which Na^+, Cl^-, urea and NH_4^+ are concentrated, is a crucial component of water and acid base balance [26]. This is achieved by:

- Counter current multiplier system involving both tubules and accompanying hair pin loops of vasa recta; high cortical blood supply needed to fuel high metabolic demand; but low medullary blood flow to prevent wash out of medullary ions and hypertonicity. [31, 32]
- Recycling of urea [29, 30, 33, 34], NH_4^+ [35, 36], Na^+, Cl^-, and K^+ to descending tubular loops of Henle [26] and medulla.

<u>**Production of Hypertonic Medulla**</u>

This contains high concentrations of Na^+, Cl^-, urea, NH_4^+ - NH_3 and K^+. Both descending and ascending loops of Henle and accompanying vasa rectae form a counter current multiplier system and with collecting ducts provide increasing osmolality from cortex to medulla. This enables excretion of dilute or highly concentrated urine. Isotonic fluid enters the descending Loop of Henle from proximal tubules. (Figure 8)

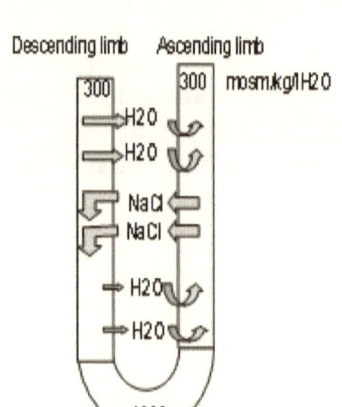

Water without NaCl is reabsorbed in the descending limb of a loop. This increases tubular fluid tonicity towards the bend. In direct contrast thick ascending limbs are permeable to NaCl but not to water. NaCl is reabsorbed without water in ascending limbs which results in increasingly dilute fluid as tubules ascend.

Figure 8. Model showing operation of counter current multiplier system.

The selective exchange of NaCl and water between two limbs running in parallel but in opposite directions.

This effect is multiplied because NaCl reabsorbed from ascending limbs passes into descending limbs which contributes to tonicity as the bend is approached; while water reabsorbed from descending limbs enters ascending limbs contributing to dilution of their fluid. Vasa recta blood vessels accompanying loops act in a similar but opposite manner, so that water is carried away to the cortex while NaCl and urea enters descending loops. This increases tonicity in the bend of arterioles in the medulla. Thus differential exchange of fluid travelling in opposite directions multiplies concentration at tips of loops.

Urea transporters in the inner, but not outer or cortical medullary ducts, reabsorb urea into the medulla stimulated by ADH [29, 33, 34]. Urea is recycled so that it is trapped in the medulla: the medullary urea moves into descending limbs loops of Henle and the descending limbs of vasa recta and recirculates. (Figure 9)

Tonicity increases from hypotonicity in the cortex to 1200-1400 mOsmol/kg H_2O at the papillary tip, under the influence of ADH, as a result of differential reabsorption of solute, water and urea in tubular fluid along nephrons; and the multiplier effect of tubular fluid and blood moving in opposite directions in two adjacent loops.

In ascending limbs of loops of Henle sodium chloride absorption without water dilutes tubular fluid to an osmolality less than cortex.

Further sodium and chloride is reabsorbed without water in distal convoluted tubules and collecting ducts, provided ADH is absent, so that tubular fluid osmolality decreases to ~ 50 mOsmol/kg H_2O. Further water absorption does not occur in the absence of ADH and dilutes urine to ~ 50 mOsmol/kg H_2O.

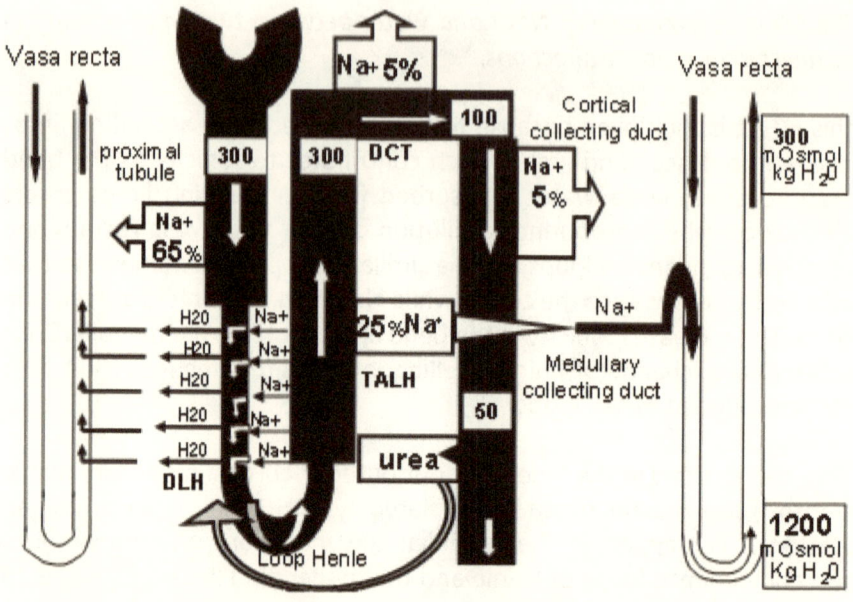

Figure 9. Model showing counter current multiplier process and recycling of urea and sodium chloride (see text).

White boxes show osmolality of tubular fluid and adjacent interstitium and percent of sodium reabsorbed in different nephron segments. Fluid in proximal tubules is approximately isotonic.

Water is reabsorbed in descending loops of Henle and increases fluid osmolality as loops descend into the medulla. In ascending limbs Na$^+$ Cl$^-$ is reabsorbed without water and tubular fluid osmolality decreases as it ascends to the cortex. Further Na$^+$ Cl$^-$ reabsorption in the distal convoluted tubule by Na$^+$ Cl$^-$ cotransporters further dilutes urine. Na$^+$ reabsorption in collecting ducts dilute urine to 50 mOsmol/kg H$_2$O provided ADH is suppressed. Four further processes contribute to medullary tonicity.

Na$^+$ (small arrows) reabsorbed in TALH is recycled into descending limbs. H$_2$o reabsorbed in descending limbs (small arrows) enters ascending limbs of vas recta thus decreasing dilution of the medulla. Na$^+$ (25%) reabsorbed in the TALH passes into descending limbs of vasa recta and increases Na$^+$ concentration in vascular loops moving into the medulla. Urea is transported from inner medullary collecting ducts and increases concentration of medullary urea. Urea is also recycled by reabsorption from medulla into descending loops of Henle. Thus, the effect of ions and water reabsorption in tubular and vascular loops, flowing in opposite directions, multiples the efficiency of achieving an increasing gradient of osmolality from cortex to medulla.

SPECIFIC NEPHRON SEGMENTS—CELLULAR MECHANISMS

Reabsorption occurs through cells, called transcellular, or between cells—paracellular.

Paracellular. Individual epithelial cells are attached to each other by a junctional complex containing proteins, called Claudins, which contain pores which open or close to selectively allow specific ions to pass, while preventing others. [37, 38]

Transcellular reabsorption and secretion require movement across two membranes: a luminal (apical) membrane adjacent to the tubular lumen and basolateral membrane adjacent to interstitial fluid and circulation and transportation across the cell. Reabsorption is achieved either passively, in response to concentration or electrical gradients, or by energy dependant active transport. Transcellular reabsorption or secretion occurs via pumps, channels or transporters.

Pumps

Pumps expend energy (active reabsorption) in moving solutes against concentration or electrical gradients. The main pump, Na^+: K^+ ATPase is responsible for 70% of oxygen used by kidneys in keeping with the importance of Na^+ reabsorption: it transfers $3Na^+$ out of cells in exchange for $2K^+$ imported into cells. Na^+: K^+ pumps are therefore responsible for maintaining both a large intracellular concentration gradient for Na^+ and negative intracellular potential (3 positives out, 2 positives in). This facilitates luminal transfer of Na^+ into tubular cells and out via basolateral membranes into surrounding interstitial fluid and capillaries. Pumps are present in abundance on basolateral membranes (adjacent to interstitial fluid) in all nephron segments except thin descending loops of Henle which are impermeable to Na^+.

Channels: ions or molecules move passively in one direction in response to concentration, electrical or osmotic gradients. Channels may be open most of the time or closed and open only in response to electrical (voltage gated) or chemical (ligand gated) change.

Transporters: move two or more molecules in the same direction, (symporters) or in opposite directions—antiporters or exchangers. Facilitated reabsorption occurs when molecules or ions are linked on a transporter in which one has a gradient promoting reabsorption-in essence hitching a ride. For example, glucose is reabsorbed with Na^+, for which there is a concentration and electrical gradient. In the diagrams of tubular function which follow:

Energy requiring pumps are shown as serrated circles.

Channels are shown as squares with an arrow.

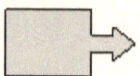

showing direction of movement.

Transporters are shown as circles.

Polarity refers to the location of pumps, channels or transporters: whether on luminal (apical) or cell membranes - (basolateral).

Membranes of tubule cells in contact with the lumen are referred to as luminal or apical; the basolateral membrane is adjacent to the interstitial fluid and peritubular capillaries.

PROXIMAL TUBULE (Figure 10)

Proximal tubules reabsorbs 70-75% of filtrate; 60-70% of filtered sodium, 55% chloride, 90% bicarbonate⁻, all glucose, amino acids and organic anions, and most calcium and phosphate.

$Na^+:K^+$ pumps provide the force for reabsorption. Na^+ is reabsorbed from the lumen by both transcellular (2/3) and paracellular (1/3) routes

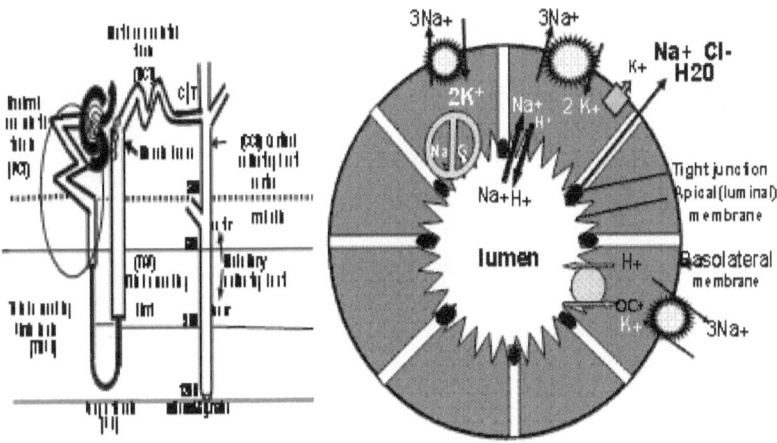

Figure 10:Proximal convoluted tubule showing tight junctions between cells, $Na^+:K^+$ pumps on basolateral membranes, $Na^+:H^+$ luminal transporters, $Na^+:glucose$ transporters(Na/G) and Na^+ Cl^- and H_2O exiting from paracellular space.

Sodium is reabsorbed from the lumen with phosphate, on NaPT2a cotransporters; with aminoacids and glucose in cotransport; and with Cl^- and HCO_3^- anions. NHE3 transporters which reabsorb Na^+ in exchange for H^+ secretion are the most important.

BICARBONATE REABSORPTION AND AMMONIUM SYNTHESIS. [39-44]

Na^+ reabsorption, in exchange for H^+ secretion, occurs via NHE transporters. 85% of the filtered HCO_3^- is reabsorbed in proximal tubules; 10% in loops of Henle and approximately 5-10% by distal convoluted tubules (DCT) and collecting ducts (CD). Na^+ is then transported from basolateral membranes of proximal tubule cells by $NaHCO_3^-$ transporters (NBC).

Na^+ reabsorption is regulated by flow sensors in cilia in apical membranes, which respond to tubular flow, and by local and systemic hormones. Angiotensin 2, acting on AT_1 receptors, increases reabsorption by NHE3. This is opposed by dopamine, synthesised locally, which inhibits AT_1 receptors and decreases numbers and activity of NHE3 on apical membranes.

There is a threshold for filtered HCO_3^- reabsorption, called Tm (Tm = maximum HCO_3^- reabsorption), which maintains serum HCO_3^- at normal levels ~ 24 mmol/L. When the threshold is exceeded, as a result of high dietary base intake, HCO_3^- is not reabsorbed beyond Tm). This threshold is increased by sodium depletion, raised pCO_2, aldosterone, angiotensin II and severe K^+ deficiency. The Tm HCO_3^- is decreased by volume expansion and low pCO_2.

Volume depletion increases proximal tubule Na^+ reabsorption by stimulating the Renin- Angiotensin Sympathetic system (RAS) and circulating catecholamines; and by causing low tubular flow. This increases exchange of Na^+ for H^+ on NHE exchangers and reabsorption of sodium with HCO_3^- through basolateral membranes. Filtered, HCO_3^- is not reabsorbed directly but combines with H^+, secreted by NHE3, to form $H_2CO_3^-$. (Figure 11).

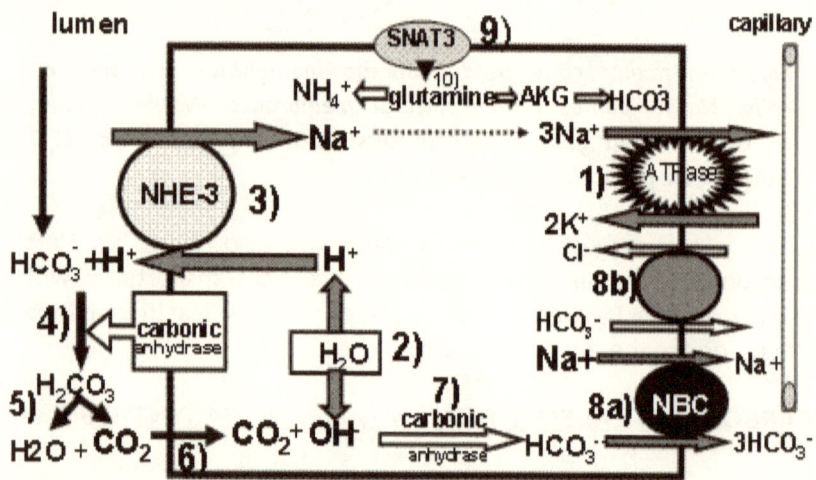

Figure 11: *Proximal tubule cell in acid base balance. Numbers correspond to numbers in text below. AKG = ∝ ketoglutarate. Oval clear circle =Na^+:H^+ exchanger (NHE-3).Oval black circle = Na^+:$3HCO_3$ transporter (NBC) and grey circle = Cl:HCO_3^- exchanger. Serrated Oval circle = 3 Na^+:$2K^+$ ATPase pump.*

1. Na^+:K^+ pumps move 3 Na^+ from the cell in exchange for 2 K^+ thus generating negative intracellular potential and low cellular Na^+.
2. Dissociation of H_2O generates H^+ ions,
3. H^+ is secreted into the lumen in exchange for Na^+ via Na^+:H^+ exchangers- (NHE3) secondary to the Na^+ gradient created in 1).
4. H^+ ions in the lumen react with filtered HCO_3^- on the brush border of tubular cells to form $H_2CO_3^-$ accelerated over 500 times by carbonic anhydrase. $H + HCO_3^- \longleftrightarrow H_2CO_3$
5. Luminal H_2CO_3 rapidly dissociates into CO_2 and H_2O.

6. CO_2, which is lipid soluble, rapidly diffuses into the tubule cell.
7. CO_2 reacts with the OH^- remaining from dissociation of water. The reaction is accelerated by intracellular carbonic anhydrase.
8. a) HCO_3^- is reabsorbed with Na^+ on $Na^+:3HCO_3^-$ transporters (NBC) through the basolateral membrane into the interstitial fluid and circulation or transported by $HCO_3^-:Cl^-$ exchangers (NBC) (8b). NBC is up regulated in response to metabolic acidosis and potassium depletion.

The net result is reabsorption of filtered $NaHCO_3$ by this indirect process. Most HCO_3^- reclamation is due to transcellular coupling of $Na^+: H^+$ exchangers (NHE-3) and $H^+: ATPase$ pumps with basolateral $Na^+: HCO_3^-$ (NBC) cotransporters.

The proximal tubule also plays a key role in production of new HCO_3^- (regeneration) by distal tubules. It does this by synthesis of $NH_4^+ + HCo_3^-$. Glutamine is synthesised by cells in a specific anatomic location in the liver. Synthesis increases during metabolic acidosis and decreases during alkalosis. [41, 42]

9. Glutamine is absorbed into proximal tubule cells by specific (SNAT 3) transporters. [43]
10. Glutamine is converted to NH_4^+ and HCO_3^- catalysed by α ketoglutarate In proximal tubule cells.

$$Glutamine \longrightarrow NH_4^+ + HCO_3^-$$

NH_4^+ is secreted into the lumen by taking the place of H^+ on the NHE3 $(Na^+: H^+)$ exchangers.

Chloride. [8, 10, 21, 45]

Most HCO_3^- has been reabsorbed when fluid reaches distal S2S3 segments of proximal tubules. Sodium is now reabsorbed with $Cl^-: Na^+:H^+$ exchangers works in tandem with chloride-base exchangers. The base, bicarbonate, formate or oxalate is recycled across luminal membranes so that in effect Na^+ is reabsorbed with Cl^-. Formate is recycled by combining with H^+, secreted by NHE exchangers, to form formic acid, which is lipid soluble and diffuses back into cells [21]. Chloride is also reabsorbed with sodium in co-transport with K^+ or in exchange with another anion. Chloride exits basolateral membrane via Cl^- channels and accompanies Na^+ to maintain electroneutrality.

Water.

Water is mainly reabsorbed by the paracellular route in response to the osmotic gradient secondary to NaCl reabsorption and to a lesser extent transcellularly by Aquaporin 1 water channels in luminal and basolateral membranes.

Urea.

Filtered urea, which is lipid soluble, diffuses from lumen into cells passively, so that only 40-50% of the filtered load is reabsorbed. The gradient for reabsorption is provided by NaCl and water reabsorption which increases urea concentration in tubular fluid. Thus an increase in Na^+ reabsorption from hypovolaemia increases urea reabsorption.

Glucose and aminoacids.

Glucose and amino acids are reabsorbed linked with Na^+ in which both are transported in the same direction (facilitated reabsorption) using the gradient for Na^+ provided by $Na^+ K^+$ pumps. Glucose exits from basolateral membranes via Glut1 and Glut 2 transporters.

Urate.

Urate is reabsorbed by a urate:OH^- or urate:HCO_3^- antiporter (transport in opposite directions) in the S3 segment of proximal tubules, linked to Na^+ transport, and exits from basolateral membranes by facilitated diffusion or in exchange for Cl^-. Thus volume depletion promotes urate reabsorption and hyperuricemia. The S2 segments of proximal tubules then secrete urate through basolateral membranes by anion exchangers in exchange for citrate intermediates. All except for 6-12% of urate is reabsorbed. The reason for initial reabsorption followed by secretion and then reabsorption is uncertain.

Organic cations and anions.

are not filtered, but are secreted by entering tubule cells from basolateral membranes. Organic anions eg (loop diuretics, thiazide diuretics and urate) are secreted into proximal tubules (S2 segment) via organic anion exchangers. Organic cations (amiloride, creatinine, ranitidine, trimethoprim, and quinine) are secreted into the lumen by H^+ cation antiporters, driven by the H^+ gradient generated by NHE exchangers.

Tubular secretion of creatinine is reversibly inhibited by other cations such as trimethoprim—serum creatinine may increase, but without changing GFR and may be misinterpreted.

Phosphate reabsorption. [46-51]

80-95% of phosphate is reabsorbed by NPT2 cotransporters, predominantly NPT2a, which carry phosphate from membranes into cells. The negative potential and Na^+ gradient produced by Na^+: K^+ pumps provide the force for reabsorption. Transporters are normally contained in vesicles within cell cytoplasm. A low phosphate diet [48] or phosphorous deficiency causes transport of NPT2a vesicles to cell membranes where they increase phosphate absorption. PTH and FGF23 [49-51] cause internalisation of NPT2a vesicles followed by their lysosomal degradation thus inhibiting phosphate reabsorption. (Figure 12) Phosphate moves from the tubule to basolateral membranes and then to circulation down its electrochemical gradient.

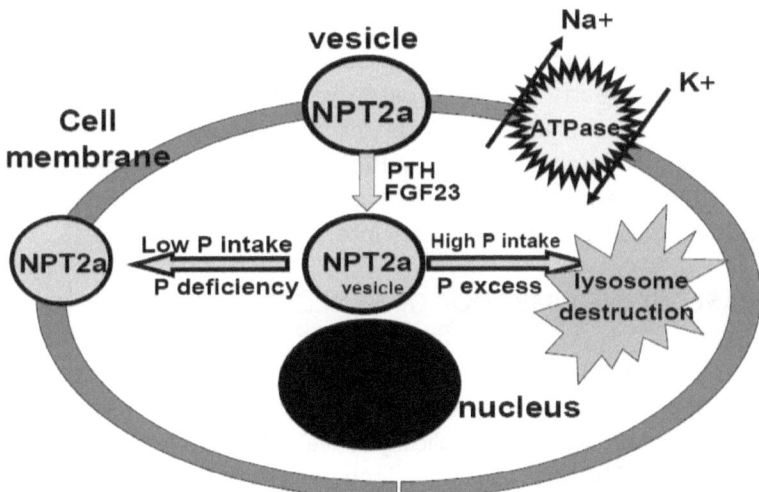

Figure 12: Tubular Phosphorus is reabsorbed by NPT2a cotransporters located on luminal cell membranes. Transporters are normally contained in vesicles within cells. Low phosphate diet or phosphate deficiency causes transport of NPT2a vesicles to cell membranes to increases phosphate reabsorption. PTH and FGF23 cause internalisation of NPT2a transporters by moving them into vesicles for lysosomal destruction [46-48]. Thus PTH and FGF23 decrease phosphate reabsorption and enhance phosphaturia.

Calcium.

60% of calcium is reabsorbed passively in proximal tubules by the paracellular route due to its increasing concentration as sodium, chloride and water are reabsorbed. Volume depletion therefore increases calcium as well as sodium reabsorption.

Magnesium.

All ionised Mg^{2+} (70-80%) is filtered and 20% of filtered Mg^2 is reabsorbed in proximal tubules.

Citrate [52] 65-90% of filtered citrate is degraded in proximal tubules. 1 mEq of citrate generates 3 HCO_3^- anions. Uptake occurs via luminal 3 Na^+: 1 citrate $^{2-}$ cotransporters.

THIN DESCENDING LIMB LOOP OF HENLE.

Twenty five percent of filtrate enters thin descending loops of Henle. Their main function is reabsorption of water, without solute, so that tubular fluid tonicity increases as it descends into the medulla. Its main role is to participate in the counter-current multiplier process which generates and maintains high medullary tonicity. Urea, Na^+ and K^+ are also recycled into descending limbs from the medullary interstitium.

THICK ASCENDING LIMB LOOP OF HENLE (TAL). (Figure 13)

Thick ascending limbs, in contrast to thin descending limbs, are impermeable to water but permeable to Na^+ and Cl^- which are reabsorbed. Thick ascending limbs (TAL) contain highly metabolically active cells and a high concentration of Na^+:K^+ pumps. The thick ascending limb has 3 main functions:

- Reabsorption of 25% of filtered Na^+.
- Contribution to generation and maintenance of medullary hypertonicity.
- Dilution of tubular fluid.
- Reabsorption of Ca^{2+}, Mg^{2+} and NH_4^+.

Luminal sodium, potassium and chloride are reabsorbed by *Na^+: K^+:2Cl^-* transporters, but <u>water is not reabsorbed</u>. Na^+ and Cl^- are also reabsorbed by NaCl transporters which are also inhibited by loop diuretics [22]. In addition to transfer into the circulation Na^+ also moves into thin descending limbs of loops of Henle. This increases the concentration of tubular fluid as loops descend into the medulla and is a multiplier system due to recycling of solute from ascending to descending limbs. The vasa recta blood flow accompanying loops flows in the opposite direction so that water reabsorbed from the descending limbs of loops of Henle moves into vasa recta taking blood away from the medulla. A small solute gradient difference is therefore multiplied. Sodium and urea are recycled into descending tubules.

As fluid ascends to the cortex in thick ascending limbs (TALH) it becomes increasingly dilute and reaches an osmolality of ≈ 300mosm/kg water. In addition TALH reabsorbs ~20% Ca^{2+}, 70% Mg^{2+} and NH_4^+ via the <u>paracellular route</u> driven by the positive lumen potential generated by K^+ recycling into the lumen: the concentration of K^+ is much lower than Na^+ in tubular fluid so that $Na^+K^+2Cl^-$ cotransporters would cease to function as luminal K^+ is reabsorbed. K^+ is recycled from cell to lumen by 2 types of K^+ channels: one of low conductance with high open probability; and a high conductance K^+ channel of low open probability, which opens in response to cell swelling—an important mechanism which regulates cell swelling. [24, 53]

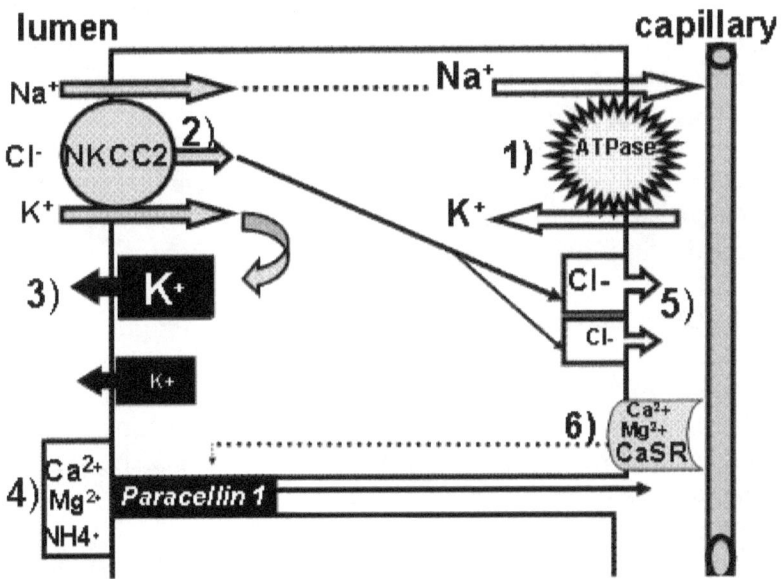

Figure 13: *Cell actions in thick ascending limb: NKCC2 is Na^+: K^+: $2Cl^-$ cotransporter. Numbers in figure correspond to those in text.*

1. *Na^+:K^+ pumps create low sodium concentration and negative intracellular potential.*
2. *This drives NKCC2 cotransporters to reabsorb Na^+, K^+ and Cl^-*

3. *K⁺, of low concentration in the tubular lumen, is recycled into the tubular lumen by K⁺ channels to provide K⁺ for NKCC2 cotransporters to function.*

4. *Recycling K⁺ produces a positive lumen which promotes passive reabsorption of Ca²⁺ and Mg²⁺ by the paracellular route (between cells) facilitated by Paracellin 1.*

5. *Cl exits through Cl channels on basolateral membranes and Na⁺ via Na⁺:K⁺ pumps.*

6. *CaSR (Ca²⁺ Mg²⁺ sensing receptor) controls paracellin related reabsorption of Ca²⁺ and Mg²⁺ by decreasing activity of K⁺ channels which decrease lumen positivity.*

Movement of both Mg^{2+} and Ca^{2+} through tight junctions in the paracellular space is facilitated by paracellin 1 (Claudin 16) [54-56] in response to hypocalcaemia or hypomagnesaemia. Stimulation of CaSR (Ca^{2+}:Mg^{2+}sensing receptor) activates K⁺ channels. Increase in the positive potential of the lumen increases the driving force for Ca^{2+} and Mg^{2+} reabsorption. On the other hand hypercalcaemia inhibits CaSR which decreases the number and or activity of K⁺ channels. This decreases the lumen positive potential which in turn decreases paracellular Ca^{2+} and Mg^{2+} transport. Decrease in availability of K⁺ also interferes with action of NKCC2 transporters and decreases Na^+Cl^- reabsorption. Thus <u>hypercalcaemia or a mutation which decreases function of CaSR</u> causes natriuresis. The latter is a cause of Barrters syndrome. Natriuresis protects the kidney from the effects of hypercalciuria and is an important protective function of CASR during hypercalcaemia. It does this by inhibiting NaCl reabsorption and therefore diluting Ca^{2+} in tubular fluid,

DISTAL CONVOLUTED TUBULE.

The distal convoluted tubule begins where the TAL makes contact with the afferent arteriole of its glomerulus (juxtaglomerular apparatus). Fluid entering the DCT has an osmolality of 300mosm/kg/ H_2O.This segment is relatively impermeable to water and has 2 main functions:

- Reabsorption of ~ 5% filtered NaCl without water. This further dilutes tubular fluid to approximately 50-100 mosm/kg/H_2O provided ADH is suppressed.
- Fine tuning of Ca^{2+} and Mg^{2+} by transcellular reabsorption.

Na⁺ is reabsorbed with Cl⁻ on NaCl cotransporters without water, In the absence of ADH, as a result of the gradient generated by Na⁺:K⁺ pumps. This further dilutes urine to~ 50-100 mOsm/kg/H_2O).

Ca²⁺ and Mg²⁺ are reabsorbed by the transcellular but not paracellular route in the DCT. Ca²⁺ (~10%) is reabsorbed from the lumen via Ca²⁺ channels (TRPV5)[55-58]; is transported across the tubule cell by a Ca²⁺ binding protein, Calbindin, followed by extrusion into interstitial fluid and circulation by 3 Na⁺/Ca²⁺ exchangers (NCX1) and Ca²⁺ ATPase pumps. [56]

A Ca²⁺: Mg²⁺ sensing receptor (CaSR) on the capillary side of the TAL controls both Ca²⁺ and Mg²⁺ reabsorption. Calcium excretion is regulated by PTH and 1; 25(OH)₂D₃. Calcitriol (1;25(OH)₂D₃) stimulates Ca²⁺ binding protein synthesis (Calbindin) in distal tubular cells and promotes luminal Ca²⁺ absorption by Ca²⁺ channels. [55-58] Klotho, the 'antiageing' hormone, stimulates Ca²⁺ uptake by glycosylating and stabilising TRPV5 Channels on luminal membranes. [58]

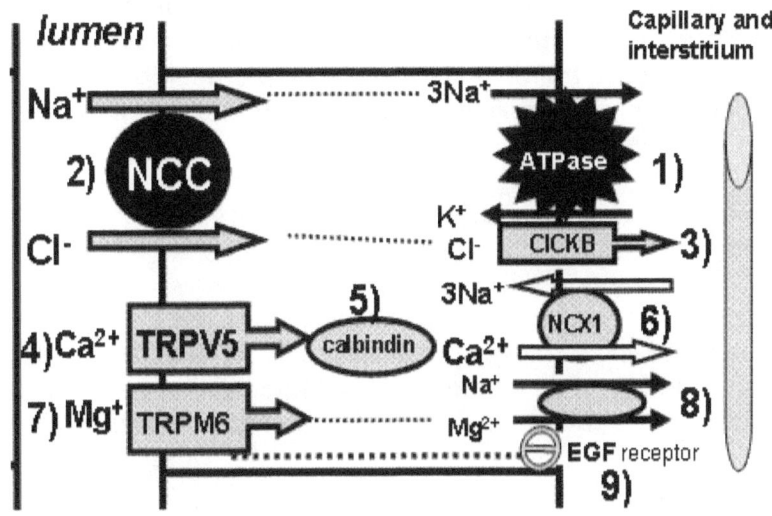

Figure 14: *Main actions of the distal convoluted tubule cell. Numbers in the diagram correspond to explanation below.*

1. *Na⁺:K⁺ ATPase pumps create low Na⁺ concentration and negative intracellular potential,*
2. *This promotes reabsorption of sodium and chloride by Na⁺ Cl⁻ transporters (NCC).*
3. *Cl⁻ exists by Cl⁻ channels (ClCKB) and Na⁺ via Na⁺ K⁺ pumps (1).*
4. *Ca²⁺ enters cell via calcium channels, TRPV5, (transient receptor protein vanilloid 5).*
5. *Ca²⁺ is transported across cell by calbindin, a Ca²⁺ binding protein.*
6. *Ca²⁺ exits the basolateral membrane on Ca²⁺: 3 Na⁺ exchangers (NCX1).*

7. *Mg²⁺ enters cell by TRPM6 (transient receptor protein melastin 6) channel.*
8. *Magnesium exits the basolateral membrane on Na⁺:Mg²⁺ exchangers.*
9. *Stimulation by epidermal growth factor (EGFR) receptor is important for optimum function of TRPM6.*

Na$^+$ and Ca^{2+} reabsorption are inversely related. Blocking NaCl transporters by thiazide diuretics increases Ca^{2+} reabsorption and causes hypocalciuria. Several reasons are suggested for this: [56]

*   Volume depletion causes a marked increase in proximal tubule Ca^{2+} reabsorption. [56]
*   Volume depletion decreases availability of intracellular Na$^+$ for continued action of Na$^+$:K$^+$ pumps. This stimulates Na$^+$:Ca^{2+} exchangers on basolateral membranes which increase intracellular Na$^+$.
*   Blockage of Na$^+$ entry into cells by thiazide diuretics and continued Na$^+$ transfer out, from action of Na$^+$:K$^+$ pumps, hyperpolarises the cell (intracellular more negative) which stimulates Ca^{2+} uptake by TRPV5 Ca^{2+} channels [56].

Approximately 10% of magnesium is reabsorbed actively through TRPM6 channels and exits the cell via Na$^+$:Mg^{2+} exchangers. [61, 62]

Thiazide diuretics, which block NaCl transporters, decrease further dilution of tubular fluid and increase calcium reabsorption. Gitelman syndrome, due to a loss of function mutation of Na: Cl transporters, simulates the action of thiazides but causes more pronounced hypomagnesaemia.

CORTICAL COLLECTING DUCTS. [63-71]

The cortical collecting ducts have two main types of cell: Principal cells and intercalated cells.

<u>**Principal cells.**</u> (Figure 15)

These are present in the connecting tubule, cortical collecting duct, and inner and outer medullary collecting ducts. Their main roles are:

*   Fine tuning of Na$^+$ reabsorption (2-3% Na$^+$ reabsorption).
*   Secretion of K$^+$.
*   Reabsorption of water in response to ADH.

Potassium channels have a common evolutionary basis in cell membranes. They are important for stabilisation of cell membrane potential, volume control and K^+ excretion. [22, 53, 64] Two K^+ channels have been identified in luminal membranes: normal flow rate channels with high open probability (ROMK) and high flow (Maxi.K) conductance channels with low open probability. The low conductance channel is always open whereas the fast conducting channel is activated when high loads of potassium require excretion or cell swelling occurs from rapid transfer of fluid from lumen into tubular cells. [53, 64] Cortical Collecting Ducts (CCD) have high membrane conduction which results in high excretion rates of K^+. Hyperkalaemia increases both channel activity and density and are a major control mechanism for K^+ excretion independent of aldosterone. [53, 64]

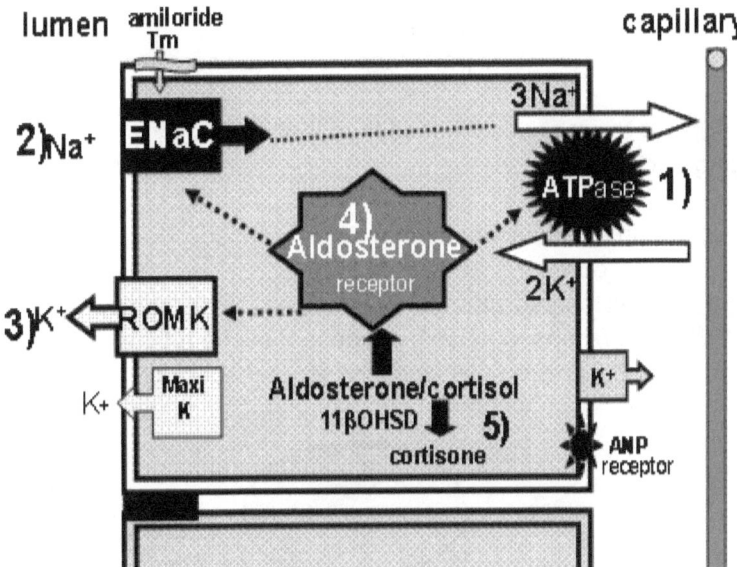

Figure 15: *Actions of Principal Cell in Collecting Duct. (water reabsorption is not shown). Numbers correspond to explanation below.* ENaC = sodium channel. ROMK = K+ channel—high open probability. Maxi K = K+ channel—high flow conductance channel. Tm = trimethoprim- inhibits ENaC. ANP = Atrial natriuretic peptide. II β OHSD= 11β hydroxysteroid dehydrogenase type 2.

1. Na+: K+ pumps generate negative intracellular and lower Na gradient within cells.
2. This increases Na+ entry across the luminal membrane through sodium channels—EnaC [63] .and increases the negative potential in the lumen.

3. *K⁺ moves into the tubular lumen through K⁺ channels in response to the negative lumen potential created by Na⁺ reabsorption. Na⁺ exits and K⁺ enters cells via Na⁺: K⁺ ATPase pumps as in 1.*
4. *The aldosterone receptor stimulates activity of ENaC channels, K⁺ channels and Na⁺: K⁺ pumps.*
5. *Cortisol, which acts with equal affinity to aldosterone on the receptor, is converted to inactive cortisone by 11 β hydroxysteroid dehydrogenase II before it can act.*

Maximum K⁺ secretion requires a high flow rate in the lumen to decrease the high lumen K⁺ concentration which results [65]. Low flow decreases K⁺ excretion. Aldosterone increases activity of Na⁺ channels, Na⁺ K⁺ pumps, H⁺ ATPase pumps and ROMK potassium channels to promote K⁺ excretion. Progesterone secretion is increased during potassium deficiency, acts on H⁺: K⁺ exchangers in distal tubules and may be a potassium conserving hormone.

It is important to emphasise that sodium is absorbed by 2 mechanisms in collecting ducts. (Figure 16)

*   Electroneutral, accompanied by Cl⁻ reabsorption through the paracellular route.
*   Electrogenic: reabsorption of Na⁺ without an accompanying anion [22, 23, 66]. This results in negative potential in the tubular lumen which promotes K⁺ secretion—in exchange for reabsorbed Na⁺.

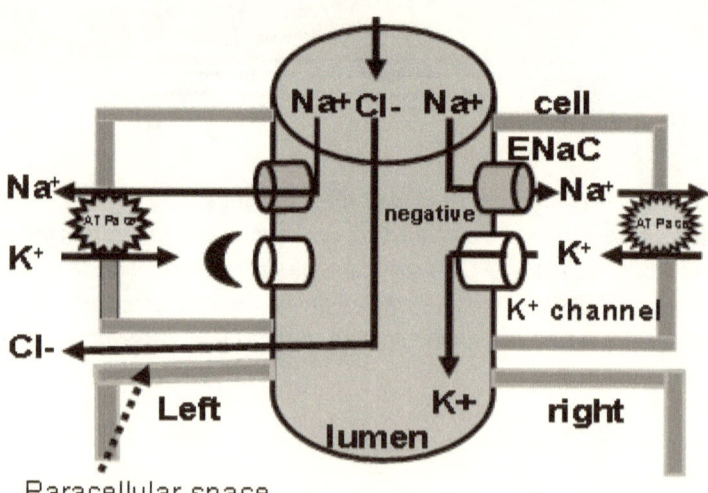

Figure 16: *Showing electroneutral, left side, and electrogenic (right side) Na⁺ reabsorption.*

In electrogenic reabsorption (right side) Na⁺ is reabsorbed through the Na⁺ channel (ENaC) and K⁺ is secreted (exchanged) in response to the negative luminal potential created by Na⁺ reabsorption. In electroneutral (left side) reabsorption Na⁺ is reabsorbed with an anion, usually Cl⁻, which is reabsorbed through the paracellular space.

It is important to emphasise that K⁺ secretion only occurs as a result of electrogenic Na⁺ reabsorption - Na⁺ reabsorbed without an anion. Even during a NaCl poor diet, as occurred in the past, there was a need to deliver 1mmol Na⁺ to the cortical collecting duct for excretion of each 1mmol of K⁺ [66].

Potassium secretion is driven by both aldosterone and high extracellular K⁺ concentration [67-70]. K⁺ stimulated aldosterone secretion is independent of sodium balance, intravascular volume or renin secretion [71]. Moreover an increase in dietary K⁺ increases K⁺ excretion independent of aldosterone [68]. Ingestion of potassium is also sensed in the gastrointestinal tract and increases renal excretion.

Aldosterone, secreted by the adrenal zona glomerulosa, is stimulated by both Angiotensin II and directly by raised serum K⁺. Renin, secreted by juxtaglomerular cells in afferent arterioles, in response to arterial underfilling or low renal perfusion pressure, stimulates synthesis of Angiotensin II.

Aldosterone binds to receptors on principal cells, transfers to the nucleus and following several intermediate steps has 4 main actions (figure 15). Aldosterone increases:

- Activity of sodium channels—ENaC.
- Activity of Na⁺:K⁺ pumps on basolateral membranes
- Activity of K⁺ channels.
- Activity of H⁺ ATPase pumps in α intercalated cells. [70]

This increases Na⁺ entry across luminal (apical) membranes; increases Na⁺ transport from basolateral membranes by Na⁺: K⁺ pumps; increases K⁺ efflux by potassium channels; and H⁺ secretion by H⁺ ATPase pumps.

The aldosterone receptor responds to both cortisol and aldosterone. Cortisol which is present at >1000 times the concentration of aldosterone (μmol compared to nmol amounts) would, if allowed to act, result in severe sodium retention. However cortisol is inactivated to cortisone [22]

by an enzyme 11 β-hydroxysteroid dehydrogenase II before it can occupy
the receptor.

In the absence of hypovolaemia aldosterone principally acts as a potassium
regulating hormone [22].When hypovolaemia is present increased proximal
tubular reabsorption of $NaHCO_3^-$ and NaCl decreases sodium delivery
to distal nephrons to exchange with K^+ so that aldosterone stimulated
potassium secretion does not occur. Antidiuretic hormone (ADH)
increases activity of Na^+ and K^+ channels and facilitates K^+ secretion and
Na^+ reabsorption under conditions of decreased water flow down tubular
lumens. Progesterone increases reabsorption of K^+.

ANP binds to a specific receptor on the basolateral membrane, closes
EnaC channels by activating adenyl cyclase, and promotes Na^+ excretion.
NSAIDs, ACE inhibitors, cyclosporine A and heparin impair aldosterone
release or action. Amiloride and trimethoprim interfere with function of
ENaC sodium channels, decrease Na^+ reabsorption and thus K^+ excretion.

Inner Medullary Collecting Duct (IMCD) and medullary interstitiium
resist extreme changes is osmolality and pH [32]: urine becomes highly
concentrated or dilute and highly acid or alkaline.[29, 30]These are responsible
for transport of urea into the medulla. This increases medullary osmolality
to 1200-1400 mOsmol/kg H_2O at the papilla. Urea is transported into
the medulla by urea transporters stimulated by ADH [33] and reaches a
concentration on the tip of the papilla of 400-900 mmol/L. Urea is trapped
in the medulla and recycled several times before excretion: the TALH, DT
and CCD are poorly permeable whereas thin descending limbs of Henle
and medullary collecting ducts are highly permeable. Thus urea passes
into descending loops of Henle and back into the CD. Urea is trapped in
the inner medulla because the structural arrangements of nephrons and
vasa rectae minimise removal. [30, 31]

WATER REGULATION. [, 26, 28, 72]

In the absence of ADH secretion collecting ducts remain impermeable to
water and dilute urine of ≈50 mOsmol/kg H_2O is passed. In the presence
of ADH water is reabsorbed by principal cells along the entire length of
the CD and results in maximum urine osmolality of 1200-1400 mosmol/
kgH_2O.

Thus daily excretion of 600mmol solute can be excreted in 12L urine at 50
mOsmol/kgH_2O or 500mls urine at 1200 mOsm/kgH_2O.

Mechanism of action of ADH

ADH is secreted from the posterior pituitary following stimulation by either osmoreceptors or volume sensing receptors in the hypothalamus. ADH is delivered to the basolateral membrane of collecting duct principal cells where it locks onto ADH receptors. This activates a G protein in the membrane followed by cyclic AMP formation from ATP. This in turn activates a protein kinase which causes Aquaporin water channels to move from cytosol to the luminal membrane. Reabsorbed water leaves tubular cells and enters the circulation by Aquaporin 3 and 4 channels in basolateral membranes. (Figure 17)

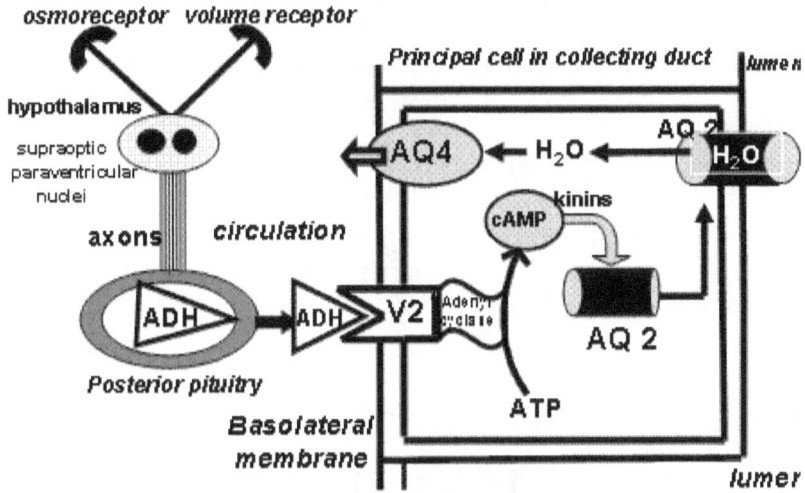

Figure 17. Mechanisms of Water reabsorption by Principal cell.

Tonicity and hypovolaemia are sensed by osmoreceptors and volume receptors in the hypothalamic paraventricular and supraoptic nuclei. These generate electrical impulses which travel down axons and depolarise membranes of the terminal axon bulb. This stimulates release of ADH into the circulation.ADH binds to a receptor, V2, on the basolateral membrane of collecting ducts. This initiates a series of changes which lead to water channels (Aquaporin 2), normally present in cytoplasm, moving to tubular luminal membranes where they transport water into the cell. Water is then reabsorbed from the basolateral membrane into the circulation by Aquaporin 4 water channels.

ADH also contributes to water reabsorption by:

- Increasing NaCl reabsorption in thick ascending limbs thus facilitating the counter current multiplier process.
- Increasing permeability of inner medullary collecting duct to urea.

INTERCALATED CELLS. [12, 13 34, 73-77)]

These are present in connecting tubules (CNT), cortical collecting ducts (CCD) and outer medullary collecting ducts. Alpha, but not beta intercalated cells, are present in inner medullary CDs. The action of α and β intercalated cells are shown in the following diagrams. They have a similar structure but are mirror images in polarity and function: the H^+ ATPase pumps and $K^+:H^+$ pumps are located on luminal (apical) membranes of α cells, but basolateral membranes of β cells. Their main function is acid-base balance. They differ in that α cells also reabsorb K^+ and β cells reabsorb Cl^- independent of acid-base balance.

α INTERCALATED CELL (αfor acid).

Note: operation of Cl^- :HCO_3^- exchangers are linked to excretion of NH_4 Cl. The main method of acid excretion is achieved by excretion of NH_4 Cl rather than H_2Po_4.

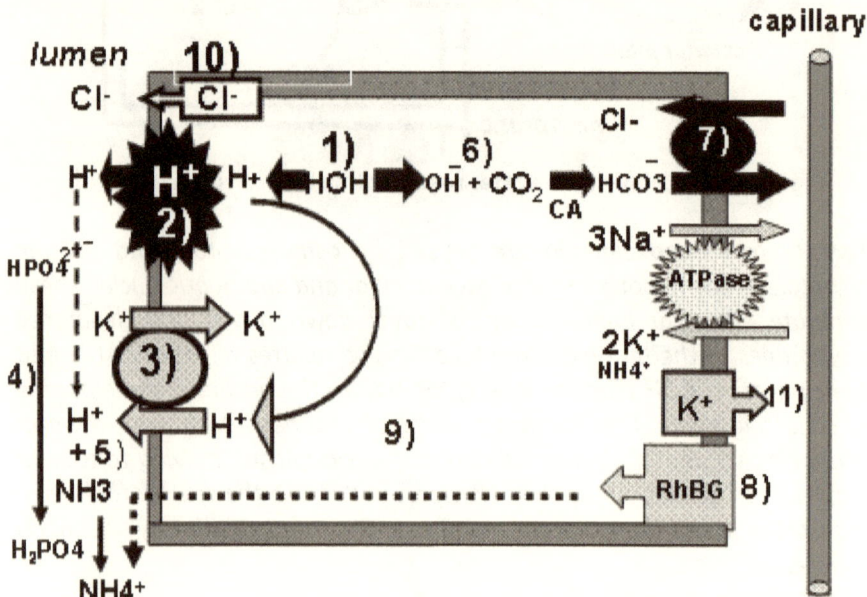

Figure 18. Intercalated α cell of the distal tubule. Numbers correspond to explanation in text.

1. H^+ and OH^- ions are generated from dissociation of H_2O
2. H^+ is secreted by proton (H^+ ATPase) pumps or
3. In exchange for K^+ on $H^+:K^+$ ATPase exchangers.
4. H^+ either combines with HPo_4^{2-} to form $H_2Po_4^-$.
5. or with NH_3 to form NH_4^+. Formation of non lipid NH_4^+ prevents its back leak into the cell.
6. Cellular CO_2 combines with OH^-, remaining from dissociation of H_2O, to form HCo_3^- catalysed by carbonic anhydrase.: $CO_2 + OH^- = HCO_3^-$
7. HCO_3^- exits the cell on $Cl^-:HCO_3^-$ exchangers.
8. NH_4^+ enters the cell by NH_4^+ transporters, (RhBG), or by substituting for K^+ on $Na^+ K^+$ pumps or basolateral $Na^+:K^+:2Cl^-$ transporters (not shown).
9. NH_4^+ enters the tubular lumen by NH_4^+ transporters.
10. Cl^- enters tubular lumen to accompany NH_4^+ via Cl^- channels.
11. Potassium exits cells to interstitium in K^+ channel.

The reverse process occurs in β (β for base) cells: HCO_3^- formed from dissociation of H_2CO_3 is transported into the lumen while H^+ and Cl^- ions are reabsorbed into interstitiium and circulation. Cl^- is reabsorbed through the lumen by $Cl^-:HCO_3^-$ exchangers or Cl^- anion exchangers associated with a protein Pendrin.(Figure 19)

$Cl^-:HCO_3^-$ exchange operates in tandem with basolateral chloride channels. [78]

β cells have an important additional function of reabsorbing luminal Cl^- to accompany Na^+ reabsorbed by Principal cells. They do this by a chloride –anion exchanger called Pendrin: this can exchange Cl^- for HCO_3^- or formate.and potentially decrease Na^+ exchange for K^+ in principal cells during potassium deficiency.

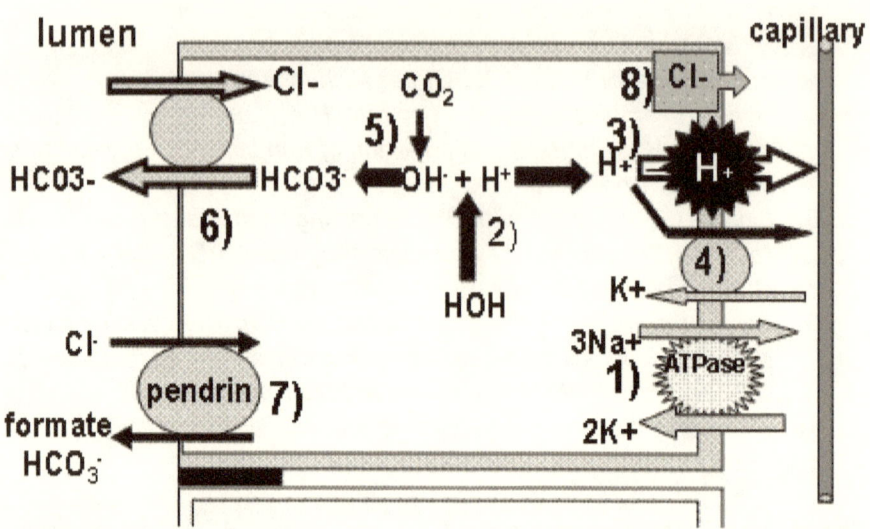

Figure 19: ꞵ intercalated cell.

The structure and function are the mirror image of intercalated cells. H^+ is transported into the circulation and HCo_3^- secreted into the tubular lumen in exchange for Cl^- which is reabsorbed.

1. *Na^+: K^+ pumps create Na^+ and negative potential gradients.*
2. *H^+ and OH^- ions are generated from dissociation of H_2O.*
3. *H^+ is transported through basolateral membranes by H^+:ATPase pumps.*
4. *or H^+:K^+ exchangers.*
5. *Co_2 combines with OH^-, remaining from dissociation of H_2O, to form HCo_3^-*
6. *Cl^- enters cell from the lumen by Cl:HCO_3^- transporters and HCO_3^- enters lumen.*
7. *or Cl^- is reabsorbed in exchange for formate or HCO_3^- by anion exchangers (pendrin).*
8. *Cl^- exits through chloride channels in basolateral membranes.*

α Cells are also important in K^+ reabsorption: when deficiency is present they increase K^+ exchange with H^+ on H^+:K^+ exchangers. This may be stimulated by progesterone. K^+ then exits from basolateral membranes via K^+ channels. H^+ excretion increases and results in acid urine. Thus H^+:K^+ and H^+:ATPase pumps respond selectively to chronic hypokalaemia and acidosis.

In conclusion the kidney has two major roles in acid base balance:

- The reclamation (reabsorption) of filtered HCO_3^- in proximal tubules. This occurs by the indirect process of converting filtered HCO_3 into H_2CO_3 by secreted H^+ ions accelerated by carbonic anhydrase. H_2CO_3 forms H_2O and CO_2. CO_2 is rapidly absorbed into cells and is reconverted into HCO_3^- and H^+ facilitated by cytosolic carbonic anhydrase. [39, 40]
- Synthesis of new HCO_3^-: Glutamine, synthesised by the liver, is broken down to NH_4^+ and HCO_3^- by proximal tubule cells.

If an excess of bicarbonate is present from dietary sources NH_4^+ is reabsorbed from basolateral membranes of proximal tubules, transported to liver and metabolised to urea and H^+ which consumes HCO_3^-. [35]

When excess acid requires excretion NH_4^+ is secreted into proximal tubular lumens by taking the place of H^+ on Na^+: H^+ exchangers. It is reabsorbed from the lumen of thick ascending limbs loops of Henle by taking the place of K^+ on Na^+:K^+:$2Cl^-$ transporters and is transported into the medulla. NH_4^+ dissociates into NH_3 and H^+ in the medulla. NH_3, which is lipid soluble, diffuses into the lumen of α cells.

Alpha intercalated cells of distal tubules secrete H^+ ions which combine with HPO_4^{2-} and NH_3 in the tubular lumen. The combination of NH_3 with H^+ forming NH_4^+ 'fixes' H^+ ions and enables excretion of large amounts of H^+ in maximally acid urine. (pH4.4). Alternatively NH_4^+ is transported into alpha intercalated cells by RhBG or RhBC channels or enters cells by taking the place of K^+ on Na^+:K^+ pumps on basolateral membranes.

NH_4^+ is transported from α cells into the tubular lumen by RhBG transporters and combines with Cl^-. NH_4^+, which combines with Cl^-, is the most important method for H^+ excretion and is capable of reaching 300 mmol in a severe acidosis compared to only 80 mmol for titratable acid, as H_2PO_4.

Net Acid Excretion = H2PO4- + NH4 Cl minus free HCO3-

It is equivalent to net HCO_3^- generated and requires both adequate NH_4^+ generation from glutamine by proximal tubules and H^+ secretion by distal tubules.

Conceptually the most important reason for NH_4^+ production and excretion is to excrete Cl^- without Na^+ thus increasing the SID (strong ion difference) predominantly Na^+ minus Cl^-. (Chapter 6)

Depending on whether there is dietary alkaline or acid load—or disordered acid-base balance:

- The liver synthesises glutamine in response to acidosis; or in alkalosis converts it to urea plus H^+ which combines with HCO_3^- to form H_2CO_3. This forms CO_2 which is eliminated.
- If glutamine is converted to NH_4^+ and HCO_3^- in the kidney, NH_4^+ can be reabsorbed into the circulation for metabolism in the liver or can be secreted into the tubular lumen to combine with Cl^-. This generates HCO_3^-.

SUMMARY

Approximately 100-120mL of protein free fluid is filtered each minute and 150,000mL each day.

All except for 300 mL can be reabsorbed including most electrolytes. The main driving force for reabsorption is activity of Na^+: K^+ pumps on basolateral membranes which provide both negative electrical potential and low intracellular Na^+ concentration. This drives sodium reabsorption.

All HCO_3^- and 65 % of filtered NaCl and water are reabsorbed isosmotically in proximal tubules. The majority of Ca^{2+}, phosphate, 90% HCO_3^- and all amino acids and glucose are reabsorbed in proximal tubules while organic acids and bases are secreted into luminal fluid.

Water reabsorption, solute and urea transfer into descending loops of Henle, increases osmolality of tubular fluid as the loop descends into the medulla. The thick ascending loop (TALH) is impermeable to water and reabsorbs 20-30% NaCl via $Na^+K^+2Cl^-$ transporters. Thus tubular fluid osmolality decreases as TALH ascends to the cortex.

The descending and ascending tubular loops and vasa recta work as counter current multipliers by exchanging solute and water in parallel loops travelling in opposite directions. Urea, transported from inner medullary collecting ducts, also recycles to the medulla and contributes to medullary hypertonicity.

Ca^{2+} and Mg^{2+} are reabsorbed in the TALH by the paracellular route, promoted by a positive lumen potential generated from K^+ recycling.

Distal convoluted tubules are responsible for 5-10% reabsorption of Na^+ by electroneutral Na^+Cl^- cotransporters, without water, and thus further dilute tubular fluid to 50-100mosm/kg/H_2o. The DCT also 'fine tunes' Ca^{2+} and Mg^{2+} reabsorption by the transcellular route stimulated by $Ca^{2+}:Mg^{2+}$ sensors (CaSR) on basolateral membranes.

Collecting ducts contain 2 main types of cell: principal and intercalated. The main actions of principal cells are:

- Fine tuning Na^+ reabsorption via ENaC channels in exchange for K^+ which is secreted into luminal fluid and then excreted.
- Secretion of K^+.
- Water reabsorption.

Aldosterone facilitates Na^+ reabsorption and K^+ secretion by:

- Increasing numbers and activity of ENaC apical sodium channels and H^+ ATPase pumps.
- Increasing activity of luminal K^+ channels.
- Increasing activity of $Na^+:K^+$ pumps in principal cells and H^+ ATPase pumps in α intercalated cells.

Water is reabsorbed through water channels in collecting ducts which are inserted into luminal membranes stimulated by ADH.

Intercalated cells have similar structure but opposite polarity and function: α Intercalated cells secrete H^+ ions into the tubular lumen, via proton (H^+) ATPase pumps or $H^+:K^+$ exchangers ; β cells reabsorb H^+ (and thus excrete HCO_3^-). Intercalated cells fine tune acid-base balance.

In addition βcells reabsorb chloride to accompany Na^+ transported into the lumen by principal cells rather than in exchange for K^+; and α cells reabsorb K^+ by exchange with H^+ when dietary K^+ is low or K^+ deficiency exists. Thus both α and β cells play a role in potassium homeostasis.

Thus with infinite complexity the red wine of Shiraz is turned into urine

REFERENCES:

GENERAL

1. Dinesen I. Seven Gothic Tales. *N.Y. Modern Library.* 1939.
2. The Urinary System p 961-1005 in Fundamentals of Anatomy and Physiology. Ed. Martini FN, 1998. Prentice Hall International Inc.
3. The Urinary System p 482-527 in Human Physiology From cells to Systems. Ed. Sherwood L, 2001. Brooks/Cole.
4. The Kidney p352-366 in Pharmacology. Ed. Rang HP, Dalem M, Ritter JM, Moore PK. 5th Ed.2007. Elsevier
5. The Urinary System p737-878 in Medical Physiology. Updated Edition.2005 Ed. Boron WF, Boulpaep EL, Elsevier Saunders.
6. Renal function and Fluid and Electrolytes. P 565-579 in Pathophysiology. 5th Edition.1998 Ed. Porth CM, Lippincott.
7. The Urinary System and Homeostasis p 992-1035 in Principals of Anatomy and Physiology. Ed. Tortora GJ, Derrickson B. 11th Edition.2003. John Wiley and Sons.
8. Renal Physiology p1-138 in Clinical Physiology of Acid-Base and Electrolyte Disorders. 5th Edition.2001 Ed. Rose BD, Post TW, McGraw Hill.
9. Urine formation by the Kidney p291-326. Urine function by the Kidney p327-347. Regulation of extracellular fluid osmolality p348-364 in textbook of Medical Physiology. Ed. Guyton AC, Hall JE. 11th Edition.2006. Elsevier Saunders.
10. Normal Anatomy, Physiology and metabolism of the Kidney p3-160. Sansom SC, Shigaki M, Giebisch G Potassium Homeostasis. in Textbook of Nephrology. Ed. Massry SG, Glassock RJ. 4th Edition.1996 Lippincott, Williams and Wilkins.
11. Renal circulation and Glomerular Haemodynamics p3-57 in Renal and electrolyte Disorders. Ed. Schrier RW. Sixth Ed. Lippincott, Williams and Wilkins 2003.
12. The Kidney 5th Edition. Ed. Brenner BM, 1996. WB Saunders.
13. Diseases of the Kidney and Urinary Tract. Ed. Schrier RW. 7th Edition 2001. Lippincott, Williams and Wilkins.

SPECIFIC

14. Eaton SB, Konner RM. *Paleolithic Nutrition.* 1985, New Engl J Medicine **312**:283-289.
15. Kurlansky M. Salt—A World History. *Vintage.* 2003.

16. Jaimes EA, Tian R-X, Pearse D, Raij L. Up regulation of glomerular Cox-2 by Angiotensin II: Role of reactive oxygen species. *Kidney Int.* 2005, **68**:2143-2153.

17. Tichtenoth DO, Marhauer V, Tsikas D, et al. Effects of specific Cox-2 inhibition on renin release and renal systemic prostanoid synthesis in healthy volunteers. *Kidney Int.* 2005, **68**:2197-2207.

18. Wang X, Armando I, Upadhyay K et al. The regulation of proximal tubular transport in hypertension: an update. *Current Opinion in Nephrology and Hypertension.* 2009, **18**:412-420

19. Knepper MA, Brooks HL. Regulation of the sodium transporters NHE3, NKCC2 and NCC in the kidney. *Current Opinion in Nephrology and Hypertension.* 2001, **10**:655-659.

20. Stokes JB. Disorders of the epithelial sodium channel: Insights into the regulation of extracellular volume and blood pressure. *Kidney Int.* 1999, **56**:2318-2333.

21. Manoocher S. Molecular physiology of the renal chloride-formate exchanger. Current Opinion Nephrol and Hypertension. 200110:677-683.

22. Giebisch G, Wang W. Potassium transport: From clearance to channels and pumps. *Kidney Int.* **49**:1624-1631.1996

23. Kamel SK, Halperin LM, et al. Disorders of Potassium Balance p 999-1037 in The Kidney. Ed. Brenner BM, 1996.

24. Peterson LN, Levi M. Disorders of Potassium Metabolism. P171-215 in Renal and Electrolyte Disorders. 6th Edition. 2003 Ed. Schrier RW. Lippincott, Williams and Wilkins.

25. Jamieson RL. Potassium Recycling. *Kidney Int.* 1987, **31**:695-703.

26. Sands JM, Kokko JP. Countercurrent system. *Kidney Int.* 1990, **38**:659-699.

27. Nielsen S, Knepper MA, Hwan Kwon T, Frokiaer J. Regulation of Water Balance, Urine Concentration and Dilution p109-134.in Renal and Electrolyte disorders. Ed. Schrier RW. 2003 Lippincott, Williams and Wilkins.

28. Robertson G, Berl T. Pathophysiology of Water Metabolism p873-928 in Brenner and Rector's The Kidney. Ed. Brenner RB, 1996 Saunders Coy.

29. Lise Bankir. Urea and the Kidney. Ch.14 p571-596 in The Kidney. Ed. Brenner BM. 5th Edition 1996. WB Saunders.

30. Madsen KM, Clapp WL, Verlander JW. Structure and function of the inner medullary collecting duct. *Kidney Int.* 1988, **34**:441-454.

31. Chou S-Y, Porush JG, Faubert PF. Renal medullary circulation: Hormonal Control. *Kidney Int.* 1990, **37**:1-13.

32. Brezis M, Rosen S. Hypoxia of the renal medulla—Its implications for disease. *NEJM.* 1995 *332*:647-655.

33. Sands Jeff M. Renal urea transporters. *Current Opinion in Nephrology and Hypertension*. 2004, **13**:525-532.

34. Fenton RA. Urea transporters and renal function: lessons from knockout mice. Current Opinion Nephrol Hypertension.**17** 513-518 2008

35. Zoubida K, Szutkowska M, Vernimmen C, Bichara M. Renal handling of NH_3/NH_4^+ recent concepts. *Nephron Physiology*. 2005, **101**:77-81.

36. Good D, Carlton R, et al. Transepithelial ammonia concentration gradients in inner medulla of the rat. *Amer. J. Physiol*. 1987, **252**:F491-F500.

37. Angelow S, Yu ASL. Claudins and paracellular transport: an update. *Current Opinion in Nephrology and Hypertension*. 2007, **16**:459-464.

38. Yu ASL. Paracellular solute transport: more than just a leak. *Current Opinion in Nephrology and Hypertension*. 2000, **9**:513-515.

39. DuBose TD. Reclamation of filtered bicarbonate. *Kidney Int*. **8**:584-589. 1990

40. Soleimani M, Burnham CE: Physiologic and molecular aspects of the Na^+: HCo_3^- cotransporter in health and disease processes. *Kidney Internat*. **57**:371-384, 2000.

41. Atkinson Daniel E, Bourke Edmund. Metabolic aspects of the regulation of systemic pH. *Amer. J. Physiol*. 1987, **21**:947-956.

42. Vinay P, et al. Regulation glutamine metabolism in Dog Kidney in vivo. *Kidney Int*. 1986, **29**:68-79.

43. Ibrahim H, Lee YJ, Curthoys NP: Renal response to metabolic acidosis: Role of MRNA stabilization. *Kidney Internat*. **73**:11-18, 2008.

44. Good DW, Carlton RC, Dubose T. Transepithelial ammonia concentration gradients in inner medulla of the rat. *Amer. J. Physiol*. 1987, **252**:F491-F500.

45. Gerardo Gamba. Electroneutral chloride—coupled cotransporters. *Current Opinion in Nephrology and Hypertension*. 2000, **9**:535-540.

46. Popovtzer MM. Disorders of calcium, phosphorus, vitamin D and parathyroid hormone activity. P 216-277 In: Schrier RW, ed. Renal and electrolyte disorders. 6th Ed. Philadelphia: Lippincott Williams and Wilkins. 2003,.

47. Kayne LH, Pham P-CT, Pham P-TT, Lee DB. Phosphate metabolism. In: Massry SG, Glassock RJ, eds. Massry and Glassock's Textbook of Nephrology. 4th Edition. Philadelphia: Lippincott, Williams and Wilkins, 2001, 355-379.

48. Miyamoto KI, Itho M. Transcriptional regulation of the NPT2 gene by dietary phosphate. *Kidney Int*. 2001, **60(2)**:412-5.

49. Fukagawa M, Nii-Kono T, Kazama JJ. Role of fibroblast growth factor 23 in health and in chronic kidney disease. *Current Opinion in Nephrology and Hypertension*. 2005, **14 (4)**:325-9.

50. Prie D, Beck L, Urena P, Friedlander G. Recent findings in phosphate homeostasis. *Current Opinion in Nephrology and Hypertension*. 2005, **14(4)**:318-24.

51. Berndt TJ, Schiavi S, Kumar R. "Phosphatonins" and the regulation of phosphorus homeostasis. *Amer. J. Physiol. Renal Physiol*. 2005, **289**:F1170-F1182.

52. Hamm LL. Renal handling of citrate. *Kidney Int*. 1990, **38**:728-735.

53. Wang WH. Renal potassium channels: recent developments [molecular cell biology and pathology of solute transport]. *Current Opinion in Nephrology and Hypertension*. 2004, **13**:549-555.

54. Rouse D, Suki WN. Renal control of extracellular calcium. *Kidney Int*. 1990, **38(4)**:700-8.

55. Lambers TT, Bindels RJ, Hoenderop JG. Coordinated control of renal Ca_2+ handling. *Kidney Int*. 2006, **69(4)**:650-4.

56. Mensenkamp AR, Hoenderop JG, Bindels RJ. Recent advances in renal tubular calcium reabsorption. *Current Opinion in Nephrology and Hypertension*. 2006, **15(5)**:524-9.

57. Peng JB, Hediger MA. A family of calcium-permeable channels in the kidney: distinct roles in renal calcium handling. *Current Opinion in Nephrology and Hypertension*. 2002, **11(5)**:555-61.

58. Topala CN, Bindels RJM, Hoenderop JG. Regulation of the epithelial calcium channel TRPV5 by extracellular factors. *Current Opinion in Nephrology and Hypertension*. 2007, **16(4)**:319-324.

59. Huang C, Miller RT. Regulation of renal ion transport by the calcium-sensing receptor: an update. *Current Opinion in Nephrology and Hypertension*. 2007, **16**:437-443.

60. Blanchard A, et al. Paracellin-1 is critical for magnesium and calcium reabsorption in the human thick ascending limb of Henle. *Kidney Int*. 2001, **59**:2206-15.

61. Yu ASL. Evolving concepts in epithelial magnesium transport. *Current Opinion in Nephrology and Hypertension*. 2001, **10**:649-653.

62. Chubanov V, Guderman T, Schlingmann KP. Essential role for TRPM6 in epithelial magnesium transport and body magnesium homeostasis. *Eur. J. Physiol*. 2005, **451**:228-234.

63. Gamba G. Molecular biology of distal nephron sodium transport mechanisms. *Kidney Int*. 1999, **56**:1606-1622.

64. Giebisch G. Renal potassium channels: function regulation and structure. *Kidney Int*. 2001, **60**:436-415.

65. Cheema-Dhadli S, et al. Requirements for a high rate of potassium excretion in rats consuming a low electrolyte diet. *J. of Physiol*. 2006, **572**:493-501.

66. Halperin ML, et al. Control of potassium excretion: a Paleolithic perspective. *Current Opinion in Nephrology and Hypertension*. 2006, **15**:430-6.

67. Field MJ, Giebisch GJ. Hormonal control of renal potassium excretion. *Kidney Int.* 1985, **27**:379-87.

68. Rabinowitz L. Aldosterone and potassium homeostasis. *Kidney Int.* 1996, **49**:1738-42.

69. Sugarman A, Brown RS. The role of aldosterone in potassium tolerance: Studies in anephric humans. *Kidney Int.* 1988, **34**:397-403.

70. Garg LC, Narang N. Effects of aldosterone on NEM-sensitive ATPase in rabbit nephron segments. *Kidney Int.* 1988, **34**:13-17.

71. Cox M, Sterns RH, Singer I. The defence against hyperkalaemia: the roles of insulin and aldosterone. *NEJM.* 1978, **299**:525-32.

72. Nielsen S, Agre P. The Aquaporin family of water channels in kidney. *Kidney Int.* 1995, **48**:1057-1068.

73. Massry SG, Glassock RJ. Acid-Base Metabolism p 391-396 in Massry and Glassock's Textbook of Nephrology. Fourth edition 2001.Eds Massry SG; Glassock RJ.Lippincott, Williams and Wilkins.

74. Alpern RJ, Rector FC. Renal acidification mechanisms in The Kidney 5 ed p408-471. Ed. Brenner BM.1996. WB Saunders.

75. Boron WF, Boulpaep EL, et al. Transport of Acids and Bases p845 in Medical Physiology. Ed. Boron WF, Boulpaep EL. Updated Edition. 2005 Elsevier Saunders.

76. Kurtzman N. Disorders of distal acidification. Kidney International 1990, **38**:720-727.

77. Batlle D, Flores G. Underlying defects in Renal Tubular Acidosis. *Amer. J. Kidney Dis.* 1996, **76**:896-915.

78. Eladari D, Chambrey R, Frische, MV et al. Pendrin as a regulator of ECF and blood pressure. Current Opinion Nephrol Hypert 2009.18:356-362.

WATER BALANCE AND DISORDERS OF WATER [1-8]

Myself when young did eagerly frequent
Doctor and saint and heard great argument
About it and about but evermore
Came out by the same door as in I went.
                    Rubiyat of Omar Kyham.

The amount of body sodium determines extracellular volume (ECV). Water balance, the amount of water in relation to solute, predominantly Na^+ and K^+, determines the concentration of solute in body fluid compartments and thus the serum sodium level and tonicity. The concentration of solute, extracellular sodium and cell potassium both decrease if net gain of water occurs without solute. On the other hand an increase or decrease in isotonic saline, (sodium and water in the same concentration as occurs in extracellular fluid), is confined to the ECV and does not change tonicity or serum sodium.

Each compartment contains ions which are mainly confined to that compartment: Na^+ in extracellular and K^+ in intracellular fluid. Increase in impermeable ions in one compartment exerts an osmotic pressure, which causes transfer of water from the other compartment until osmotic pressure equalises across membranes. If solute is freely permeable, such as urea, its concentration rapidly equalises across membranes, does not change tonicity or cause movement of water.

Osmolality.

The osmolality of a solution is the sum of the total number of particles per litre of solvent, essentially water, <u>regardless of permeability across membranes</u>. Solutes, molecules which are soluble in water, contribute to osmolality depending on the extent of their dissociation.

NaCl	$\leftrightarrow$	$Na^+ + Cl^-$	= 2 particles.
$CaCl_2$	$\leftrightarrow$	$Ca^+ + Cl^- + Cl^-$	= 3 particles.
Urea	$\leftrightarrow$	Urea	= 1 particle.

Molecules which are insoluble in water, such as lipids, do not contribute to osmolality. Osmolality of extracellular fluid equals the sum of their solutes multiplied by their dissociation.

$$= Na^+ + K^+ + Ca^{2+} + Mg^{2+} + Cl^- + HCO_3^- + Phosphate^- + albumin^- + So_4^{2-} + organic$$
$$acids^- + glucose\ (mmol/L) + urea\ mmol/L$$

To satisfy electroneutrality cations must equal anions: therefore serum osmolality equals double total cations or double total anions plus non ionised solutes such as glucose and urea. These are not doubled because they are single particles.

Serum osmolality = 2 x $(Na+K^+ + Ca^{2+} + Mg^{2+})$ + Glucose (mmol/L) + urea (mmol/L).

However 50% of serum Ca^{2+} and 30% of Mg^{2+} are bound to albumin and are not free in solution. There are two further factors which influence osmolality:

- Sodium chloride and sodium bicarbonate in serum are not completely dissociated: approximately 93%-94% are dissociated and 7% are not dissociated.
- Osmolality applies to and is measured in serum water. However serum contains 93% water and 7% solids: mainly lipids and protein which do not contain solute.

In estimating osmolality from serum sodium the 93% water factor approximately cancels the 93% dissociation factor (explained further under pseudohyponatremia.) Therefore plasma osmolality can be estimated by doubling serum Na^+ (to take anions into account) and adding serum glucose and urea in mmol/L.

Estimated osmolality   = | **(2 x Na) + glucose + urea (mmol/L)** |

Approximately   = 2 X 140 + 5 + 4 = <u>289 mOsmol/kgH$_2$O.</u>

This is similar to the normal measured plasma osmolality of ~289 (– 10) mOsmol/kg H$_2$o. Estimated and measured osmolality have a close correlation over large variations in plasma sodium. <u>Estimated osmolality</u> (including urea) can be compared with plasma osmolality measured by freezing point depression. This should be measured on plasma rather than serum and ideally with minimal use of tourniquet.

<u>Measured—estimated osmolality = < 15</u>

An osmolal gap greater than 15 suggests that an unmeasured solute is present in plasma, for example, alcohols or ethylene glycol– sometimes an important clue to poisoning.

Tonicity

Tonicity (also called effective osmolality) of a solution depends on the total concentration of solutes that exert an osmotic force across a semipermeable membrane and thus induce transmembrane movement of water. [9-11] Solutes which are freely permeable across cell membranes, such as urea and alcohols, increase osmolality but do not change tonicity, induce transfer of water or change cell size: they can be considered as ineffective solutes. [9-11]

Total osmolality = effective osmolality (tonicity) + ineffective osmolality

or rearranging the equation

Effective serum osmolality (tonicity) = total osmoles—ineffective osmoles.

Effective serum osmolality (tonicity) $\cong$ (2 $\times$ serum Na^+) + glucose mmol/L.

An increase in extracellular tonicity causes cells to shrink; decrease causes cells to swell.

Glucose is partly confined to extracellular fluid and exerts an osmotic force until it is metabolised or moves into cells. It draws water out of cells until osmolality equalises between cells and extracellular fluid. This decreases extracellular sodium concentration. [10] It acts as a 'partly' effective osmol.

Plasma sodium, rather than plasma osmolality or tonicity, is usually measured in everyday practice. Two corrections should be made if it is used as an indicator or surrogate for tonicity (effective osmolality).

- Half serum glucose above normal should be added. Only half serum glucose is added because glucose, which is unionised, contributes one particle whereas Na^+ has accompanying anions in its contribution to osmolality. Alternatively, effective serum osmolality can be estimated by doubling serum sodium and adding glucose in mmol/L.
- Allowance should be made for increase in the solid insoluble component of serum.

Serum contains 93% water, which contains all the Na^+ plus accompanying anions, and 7% insoluble solids which do not contain sodium (Figure 1).

Thus an increase in the solid component of serum, for example protein in multiple myeloma or lipids in hypertriglyceridemia, increases the solid component of serum and dilutes serum sodium. This is called pseudohyponatraemia because it does not change osmolality or reflect water balance. [12]

Pseudohyponatraemia [12] (Figure 1)

If a solution with plasma sodium of 140mmol/L was measured in 1L of plasma water rather than 1L of plasma the Na^+ concentration would be 140 ÷ 0.93 = 150.5 mmol/L in plasma water. This is because the non solute, solid component of plasma, which is sodium free, is 7% (Figure 1).

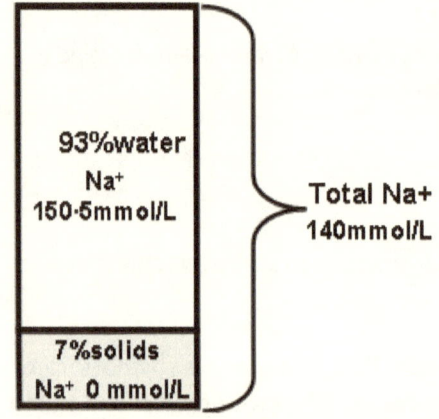

Figure 1. Na^+ concentration in water and non solute components of plasma to show the mechanism of pseudohyponatraemia.

Plasma contains 93% water and 7 % non solute solids. If serum Na^+ is 140 mmol/L and all sodium is present in serum water and none in serum solids the Na+ concentration in serum water is 140/0.93 = 150.5 mmol/L

Pseudohyponatraemia is a laboratory artefact: it does not occur if serum sodium is measured in the water phase of serum by an ion selective electrode compared to measurement of sodium in the total volume of serum (containing both water and solid components) by flame photometer.

Hypertriglyceridemia does not cause significant pseudohyponatraemia unless serum is lactescent—usually reported by the laboratory. Hypercholesterolaemia does not cause lactescence but is rarely sufficiently raised to cause pseudohyponatraemia. Serum Na^+ decreases by approximately 1.5mmol/L for each 1000mg/dL (12mmol/L) increase in serum triglyceride. [13]

Serum sodium decreases by 0.7mmol/L for each gram of monoclonal protein. Another quoted rule of thumb is to multiply the increment in serum protein above 8g/dL by 0.25 to correct serum sodium in order to reflect water balance or tonicity. [14] Osmolality measured by freezing point depression gives a better indication of water balance if pseudohyponatraemia is present, provided serum urea is normal.

Correction for an elevated serum glucose and water balance

Elevated serum glucose increases osmolality by its molal concentration above normal and causes transfer of water from cells to extracellular fluid until transcellular tonicity equalises. Half glucose above normal is added to serum Na^+ if sodium is used as an indication of current plasma osmolality. [10]

However, although this correction indicates current plasma osmolality, it does not accurately reflect total body osmolality (combined intracellular and extracellular osmolality) or water balance: when glucose normalises water re-enters cells from extracellular fluid, decreases extracellular volume and increases plasma osmolality; while cell volume increases and cell tonicity decreases. A change in extracellular glucose is shared by total body water (TBW) rather than ECV alone.

It has therefore been suggested that a correction factor should be applied to serum sodium to estimate what serum sodium will become following normalisation of elevated serum glucose—considered to reflect water balance more accurately than estimated plasma osmolality.

Katz [15] suggested a correction factor to reflect water balance: 1.6mmol is added to serum sodium for each 100mg/dL (5.6mmol/L) increase in serum glucose above normal. This was derived theoretically and based on several assumptions. The assumption that glucose was entirely confined to extracellular fluid was flawed because glucose enters cells in brain, heart and 50% of skeletal muscle by non-insulin mediated glucose uptake.

A factor to correct serum Na^+ to reflect water balance, derived experimentally in healthy volunteers, varied between 1.6-2.4mol for each 5.6mmol increase in serum glucose, depending on the severity of hyperglycaemia. [16] This may not be relevant in diabetic patients with hyperglycaemia of longer duration; and the use of hypotonic saline in the experiment may have distorted the results.

Using correction factors, however, lacks reliability; is of questionable relevance and rarely changes management because:

- Distribution of glucose varies within specific organs.
- The correction factor may vary widely depending on both the severity and duration of hyperglycaemia and severity of associated volume depletion.
- Estimates of total body water (TBW) and extracellular volume (ECV) based on body weight are inaccurate. [17] Marked variations of urinary

solute output during treatment changes serum Na⁺ independently of correction factors.

- Response of osmoreceptors is dependent on serum sodium rather than serum osmolality corrected for glucose. [18]
- Potassium depletion influences osmolality: on treatment with potassium extracellular osmolality increases from K⁺: Na⁺ exchange.
- Adaption of brain to changes in tonicity is difficult to predict.
- Hypotonicity or Hypertonicity should be corrected slowly, regardless of the level of serum glucose or tonicity, unless symptoms are severe, because brain cells may have adapted to the abnormal tonicity.

Role of Potassium in Total Body Osmolality

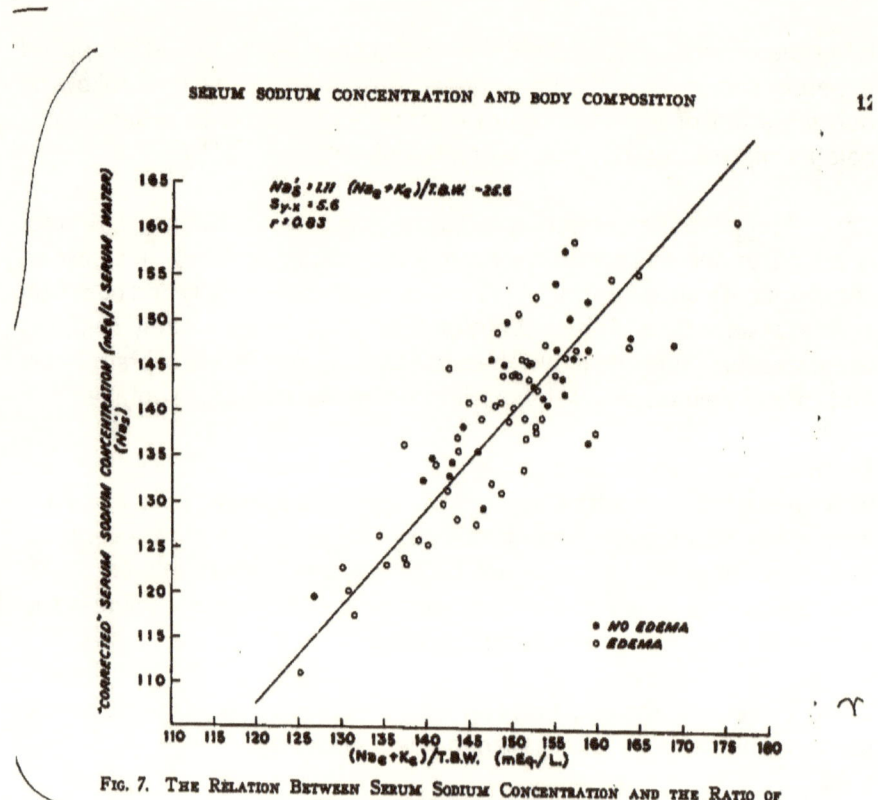

FIG. 7. THE RELATION BETWEEN SERUM SODIUM CONCENTRATION AND THE RATIO OF (Na₊ + K₊)/TOTAL BODY WATER

Figure 2. *Relation between plasma water, Na⁺ concentration and the ratio of (Na_e⁺ and K_e⁺/TBW, (Edelman I, Leibman J, O'Meara MP, Birkenfeld L, J. J Clin Invest 37:1236.1958. Copyright. American Society for Clinical Investigation. By permission.*

Figure 2 illustrates the contribution of K^+ to osmolality. Administration of an equivalent amount of either Na^+ or K^+ changes osmolality by the same amount unless or until renal excretion of these ions or water occurs.

The effective osmolality of intracellular fluid is the same as extracellular fluid because water moves freely between them. Na^+ and K^+ are the major exchangeable ions in solution in each case. Therefore effective osmolality of total body water and plasma is approximately:

$$2(Na_e^+ + K_e^+) / TBW \text{ (e = exchangeable).}$$ [19]

Doubling the exchangeable Na^+ and K^+ accounts for accompanying anions.

This should be taken into account in patients with hyponatraemia or hypokalaemia. For example infusion of 1L of normal saline with 40 mmol KCl added delivers a hypertonic fluid of 384 mOsmol/kgH$_2$O ($2 \times (154 + 40)$ and initially increases plasma tonicity.

External losses of K^+ are buffered by cells to limit the change in resting membrane potential which is mainly due to the intracellular K^+/extracellular K^+ ratio. The main mechanism involves exchange of intracellular K^+ for extracellular Na^+. Loss of total body K^+ decreases total body osmolality if external losses of water are discounted. Whether hypotonicity develops depends on net water changes.

If K^+ is retained, following potassium administration in a potassium depleted patient, it contributes to osmolality and also to extracellular sodium as Na^+ moves out of cells in exchange for K^+. This is important in patients with heart failure and in correction of hypotonicity associated with hypokalaemia because hypotonicity may be corrected too rapidly.

The account given is a clinically relevant simplification of a more complex process. The following gives a more detailed, but abbreviated account, of the variables involved in determining plasma sodium [20] but is of low practical importance to clinicians and can be bypassed.

*Edelman showed that the Na^+ concentration in plasma water was linearly correlated with the **total exchangeable (Na^+_e) plus total exchangeable K^+ (K_e) divided by the total body water (TBW).***

Edelman's equation was Na^+ in plasma water __(Na+(pw)) = mx + b__: (the independent variable __x__ is $Na^+_e + K^+_e/TBW$, m is the slope and b is the intercept in the graph relating Na^+ in plasma water to exchangeable $Na^+ + K^+$ in total body water: m=1.1 and b=25.6

This gives: **$Na^+(pw) = 1.11 (Na^+_e + K^+_e)/TBW - 25.6$** [19]

This has been simplified to:

$$\textbf{Plasma } Na^+ = Na^+_e + K_e/TBW$$

This emphasises the important contribution of K^+ to osmolality.

Variables, other than $\textbf{Na}^+_e, + \textbf{K}^+_e,$ $\textbf{total body water}$, which influence plasma Na^+ because of their effect on m (slope) and b (intercept) are [20]:

- *Average osmotic coefficient of sodium salts in plasma (dissociation is not complete). Dissociation of $Na^+Cl \sim 93\%$; $Na^+HCo_3 \sim 96\%$. Therefore the average Na^+ anion⁻ dissociation is ~94%.*
- *The ratio of sodium in plasma (water and solids) compared to plasma water alone is 0.93.*
- *Thus the dissociation factor and plasma water-plasma factor approximately cancel.*
- *The Gibbs Donnan effect alters distribution of Na^+ and Cl^- in plasma compared to interstitial fluid because negative charges on protein attract Na^+. [Na^+pw] =152.7 mmol/L compared to [Na^+ interstitial fluid] which is 145.1 mmol/L; [Cl^- pw] =117.4 mmol/L compared to [Cl^- interstitial fluid] which is 119.9 mmol/L.* [20]
- *Non Na^+ and non K^+ osmoles: Ca^{2+}, Mg^{2+}, Cl^-, HCO_3^-, Phosphate⁻, organic anions, organic cations and glucose.*
- *Transcellular fluxes of Na^+, H^+, K^+ which occur in electrolyte fluid disturbances.*
- *The osmotically inactive component of Na^+_e and K^+_e.*

There is evidence that osmotic inactivation of Na^+_e occurs in subjects with net positive sodium balance and in animal models.(chapter 2 and 5)

In clinical practice the effect of potassium and glucose on plasma Na^+ are important. The practical importance of other variables, given above, is uncertain: Suggestions that more accurate quantitation of water balance, described above, is clinically important is questionable because:

- Tonicity should be corrected slowly independently of its severity and the speed of correction should depend on assessment of whether brain adaption to hypotonicity has occurred.
- Slow correction of tonicity disturbances in either direction does not require more sophisticated analysis compared to monitoring serum sodium levels.
- Ongoing losses of water (renal and insensible water loss) and electrolytes in urine are variable, but more important, and difficult to estimate.
- Urine losses of K^+, may or may not affect serum osmolality, depending on whether their source is endogenous or exogenous: [21, 22]
- Many variables described above are not routinely measured or available (e.g. normal total body water, exchangeable sodium and potassium.
- Plasma osmolality can be measured accurately by the laboratory and effective osmolality estimated.

Renal Free Water Excretion

Determination of free water excretion has traditionally been carried out by measuring urine osmolality and relating this to serum osmolality. [23] For example, if calculated serum osmolality is 290 mOsm/kg H_2O and urine osmolality 580 mOsm/kgH_2O, urine volume can be conceptualised as composing 500mL containing 290 mOsm/kg/H_2O, equal to plasma osmolality, and 500mL of free water clearance. Basing deductions of free water excretion on urine osmolality is flawed for 3 reasons:

- Urea, which has a considerable contribution to urine osmolality, is an ineffective osmole: it does not change tonicity because it is freely permeable between cells and extracellular fluid. For example, if daily urine and urea output are 500 mL and 600 mmol/day respectively, urine osmolality is 1200 mOsmol/kgH_2O without a contribution from sodium or potassium. Despite high plasma osmolality free water excretion or urinary dilution may be normal.
- Urea may not obligate excretion of water depending on the ratio of urea to non urea solutes (NUS). [24-26] Urea is an ineffective urine osmole during high rates of sodium and potassium excretion but is an effective osmole (obligates water excretion) when urine electrolyte excretion is low. [26]
- The amount of urea excreted is highly variable depending on diet, nutritional state, presence of hypovolaemia and several other variables.

When urine has low concentration of (Na^+ + K^+) urine osmolality may be high, mainly due to urea: for example free water excretion may be normal during hypovolaemia or cardiac failure despite high urine osmolality.

- NH_4^+ is the principal non urea osmole in starvation and diabetic ketoacidosis, as NH_4 ßhydroxybutyrate, rather than NaCl.

Therefore urine solute excretion is best expressed as:

$$2 \times \text{(urine } Na^+ + K^+)$$

This is a simplification (as for total body osmolality described earlier).

The urine is isonatric (does not change plasma Na^+) when:

[Na+ + K^+] urine = [Na^+ plasma + 23.8/1.63 = 0.97 plasma Na^+ + 23.1] **(20)**.

This more complicated formula is of questionable practical importance.

Potassium however only influences body tonicity and free water excretion when it is derived endogenously. During normal potassium balance dietary potassium may not influence free water excretion or tonicity. [22]

When urine Na^+ and K^+ concentration are low urine osmolality may be either high or low depending on the concentration of urea and other solutes. Osmolality of urine may be either low or high in severe sodium depletion, contrary to information in some publications, although urine Na^+ is very low. [27, 28]

Thus there are no normal values for maximum urine osmolality under conditions of water deprivation. Urine osmolality is high, ~ 1200mOsm/kgH$_2$o, when urea and electrolyte excretion are approximately equal under conditions of water deprivation. When either predominates urine osmolality is less. [25, 26]

Adaption to Disturbances of Tonicity [29-33]

Disturbances of extracellular tonicity cause cells to shrink when tonicity increases and swell when tonicity decreases. Changes in cell volume, not changes in osmolality compromise cell function. The ability to regulate cell volume is present in all cells in virtually all species. [29-31] The regulatory process has a sensor, which monitors cell volume, and a signalling cascade which stimulates loss or gain of osmoles to restore cell volume towards normal.

This mechanism is especially important in brain because of its enclosure within a rigid skull. Endothelial cells lining capillaries in the brain have tight junctions, composing the blood brain barrier, which limit movement of water and solutes. [32, 33] Tight junctions interface with glial cells which contain Aquaporin 4 and Aquaporin 1 water channels through which water leaves and enters. [34-36] An animal model, without Aquaporin 4 water channels, is resistant to hypotonicity [37, 38] and protects neurones from swelling from hyponatraemia. [37] Glial cells adapt to hypotonicity and counteract swelling by decreasing osmolality in the following sequence. [29-32, 33]

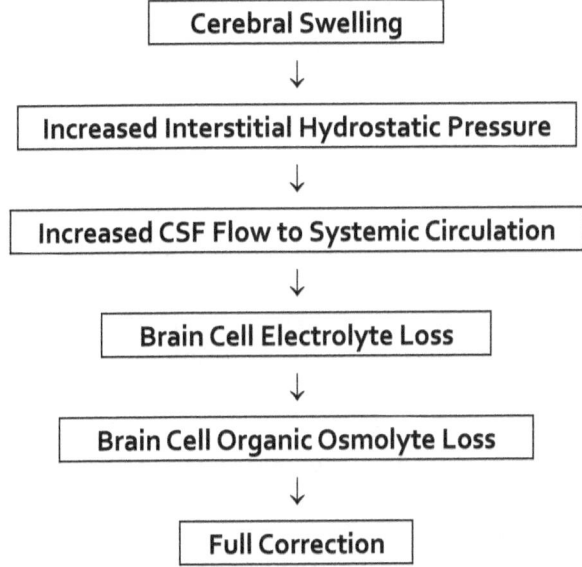

Figure 3:   Simplified model of brain cell adaption to hypotonicity.

Back flow of interstitial fluid occurs from brain to cerebro-spinal fluid and then to the systemic circulation through arachnoid villi. Increase in cell volume (stretch) stimulates Na^+: K^+ pumps, Cl^- and K^+ channels within minutes to transfer Na^+ and K^+ from cells. Potassium channels (with low open probability) and Cl^- channels open in response to cell swelling and regulate cell water. Na^+, K^+ and Cl^- losses are complete within seven hours. Activity of Na^+: K^+ pumps are crucial for this process. This is compromised by hypoxia, hypokalaemia and female sex hormones and increases vulnerability of women to hyponatraemia. [38]

This is followed by loss of uncharged organic osmoles, [31] such as aminoacids, polyphenols and myoinisotol, because losses of cell electrolytes compromise cell function. They eventually comprise the major cellular adaption which limits cell swelling. However cellular loss of organic osmoles takes longer to occur because synthesis of transporters is required for their transfer into or out of cells. [37] Brain osmolytes have been shown to change by as much as 50% on MRI. [39] The increase in water content of rat brain was only 40% of that predicted by fluid depletion and plasma sodium levels after six hours. [40] The brain undergoes less swelling from hypotonicity than other tissues. Cellular adaption to hypertonicity follows a similar process but involves gain of osmolytes :[33] cerebral contraction lowers cerebral interstitial pressure and promotes fluid movement into dehydrated brain. This is followed by cellular uptake of Na^+, K^+ and Cl^- as cell shrinkage activates Na^+: K^+ :2Cl cotransporters, Na^+: H^+ and Cl^-: HCO_3^- exchangers. Following this organic osmolytes move into cells via transporters and can be identified by nuclear magnetic resonance spectroscopy. [41]

In conclusion:

The sum of Na+ and K+ in TBW determines tonicity and reflects water balance. Water balance or tonicity is estimated by measurement of plasma sodium or osmolality because these can be sampled easily compared to cellular tonicity. Both estimations require corrections:

Osmolality should have serum urea, in mmol/L above normal, subtracted to reflect effective osmolality or tonicity.

Serum Na+ may require 2 corrections: for the effects of an increase in serum solids (pseudohyponatraemia); and addition of half serum glucose above normal, in mmol/ L, to serum sodium. However this correction gives an inaccurate indication of cellular tonicity or water balance because water re-enters cells when serum glucose normalises.

Low 'corrected' serum Na+ indicates an excess of water whereas high serum Na+ indicates deficiency of water. Hypokalaemia influences water balance: correction of potassium deficiency results in cellular transfer of Na+ to the extracellular fluid in exchange for K+.

Assessment of the renal capacity to excrete free water should be estimated by measurement of combined urine ($Na^+ + K^+$) concentration rather than urine osmolality.

Changes in tonicity are harmful because cell volume changes. This is defended by cellular gain or loss of ionic and organic osmolytes.

Cellular adaption is a temporary solution to tonicity disturbances. This is followed by excretion or retention of free water by the kidney.

> **Maintenance of Normal Tonicity**

Excretion of excess water is an essential function in organisms that moved from primeval seas to fresh water. Conservation of water also became vital on moving to land. Water regulation is governed by:

- Thirst.
- Renal dilution and concentration.

ADH (antidiuretic hormone) (AVP) secretion or inhibition is vital for this process. [42, 43]

Renal dilution and concentration.

Dilution of tubular fluid occurs in thick ascending limbs loops of Henle (TALH) and distal convoluted tubules (DCT). Water concentration occurs from water reabsorption in collecting ducts (CD), which are normally impermeable to water, but which become permeable from the action of ADH. The kidney can excrete urine with an osmolality between 50 to1400 mOsmol/kgH$_2$O in response to tonicity signals. This is achieved by:

Producing and maintaining a gradient of increasing osmolality, from cortex to medulla, due to urea, NaCl, and other ions, involving a countercurrent process.

Reabsorption of ions, predominantly Na$^+$ and Cl$^-$ without water, from thick ascending loops of Henle (TALH) and distal convoluted tubules (DCT), which produce dilute tubular fluid from isotonic glomerular filtrate.

Either excreting dilute urine by maintaining impermeability of collecting ducts to water; or concentrating urine by increasing permeability of collecting ducts by the action of ADH (AVP). This promotes tubular fluid water reabsorption into a hypertonic medulla.

Approximately 65% of glomerular filtrate is reabsorbed in proximal tubules, leaving 30% of isotonic fluid to enter descending limbs of loops of Henle. Descending limbs loops of Henle DLH) are permeable to water but not to solute. Thus water reabsorption, without solute, increases tubular fluid concentration as the bend of the loop descends into the medulla. (Fig 4)

In contrast thick ascending limbs of loops are permeable to Na^+ and K^+, via $Na^+:K^+:2Cl$ transporters, but not to water. Sodium and chloride are reabsorbed into medullary interstitiium and re-enter descending limbs of the loops of Henle (DLH) so that tubular fluid increases in concentration as bends of loops are approached. This is in effect a multiplier system due to recycling of solute from ascending to descending limbs.

The vasa recta blood flow accompanying loops flows in the opposite direction so that water reabsorbed from DLH moves into the vasa recta taking blood away from the medulla, thus avoiding its dilution; and NaCl reabsorbed from ascending limbs enters the vasa recta descending into the medulla which increases medullary concentration. Urea is transported into the medulla from inner collecting ducts, stimulated by ADH, and is recycled by transport into DLH and leads to high urea concentration in the medulla.

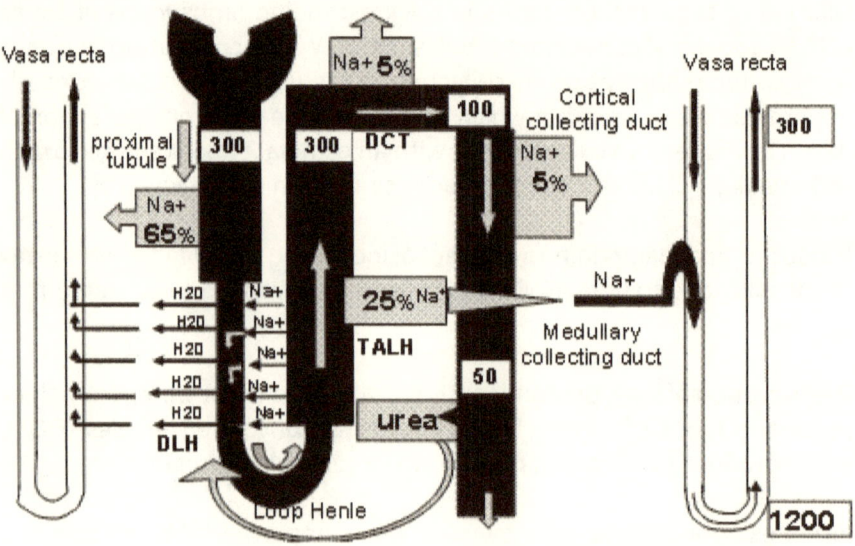

Figure 4: Process of urinary dilution. White boxes show osmolality of tubular fluid. Grey boxes show percent of sodium reabsorbed in different nephron segments. DLH =Descending loop Henle; TALH = thick ascending limb loop of Henle; DCT=distal convoluted tubul.e

Fluid in proximal tubules is isotonic. Water is reabsorbed without Na^+ in descending limbs, loops of Henle(DLH), thus increasing tubular fluid osmolality as loops descend into the medulla. NaCl is reabsorbed without *water in ascending limbs (TALH) and decreases tubular fluid osmolality as they ascend to cortex. Further NaCl reabsorption without water in distal convoluted tubules by NaCl cotransporters and in collecting ducts further dilutes urine to 50 mOsm/kg water provided ADH secretion is absent. Cortical osmolality reaches 300 mOsmol/kgH$_2$O and progressively increases to a maximum of 1200 mOsmol/Kg water, if ADH is secreted, as fluid moves down collecting ducts to medulla. The following also contribute to high medullary osmolality. Na$^+$ (small arrows) reabsorbed in the TALH is recycled into descending limbs loops of Henle and into descending limbs of vasa recta (right hand side of figure) thus increasing Na$^+$ concentration in vascular loops descending into the medulla. H$_2$O reabsorbed in descending limbs (small arrows) enters ascending limbs of vas recta, which takes water away from the medulla and decreases its dilution. Urea transported out of inner medullary collecting ducts increases concentration of urea in the medulla. Urea is also recycled by reabsorption into the DLH. Thus, the effect of ions and water reabsorbed in tubular and vascular loops flowing in opposite directions multiplies the efficiency of achieving an increasing gradient of osmolality from cortex to medulla.*

A small solute gradient difference is therefore multiplied: sodium and urea are recycled to the descending loops of Henle and into interstitiium of the medulla. This reaches an osmolality of 1200-1400 mOsm/kg/H$_2$o.

Fluid ascending to the cortex in thick ascending limbs of loops of Henle (TALH) becomes increasingly dilute as Na$^+$ and Cl$^-$ are reabsorbed without water. Tubular fluid reaches an osmolality of 100-300 mOsm/kg water in renal cortex. Further sodium is reabsorbed without water in distal convoluted tubules and collecting ducts, via Na$^+$Cl$^-$ transporters, provided ADH is suppressed. This dilutes tubular fluid to approximately 50 mOsmol/kgH$_2$O. If ADH is present tubular osmolality equilibrates with cortical osmolality: ≈300 mosmol/kg H$_2$O. Distal convoluted tubules (DCT) and collecting ducts remain impermeable to water, in the absence of ADH, which leads to excretion of dilute urine. Collecting duct permeability to water increases in response to an increasing concentration of ADH. Tubular fluid is progressively concentrated and achieves maximum osmolality of 1200mOsm/kg/H$_2$o at the papilla: Figure 4.

ADH (AVP). [42-44]

ADH (AVP) is produced in the supraoptic and paraventricular nuclei of the hypothalamus, moves down the axons of the supraopticohypophyseal tract and is stored in the posterior lobe of the pituitary.

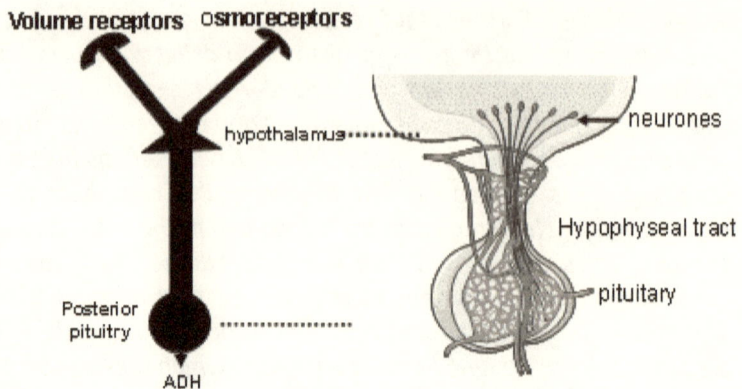

Figure 5. Volume and pressure receptors in the hypothalamus stimulate synthesis of ADH in specialised neurones and its release. ADH (vasopressin) passes down blood vessels of the hypophyseal tract to the posterior pituitary. (Produced using Servier medical art.)

Cells in the hypothalamus, called osmoreceptors, sense an increase in tonicity if water deficiency occurs and stimulate ADH secretion from the posterior pituitary. Electrical impulses, generated in paraventricular and supraoptic hypothalamic nuclei, travel down axons, depolarise the membrane of terminal axon bulbs which release ADH into capillaries

The set point (the minimal serum osmolality which stimulates ADH secretion) is between 275 -290 mOsml/kgH$_2$O.This is highly variable and probably genetically determined. The most potent stimulus to ADH secretion is effective osmolality: 1% increase in tonicity stimulates ADH secretion. There is a strong correlation between plasma osmolality and ADH secretion. [42] However the rate of change is important. Each unit increase of serum ADH increases urine osmolality by approximately 250 mOsmol/kgH$_2$O.

Osmoreceptors, which are outside the blood brain barrier, respond to shrinking or swelling of cells—tonicity (effective osmolality) but not to plasma sodium or osmolality *per se*. For example, although urea increases osmolality, it does not stimulate ADH release because it passes rapidly into cells and does not change tonicity.

Glucose is impermeable, is mainly confined to extracellular fluid, and thus exerts an osmotic effect. However it does not stimulate ADH secretion in healthy adults or in insulin treated diabetic patients because insulin promotes rapid transfer of glucose into osmoreceptor cells. This equalises glucose concentration across osmoreceptor membranes.[42, 43] Indeed it may decrease ADH secretion because hyperglycaemia decreases serum sodium. However It stimulates ADH release in diabetics who have insulin withheld. [42, 43] Thus insulin is required for uptake of glucose into osmoreceptor cells: in its absence an elevated glucose causes these cells to shrink and signal the release of ADH.

Non osmotic stimulation of ADH.

Several non osmotic stimuli cause secretion of ADH but are less potent [42, 43] For example, a 5-10 percent decrease in vascular volume stimulates ADH secretion. [42-44] However, as volume depletion progresses, stimulation by non osmotic receptors exceeds osmotic stimulation so that water reabsorption increases progressively if water intake continues.

McCance [45] showed that healthy sodium depleted male volunteers, who were allowed to drink water ad libitum, continued to excrete free water and maintain normal serum sodium until a deficiency of approximately 3L of saline developed. Delayed water diuresis developed initially but further volume depletion caused water retention and hyponatraemia. This may not occur if salt depletion occurs slowly. [46]

The secretion of ADH shows a steep linear relation with osmolality as it rises. In volume depletion ADH secretion shows little increase until hypovolaemia reaches 5-10 % of body weight. [1, 4]

Nausea, vomiting, anxiety, stress, hypoxia, pain, psychiatric disorders, hypotension, angiotensin II and some drugs increase ADH secretion sufficiently to decrease free water excretion. [42, 43] The set point for secretion is altered in pregnancy: ADH is secreted at lower tonicity which influences the concentration- dilution process in the kidney.

Mechanism of action of ADH. Figure 6.

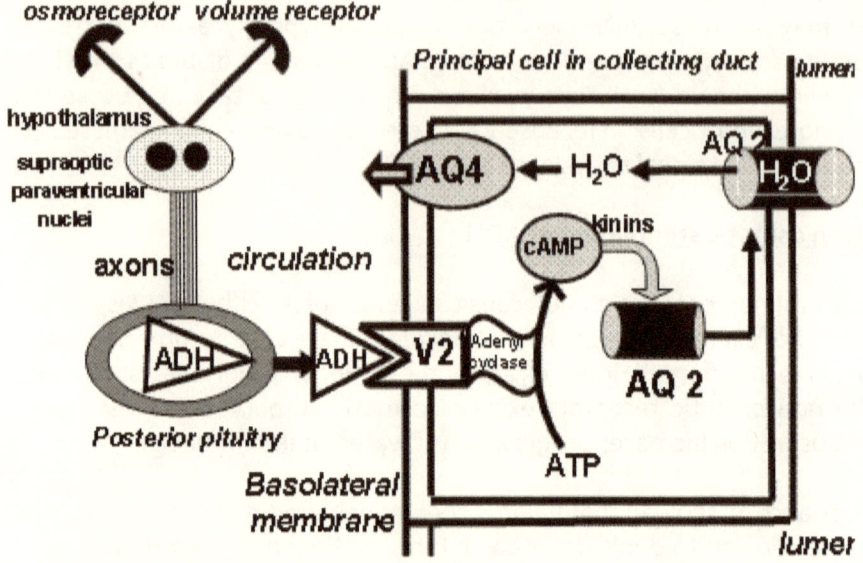

Figure 6: Model of secretion and action of ADH on collecting ducts. Tonicity and hypovolemia, sensed by hypothalamic osmoreceptors and volume receptors, generate electrical impulses in hypothalamic paraventricular and supraoptic nuclei. These depolarise membranes of terminal axon bulbs which release ADH into the circulation. ADH binds to a receptor (V2) on basolateral membranes of principal cells of collecting ducts. This initiates a series of changes which lead to water channels, Aquaporin 2 (AQ2), normally present in cytoplasm, moving to tubular apical (luminal) membranes where they transport water. Water is then transported in Aquaporin 2 channels to the basolateral membrane where Aquaporin 4 water channels transport water into the circulation.

Collecting ducts are normally impermeable to water. ADH increases their permeability so that water is reabsorbed into the hypertonic medulla. Water is carried away by ascending limbs of vasa recta thus decreasing wash out of medullary hypertonicity.

ADH acts by binding to (V_2) receptors on basolateral membranes of collecting duct principal cells and stimulates cAMP formation from ATP by activating adenyl cyclase. Both cAMP and medullary hypertonicity stimulate synthesis of Aquaporin2 (AQ2) water channels. Phosphorylation of AQP2 by protein kinase A (PKA) and reorganisation of the actin cytoskeleton is important for trafficking of AQ2 to luminal membranes. [34]

Aquaporin 4 water channels transport water through basolateral membranes into medullary interstitiium and circulation.

ADH also increases permeability of outer medullary collecting ducts to urea by causing insertion of transporters (VRUT) into luminal membranes. This further increases medullary hypertonicity and facilitates water reabsorption. Urea is recycled to medulla by counter current exchange with descending limbs of vasa recta and to descending limbs of loops of Henle. Thus urea and Na⁺ are recycled to the medulla while water is transferred to cortex. There are several determinants, apart from ADH.

Delivery of Na+ Cl- to the distal diluting segment (TAL and DCT). [1-4]

The volume of fluid reaching bends of ascending loops of Henle, where NaCl is reabsorbed without water, sets the upper limit for water excretion. Decrease in GFR or increase in proximal tubular reabsorption of sodium or both decrease sodium and water delivery to distal tubules sufficiently to limit excretion of water. For example, if GFR decreases to 10mL/min from renal failure, delivery of fluid to distal tubules, normally one fifth of GFR, may be only 2.8 L daily.

$$10mL/min \times 1440(minutes/day) \times 0.2 = 2.88L$$

Therefore, water intake in excess 2.88L + insensible water minus water derived from food may cause hyponatraemia whereas 12-20L of water can be excreted by normal subjects.

Low cardiac output, from effective hypovolaemia or cardiac failure, decreases GFR and stimulates angiotensin 2 secretion which causes efferent arteriolar constriction. Both mechanisms increase the filtration fraction which in turn increases proximal tubular fluid oncotic pressure. This increases proximal reabsorption of Na⁺ and Cl⁻. Decrease in GFR and increase in proximal tubule sodium reabsorption decreases delivery of Na⁺ and Cl⁻ to TALH and DCT to enable maximum urinary dilution to occur. A low dietary intake of sodium chloride also limits delivery to the TAL (ascending loop of Henle) to enable maximum urinary dilution—one mechanism of hyponatraemia in beer potomania.

Decrease in sodium delivery to the thick ascending loop (TAL), where reabsorption of ions without water occurs, also decreases medullary hypertonicity and limits maximal concentration of urine.

Medullary Blood Flow.

An increase in blood flow may wash out medullary hypertonicity.

Decreased medullary urea concentration.

Low protein, but adequate calorie diet, decreases medullary urea concentration and limits maximal urine concentration [47]. Fasting impairs urinary concentration by down regulating Aquaporin 2 receptors [42, 43] and by decreasing medullary tonicity. [47]

The ratio of urine urea to non-urea solutes determines the maximum osmolality of urine. Urea does not obligate water excretion if ($Na^+ + K^+$) excretion are high. The second main component of water regulation is thirst:

THIRST. [42, 43]

The hypothalamic thirst centre (figure 7) is stimulated by hypertonicity, volume depletion, hypotension, angiotensin II, hypokalaemia and other mediators. Thus volume depletion not only stimulates ADH secretion, but also thirst, even when hypotonicity is present.

However the threshold (~290-295 mOsml/kg water) at which thirst is stimulated is higher than for ADH stimulation. Urea and glucose are ineffective in stimulating thirst. [42- 44] The elderly, compared to younger persons, have decreased osmolar responsiveness to thirst, but not to ADH secretion. [48, 49].Thirst is also influenced by oropharyngeal and upper gastrointestinal receptors that respond in the process of drinking: a satiety mechanism during drinking briefly suppresses water intake.

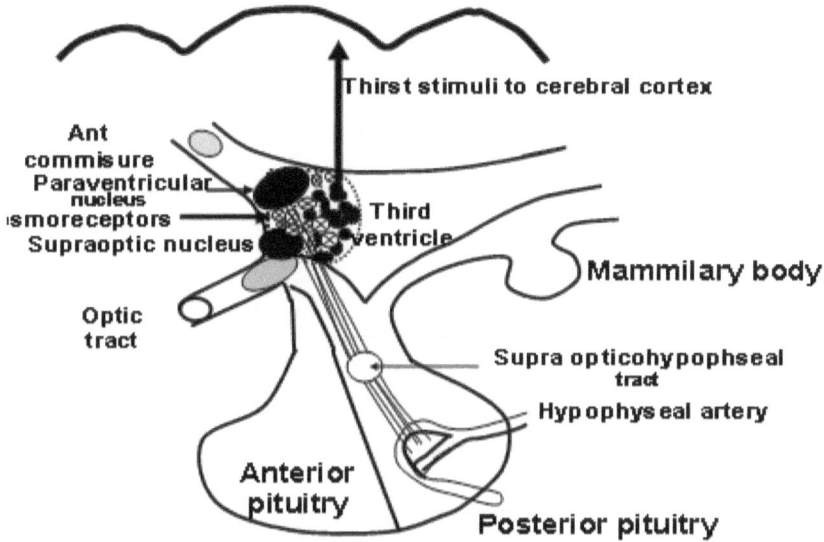

Figure 7: Osmoreceptors (circle with cross) and thirst receptors (black circles) overlap in the hypothalamus. Osmoreceptors signal to paraventricular and supraoptic nuclei and thirst centre relays to the cortex.

In conclusion: Provided serum glucose and lipids are considered serum sodium reflects exchangeable $Na^+ + K^+$ relative to total body water and thus tonicity.

Abnormalities of serum Na^+, in the absence of hyperglycaemia, hyperproteinemia and hypertriglyceridemia, indicate a disturbance of water balance is present. This may occur in the setting of normovolemia, euvolaemia or hypervolemia. Water balance requires:

* Intact thirst mechanism and access to water.
* Renal variation of urinary concentration which requires:

   Normal renal function.
   Appropriate ADH secretion.

Disorders of water balance, either hypertonicity or hypotonicity, are rarely due to either under or over consumption of fluids alone because the normal kidney can excrete between 300mL-20L water each day without a change in tonicity ;and thirst increases water intake.

Adjustments to disturbances of water balance are shown in Figure 8.

Changes in Water balance

↓

Renal concentration/dilution + /- Water intake

	Hypertonicity	*Hypotonicity*
Water intake	Increased	variable
Thirst	Increased	variable
ADH	turned on	turned off
Renal Response	Maximum urine concentration	Minimum urine concentration

▼

Failure of osmotic regulation

▼

Ionic loss/gain

▼

Organic osmolyte loss/gain

▼

Regulation of receptors

Figure 8: Adjustment to disturbances of water balance. During hypotonicity water intake may be inappropriately normal or increased and maintenance of normal tonicity relies on suppression of ADH secretion.

HYPERTONICITY

Hypertonicity indicates that an absolute deficiency of total body water is present, compared to solute, and thus free water deficiency. This occurs from hypernatraemia or less commonly <u>impermeable solutes,</u> such as glucose, which remain confined to extracellular fluid and increase its tonicity.

Half plasma glucose above normal should be added to plasma Na^+ if this is used as an index of plasma tonicity. Thus if a patient has plasma Na^+ of 130mmol/L and plasma glucose of 55mmol/L, 25mmol/L should be added to the plasma Na (1/2 x (55-5)) to give plasma sodium, corrected to reflect tonicity, of 155 mmol/L.

<u>Corrected plasma Na^+ = plasma Na^+ + ½ serum glucose above 5 mmol/L</u>

However, correction for glucose does not necessarily reflect water balance as discussed previously. Alternatively the plasma osmolality can be estimated by doubling plasma Na^+, to account for accompanying anions, adding 10 and the serum glucose in mmol/L above normal. (10 is for the contribution of potassium, ionised calcium, and magnesium plus their accompanying anions)

<u>Estimated osmolality = (2 x Na) + 10 + glucose (mmol /l)</u>

Hypertonicity leads to:

- <u>ADH secretion from osmoreceptor stimulation. This increases collecting duct permeability to water</u>
- <u>Stimulation of thirst.</u>

Causes of hypertonicity and hypernatraemia.

Non renal losses of hypotonic fluids: gastrointestinal, sweat, lungs.

Renal losses of hypotonic fluids: failure of renal concentration.

Failure of AVP secretion—hypothalamic disorders—(central diabetes insipidus).

Dysfunction of the hypothalamic thirst centre.

Limitation of access to water.

Rarely ingestion of or administration of intravenous hypertonic fluids, osmotic diuretics or near drowning in salt water.

Table 1: *Causes of hypertonicity (increased effective osmolality)*

Thirst is a very compelling symptom, although it is slightly less sensitive in elderly.[48, 49] Therefore, even when a severe impairment in concentrating urine is present, adequate access to water prevents development of hypernatremia. Polyuria, nocturia and polydipsia occur instead and in some cases hydronephrosis and renal dysfunction. In young infants and children with Diabetes insipidus inadequate access to water may cause hypernatremia and mental retardation.

LOSSES OF HYPOTONIC FLUID.

Physiological Losses or Gain of Hypotonic Fluids.

Insensible water loss (IWL) under basal conditions is approximately 1L: [50, 51] 50% each from evaporation from lungs and skin[52] although others have found that losses were 60% from skin and 40% from lungs[51]. Insensible water loss increases when humidity is low, environmental temperature high, during fever, increased catabolism, increases in activity and raised pulmonary ventilation. [51-53] Pulmonary water loss decreases to zero when atmospheric humidity exceeds 98 %. [50, 53] Clothing decreases losses from skin. [53]

Sweating results in loss of hypotonic fluid containing up to 60mmol NaCl depending on acclimatisation. [54] In severe physical activity between 480mL - 840mL/hour may be lost. [55]

Water is gained from food as preformed water (the water content of food) and water of oxidation (WOx) when food is oxidised. Average water in <u>preformed food</u> on a normal diet is approximately 700-1000mL (meat without fat contains 75%, fruit and vegetables 60-90% water).

<u>Water from oxidation</u> (**Wox**) of fat protein and carbohydrate provides approximately 300-350mL water per day. [51]

In starvation muscle provides 75% preformed water per gram of muscle catabolised plus water of oxidation of protein and fat. Fat provides mainly water from oxidation (WOX) because it has low (10%) water content. Glycogen metabolism provides water from its oxidation plus 3-4mL of water bound to each gram of glycogen. [56] On average, the body produces 300-500mL of water daily in starvation: from preformed water, plus water of oxidation from fat, protein and glycogen catabolism. [51]

The sum of water produced from water in food and its oxidation approximately equals the insensible water loss from skin, lungs and stool in the absence of activity, raised body temperature and sweating. [57]

Insensible Water Loss $\cong$ Preformed Water (in food) + Wox

Water balance, in the absence of activity, is mainly due to the difference between the volume of fluid intake and volume of urine excretion. Water restriction alone may not increase serum Na^+ in the treatment of hyponatraemia unless restricted to less than 500 mL.

PATHOLOGICAL LOSSES OF HYPOTONIC FLUID OR INTAKE OF HIGH SOLUTE CONTAINING FLUIDS.

<u>Losses from skin and lungs.</u>

Loss of water increases from lungs when ventilation increases; from skin from burns; from lungs and skin during fever and when activity levels are high.

<u>Diarrhoea and Vomiting.</u> (Chapter 12)

Losses of fluid from diarrhoea and vomiting cause less ($Na^+ + K^+$) than water loss. Hypovolaemia stimulates thirst. Thus hypernatremia rarely occurs unless access to water is limited: this occurs in infants who rely on another person to respond appropriately to their water needs; the elderly with dementia, dysphasia, stroke or who fall and cannot get up; those with neurological disorders; and post-operative patients.

Severe vomiting may also limit ingestion of water. However in practice this rarely causes severe hypernatraemia.

Hypernatremia was common in infants fed with formulas or fluids containing high concentrations of electrolytes in the past, especially if vomiting occurred. [28] Breast feeding gives considerable protection against hypernatremia [27] because breast milk contains only 5.0-6.0 mmol/L of sodium and contributes only one third the solute load than does cow's milk. [28, Committee on Nutrition-American Academy of Pediatrics report 1957]

Osmotic laxatives or lactulose, taken for hepatic encephalopathy, cause greater losses of water than solute from the gastrointestinal tract.

Post-operative patients,

Postoperative patients who cannot take fluids orally are also at risk of hypernatremia, but hyponatraemia is much more common because of excretion of urine of high tonicity, secondary to increased ADH secretion, and the policy of encouraging oral fluid intake.

High Sodium Intake.

Intravenous administration of hypertonic sodium bicarbonate (now abandoned), especially following cardiac arrest, caused hypernatremia in the past. The addition of KCl to normal saline predisposes to hypernatremia because the fluid infused is hypertonic. For example, addition of 40 mmol KCl to 1L saline-containing 150 NaCl mmol/L, a popular premixed solution, results in a concentration of 190 mmol/L of sodium plus potassium or an osmolality of 380 mOsm/kg water. Administration of hypertonic saline, increasingly used in patients with cerebral oedema, trauma or other cerebral conditions, may cause hypernatremia. Hypernatremia has rarely occurred from excessive salt ingestion [58] but was more common in infants in whom administration of fluids during diarrhoea were prepared at home. [28]

DEFECTIVE RENAL CONCENTRATION.

Urinary Water Losses depends on:

Water intake.
Secretion of ADH (AVP).
Adequacy of renal concentration.
Solute load.

Congenital Nephrogenic Diabetes Insipidus. [59-61]

Several affected children now survive to become adults. Mutations in the V2 (ADH) receptor (AVPR2) (~90%) or the Aquaporin 2 receptor gene (10%) are responsible. [59, 60] Mutations in the ADH receptor gene are usually sex linked disorders only fully expressed in males; mutations in the gene encoding Aquaporin 2 channels causes autosomal and recessive forms of Hereditary Nephrogenic Diabetes Insipidus. Hypernatremia, polyuria, polydipsia, hydronephrosis and ureteral reflux, which develop secondary to over distension of the bladder, commonly, occur in infancy. Mental deficiency may result from episodes of hypernatremia. The V2 receptor also mediates release of factor VIII and von Willebrand's factor from endothelial cells and may cause coagulopathy and vasodilatation.

Polyuria also occurs in Bartter's syndrome and rarely in disorders of urea transporters because generation of the medullary concentration gradient is defective. (Chapter 14)

Acquired Nephrogenic Diabetes Insipidus. [1, 2, 4, 7, 61]

Chronic Renal disease - especially involving the medulla -
   Medullary cystic disease, interstitial nephritis, polycystic disease, Sjogren's syndrome, ureteral obstruction.
Drugs – various, especially Lithium, Demeclocycline, diuretics (especially loop diuretics)
Sickle Cell disease
Hypercalcaemia, Hypokalaemia
Glycosuria, osmotic diuretics
Low protein, intake – decreased medullary urea
Release of ureteral obstruction
Rare causes of Polyuria
   Transient polyuria of pregnancy.
   Polyuria during supraventricular tachycardia.

Table 2: Causes of Acquired Nephrogenic Diabetes Insipidus

Osmotic diuresis.

Osmotic diuresis increases flow down renal tubules during high rates of solute load. This decreases tubular sodium concentration and increases water loss. This occurs in severe diabetes from hyperglycaemia; in hypercatabolic states from increased formation of urea; and from administration of osmotic diuretics such as mannitol. Urine osmolality approaches that of plasma at very high flow rates. [51]

Diabetic Ketoacidosis and Hyperglycaemia.

Hyperglycaemia causes greater loss of water than Na^+ plus K^+ from osmotic diuresis until GFR decreases severely.

Hyperglycaemia causes less cellular dehydration than hypernatremia because glucose moves into brain, liver and muscle (50%) by non-insulin mediated uptake and hyperglycaemia is less potent in stimulating both thirst and ADH secretion than hypernatremia. [42,43] However hypertonicity is uncommon unless access to water decreases from conditions such as stroke, dementia, or decreased mobility.

Low protein intake. decreases urea formation and interferes with generation of medullary tonicity as discussed previously.

Drugs. Diuretics, especially loop diuretics, decrease renal concentration but rarely, if ever, cause hypernatraemia.

Lithium. is a common cause of Diabetes insipidus in developed countries, occurring in up to 20% of chronic users, but is usually mild. Lithium inhibits ADH stimulated translocation of cytoplasmic Aquaporin 2 channels to apical (luminal) membranes and acts on urea transporters. [62]. Amiloride, which inhibits lithium uptake by sodium channels (ENaC), may decrease the inhibitory effect of lithium on water reabsorption.[62, 63] Amiloride, 10 mg daily for 6 weeks, increased maximum urine osmolality and AQ 2 excretion in a small randomised controlled trial.[63] The concentration defect may become irreversible with continued use beyond two years. [62] Diagnosis may be long delayed. Polyuria, rather than hypernatraemia, develops unless access to water is decreased.

Hypercalcaemia and hypokalaemia. interfere with renal concentration and are discussed in the chapters on Calcium and Potassium respectively.

Intrinsic renal disease and ureteral obstruction.

Renal diseases affecting the medulla decrease medullary tonicity and limit maximum urine concentration and dilution. (chapter 15)

AVP deficiency—(central) diabetes insipidus) [1, 4,42, 43]

Several diseases involving the osmoreceptor, hypothalamic nuclei and hypophyseal tract cause partial or complete Diabetes Insipidus. Damage below the median eminence or removal of the pituitary gland usually only cause transient polyuria because secretion of ADH continues from the hypothalamic median eminence via portal capillaries.

<u>PRIMARY</u>: Familial (autosomal dominant) and Idiopathic.

<u>SECONDARY</u> Involving the hypothalamus and or pituitary gland.

Following Head Trauma.

Supra or intrasellar tumours—Primary and metastatic (eg Craniopharyngioma).

Post partum pituitary necrosis, severe shock.

Post hypophysectomy, other neurosurgery.

Granulomas and infiltrations—sarcoidosis, tuberculosis, hemochromatosis, eosinophilic granuloma.

Brain infection—meningitis, encephalitis, syphilis.

Cerebro-vascular disorders.

Drugs.

Vasculitis and autoimmune disease.

Table 3: *Causes of ADH (AVP) deficiency.*

The most common causes of AVP (ADH) deficiency are idiopathic (30%); neurosurgery, especially following removal of Craniopharyngioma; other cerebral tumours; head trauma; infiltrative diseases, especially Histiocytosis X; and autoimmune disease. Autoimmune disease causes infiltration of the pituitary stalk with lymphocytes. Idiopathic Diabetes insipidus is rarely due to autosomal dominant inheritance of the gene encoding Preprovasopressin-neurophysin 2, the precursor of ADH (AVP).

Neurosurgery for craniopharyngioma causes abnormal ADH secretion in three phases: [7]

*   Polyuria from hypothalamic dysfunction ~5 days.
*   Antidiuresis—slow release of stored ADH.
*   Permanent diabetes insipidus.

Most patients maintain water balance because thirst is intact and present with polyuria and polydipsia. Hypernatremia occurs if access to water decreases or thirst is impaired from adjacent hypothalamic thirst centre involvement. Anterior pituitary involvement may cause cortisol and thyroid deficiency.

DYSFUNCTION OF THE THIRST CENTRE

Thirst, in response to hypertonicity, decreases with ageing and may contribute to hypernatremia.[48, 49] Lesions in proximity to the hypothalamus may lead to dysfunction of the thirst centre. ADH secretion may be appropriately high. However alteration in the sensitivity of the osmoregulatory system may also occur so that ADH levels are inappropriate for plasma tonicity. Both ADH and thirst centre may be involved together because of their proximity. Hypernatremia due to involvement of the thirst centre is rare. Sarcoidosis may cause both decrease in ADH secretion and dysfunction of thirst. [64] Chronic hypernatremia, despite normal access to water or absence of thirst, should suggest the diagnosis. Forced drinking corrects the disturbance. However, this is ineffective if the threshold for osmoreceptor stimulation is increased, so that a higher level of plasma sodium is required to stimulate both thirst and ADH secretion—called Essential Hypernatremia. [4, 43]

Hypernatraemia in hospitalised patients. [65-68]

Patients who develop hypernatremia in hospital are usually elderly, have decreased access to water and or increased fluid losses, but are given an inadequate amount of hypotonic fluids[65]. Renal concentration is defective due to use of loop diuretics or solute diuresis. Thus hypernatremia is often iatrogenic. [65]

Post operative hypernatremia, although less common than hyponatraemia, depends on the type of operation, [66] patients age and composition and volume of fluid given. On presentation to hospital hypernatremia occurs most commonly in elderly, especially from nursing homes and in those who have difficulty in accessing water, such as the frail elderly [66] or mentally handicapped. [67] Reduced thirst contributes to hypernatremia but by itself, is an uncommon cause. Hypernatremia is common in Intensive Care units, occurring in 5% of patients in one hospital, [68] and in those with neurological disorders. [51]

Severity of Renal Concentration Dysfunction.

On an average diet 600 mosmol of solute are excreted. The obligatory urine volume required to excrete this depends on the maximum achievable urine osmolality: this is 12L at a urine osmolality of 50 mosmol/kgH$_2$o or 500mL at the maximum osmolality achievable of 1200 mosmol/kgH$_2$o. The volume of urine obligated is disproportionately higher at low osmolality: an increase in maximum urine osmolality from 50 to 300 mosmolkgH$_2$O changes obligatory urine volume from 12L to 2L whereas a change in maximum urine osmolality of 300 to 600 mosmol/kgH$_2$O changes urine volume from 2L to 1L. This is important in management.

DIAGNOSIS.

This involves the differential diagnosis of both hypernatremia and polyuria in cases in which extra water intake is sufficient to prevent hypernatremia. The acquired renal causes of defective urinary concentration, which usually cause mild-moderate polyuria, nocturia or urinary incontinence, are usually obvious from clinical data. Lithium however may cause severe polyuria and even hypernatremia.

Patients with Central Diabetes insipidus, Nephrogenic Diabetes insipidus and Compulsive water drinking usually present with polyuria. The differential diagnosis between Compulsive water drinkers, in whom excess water intake suppresses ADH, and Central Diabetes Insipidus, in whom ADH secretion is defective, can be difficult because Diabetes insipidus may be partial and Compulsive water drinkers may have a blunted response to ADH. Important clues in the differential diagnosis are: [7]

- Onset of Central diabetes insipidus is often sudden and polyuria more severe compared to compulsive water drinkers and nephrogenic diabetes insipidus.
- Nocturia is often less in compulsive water drinkers who usually cease drinking at night.
- Preference for cold water is characteristic of Central Diabetes Insipidus.
- Compulsive water drinkers usually have underlying psychiatric disease. [7]

The best diagnostic test is to restrict water for 16-18 hours and carefully monitor plasma sodium (or osmolality), urine osmolality (hourly), thirst, weight and access to water. Diagnosis of Compulsive water drinking is probable if adequate urine osmolality is achieved (>600-800mOsm/L). Continued low urine osmolality while plasma osmolality rises is usually diagnostic of Central Diabetes insipidus. If urine osmolality remains low, ADH is given. This increases urine concentration further in Central Diabetes insipidus but not in Nephrogenic Diabetes insipidus. Urine osmolality is measured every 30 minutes for 3 hours following ADH or Desmopressin (dDAVP). ADH should not increase osmolality in nephrogenic diabetes insipidus.

SYMPTOMS. [1, 4, 7, 28, 59]

Symptoms depend on serum Na$^+$ and on the rapidity of development of hypertonicity because this limits brain adaptation. Severe thirst, irritability, agitation and confusion are early symptoms. Muscle twitching, seizures and coma occur later. Mucous membranes are dry or parched and pulse rapid.

Loss of cerebral volume may stretch veins connecting brain to the dura and cause subdural haemorrhage. Engorged vessels, capillary rupture, parenchymal, subarachnoid and subdural haemorrhage may be present at autopsy.

Laboratory tests show hypernatremia, an increase in serum urea greater than serum creatinine (urea: creatinine ratio >60; each in mmol/L); and urine shows decrease in sodium as water depletion increases. [51]

<u>Significant hypovolaemia and its manifestations do not occur because most of the deficit is borne by cell water.</u>

Water depletion alone does not cause significant hypovolaemia or signs of interstitial fluid depletion such as tongue furrowing, diminished skin turgor or sunken eyes (chapter 5). Misinformation continues to occur because of the failure to separate saline from free water depletion. An increase or decrease of water without losses of solute causes a small change in extracellular and plasma volume.

For example one third of the TBW is extracellular and 2/3 intracellular. The plasma volume, normally 3L in a 70 kg male, is approximately ¼ of the extracellular volume. Thus for every 1L deficit of water the change in plasma volume is:

<u>1/3 x ¼ x 1L = 0.083L.</u> or 0.83L for a 10L change in water without solute.

Free water loss of 3L decreases intracellular fluid 2 L and extracellular fluid 1 L- 750 mL from interstitial fluid and 250 mL from plasma volume (ratio 3:1).Thus plasma volume decreases by 250mL for a loss of 3 L free water or 500 mL for a loss of 6L of free water. The small change in plasma volume does not cause manifestations of hypovolaemia or interstitial fluid depletion. Moreover plasma volume decreases less in water depletion because an increase in plasma protein attracts water back into the vascular compartment [51]. Coexisting sodium depletion should be suspected if hypotension or other signs of interstitial depletion are present.

TREATMENT OF HYPERNATRAEMIA (HYPERTONICITY)

This involves:

- Treatment of hypernatremia itself.
- Treatment of associated volume depletion.
- Treatment of the cause.

Hypertonicity should be corrected slowly because brain cells may have adapted. Thus brain cell tonicity may be relatively normal depending on the duration of hypertonicity. Rapid infusion of hypotonic fluids may cause cerebral oedema. Complete correction should take 24-72 hours, depending on severity, although this is not based on randomised controlled trials. Severe symptoms of hypernatremia suggest cerebral adaption is incomplete and initial correction can be more rapid. Formulas used to calculate free water required for correction are usually unnecessary and potentially flawed because of:

- Inaccuracy in estimation of normal total body water (TBW) especially in obese or elderly patients.
- Variations in associated sodium depletion and hypovolaemia.
- Variations in ongoing insensible water and saline losses.
- The need to correct associated saline losses rapidly.

Osmolality should be decreased slowly by judicious selection of fluid composition and repeated plasma sodium measurements.

The (free) water deficit can be estimated if water is lost without solute The total solute remains the same as before water loss but is contained in a smaller volume of water.

Estimated TBW x normal Serum Na^+ = Present TBW x present Serum Na^+.

Rearranging the equation:

Present TBW = normal estimated TBW x normal serum Na^+ / present Serum Na^+.

Water Deficit = Normal TBW—Present TBW.

Eg—in a young non obese 60kg female with plasma Na+ of 160mmol/L:

Estimated normal total body water (TBW) = 60 x 50% = 30L

Present TBW = 30 x 140/160 = 26.25L

Water Deficit = 30-26.25 = 3.75L

The approach to therapy in hypernatremic patients is mainly governed by associated <u>saline and potassium depletion</u>. Hypernatremia indicates that (free) water deficiency is present. <u>It does not indicate whether sodium depletion or hypovolaemia is also present or their severity.</u> Saline depletion may more severe than free water depletion in a patient with hypernatremia. Hypovolaemia may require rapid correction until urine output is normal, compared to osmolality disturbances, which should be corrected slowly. Administered K^+ also contributes to osmolality.

$$\underline{Osmolality = 2(Na^+ + K^+)/TBW}$$

Isotonic electrolyte fluid such as saline should be given rapidly until urine output is adequate (30-50mls/hour) if volume depletion is associated, as it usually is. Giving 0.45% saline—averaging the saline and free water deficit is irrational because saline deficiency should be treated rapidly but free water deficiency slowly.

Low electrolyte containing fluids, such as 5% dextrose water, ½ normal saline or oral water should be given to patients without volume depletion <u>to correct hypertonicity slowly.</u>

<u>The type of fluid used and rate of administration depend on the estimation of associated saline, volume and K^+ depletion.</u>

<u>Specific treatment of the cause of hypertonicity and polyuria.</u>

<u>Central Diabetes Insipidus.</u>

Acute—Subcutaneous aqueous Vasopressin (Pitressin) with a short duration of action allows better control. This acts on both V1 and V2 receptors.

dDAVP [69] (Desmopressin acetate) is a synthetic analogue which mainly acts on V2 receptors and has 2 main advantages:

- Decrease in vascular constriction compared to AVP(ADH).
- Longer half life which enables dosing of only 1-2 times /day.

It is available in 3 forms: subcutaneous, intravenous injection and as an intranasal spray.

Chronic: The nasal spray of dDAVP) 10/ug-20/ug 8-12 hourly, has a prolonged (6-24 hour) action with minimal vasopressor activity. [69]

An increase in blood pressure, nausea, headache, nasal congestion and abdominal cramps are uncommon and dose related. Excessive water intake can cause hyponatraemia. Therefore patients should be cautioned to avoid excessive fluids and rely on thirst to gauge fluid requirements.

Reduction of solute load by low sodium diet or thiazide diuretics may be effective in partial diabetes insipidus and Carbamazepine may decrease polyuria.

Primary Nephrogenic Diabetes Insipidus

An improvement can be achieved by low sodium diet or decrease in sodium delivery to distal nephrons by producing mild sodium depletion. Thiazide diuretics, which do not interfere with urinary concentration, are partially effective.

Lithium Associated Diabetes Insipidus.

This is ameliorated by treatment with amiloride, which acts on ENaC channels of principal cells, to decrease lithium uptake [62, 63]. However continuing lithium may result in irreversibility.

HYPOTONICITY

Hypernatremia indicates that both hypertonicity and hyperosmolality are present. However hyponatraemia may occur in association with:

Hypotonicity.

Normal tonicity due to dilution of plasma by elevated non-solutes such as protein or lipid (Pseudohyponatremia) or glucose.

High tonicity: from coexisting elevation of serum glucose.

Hyperosmolality—due to coexistent elevation of glucose or urea.

Hypotonicity indicates that an excess of free water relative to effective solutes is present: an amount of (free) water in excess of physiological saline.

It is important to emphasise that hypotonicity refers to plasma and extracellular hypotonicity. This can be associated with cellular hypertonicity if a non permeable solute such as glucose results in transfer of cellular water to extracellular space: this results in extracellular hypernatraemia but cellular hypertonicity.

Plasma Na$^+$ does not give an indication of sodium status, the presence of saline deficiency or excess or volume status: Hyponatraemia may occur in association with euvolaemia, hypovolaemia or hypervolemia.

Hypotonicity can only develop if intake of water is greater than the capacity to dilute urine. An extremely rare exception may be the excretion of hypertonic urine due to thiazide diuretics. [7] Man has a huge capacity to excrete water: in normal adults up to 20L a day without change in serum sodium levels. [70, 71] Two factors are necessary to excrete free water:

• Adequate delivery of solute to distal diluting sites –thick ascending loops of Henle and distal convoluted tubules. Distal diluting tubules are functioning adequately so that free water can be generated by sodium chloride reabsorption without water.
• ADH is suppressed.

Adequate delivery of sodium to distal tubules depends on normal renal perfusion and function. Decrease in GFR and efferent arteriolar constriction cause an increase in filtration fraction. This results in a higher concentration of protein and colloid oncotic pressure in blood surrounding proximal tubules and increases proximal tubule sodium reabsorption. Decrease in GFR and increase in sodium reabsorption in proximal tubules decrease solute delivery to distal diluting tubules.

Table 4 shows the causes of hyponatraemia based on the principal mechanism.

In practice hypotonicity usually has multiple causes. It is however clinically useful to consider the causes of hypotonicity in the following groups:

* Decrease in effective cardiac output and/or arterial underfilling for example from sepsis.
* Renal dysfunction—global or local—dysfunction of the distal diluting segment.
* Unsuppressed ADH secretion without hypovolaemia or cardiac failure.
* Polydisia.

Effective Hypovolaemia.

    Hypovolaemia

    Increase in venous capacitance.

    Obstruction to venous return.

    Arterial vasodilatation.

Cardiac Disorders.

    <u>Muscle:</u> localised loss (infarction) or global dysfunction (cardiomyopathy).

    <u>Obstruction</u>—pulmonary embolism or <u>Valve Dysfunction.</u>

Primary Renal Causes

    Global—acute or severe chronic intrinsic renal failure.

    Selective dysfunction of the distal diluting segment—Thiazides.

    Renal artery stenosis.

    Hereditary: gain of function mutations of V_2 receptors.

<u>Unsuppressed ADH Secretion not due to arterial underfilling</u> or low cardiac output.

    Drugs.

    ADH secreting tumours.

    Central nervous system disorders.

    Acute psychosis.

    Hypothyroidism, Hypopituitarism, Addison's disease, Acute Porphyria.

    Pulmonary disorders.

    Post operative state.

    Pain, nausea, anxiety, stress.

    AIDS.

    Physical exercise.

    Renal artery stenosis.

Primary Excessive Water Intake.

    Primary polydipsia.

    Water ingestion with decreased solute intake—beer potomania.

    Sodium free irrigant solutions or enemas.

    Marathon runners or extended physical work with continued water intake.

    Fresh water immersion (drowning).

    Encouragement or orders to increase oral fluids intake (push fluids).

Inappropriate administration of intravenous hypotonic fluids.

Table 4: Diseases causing hypotonicity based on <u>principal</u> mechanism. In practice hypotonicity usually occurs from several mechanisms. [1, 4, 8, 42]

> **Decrease in Cardiac Output or arterial underfilling (chapter 5)**

Cardiac output may be relatively normal, but may not fill the arterial system adequately, due to an increase in its capacity from arterial dilatation. [75, 76] This hypothesis explains the development of hyponatraemia in such diverse disorders as hypovolaemia, cardiac failure, liver cirrhosis and pregnancy. [76] Thus arterial underfilling may be due to either arterial dilatation or decrease in cardiac output. Arterial under filling activates the sympathetic nervous system, the renin angiotensin aldosterone system, stimulates ADH secretion and thirst and decreases GFR. [76]

Decrease in CO may be due to pump failure or effective hypovolaemia.

The term effective hypovolaemia is used to emphasise the most common cause—losses of blood, colloid and/or saline but 'effective' is used to include less common causes of under filling of the heart : decreased venous return from acute sympathetic paralysis from cervical cord transection; increase venous capacity from drug overdose; and obstruction to venous return from pericardial effusion, positive pressure ventilation and tension pneumothorax. In these disorders increasing volume by saline infusion is often beneficial. (Chapter 5)

Transient severe cardiac dysfunction, hypovolaemia from an increase in capillary permeability and vascular dilation, leading to low cardiac output, frequently occur in severe sepsis.

Congestive Cardiac Failure. [75-79]

This is a common cause of hyponatraemia in and outside of hospital [74-78]. Right-sided heart failure due to pulmonary hypertension also causes hyponatraemia. [79] Hyponatraemia is associated with a poor prognosis in both congestive and right sided heart failure. [76, 77, 79]. There are several causes of hyponatraemia in heart failure:

* Low cardiac output causes low GFR.
* Increased proximal tubular sodium reabsorption.
* Activation of the sympathetic nervous system, renin angiotensin aldosterone system and ADH release. These mechanisms decrease sodium delivery to distal nephrons which interfere with urinary dilution; and unsuppressed ADH secretion increases water reabsorption from collecting ducts.

* Diuretics—Thiazide and Loop diuretics cause sodium depletion; and thiazide diuretics interfere with urinary dilution by acting on distal convoluted tubules.
* Increase in ADH secretion from a low cardiac output stress and hypotension.
* Increase in thirst from arterial underfilling.
* Stimulation of atrial natriuretic peptide secretion—a minor role.

Primary Renal Causes.

Hyponatraemia rarely occurs from renal failure alone until GFR falls below 30ml/min. In both acute and chronic renal failure delivery of sodium to distal tubules to enable dilution decreases. For example, if GFR is 10mL/min and delivery of fluid to distal tubules is normally one fifth (0.2) of GFR, only 2.8 L of fluid is delivered to the distal tubule each day:

10mL/min x 1440(minutes/day) x 0.2 =2.88L

Therefore water intake in excess of 2.88L plus insensible water loss (total 3.88L) causes hyponatraemia whereas 12-20L of water can be excreted by normal subjects.

Renovascular Hypertension. [80-83]

This is usually associated with severe renal artery stenosis The ischemic kidney increases renin secretion. High blood pressure increases sodium loss from the normal kidney—called pressure natriuresis. Hyperaldosteronism, secondary to hypovolaemia, increases renal potassium loss from $Na^+:K^+$ exchange. Thus hypertension, severe sodium depletion, hyponatraemia and hypokalaemia may result.

Diuretics. [84-88]

Diuretics are common causes of hyponatraemia and have been considered the most common cause of community-developed hyponatraemia. [88] Thiazide diuretics and indapamide cause the majority of cases. Loop diuretics are responsible for a small minority– 6% in one series. [85]

Loop diuretics impair medullary hypertonicity because they inhibit $Na^+ Cl^-$ reabsorption in thick ascending limbs of loops of Henle. Thiazide diuretics act on distal convoluted tubules in the cortex and do not interfere with medullary hypertonicity or water reabsorption in collecting ducts. Thiazide diuretics may cause hyponatraemia, in the absence of hypovolaemia, whereas loop diuretics rarely do. Indeed loop diuretics are administered to increase free water clearance in patients with the 'Syndrome of inappropriate ADH'.

Loop diuretics.

Loop diuretics decrease both urinary concentration and dilution and usually only cause hyponatraemia if severe volume depletion or low cardiac output develops. [88]

Loop diuretics do not affect dilution in distal convoluting tubules or wash out medullary hypertonicity. [88]

Thiazide Diuretics (and Indapamide) –(chapter 14).

Thiazides and indapamide act on distal convoluted tubules in renal cortex and do not wash out medullary hypertonicity. They are common causes of hyponatraemia and may cause death. [85-87]

Women, especially post menopausal, [86] are much more commonly affected than men and most are reported to present within two weeks of starting treatment. [85] This is contrary to the authors experience. Factors other than the action of thiazide diuretics on the distal convoluted tubule play a role in thiazide associated hyponatraemia. In one review 72% had one or more of: [85]

- Unsuppressed ADH.
- Hypokalaemia.
- Polydipsia.
- Hypovolaemia from electrolyte loss.

Serum ADH was abnormally elevated in all cases in which it was measured during hyponatraemia associated with thiazide diuretics. [84]

In an elegant experiment Friedman et al [87] tested patients, who had previously developed hyponatraemia on thiazide diuretics, with a single dose of thiazide-amiloride. Water was allowed ad libitum. Hyponatraemia developed again, but not in young or old controls, who had taken thiazide diuretics in the past without developing hyponatraemia. My personal observations suggest that patients may present after prolonged use and factors, other than the effect on the distal convoluted tubule, are often implicated in hyponatraemia:

• Infection, for example urine infection, may cause ADH secretion secondary to vascular dilatation and arterial underfilling.
• Recommendations to "push" fluids especially in those with recurrent urinary infections.
• Stress, nausea and vomiting which increase ADH secretion.

Use of Thiazide diuretics are frequently denied by women with eating disorders and older women who mistakenly volunteer that they are on Avapro (Irbesartan) or Coversyl (Ramipril) rather than Avapro plus (Irbesartan, Thiazide) or Coversyl Plus (Ramipril, Indapamide).(Personal observations)

Thiazide diuretics should be stopped before surgery because they predispose to post operative hyponatraemia.

In conclusion hyponatraemia due to thiazide diuretics are not solely due to their effect on the distal diluting segment of the kidney but have several other causes: polydipsia, hypovolaemia, arterial underfilling from sepsis, and unsuppressed ADH secretion.

Medications Apart From Diuretics. [88, 89]

Medications, apart from thiazide diuretics, cause hyponatraemia by several different mechanisms. (Table5).Enormous numbers of medications have been reported to predispose to hyponatraemia. [88] Thus all medications should be considered potential causes.

Simulate ADH action.	DDAVP. [90] Oxytocin. [91-93]
Enhance ADH release.	Chlorpropamide, Carbamazepine. [94, 95]
Potentiate renal response to ADH.	Chlorpropamide. NSAIDs,
	Cyclophosphamide·
Volume Depletion—Medullary Washout.	Loop diuretics. [89]
Action on DCT (+ADH).	Thiazide diuretics. Indapamide. [84-88]
Arterial Vasodilators: arterial underfilling.	ACE Inhibitors. A2 receptor blockers. [89]
Uncertain Cause (?↑ ADH secretion).	Selective serotonin reuptake inhibitors. [96-99]
	Ecstasy. [100-101] Clozapine. Phenothiazine. Antiepileptic Drugs.

Table 5: Causes of hyponatraemia due to Drugs—modified from references 88 and 89. (DCT=distal convoluted tubule.)

Water retention and hyponatraemia is hazardous in those taking Desmopressin (dDAVP) [90] for Diabetes insipidus or Von Willebrand's' disease .dDAVP given for Diabetes Insipidus should be accompanied by advice to avoid excessive drinking and that water intake should be governed by thirst. [89]

Oxytocin, which has similar molecular structure to ADH, given for inducing labour, may cause hyponatraemia in both mother [91-93] and baby [93] -called transplacental hyponatraemia. In a randomised study the serum sodium was significantly lower in those given oxytocin in dextrose water compared to oxytocin in normal saline. [9]

Carbamazepine is a relatively common cause of drug related hyponatraemia [88, 94, 95] and was the third most common class of drugs associated with hyponatraemia in one retrospective review. [95] Serum ADH levels were inappropriately raised in one reported case. [94] Hyponatraemia correlates with the dose and serum concentration of Carbamazepine. [89]

Selective Serotonin Reuptake Inhibitors. [95-99]

Selective serotonin reuptake inhibitors (SSRI) are commonly associated with hyponatraemia: [95] a reported incidence of 12 % [95] and 1 in 200 elderly people treated per year with fluoxetine or Paroxetine. [96] Most cases occurred within 3 weeks of treatment. Risk factors for SSRI associated hyponatraemia are older age, [95-98] female gender, concomitant use of diuretics, low body weight and pre-existing lower initial serum sodium concentration. [98]

Other medications, taken in addition to SSRI's, and the presence of comorbid disease make attribution of the cause of hyponatraemia uncertain. However rechallenge results in recurrence in approximately 60 %. [99] Moreover most cases of hyponatraemia develop soon after treatment is started. [99] Serotonin may stimulate ADH secretion. [99]

Ecstasy, [100,101] MDMA (3, 4—methylenedioxy methamphetamine) is an important cause of hyponatraemia because of its common use as a recreational drug. Misdiagnosis is common because confusion and bizarre behaviour may be attributed to the drug itself rather than hyponatraemia.

The role of elevated ADH levels in causing drug related hyponatraemia is uncertain because serum levels have rarely been measured at the time patients present with hyponatraemia. In cases where serum ADH was measured during hyponatremia levels have usually been unsuppressed.

Post operative hyponatraemia. [102-107]

This previously common and dangerous cause of hyponatraemia in adults [102-106] and children [107] has decreased following avoidance of routine intravenous hypotonic fluids following operation. This was, captured in an editorial in the British Medical Journal:

"Post operative hypotonic fluids have no place in the modern practice of Medicine." [104]

Use of hypotonic, rather than isotonic fluids, were promoted in the past from concern to avoid pulmonary oedema. However post-operative pulmonary oedema is rare and has many causes other than sodium overload. [108] Post operative hyponatraemia is more common and more serious in females, especially if Menstruant: [105] in one review 33 of 34 patients who died or had permanent brain damage were female and 76% were Menstruant. [105] The relative risk in females compared to males was 28:1.

Post operative hyponatraemia has a poor outcome because it develops acutely and is often diagnosed late. In a review of 260 reported cases from 1935-1992 21% had permanent brain damage or died. [105] Respiratory arrest is common before treatment and may occur abruptly, without warning, in adults and children.

The principal causes of post operative hyponatraemia are: increase in ADH secretion [102,104-107] stimulated by stress, pain, nausea, vomiting, anaesthesia, hypovolaemia and drugs. Serum ADH was increased in all patients in whom it was measured in one review. [102] In women undergoing gynaecologic surgery maximum combined urine $Na^+ + K^+$ concentration was $294(\pm 9)$ mmol/L for a variable time postoperatively—a tonicity that is almost double that of sodium concentration in normal saline [106]. Administration of each 1L NS resulted in generation of 500mls of free water. Thus even intravenous normal saline can result in hyponatraemia by a process of desalination. [106] Serum Na^+ of 115mmol/L and severe confusion developed in a young woman, following administration of 3L NS daily without oral water for six days (personal observations).

Administration of, or advice, to take hypotonic fluids.

Although use of parenteral postoperative hypotonic fluid administration has declined nursing staff often pressure patients to take oral fluids which results in hyponatraemia (personal observations).

Post operative hyponatraemia is also common in children [107,109-113] because of reluctance to use isotonic fluids from fear of the development of hypernatremia; and the slavish adherence for incorporating generous allowances for maintenance fluids. [111] Popular regimes for maintenance fluids are based on flawed data from healthy children reported over 40 years ago and do not make allowances for increased ADH secretion in hospitalised children [110,114] due to hypovolaemia, nausea, pain, stress, anxiety, the effects of drugs and comorbidity. Moreover Insensible water loss may be low from inactivity and high humidity ; while water released from breakdown of cells, water of oxidation and from breakdown of glycogen may increase. [114]

Fluid resuscitation with hypotonic fluids, which was often carried out in the past, has also led to death. [28]

A systematic review showed that the odds of hyponatraemia were 17 times higher in children receiving hypotonic fluids. Traditional guidelines for maintenance fluids are inappropriate, [109] hypernatremia is rare, but deaths from hypotonicity continue to occur. [109] Prescription of hypotonic fluids by anaesthetists has been reported and places children at risk. [110]

Hypotonic fluids, containing Glycine, which is subsequently metabolised, for prostate surgery [72,115] and for irrigation in hysteroscopy [116] are rare perioperative causes of hyponatraemia.

Prolonged physical activity and marathon runners. [117-127]

Exercise-associated hyponatraemia is the most common serious complication of endurance exercise. [117,120]This is important given that it usually affects young subjects and has been reported to occur in between 0.3-10 %[118] of those undertaking prolonged physical activity.

Hypotonicity occurred in 18% of those participating in a New Zealand Iron Man event, 29% in the Hawaiian Iron Man event [118] and 1.3% of those completing the Boston marathon. [119] Severe hyponatraemia (serum Na^+ <120mmol/L) occurred in 0.6% of the latter.

Females are more commonly and severely affected than are males [120-122]. The underlying contributory factors are shown in Table 6:

- Increased ADH levels [117,118,120,121,123-125], possibly due to cytokines [123,125] from the stress of physical activity and possibly arterial underfilling.

- Ingestion of regular (often hourly) hypotonic fluids.[124-127]

- Hypovolaemia. [117,120]

- Weight gain during the event. [118,123,124]

- Long racing time. [118,120,124,126]

- Low body mass index—probably reflecting low TBW.

- Use of non-steroidal antiinflammatory drugs. [120-122]

- Female gender. [120,121,123,126]

Table 6: Causes and risk factors in marathon associated hyponatraemia.

Military training, especially in new recruits, has caused severe hyponatraemia and death. [128,129] Hyponatraemia is common among backpackers in National Park desert areas.

Water intake in excess of need, in combination with unsuppressed ADH secretion, is the most important cause of hyponatraemia in marathon runners, Back Packers and other forms of physical activity, Marked elevations of serum ADH levels were reported in Marathon runners in whom levels were measured, regardless of whether hyponatraemia was present. [117] Hypovolaemia also contributes by stimulating ADH secretion and by decreasing sodium delivery to distal (diluting) tubules. [117] Although serum ADH levels are not abnormally raised in all cases, levels may suppress soon after completion of a marathon at the time they are measured and therefore give a misleadingly low indication of frequency.

It is important to emphasise that less insensible water loss occurs when humidity is high than low. [51-53] Indeed insensible water loss from lungs is essentially absent when humidity is 100 %. [50, 53] Sweating may also cause hypovolaemia from sodium depletion and contribute to hyponatraemia. [120,127] Although sweat is hypotonic it contains more NaCl (25-50mmol/L) than sports drinks. Endogenous water is also derived from the utilisation of glycogen: from the hydration shell and from its oxidation. This may amount to 3L in a 70kg man who utilises most of his glycogen stores. [57,127] Insensible water loss may roughly equal water derived from endogenous metabolism. [127] There are two contributory factors implicated in the frequency of hyponatraemia due to prolonged physical activity:

- Promotion of sports drinks by corporations—especially those sponsoring marathons. [120,130,131]
- Inappropriate guidelines by sports associations and organisations, such as the United States Military [126] which are not based on evidence.

More recent guidelines emphasise that thirst should guide replacement and that fluid consumption should be limited to avoid weight gain. [130]

Hyponatraemia following marathons has led to manifestations of cerebral oedema, seizures, [117,120-122] pulmonary oedema [122,132] and death. [120] Hyponatraemia may be misdiagnosed as dehydration and lead to inappropriate treatment with hypotonic fluids [122]. Hyponatraemia may also worsen following completion of the race because of delayed absorption of gastrointestinal fluid. [133] Urgent treatment has been recommended, [121,123,133] including administration of a bolus of 3% NaCl over 10 minutes to raise serum Na^+ by 2-3mmol/L. [120]

POLYDIPSIA. [134-138]

Many patients with severe polydipsia have underlying psychiatric disease such as Schizophrenia. [134-136] Both polydisia and inappropriately suppressed ADH are responsible. Increased serum ADH levels were demonstrated in experimentally induced psychosis in Schizophrenic patients [136] and in spontaneous psychosis accompanied by self-induced water intoxication. [138] The proximity of both ADH secreting neurones and thirst centre to the limbic system may be important. Seizures are common in Schizophrenic patients with compulsive water drinking whereas osmotic demyelination is reportably rare. [137] Late treatment increases mortality. Rapid correction of symptomatic hyponatraemia has been recommended.

Friedman [87] showed that polydipsia was an important cause in those who developed hyponatraemia from thiazide diuretics.

Beer potomania. is due to a combination of excessive water intake combined with low sodium and solute intake which decreases sodium delivery to distal tubules to enable urine dilution. [139-142] In a review of 22 cases common manifestations were hyponatraemia (mean serum Na^+ 108 mmol/L), hypokalaemia, low blood urea, mild neurological symptoms, low urinary sodium concentration and brisk water diuresis in response to solute intake. [140] Solute excretion is normally between 500-900 mmol/L per day on a normal diet. Beer contains minimal sodium and protein. If solute excretion were only 100 mmol/L day water intake in excess of 2L could lead to hyponatraemia. [140]. Beer drinkers take in large amounts of water and low solute load; they may develop sodium depletion from low dietary intake and vomiting; and nausea causes ADH secretion. Rapid spontaneous correction of hyponatraemia, following hospitalisation and subsequent development of osmotic demyelination is an important hazard. [140]

A similar condition occurs in infants who continue to breast feed "on demand" during episodes of diarrhoea. [27] Breast milk contains only 5-6 mmol Na^+, 10mmol K^+ per litre and only one third the solute load than cow's milk. [143] Thus large quantities of water, containing low solute content, are ingested compared to the much larger losses of sodium and potassium in diarrhoeal stool. This could be called 'breast milk potomania'!

Endocrine and metabolic causes.

Glucocorticoids facilitate water excretion by suppressing ADH mRNA, which inhibits ADH synthesis, and by increasing glomerular filtration rate. Unsuppressed ADH secretion occurs in hypopituitarism [144] and as a contributing factor in Addison's disease.

Both hypovolaemia from saline loss and inadequate suppression of ADH secretion by cortisol contribute to hyponatraemia in Addison's disease. Severe hyponatraemia occurs in mitochondrial encephalomyopathy [146] and acute intermittent Porphyria in association with unsuppressed ADH secretion. [32] Increased ADH secretion may be the cause of hyponatraemia in hypothyroidism. [145]

Pulmonary disorders.

Hyponatraemia is common in pneumonia, [147,148] other chest infections [148,149] and tuberculosis [150] and is associated with an increase in mortality. [148] Unsuppressed serum ADH levels occurred in all patients in one observational study. Chest infections were a more common cause of "Inappropriate ADH syndrome" than carcinoma of the lung. Serum ADH elevation was transient and rapidly normalised. [148] Delay in measurement may give a misleading indication of frequency. Hypoxia worsens the adverse effects of hyponatraemia. [151]

AIDS.

Hyponatraemia is common and due to multiple causes: [152] elevated ADH, volume depletion and pseudohyponatremia from hyperglycaemia and hyperlipidemia.

Central nervous system disorders. [72-75,153]

Increased ADH secretion is common in many disorders of the central nervous system. Hypotonic solutions should be avoided in those with head injury, brain tumours, subarachnoid haemorrhage and other brain disorders. Unsuppressed ADH secretion should be differentiated from cerebral salt wasting because treatment is different.

Cerebral Salt Wasting Syndromes. [154-157]

Cerebral salt wasting, a highly controversial topic, is due to excessive urinary losses of Na^+ and Cl^- in absence of a known cause for excretion and is associated with a cerebral condition.

Common causes are subarachnoid haemorrhage, brain trauma, brain tumours and chronic meningitis. [154-157] Hyponatraemia may or may not be present. The diagnosis should not be made unless the following are met: [154]

Deficiency of sodium or hypovolaemia is present.

Known stimuli to sodium loss, such as hypoaldosteronism or intrinsic renal disease are absent.

Urinary sodium loss is increased.

Response to correction of sodium depletion is beneficial. [154]

Differentiation from the syndrome of Inappropriate ADH section, which is common in cerebral conditions, is difficult but important, because water restriction in cerebral salt wasting is detrimental. Urine sodium concentration is raised in both conditions. Natriuretic peptides are elevated in aneurysmal subarachnoid haemorrhage and cause renal sodium loss. [156] The diagnosis of cerebral salt wasting is difficult because the sensitivity of the clinical diagnosis of sodium depletion or hypovolaemia is low. Both cerebral salt wasting and excessive ADH secretion may coexist and make diagnosis even more difficult. Thus a trial of saline infusion may be necessary—with careful monitoring of serum Na^+ levels.

Hospitalised patients.

Hyponatraemia is the commonest electrolyte disorder in clinical practice and in hospitalized patients [158-161] and is more common in elderly patients and those with pre-existing asymptomatic hyponatraemia. [95] Mortality is increased. [95,160] Unsuppressed ADH secretion occurs in the majority: [159,160] 97% in one observation study. [160] Drugs, especially thiazide diuretics, surgery, use of hypotonic fluids [141] and previous hyponatraemia are risk factors. [95]

Common causes are congestive cardiac failure, [95,158] hypovolaemia, [95,160] thiazide diuretics, [95] serotonin reuptake inhibitors, [95] pneumonia [95,149,158,159,162] and liver cirrhosis [158] whereas small cell carcinoma of the lung is a rare cause. Hyponatraemia developing in hospital is often iatrogenic. [161] The risk for recurrence of hyponatraemia is high when patients leave hospital. [95]

SYNDROME INAPPROPRIATE ADH SECRETION (SIADH)

Bartter and Schwartz defined the term 'Syndrome Inappropriate ADH' (SIADH) in a key paper in 196 7 [163] and suggested the following criteria for diagnosis:

- Hyponatraemia is due to hypotonicity—excludes pseudohyponatraemia.
- Continued high renal Na^+ excretion occurs.
- Volume depletion is absent.
- Urine osmolality is inappropriate for hypotonicity.
- Renal and adrenal function are normal.

They initially described <u>chronic</u> rather than <u>acute</u> inappropriate ADH secretion from small cell carcinomas. However even in this syndrome plasma sodium and urinary sodium concentration vary because of variations in the level of adaption, sodium and water intake. Urinary sodium decreases to <20mmol/L in some cases and fractional excretion of sodium (FENa) to less than 0.5 %. [164]

<u>Adaption</u> to prevent brain swelling by loss of brain electrolytes, followed by osmolyte loss, has been described previously but involves 2 further processes.

Increase in ECV (extracellular volume) from water retention increases Na^+ excretion and may decrease serum $Na.^+$ levels.[165] Natriuretic peptides are increased in patients with the syndrome of Inappropriate ADH and in normal subjects who ingest water. Low sodium intake from nausea may contribute. Natriuresis returns ECV towards normal [165,166]. This explains the absence of oedema. Potassium, transferred from cells as part of the adaption process, is excreted.

Action of Aquaporin channels or V_2R receptors decreases from down regulation.[166] The complete process is summarised in figure 10. The body as a whole regulates extra and intracellular volume towards normal by secondary natriuresis from an expanded ECV and from renal loss of K^+ transferred out of cells. A steady state occurs when both intracellular and extracellular volume normalise but the solute content of <u>both</u> decrease.

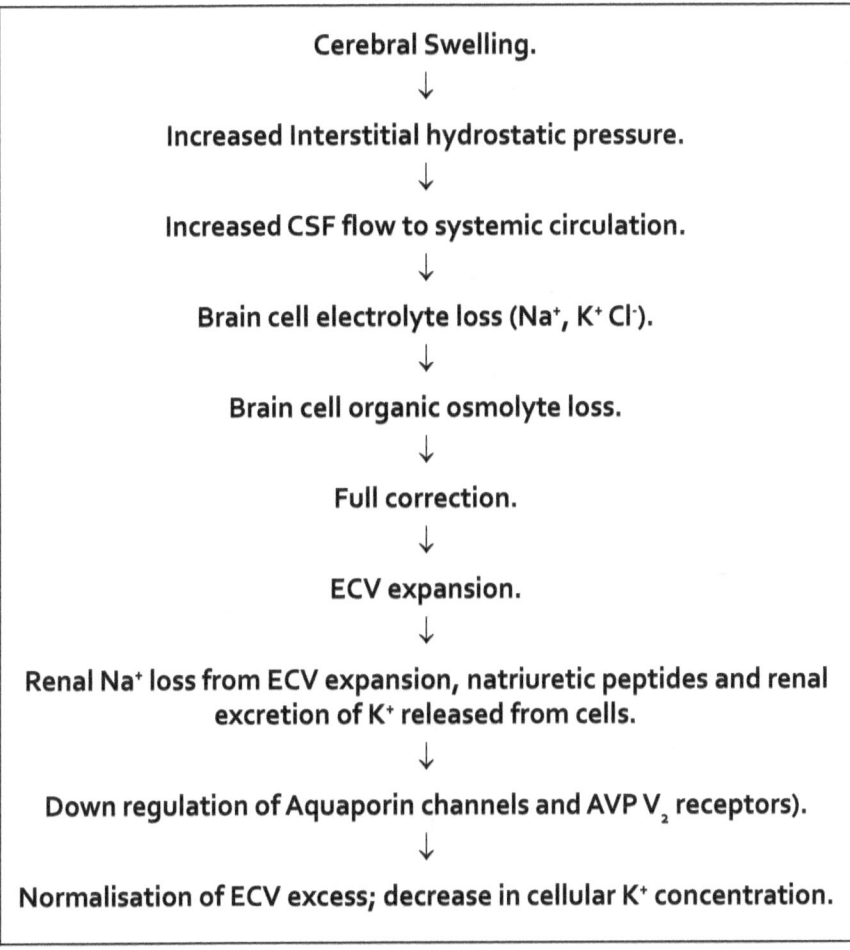

Figure 9: Showing process of adaption to chronic ADH secretion.

Urine Na^+ should be high in the SIADH because hypovolaemia is characteristically absent. In practice there is considerable overlap with sodium depletion. During a low sodium intake, or low urine output, (reflected by a high urine creatinine/plasma creatinine ratio), the FeNa may be low (<0.5%) in the SIADH.[164] The combination of FeNa<0.5% and fractional excretion urea (Fe urea) improves prediction of the response to n saline infusion. [164] However during low urine output (antidiuresis), reflected in a urine Cr/plasma ratio of more than 140, the FeNa is <0.15 % and the Fe urea <45 % in Na^+ depletion. [164]

Urine Na^+ concentration may decrease to low levels, despite SIADH, because of the development of euvolaemia, a decrease of dietary salt intake, losses of salt from diarrhoea or vomiting and arterial underfilling from infection. [165]

The degree to which hyponatraemia or solute depletion occurs depends on the cause, rapidity of development, water intake during the process and differences in adaption. Down regulation of Aquaporin 2 may be mediated by intrarenal (paracrine factors) associated with increased intramedullary blood flow [165] and Angiotensin2. Non-steroidal antiinflammatory drugs blunt escape. [165] Four variations have been described in the SIADH: [166]

Type A. Erratic fluctuations of serum ADH levels occur during hypertonic saline infusion unrelated to plasm Na^+ levels. Urine osmolality is "fixed".

Type B Serum ADH level is raised but less than type A and does not change following administration of 3% saline until serum Na^+ becomes normal. The level then rises appropriately in relation to the extent of hypoosmolality.

Type C (reset osmostat). Serum ADH and urine osmolality are low when hyponatraemia is present but during 3% saline infusion serum ADH increases inappropriately before hyponatraemia is corrected.

Type D may not be due to inappropriate ADH secretion.

The SIADH is therefore a heterogenous disorder with varying patterns of ADH release, volume status and water intake.

The term Inappropriate ADH syndrome causes more confusion than clarity and promotes inappropriate treatment. The term was introduced by Bartter and Schwartz [163] to describe the pathogenesis of hyponatraemia due to chronic ectopic secretion of ADH from small cell bronchogenic carcinoma. The term itself is inappropriate because:

Nearly all patients, hospitalised with acute hyponatraemia, have raised serum ADH levels [148,158, 160]—97% or over in one study. [160] Ectopic ADH secretion is a rare cause.

Serum ADH is raised in the majority of disorders causing hyponatraemia where levels have been measured: thiazide diuretics [85]; psychotic patients with compulsive polydipsia; [136,138] postoperative patients (100%);[102]

patients with chest infections; [148] (100%) marathon runners; [123] and heart failure. [76] Indeed the frequency of raised serum ADH levels is probably higher than has been reported because suppression of previously raised ADH secretion may occur soon after presentation: following treatment of hypovolaemia, psychosis, heart failure, chest infections, cessation of causal medications, reduction of polydipsia, physical activity and resolution of nausea or pain.

- Hyponatraemia due to unsuppressed ADH secretion is usually of short rather than chronic duration and often resolves rapidly following admission.
- Multiple causes are probably present in most cases of hyponatraemia. [152, personal observations] Nearly all have elevated serum ADH levels and have varying degrees of polydipsia greater than need; and many have low effective cardiac output or arterial underfilling. For example those with thiazide related hyponatraemia may have:

    - Raised serum ADH levels. [87]
    - Polydipsia. [87]
    - Decrease in action of Na^+Cl^- transporters in the DCT due to thiazide diuretics.
    - Nausea and vomiting.
    - Hypovolaemia, secondary to arterial underfilling from associated sepsis, (personal observations) or sodium depletion from vomiting or diuretics.

Patients with beer potomania may have polydipsia; low solute intake, which decreases generation of free water in renal distal tubules; sodium depletion; and unsuppressed ADH secretion from nausea and vomiting.

It is often difficult to be certain which causes are relevant in a particular patient because hypovolaemia and sodium depletion are difficult to diagnose reliably. Low urine Na^+ concentration may be present in the SIADH as discussed; serum ADH is rarely available; and unsuppressed secretion may rapidly normalise before it is measured in many patients.

When multiple causes are present each may vary in severity and contribution to the genesis of hyponatraemia. Treatment of hyponatraemia varies depending on the cause, duration—often uncertain, presence of neuropsychiatric symptoms and tendency of ADH to suppress spontaneously, but at a variable rate.

In conclusion It is inappropriate to label a biochemical test—hyponatraemia, as 'Inappropriate ADH Syndrome' when serum ADH levels are unavailable and rarely measured, but raised in nearly all cases; inappropriate is difficult to define or substantiate; multiple causes are present to a varying extent in many cases; there is a variable natural history and treatment; and urinary sodium, an important part of the diagnosis, overlaps to a considerable extent with sodium depletion. [164]

Nephrogenic syndrome of inappropriate antidiuresis. [60,167]

This recently described rare syndrome resembles the syndrome of Inappropriate ADH secretion but is due to a gain in function of the ADH signalling pathway in the kidney probably involving the V_2 receptor. ADH levels are appropriately suppressed.

In conclusion it is important to stress that:

Hyponatremia does not develop unless water is taken to a greater extent than can be excreted. Therefore nearly all cases have an element of polydipsia—water intake in the absence of need.

However water intake by itself rarely, if ever, causes hyponatraemia unless urinary dilution is abnormal because normal individuals can ingest over 20L water in 24 hours without developing clinically significant hyponatraemia. [24, 43, 70, 71] The most common cause of defective urinary dilution is unsuppressed ADH secretion.

Therefore, in the absence of severe renal failure, virtually all cases of hyponatraemia have both water intake in excess of need and unsuppressed ADH secretion. Diagnosis should focus on whether causes other than excess intake of water and unsuppressed ADH secretion are present such as hypovolaemia, cardiac failure and low solute intake.

Hyponatraemia often has multiple rather than a single cause. The diagnosis of coexisting sodium depletion is especially important given the difficulty in diagnosis and importance of treatment.

ADVICE OR ENCOURAGEMENT TO DRINK FLUIDS

An important contributory cause of hyponatraemia is advice, orders or encouragement to drink fluids in the absence of thirst.Hyponatraemia therefore commonly occurs:

* During or following prolonged physical activity-as described.
* In the perioperative period.
* During or to prevent urine infection—especially in those on diuretics (personal observations).
* Intraoperative use of hypotonic fluids, for example, in prostate and endometrial operations. [115]
* During bowel preparation for colonoscopy. [168-174]
* In preparation for ultrasound imaging. [175]

Post-operative hyponatraemia, common in the past from administration of intravenous hypotonic fluids, still occurs as a result of recommendations by nurses to push oral fluids. (Personal observations).

Thiazide diuretics are one of the commonest causes of hyponatraemia. However in my experience excessive intake of oral fluids, based on medical advice, are commonly associated (personal observations).

Severe hyponatraemic encephalopathy developed following a blood transfusion as a result of advice to drink large amounts of fluid by Blood Bank personnel. (Personal observations, reported to the Blood Bank).

Bowel preparation for Colonoscopy

Bowel preparation for surgery or colonoscopy has caused both sodium depletion [174] and severe hyponatraemia. [169-172] Although the incidence is uncommon it is important because of the frequency with which colonoscopy is performed: for example over 550,000 in Australia in 2010. Moreover it is dangerous because it develops acutely and is sometimes poorly managed. This is due to excessive water intake secondary to advice to push fluids and unsuppressed ADH secretion from nausea, stress and sodium depletion. Serum ADH levels were increased in cases in which it was measured. [169] Advice in MIMS prescribing information is: "Drink plentiful water prior to, during and after taking Picolax".The instruction leaflet given to the patient with cerebral oedema, in association with picolax ingestion, shown in figure 9, stated: "Drink as much water as possible".

Promotion of consumption of sports drinks by corporations or guidelines, which are not evidence based, are a common underlying factor in development hyponatraemia during physical activity. In addition the common advice to restrict salt intake, for health reasons, in hot humid climates, contributes to hyponatraemia by causing salt depletion in those working or involved in physical pursuits. (Personal observations).

SYMPTOMS OF HYPONATRAEMIA. [1, 7, 8, 38, 72, 74, 78,103,105,107,132,135,176-178, 189]

The severity of symptoms depends on the serum Na^+ level—although this is disputed; [86,107,176] and the rapidity of onset which limits adaption. Both are probably important. Other variables which influence severity of symptom are:

- Female gender. [38,78,86,103,105,151,176]
- Menstruation. [105]
- Hypoxia. [32,37,78,86,132,176-182]
- Hypokalaemia. [85, 177]
- Comorbid disease—Cirrhosis, malnutrition, alcohol abuse.
- Associated volume status.

Males and females may be equally likely to develop hyponatraemia but females, especially if menstruant, are at much greater risk of developing severe symptoms and death—a relative risk of 28 times in one study. [105] Causes suggested are decreased adaption by $Na^+:K^+$ pumps, possibly related to the effect of sex hormones, [78,105] or increased ADH secretion.

Hypoxia is considered an important risk factor for causing symptoms and poor outcome. This has been postulated to compromise adaption [151,179] by interfering with action of $Na^+:K^+$ pumps. [176] Raised pCO_2 is a theoretical risk, because this increases cerebral oedema by itself, and may occur in association with respiratory arrest, intubation and seizures. It is theoretically important to correct hypovolaemia, which may decrease perfusion of the brain, when raised intracranial pressure is present.

Cerebral oedema is related to plasma Na^+ when hyponatraemia occurs acutely but correlates poorly when hyponatraemia is chronic. Delays in treatment of acute hyponatraemia predispose to death and permanent brain damage. [78, 86, 103, 105, 107, 177, 178,]

Anorexia, nausea, vomiting, headache, muscle cramps, blurred vision and impaired concentration are early symptoms. [105,135,177,181] This may lead to confusion, hallucinations, bizarre behaviour, seizures, myoclonus and coma with fixed dilated pupils. Dysgeusia is a rare symptom [74]. Decorticate or decerebrate posturing indicates that respiratory arrest is imminent. [105] However respiratory arrest may occur abruptly and unexpectedly [105,107,184] and the diagnosis may be made for the first time when respiratory arrest occurs. [184] Diffuse cerebral oedema, obliteration of the sulci and herniation of the brain stem are seen at autopsy. [105,107,177,179] (Figure 10).

An important clue to diagnosis is that focal symptoms are rare.

Non cardiogenic pulmonary oedema has been described, [122,132] especially in Marathon runners. This may worsen encephalopathy and outcome because of associated hypoxaemia. Chronic hyponatraemia may appear asymptomatic. However Decaux [185] suggested that increased rates of falls occur and, although the Mini-Mental State examination scores were normal, more sophisticated tests of mental function were abnormal.

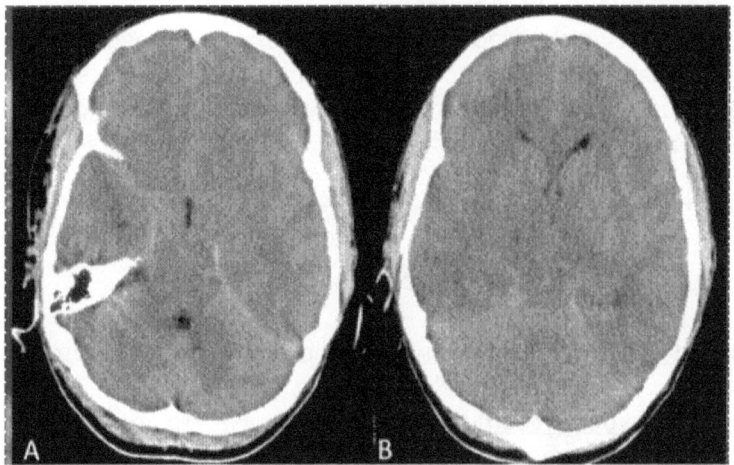

Figure 10: *Computerised tomographic scan showing severe diffuse cerebral oedema with effacement of ventricles and loss of grey-white matter differentiation due to hyponatraemia (serum Na+ 112 mmol/L). Note low density in hemispheres in contrast to relatively high density of the cerebellum. This developed acutely from excess water ingestion associated with preparation for colonoscopy.* (Prepared by Sandeep Bhuta Associate Professor Griffith University)

The amount of water intake over time also governs the severity of hyponatraemia. For example, cholera causes shock with normal or elevated serum sodium, because vomiting decreases water intake and the severity of diarrhoea decreases time for adaption. Less severe diarrhoea, in infants who continue to breast feed on demand, results in a large intake of fluid containing only approximately 5.0mmol/L Na^+, 10mmol/L K^+ and one third the potential solute load than cows milk. The gradual net loss of Na^+ and K^+ (diarrhoeal loss minus intake) results in progressive hyponatraemia which may result in a serum Na^+ of <100mmol/L. [27, 28] Free water excess and (vascular constriction) decreases the severity of effective hypovolaemia at the expense of severe hyponatraemia. [28].

Severe hyponatraemia can occur without signs of hypovolaemia in those with severe sodium depletion and be misdiagnosed as the syndrome of Inappropriate ADH secretion: considerable water retention supports the extracellular volume at the expense of hyponatraemia. In conclusion for hyponatraemia to develop, there must be both:

- Increased water intake- greater than need.
- Failure to dilute water adequately in the distal tubule- in most cases due to unsuppressed ADH secretion.

Even when ADH is elevated water intake in excess of need is required to cause hyponatraemia. Hypotonicity is uncommon in the absence of ADH secretion, because water ingestion must exceed 18-20 L per day, in order to exceed the normal capacity for urinary dilution. [24, 43, 70, 71]

INTERPRETATION OF HYPONATRAEMIA.

Does serum Na^+ indicate tonicity?

Exclude Pseudohyponatremia. Are lipids present or serum proteins elevated?

Exclude hyperglycaemia. Correct serum Na^+ to reflect osmolality by adding half serum glucose in mmol/L to the serum sodium level. To estimate water balances use a correction factor of 1.6-2.5mmol/L for each 5.8mmol/L serum glucose above normal. This is not usually helpful.

What is the volume status?—Hypovolaemia, Euvolaemia, Hypervolemia (cardiac failure). Clinical assessment of hypovolaemia is unreliable.[186] This is discussed in detail in the chapter on Oliguria, Hyponatraemia, Hypotension and Hypovolaemia. The urine sodium concentration predicts the response to saline in patients with hyponatraemia better than clinical examination or other laboratory tests. [186,187] The key manoeuvres are:

Urine electrolytes. The combined fractional excretion of sodium and urea are better in predicting hypovolaemia than urine sodium or fractional excretion of sodium alone. Calculation of urinary chloride and anion gap are occasionally useful.

* <u>Clinical assessment for heart failure</u>: jugular venous pressure, postural changes of pulse and blood pressure.
* <u>Could drugs be the cause</u>? Consider that all medications may cause hyponatraemia: thiazide diuretics and SSRI's are the most common.
* <u>What is the context</u>? For example: post operative, recent physical activity, comorbidity, sepsis, psychiatric disease, preparation for colonoscopy, eating disorder, alcoholic abuse?
* <u>Is water intake excessive? Has there been advice to 'push fluids'.</u>
* <u>Is hypertension present</u>? –Renal artery stenosis?
* <u>Is hypothyroidism, hypopituitarism or adrenal failure likely</u>?
* <u>What are other routine serum electrolytes and biochemical tests</u>?
  <u>Low serum K^+</u>: Diuretics, vomiting, diarrhoea, renal artery stenosis.
  <u>High serum K^+</u>: Adrenal failure, renal failure, K^+ sparing diuretics, rhabdomyolysis.
  <u>High serum total CO_2 (or serum bicarbonate</u>): vomiting, diuretics.
  <u>Low serum HCO_3^-</u>: Diarrhoea, renal tubular acidosis, lactic acidosis.
  <u>Elevated Anion Gap</u>: lactic acidosis, ketoacidosis, renal failure, poisons.
  <u>Low serum urea and uric acid</u>: unsuppressed ADH secretion.
* <u>What are urine electrolytes?</u> (chapter 16).
  <u>Low urine Na^+</u> (<20mmol/L): evidence of low cardiac output from hypovolaemia or cardiac failure. A considerable overlap between salt depletion and SIADH can be decreased by calculating fractional excretion (Fe) Na^+ and Fe urea on spot urine. (See urine electrolytes).

    > <u>Low urine Cl^-</u> : vomiting, hypovolaemia—(useful when urine Na^+ is increased from alkalosis).
    > <u>High urine Cl^-</u> : (+ low Na^+) acidosis from diarrhoea, diuretics, Gitelmans and Barrters syndrome.
    > <u>High urine K^+</u> (despite hypokalaemia): vomiting.
    > Urine <u>NH_4^+</u>: estimate urine NH_4^+: calculate urine anion gap= $Na^+ + K^+ - Cl^-$

  Low negative or positive urine anion gap = low NH_4^+ excretion. If systemic acidosis is present and ammonium excretion is low renal tubular acidosis is probable.
* Trial of normal saline in cases where separation of SIADH and salt depletion is difficult. If the serum sodium increases by 5 mmol/L following 2 L saline given in 24 hours sodium depletion is likely.[188]

TREATMENT

Prevention:

Avoid intravenous hypotonic fluids in hospitalized patients unless hypernatraemia occurs—especially in post operative patients. Pushing oral fluids to excess in the absence of thirst should be avoided.

- Avoid "generous" maintenance fluids, especially in hospitalized children.
- Stop thiazide diuretics before operation,
- Warn about the dangers of pushing water intake in those undertaking physical activity and emphasise the value of gauging fluid requirements by thirst.
- Warn patients with recurrent urinary tract infections and those preparing for colonoscopy about pushing fluids to excess.
- Monitor serum sodium levels, at least initially, in patients on drugs which have a high incidence of hyponatraemia, such as SSRI antidepressants and thiazide diuretics.
- Caution patients with heart failure, cirrhosis, and malnutrition about unrestricted water intake.
- Consider whether unloading is excessive when patients with heart failure develop hyponatraemia.
- Avoid thiazide diuretics in those with eating disorders and past recurrent hyponatraemia.

ACTIVE TREATMENT.

There is considerable controversy on the treatment of hypotonicity because brain damage, called osmotic demyelination or central pontine myelinosis, develops in some patients as a consequence of its correction. In many patients, especially in those with chronic hyponatraemia, brain adaption may be complete at presentation. Following adaption brain osmolytes take several days to return to normal. Thus rapid correction of hypotonicity, especially with hypertonic saline, causes brain cells to shrink. This causes osmotic demyelination (OD) Figure 11.

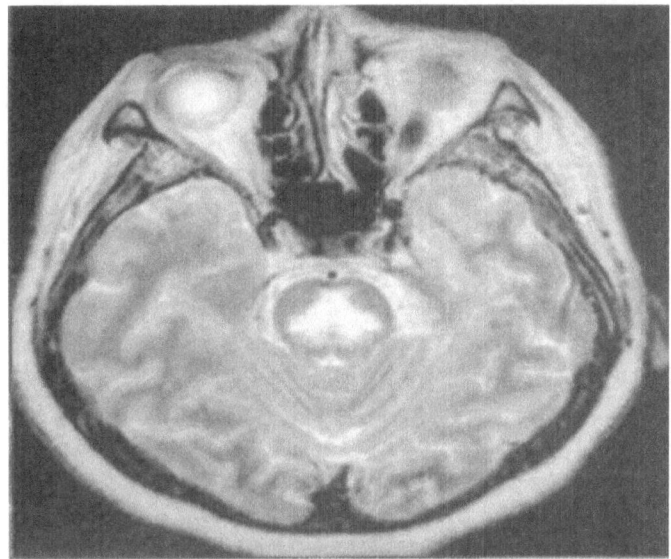

Figure 11: *MRI T2 weighted image. Osmotic Demyelination showing a characteristic hyperintense lesion in the centre of the pons.*

PATHOLOGY AND PATHOGENESIS OF OSMOTIC DEMYELINATION (OD)

Glial cells, which surround neurones within the central pons, cortex and extrapyramidal gray matter, are most susceptible to sudden osmotic change; while neurones and axons are relatively resistant.[189,190] Inflammatory changes are absent, suggesting that metabolic rather than an inflammatory cause is responsible. [189,190]

When hypoosmolality occurs in brain interstitiium glial cells rapidly lose electrolytes in response to increase in cell water (stretch). The resulting change in ionic concentration is replaced by cellular efflux of organic osmolytes which are less disruptive of cell function [31, 36]. Efflux of organic osmolytes however take days or longer to occur because of the need to synthesise transporters. [36]

When osmolality increases on treatment organic osmolytes must be transported back into cells—a process which takes days to complete. Glial cells dehydrate [189,190] if osmolality normalises too rapidly. The grid like compacted arrangement of neurones and glial cells in the pons make this region especially susceptible to both cellular swelling and shrinking and decrease in energy availability. [189,190]

A rapid increase in serum sodium may also disrupt the Blood Brain Barrier. [191]Osmoregulation, both up and down, require increased activity of Na^+ K^+ pumps which are coupled to glucose-lactate metabolism. [189,190]This may explain the susceptibility of those with malnutrition, alcoholism, hypoxia and hypokalaemia, which decrease activity of $Na^+:K^+$ pumps, to both hypoosmolality and osmotic demyelination. [189]

Osmotic demyelination was originally described in chronic alcoholics [190], in the pons alone, but is increasingly described in a large number of different conditions and outside the pons.[189-190] Osmotic demyelination is a more inclusive term than central pontine myelinosis (CPM) although the Pons is the commonest area of the brain involved.

The majority of cases reported follow correction of hyponatraemia, less commonly hypernatraemia, [192] perhaps because hypernatraemia is less common. However osmotic demyelination has been reported when serum sodium was normal; [189,190,193-196] only slightly decreased [197,198] or when corrected slowly—well within recommended guidelines. [158,197-200] In some studies only a minority of cases of OD were associated with hyponatraemia. [78] Indeed the role of hyponatraemia in the pathogenesis has been challenged [201,202] and misdiagnosis considered to be substantial [201,202]. Incidental osmotic demyelination (OD) has been found at autopsy [201] and on radiological surveys in the absence of a previous cause or past electrolyte abnormalities. [204,205]

There is general agreement that females tolerate hyponatraemia less well than males, perhaps due to the effect of sex hormones on function of Na^+ K^+ pumps. [38, 78] Whether OD is more common in women has not been established. OD is considerably more common in those with malnutrition, [189,190,201] debility, alcoholism, [190,202-204] liver disease [190,203,204]—especially transplantation,[203] but has been reported in wide variety of other diseases. [189,190]

Hypoxia is an important risk factor for hyponatraemic encephalopathy [32, 37, 78, 86, 91,132,176-182] and also for development of OD [189,190,199,201]. Indeed some consider hypoxia, by itself, a cause of OD. [204]

Hypokalaemia, especially when uncorrected before sodium infusion, is a risk factor for OD. [189, 190, 196, 198, 213] In a literature review of OD, in which both serum Na^+ and K^+ were reported, 89% of patients had hypokalaemia in addition to hyponatraemia. In 20 cases in which sequential serum K^+ were reported none had hypokalaemia corrected before correction of serum

Na^+. [198] OD has been reported to occur in patients with hypokalaemia without hyponatraemia on several occasions [196]: potassium is a crucial part of adaption to changes in cell volume from activity of Na^+:K^+ pumps. [206]In addition <u>correction of hypokalaemia results in transfer of sodium to the extracellular fluid and may not be accounted for in the assessment of sodium required in treatment.</u> KCl added to 1 L of normal saline results in a hypertonic fluid. Until K^+ is excreted it has the same quantitative effect in correcting hyponatraemia as sodium.

Risk factors for both outcome in hyponatraemic encephalopathy and development of OD are shown in Table 7:

The most important modifiable risk factors cited for the development of OD are:

*   Absence of symptoms of hyponatraemia.
*   Severity of hyponatraemia.
*   Duration of hyponatraemia—whether acute or chronic.
*   Serum sodium level.
*   Rate of correction.
*   Overall magnitude of correction within a specific time.
*   Overcorrection to hypernatremia.
*   Hypokalaemia.

Duration of hyponatraemia is important in that adaption to hypotonicity increases with time. However it is impossible to determine duration accurately in many cases. [32, 197,207, 213,] I believe the presence of severe symptoms due to hyponatraemia, rather than estimates of duration, should determine the risk of cerebral oedema and rapidity of correction.

The severity of hyponatraemia is considered an important risk factor by some but not by others. [86,107,176] The rate of correction is the most important risk for OD but this is disputed. [86, 103, 107, 205,]

	Acute Hyponatraemic encephalopathy	Osmotic Demyelination
Duration of hypotonicity	Short duration increases mortality. (36,38,74,78,103,107,178,207))	Short duration decreases risk. (38,103,197,212,213) Chronic increases OD if treated. (32,36,199,206,210,212)
Plasma sodium	Not important(86,107,176, 207,213) Important. (178)	Not important. (86,193,194,205,206,208,211)
Initial Symptoms	Increases Mortality. (76,86,103,105, 107,178,181,184,217)	Absence increases risk on correction. (189,190)
Female gender	Worse Outcome. (78,85,86,105,151,176,177)	No evidence OD is Increased. (105,206)
Hypoxia	Worsens Outcome. (32,37,78,86,132,176,182,205)	Increases risk. (179,180,182,201, 205)
Alcoholism, cirrhosis Malnutrition, Co-morbidity	Worsens Outcome. (177)	Increases OD. (189,190,197,199,202,204,212,213)
Hypovolaemia	Rapid correction does not cause OD.	OD rare from hypovolaemia Rapid correction Safe. (211)
Hypokalaemia	Worsens Outcome. (85,177)	Predisposes to OD. (189,190,195,196,198,213)
Speed of correction	Improves Outcome. (78,86,103,105,107,137,212)	Increases risk. (141,207-210,212,213,218) No increased risk. (86,103,107,137,205,216,217)
Magnitude of correction		>10-25mmol/day or overcorrection. (78,103,178,210,213,220) <10-15mmol/day rarely causes. OD(72,74,78,103,178,212)

Table 7: Factors influencing outcome and treatment in hyponatraemic encephalopathy and osmotic demyelination. OD = osmotic demyelination.

The overall magnitude of correction within a specific time period is probably more important than the initial rate of correction. [78,103,206,213] It is considered important to avoid overcorrection to normal or development of hypernatremia. Correction by less than 10-15mmol/day rarely causes OD, [72, 74, and 78,103,213] but even this is disputed.

OD has only rarely been reported in those with hypotonicity in association with hypovolaemia from severe sodium depletion. [211] An undue concern about OD may inappropriately delay correction of hypovolaemia: a survey of 12 experts in fluid electrolyte disorders indicated that all would initially treat hypovolaemia rapidly without concern about the rapidity of correction of hyponatraemia. [211]

Aggressive infusion of isotonic sodium containing fluids and rapid normalisation of hyponatraemia reduced mortality in children with diarrhoea and severe sodium depletion from over 10% to 1.3%. [28]

Most experimental OD has been produced in animals made hypotonic with water excess: [213] the cerebral interstitial fluid pressure probably increases in comparison to hyponatraemia associated with hypovolaemia in which cerebral interstitial volume and pressure probably decrease. This may facilitate cellular ionic loss. The cause of hyponatraemia may be an important risk factor.

SYMPTOMS OSMOTIC DEMYELINATION. [74,189,190,194,197,199,209,210,213,214]

The most severe symptoms are flaccid quadriplegia, pseudobulbar palsy, cranial nerve palsies, change in behaviour, lethargy, dysphagia, mutism, locked in syndrome, [189,214] respiratory depression and coma. Their frequency has been considered both rare and common. [189,190] Mid-brain involvement causes cranial nerve, including pupillary abnormalities. Pontocerebellar symptoms may be the sole manifestations [214]. Extra pontine myelinosis may cause ataxia and extrapyramidal manifestations: movement disorders such as choreoathetosis, Parkinsonism, myoclonus and catatonia have been described. [209]

Mutism, dysarthria, changes in affect, confusion and psychosis may cause a misdiagnosis as psychiatric disease. Symptoms characteristically develop 3-7 days following correction of hyponatraemia. However, osmotic demyelination can develop without symptoms and symptoms can resolve spontaneously. Symptoms may develop in a characteristic biphasic pattern: initially from cerebral oedema followed by improvement and then deterioration in 2-7 days, occasionally weeks, with general and focal symptoms due to pontine and extrapontine demyelination.

DIAGNOSIS.

Standard magnetic resonance imaging (MRI) shows symmetrical areas of pontine and extra pontine hyperintense lesions on T2 and hyperintense lesions on T1 weighted images which do not enhance with gadolinium. [214] The classical appearance is of a hyperintense trident shaped lesion in the centre of the pons with sparing of the ventrolateral pons and corticospinal tracts. (Figures 11, 12).The CT scan is less sensitive and changes may take 1-2 weeks to appear.

Much earlier abnormalities appear within 24 hours on Diffusion weighted imaging: restricted diffusion results from decrease in water in the interstitial space combined with water trapping in cells. [215] (Figure 12).

Incidentally diagnosed cases are more common since MRI has become more readily available—in both alcoholics and non-alcoholics. However some reported cases may have been due to causes other than osmotic demyelination. The EEG may show generalised slowing and protein in the cerebrospinal fluid may be slightly raised.

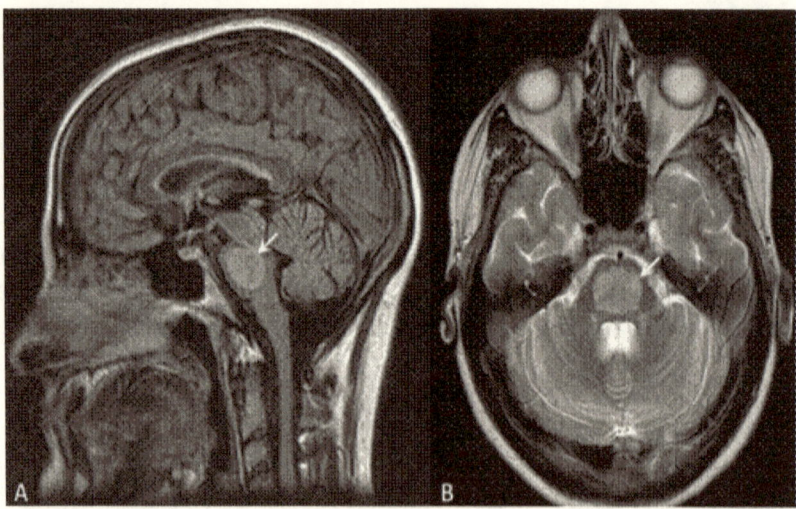

Figure 12.Sagittal FLAIR (A) and T2 weighted axial (B) images demonstrates confluent high signal in the central pons(arrows) suggestive of demyelination,typical site and imaging appearance of central pontine myelinosis. Serum Na+ 106 mmol/L;K+ 1.6 mmol/L on admission. *Serum Na+ increased 25 mmol/L in 24 hours.. (Prepared by Associate professor Sandeep Bhuto Griffith University)*

PROGNOSIS: originally considered poor, is now considered to be variable but often good and includes full recovery. [189, 190] The change in prognosis may be due to earlier diagnosis from availability of MRI and increased awareness. The prognosis may not correlate with imageing.

<u>In conclusion</u>: my experience and review of the literature suggest that acute symptomatic hyponatraemia is more common in women and is more dangerous when hypoxia and hypokalaemia coexist. Virtually all cases have unsuppressed ADH levels and polydisia in the absence of severe renal failure. Severity is related to serum Na^+ level and speed of development: rapid decrease of serum Na^+ to less than 120 mmol/L may cause severe symptoms, but gradual decrease to 100mmol/L may be asymptomatic (personal observations).

The majority of cases of OD develop in those with malnutrition, liver disease, alcoholic abuse or other severe comorbidity. OD develops in those with minimal symptoms of hyponatraemia of chronic onset which has allowed brain adaption to occur. In this setting an increase in serum Na^+ >12 mmol/L in 24 hours, especially to normal or above, <u>rather than the initial rate of correction</u>, predisposes to OD.

Hypokalaemia and hypoxia are important risk factors for its development. Hypokalaemia is especially dangerous because Na^+ leaves cells on correction of K^+ and increases serum osmolality.

OD rarely develops in the setting of severe hypovolaemia. OD usually develops within 3-7 days, occasionally longer, following initial improvement, associated with increase in serum sodium.

TREATMENT OF HYPONATRAEMIA:

'Diseases desperate grown;

By desperate appliance are removed or not at all'. W.Shakespeare

There are no randomized trials to guide therapy. An extensive number of publications address the issues involved and give recommendations for treatment which are often diametrically different and based on personal opinion, uncontrolled observations characterised by selection bias. Some emphasize the poor outcome and high mortality of delayed correction of severe hyponatraemia [78, 86,103,105,107,182,213,216,217] and consider osmotic demyelination is rare and may be due to factors other than rapid correction of serum sodium by hypertonic saline. [86, 103, 137, 142, 180, 194, 196, 205,]

Others consider that osmotic demyelination is a common and serious consequence of rapid correction of hyponatraemia. [32, 89, 90,197,207, 210,212,218] Serum sodium < 120mmol/L (10% below normal) indicates that some adaption has occurred because brain cannot increase its volume by greater than 10 %.[36] Brain cell osmolytes may take several days to regenerate. This suggests that serum sodium should not be corrected to normal for 2-3 days if chronic or asymptomatic hyponatraemia is present. Berl [213] gives an excellent review of the issues involved.

It is often difficult to be certain of the duration of hyponatraemia—whether it is acute or chronic. The severity of symptoms at presentation, regardless of other variables, should guide therapy because this suggests that adaption is incomplete and cerebral oedema present. [76,103,105,107,179,182,213] Other variables are important only because they influence this. Urgent imaging may aid in diagnosis of cerebral oedema, if the cause is uncertain, but is unlikely to be available in a timely manner.

Slow correction of acute hyponatraemia by fluid restriction alone is appropriate if cerebral symptoms are minimal. There is consensus that hyponatraemia with moderate—severe symptoms should receive initial rapid partial correction by hypertonic saline.

However recommendations for the rate of correction vary widely. This includes a bolus to increase the serum sodium by a mean of 7.4 mmol/L in 10 minutes ;[223] a correction rate of 4-5 mmol/hour [78] to as low as 0.5 mmol/hour. A recent expert review recommends correction of serum Na^+ by 1-2mmol/hour. [74]

However it is physiologically unsound to correct serum sodium by 1-2mmol/hour when cerebral oedema is present, especially in those with decorticate or decerebrate posturing or if respiratory arrest or seizures are a substantial risk.

Respiratory arrest may occur unexpectedly. [105]

Delay may result in seizures. Seizures lead to hypoxemia (Lancet 337 394 1991)—an important risk factor for outcome in both hyponatraemic encephalopathy and osmotic demyelination[179]; raised intra-cranial pressure (Brain 101 687 1978) and may cause hypercarbia and pulmonary aspiration.

Moreover serum Na^+ may decrease further following admission and increase the risk of seizures. This has been reported in marathon runners; and occurred in 38% in a recent audit of 26 consecutive patients presenting to hospital with severe euvolaemic hyponatraemia (serum Na$^+$<120 mmol/L) with confusion or seizures carried out by the author. (Unreported observations)

Administration of hypertonic saline over several hours is unsound because cerebral adaption to the hypotonic state and the onset of spontaneous water diuresis may make continuous administration both unnecessary and potentially dangerous as occurred in patients shown in figures 9 and 11.

Raised serum ADH levels occur in the overwhelming majority of patients admitted with hyponatraemia. [37,160] Rapid excretion of retained water often occurs following admission because of resolution of the causes of hyponatraemia. [76, 217, 218, personal observations] Resolution of raised ADH levels may occur for the following reasons:

- Adaption to or correction of associated hypovolaemia.
- Decrease in ADH secretion in hyponatraemic patients with psychiatric disorders.
- Decrease in the action of Thiazide diuretics which have been stopped.
- Decreased access to water in those who have taken excess water.
- Resolution of pain, stress nausea and the effects of sepsis following treatment.

Severe polyuria almost invariably followed within a short time of administration of isotonic saline to infants and children with both severe hyponatraemia (serum Na$^+$<120mmol/L) and hypovolaemia which rapidly led to normalisation of serum Na$^+$. Polyuria may occur suddenly, [207,213] especially in those with compulsive polydisia, in those with sepsis associated hypotonicity and in hyponatraemia associated with thiazide diuretics.

In my experience spontaneous water diuresis, secondary to suppression of ADH secretion, which often occurs after presentation, is a much more common cause of over rapid correction of serum sodium than use of hypertonic saline. The role of spontaneous water diuresis in correction of hyponatraemia has been emphasised by others. [207,213,218]

The rapid treatment of acute symptomatic hyponatraemia has been marginalised because of concern that OD may develop following correction of hyponatraemia with minimal symptoms. However minimal symptoms suggest that brain adaption has occurred and therefore should be treated by water restriction alone.

In view of continued advocacy by some experts to administer hypertonic saline slowly to increase serum Na^+ by 1-2 mmol/L/hour it is important to emphasise the following:

A rapid bolus to increase serum Na^+ by 5 mmol/L in 30 minutes has no more risk of causing OD than the same amount given over 5 hours but is much more likely to decrease the incidence of seizures, respiratory arrest, cerebral compression, mental changes and death. It is especially important in those whose hyponatraemia worsens after presentation. It makes physiological sense to correct hyponatraemia rapidly in the unadapted brain and turn off adaption while decreasing risk of seizures and respiratory arrest. The rapid loss of cellular water from hypertonic saline decreases cerebral oedema, improves associated hypovolaemia and probably turns off ongoing loss of brain cell osmolytes.

The author's practice is to give a bolus of hypertonic saline to raise serum Na^+ by 5mmol in 15-30 minutes, provided heart failure is absent, and repeat this if severe symptoms remain, but this is uncommonly necessary. No further hypertonic saline is given. The focus then becomes monitoring to ensure that spontaneous correction to a serum sodium levels greater than 12 mmol/L in 24 hours does not occur.

If only minimal symptoms are present, regardless of severity or duration of hyponatraemia, initial correction of hyponatraemia is not an important priority. The goal is to ensure that spontaneous correction of water intoxication, due to suppression of ADH secretion, which often follows admission, does not result in over rapid correction of serum Na^+.

If serum Na^+ increases too rapidly 5% dextrose water infusion [219] or administration of dDAVP [219-222] has been recommended to those at risk. Administration of hypotonic fluids in rats' within 12 hours of overcorrection, prevented OD. [220] Administration of 5% dextrose water, with K^+ if indicated, is simple and effective in nearly all cases.

There are few publications recommending rapid bolus infusion. Worthley and Thomas [223] used hypertonic saline over 10 minutes to increase serum Na^+ by 7.4mmol/L.

Bolus infusions of 3% saline to raise serum sodium by 3-5mmol/L were compared to anticonvulsants in children with seizures associated with hyponatraemia. The treatment was effective and safe whereas routine anticonvulsants were ineffective and associated with a high incidence of apnoeic episodes. [224]

Achinger et al recommended a bolus of hypertonic saline to increase serum sodium by 2-4mmol/L in severe cases. [183] Robertson et al [43] considered increasing serum Na by 5mmol/L rapidly was important in severely symptomatic patients. An initial bolus was recommended for severely symptomatic marathon runners with hyponatraemia, before transfer to hospital, by the Second International Exercise-Associated Hyponatraemic Consensus Development conference. [120]

Although rarely advocated for treatment of hyponatraemia hypertonic saline has been used in stroke, [226] heatstroke, [227] septic shock, [228] cerebral oedema, [229] and diabetic ketoacidosis with altered mental status, [230] increased intracranial pressure [231,232] and traumatic brain injury, [233] because of advantages compared to mannitol, [231,234] without reports of OD.

Use of loop diuretics in treatment of hyponatraemia is usually unnecessary: it is inappropriate if hypovolaemia is present and may result in an uncontrolled and variable loss of solute including potassium. However, if heart failure is present a loop diuretic, which results in dilute urine (containing 50-80 mmol/L sodium), should be used.

Hypokalaemia may be a more important disturbance than hyponatraemia. If cerebral symptoms of hyponatraemia coexist with severe hypokalaemia (serum K^+ < 2.0mmol/L). 40 mmol K^+ added to normal saline is an appropriate initial hypertonic fluid: Na^+ plus K^+ = 190mmol/L. Potassium can be added to 5% dextrose water (minimum concentration 40 mmol/L to prevent arrhythmias) if serum Na^+ increases too rapidly rather than Na^+ containing fluids. K^+ must be counted as a source of sodium. In the subject with OD in figure 12, administration of K^+ by boluses and K^+ in normal saline was the most important cause of rapid overcorrection of hypotonicity.

In practice it is often very difficult to achieve a slow smooth correction of plasma Na^+ because unpredictable free water and solute loss continues and It may even be necessary to administer free water or liberalise water restriction to avoid this.

The management of spontaneous resolution is an important part of treatment of both symptomatic (acute) and asymptomatic hyponatraemia. Ongoing urinary losses following resolution of raised serum ADH levels are a major—perhaps the main contributor to unintended increases in serum sodium levels. A decrease in urine Na^++K^+ concentration should alert to the return of the capacity to dilute urine. Measurement of urine osmolality may be misleading as discussed previously.

Urine measurement of Na$^+$ plus K$^+$ concentration is important in overall management. [235]

It is important to appreciate that saline infusion alone may be ineffective in treating water excess from unsuppressed ADH secretion: If the urine (Na$^+$ + K$^+$)concentration is 300 mmol/L each litre of normal saline results in 500 mL of urine for solute excretion and provide 500 mL of free water which further decreases plasma Na$^+$.

It is essential to correct severe volume depletion rapidly—using isotonic electrolyte fluids until urine output is adequate (≥50mL/hour). Normal saline restores volume rapidly while increasing tonicity, although marked polyuria with loss of dilute urine may occur once volume deficiency is only partially corrected. [27, 28,235]

In conclusion : severe symptomatic hyponatraemia usually indicates that cerebral adaption is incomplete and cerebral oedema present.

It is not biologically plausible to take 2.5- 5 hours to correct cerebral oedema especially if seizures are a potential risk.

A bolus of hypertonic saline should be given to increase serum sodium by 5mmol in 15-30 minutes depending on severity unless heart failure is present or a severe risk. There is no evidence that correction of serum Na$^+$ by 5 mmol in 15-30 minutes by bolus of hypertonic saline causes OD. Osmotic demyelination may be more commonly due to spontaneous water diuresis secondary to suppression of ADH secretion: from correction of low cardiac output, improvement in sepsis, stress, nausea, and cessation of causal drugs predisposing to hyponatraemia rather than infusion of hypertonic saline. [234] Correction should be slowed once symptoms resolve if necessary by oral or intravenous water or administration of dDAVP in those at risk for OD.

On the other hand hyponatraemia with minimal symptoms does not require correction acutely. Even gradual correction may not be indicated in patients with ectopic ADH secretion unless chronic therapy, to maintain higher serum sodium levels, with ADH receptor antagonists or demeclocycline, is contemplated. Although subtle neurological defects may be present in "adapted" chronic hyponatraemia [185] there is inadequate evidence that permanent brain damage results from withholding treatment. If severe hypokalaemia coexists potassium should be given early as previously described.

CALCULATION OF HYPERTONIC SALINE REQUIRED

1L 3% saline contains 513 mmol/L sodium.

Both intra and extracellular water contribute to hypotonicity in proportion to their volumes because water is freely permeable across membranes.

Estimate total body water (TBW)   :Female 45-50% ideal body weight.

Male: 55-60% ideal body weight.

Fat contains only 10% water, muscle 70-80%. Thus additional allowance should be made for adiposity with additional supporting muscle and visceral mass. The TBW also decreases with ageing.

Estimate increase in plasma Na^+ following infusion of 1L of 3% saline (513mmol/L).

$$= (513 \text{ minus plasma } Na^+) \div \text{estimated TBW} + 1.$$

TBW is used because addition of Na^+ will result in both intracellular water and extracellular water participating in change. 1L is added to TBW because of the addition of 1L of hypertonic saline.

Example: Female 60 kg (not obese); plasma Na 110 mmol/L

Estimated TBW = 60 x 50% = 30 L.

After 1L 3%hypertonic saline increase in plasma Na+   = (513 minus110) ÷ 30 + 1

= 403 ÷ 31 = 13 mmol/L

100ml will therefore correct sodium by ≈ 1.3mmol. Therefore 400mL 3% saline approximately corrects serum Na^+ by 5.2mmol/L.

However reliability of estimation of current total body water depends on the extent of accompanying saline depletion and the volume of free water excess. If the patient has no saline depletion, but 6L free water excess, then 6 L should theoretically be added to the estimated current TBW. In addition hypertonic saline is given in water whereas serum Na^+ is measured in serum which contains higher Na^+ in water than the serum level suggests. It is also important to remeasure serum Na following a bolus infusion because gastrointestinal water absorption following admission may decrease serum Na$^+$ further. This occurred in 38% of 26 consecutive patients admitted for severe euvolaemic hyponatraemia. (Unpublished audit). Alternatively the change in serum sodium for 1L of any infusion can be estimated by the following formula: [57]

$$\Delta \text{ Serum [Na}^+\text{]} = \{\text{Na}^+ \text{ infused—serum Na}^+\}/\text{TBW+1.}$$

However repeated plasma Na$^+$ measurement and monitoring should be done because of:

- Errors in estimation of TBW.
- Variations in continuing renal free water clearance and electrolyte excretion which depend on when resolution of unsuppressed ADH occurs.
- Ongoing insensible water, urine water and other losses may be difficult to estimate.
- Uncertainty surrounding the extent of cerebral adaptation prior to and duringc treatment.

If K$^+$ is added to normal saline it should be counted as sodium in estimations of the expected change in serum sodium.

The change in serum Na$^+$ can be estimated (excluding losses from diarrhoea or vomiting) by urine Na$^+$ + K$^+$ when urine is available. A more complicated formula is as follows. [21,235]

Change in serum [Na$^+$] = V x [Na$^+$ + K$^+$] inf $-$ V [Na$^+$ + [K$^+$] urine/TBW

(V = volume) [Na$^+$] [K$^+$] = concentration Na$^+$ and K$^+$/ mmol/L. inf = infused

However the influence of potassium depends on its source.

Note insensible water loss approximately=preformed water + water of oxidation from food or catabolism of tissues. Therefore serum may not decrease unless free water is restricted to <500 mL /day.

It is essential in management to account for all sources of sodium, especially potassium.

IN CONCLUSION: In severely symptomatic hyponatraemia:

- Raise serum Na^+ by 5mmol in 15-30 minutes using a bolus of hypertonic saline and repeat if symptoms remain severe.
- Assess risk factors for OD.
- Monitor urine volume and Na^+ plus K^+ concentration. Take action to limit rapid spontaneous resolution of the defect in urinary dilution, especially in those with risk factors for OD.
- If severe volume depletion is present give normal saline rapidly. This is hypertonic compared to the tonicity of the patient and increases volume but will not raise serum sodium too rapidly by itself. If heart failure is present administration of a loop diuretic is effective for both heart failure and initial correction of the serum sodium.
- Correct hypokalaemia early but anticipate its effect in increasing serum tonicity and sodium levels. Correction of severe hypokalaemia may be the most important priority.
- Strenuously avoid hypoxaemia.
- If serum Na^+ rises too rapidly or overcorrection occurs increase oral fluids or give intravenous hypotonic fluids.

If the patient is asymptomatic and does not have hypovolaemia restriction of water alone should be carried out. Water should be restricted to 500-1000 mL per day because water in food and its oxidation provides ≈ 1000 mL per day.

SPECIFIC TREATMENT OF CHRONIC HYPONATRAEMIA.

Chronic Hyponatraemia from Ectopic Inappropriate ADH Secretion.

Demeclocycline 600 = 1200 mg day (V_2 receptor antagonist) inhibits cAMP in the collecting duct and is effective in maintaining normal serum sodium levels. [236]

An important side effect is nephrotoxicity.

Furosemide inhibits free water excretion; 40mg daily was effective in a case of chronic ADH elevation. [238]

ADH Antagonists. [239-242]

These block ADH from binding to V_2 receptors of the distal nephron. The efficacy of oral ADH (Vasopressin) antagonists was evaluated in two multicentric randomised double blind placebo controlled trials in patients with euvolaemic or hypovolaemic hyponatraemia. There was a significant improvement in serum sodium levels. [241,242] The place of these drugs has not been established at the time of writing.

REFERENCES: Water Balance and Disorders

General Reading:

1.   Berl T; Schrier, RW: Disorders of Water Metabolism p1-63 in Renal and Electrolyte Disorders. Ed. Schrier RW, 2003. Lippincott, Williams, Wilkins.

2.   Massry S; Glassock R: Water and Sodium Metabolism. Part 3 Chapter 15. Textbook of Nephrology. 4th Ed. 2001 Lippincott, Williams and Wilkins.

3.   Verbalis JG: The syndrome of Inappropriate ADH Secretion and other Hypoosmolar disorders. p2511-2548. Bichet DC,Nephrogenic and Central Diabetes Insipidus p 2549-2576. In Diseases of the Kidney and Urinary Tract. Eds. Schrier RW. 2001 Lippincott Williams and Wilkins.

4.   Robertson GL; Berl, T: Pathophysiology of Water Metabolism. P 873-928. Brenner and Rectors The Kidney Ed Brenner RB; 5th Ed1996. Saunders.

5.   Yee J, Sterns RH, Bernstein P, Narins RG: Dysnatraemias. p261-275 in Water and Sodium Metabolism. Textbook of Nephrology Eds. Massry S, Glassock R. 4th ed. 2001. Lippincott, Williams and Wilkins

6.   Halperin, Mitchell, L; Goldstein MB: (Editors) Fluid, Electrolyte and Acid-Base Physiology. A problem-based approach. Hyponatraemia p253-288 WB Saunders 1994

7.   Clinical Physiology of Acid Base and Electrolyte Disorders. 285-298; 682-821. 5th Edition. 2001. Eds. Rose, BD; Post, TW. McGraw Hill.

8.   Verbalis JG, Goldsmith SR, Greenberg A et al. Hyponatraemia Treatment Guidelines 2007. Expert Panel Recommendations. *Amer. J. Med.* 120(11A):S1-S21.

Specific References:

9.   DeFronzo RA; Their D: Pathophysiologic Approach to Hyponatraemia. *Arch Intern Med.* **140**:897-902, 1980.

10.   Gennari FJ: Serum Osmolality—Uses and Limitations. *New Eng. J. Med.* **310**:102-105, 1984.

11. Oster J, Singer I: Hyponatraemia, Hypoosmolality, and Hypotonicity. *Arch Intern Med.* **159**:333-336, 1999.

12. Weisberg LS: Pseudohyponatraemia: a reappraisal. *Am J. Med.* **86**:315-318, 1989.

13. Nanji AA: Factitious Biochemical Results in Clinical medicine. *Annals RCPSC.* **15**:35-38, 1982.

14. Narins RG, Jones ER, Stom MC et al: Diagnostic Strategies in Disorders of Fluid, electrolyte and Acid-Base Homeostasis. *Amer. J. Med.* 1982;**72**:496-519.

15. Katz Murray A: Hyperglycaemia-Induced Hyponatraemia—Calculation of Expected serum Sodium Depression. *New Eng. J. Med.* **289(16)**:843-844, 1973.

16. Hillier TA, Abbott RD, Barrett EJ: Hyponatraemia: Evaluating the Correction Factor for Hyperglycaemia. *Amer. J. Med.* **106**:399-403, 1999.

17. Kashyap AS: Hyperglycaemia-Induced Hyponatraemia: Is It Time to Correct the Correction Factor. *Arch Intern Med.* **159**:2745-2746, 1999.

18. Daugirdas JT; Kronfol NO, Tzamaloukas AH Ing TS: Hyperosmolar Coma: Cellular Dehydration and the Serum Sodium Concentration. *Annals of Intern. Med.* **110(11)**:855-857, 1989.

19. Edelman I, Leibman J, O'Meara MP: Interrelations between serum sodium concentration, serum osmolarity and total exchangeable potassium and total body water. *J. Clin. Invest.* **37**:1236-1256, 1958.

20. Kurtz I, Nguyen MK: Evolving concepts in the quantitative analysis of the determinants of the plasma water sodium concentration and the pathophysiology and treatment of the dysnatraemias. *Kidney Int.* **68(5)**:1982-1993 2005.

21. Halperin ML, Skorecki KL: Interpretation of Urine electrolytes and Osmolality in the Regulation of Body fluid Tonicity. *Amer. J. Nephrol.* **6**:241-245, 1986.

22. Kamel KS, Ethier JH, Richardson RM et al: Urine Electrolytes and Osmolality: When and how to use them. *Amer. J. Nephrol.* **10**:89-102, 1990.

23. Rose BD: New Approach to Disturbances in the Plasma Sodium Concentration. *Amer. J. Med.* **81**:1033-1038, 1986.

24. Metabolic Homeostasis. Talbot, Nathan B; Richie, RH; Crawford, J: *Harvard University Press.* p16, 1959.

25. Gowrishnakar Manjula, Lenga Ilan, Cheung RYI et al: Minimum urine flow rate during water deprivation: Importance of the permeability of urea in the inner medulla. *Kidney Intern.* **53**:159-166, 1998.

26. Drescher AN, Barnett HL, Troupkou V: Water Balance in Infants during Water Deprivation. *Amer. J. Dis. Child.* **104**:366-378, 1962.

27. Kingston ME: Electrolyte Disturbances in Breast-Fed Infants with Gastroenteritis and Dehydration. *J. Pediatrics* **83**:1073, 1973.

28. Kingston M: Electrolyte and Fluid disturbances in Liberian Children. MD Thesis. London University.1974

29. McManus ML, Churchwell KB, Strange K: Regulation of Cell Volume in Health and Disease. *New Eng. J. Med.* **333(19)**:1260-1266, 1995.

30. Pasantes-Morales H, Lezama R A; Ramos-Mandujano G et al: Mechanisms of Cell Volume Regulation in Hypo-osmolality. *Amer. J. Med.* **119(7A)**:S4-S11, 2006.

31. Somero GN: Protons, osmolytes, and fitness of internal milieu for protein function. *Amer. J. Physiol.* **20**:R197-R213, 1986.

32. Kleeman CR: Metabolic Coma. *Kidney Internat.* **36**:1142-1158, 1989.

33. Strange K: Regulation of Solute and Water Balance and Cell Volume in the Central Nervous System. *J. Amer. Soc. Nephrol.* **3**:12-27, 1992.

34. Sasaki S, Noda Y: Aquaporin-2 Protein dynamics within the cell. *Curr. Opinion Nephrology Hypertension.* **16**:348-352, 2007.

35. Yamamoto Tadashi; Sasakei Sei: Aquaporins in the kidney: Emerging new aspects. *Kidney Intern.* **54**:1041-1051, 1998.

36. Sterns Richard H; Silver Stephen M: Brain Volume Regulation in Response to Hypoosmolality and Its Correction. *Amer. J. Med.* **119(7A)**:S12-S16, 2006.

37. Gross Peter: Treatment of Severe Hyponatraemia. *Kidney Intern.* **60**:2417-2427, 2001.

38. Cadnapaphornchai MA, Schrier RW: Pathogenesis and Management of Hyponatraemia. *American Journal of Medicine.* **109**:688-692, 2000.

39. Videen JS; MichaelisT, Pinto P, Ross BD: Human Cerebral Osmolytes during Chronic Hyponatraemia. A Proton Magnetic Resonance Study. *J clin investigation.* **95**:788-793, 1995.

40. Verbalis Joseph G; Drutarosky Marcia D: Adaption to chronic hypoosmolality in rats. *Kidney Internat.* **34**:351-360, 1988.

41. Lee JH, Arcinue E, Ross BD:Brief report: Organic osmolytes in the brain of an infant with hypernatraemia.NEJM **331** 439-450 1994

42. Robertson Gary L; Shelton Ronald L; Athar Shahid: The Osmoregulation of Vasopressin. *Kidney Intern.* **10**:25-37, 1976

43. Robertson Gary L; Aycinena Patricio, Zerbe Robert L: Neurogenic Disorders of Osmoregulation. *Amer. J. Med.* **72**:339-353, 1982.excretion. *Clin. Endocrinology.* **58**:1-17, 2003

44. Ishikawa San-e; Schrier Robert W: Pathophysiological roles of arginine vasopressin and Aquaporin-2 in impaired water:

45. McCance RA: Experimental sodium chloride deficiency in man. *Proc. Roy. Soc. Series B.* **119**:245, 1936.

46. Cizek LJ, Huang KC: Water Diuresis in the salt depleted dog. *Amer. J. Physiol.* **167**:413, 1951.

47. Starklint, Jørn; Bech, Jesper Nørgaard; Pedersen EB: Down-regulation of urinary AQP2 and unaffected response to hypertonic saline after 24 hours of fasting in humans. *Kidney Intern.* **67(3)**:1010-1018, 2005.

48. Phillips Paddy A, Rolls Barbara J; Ledingham JGG et al: Reduced Thirst after water deprivation in Healthy Elderly Men. *New Eng. J. Med.* **311(12)**:753-759, 1984.

49. Miller PD, Krebs RA, Neal BJ, McIntyre DO: Hypodipsia in Geriatric Patients. *American Journal of Medicine.* **73**:354-356, 1982.

50. Talbot NB, Richie RH, Crawford JD: Water loss via lungs and skin p 6. Normal limits of total body tolerance for water p18. In Metabolic Homeostasis. *Harvard Univ. Press.* 1959.

51. Zierler K: Hyperosmolality in Adults: A Critical Review. *J. Chr. Dis.* **7**:1-23, 1958.

52. Burch GE, Winsor T: The relation of total insensible loss of weight to water loss from the skin and lungs of human subjects in a subtropical climate.Amer J Med Science **209** 226-234 1945.

53. Newburgh LH; Johnston MW: The insensible loss of water. Physiological Reviews. **22**:1-17, 1942.

54. Hodson ME; Beldon I, Power R et al: Sweat tests to diagnose cystic fibrosis in adults. *Brit. Medical J. Clinical Research Ed.* **286**:1381-3, 1983.

55. Dill DB; Soholt LF; McLean DC et al: Capacity of young males and females for running in desert heat. *Medicine & Science in Sports.* **9**:137-142, 1977.

56. Olsson Karl-Erik, Saltin Bengt: Variation in Total body Water with Muscle Glycogen Changes in Man. *Acta Physiol. Scand.* **80**:11-18, 1970.

57. Barsoum NR; Leune BS: Current prescriptions for the correction of hyponatraemia and are they too simple? *Nephrol. Dial. Transplant.* **17**:1176-1180, 2002.

58. Moder KG; Hurley DL: Fatal Hypernatraemia from Exogenous Salt Intake: Report of a case and the review of literature. *Mayo Clinic Proc.* **65**:1587-1584, 1990

59. Sands, J M; Bichet, DG: Nephrogenic Diabetes Insipidus. *Annals of Intern. Med.* **144(3)**:186-194, 2006.

60. Knoers.N VAM. Hyperactive Vasopressin-Receptors and Disturbed Water Homeostasis. N Engl J Med.352:1847-1850.2005

61. Garofeanu C, Weir M, Rosas-Arellano P, et al: Causes of Reversible Nephrogenic Diabetes Insipidus: A Systematic Review. *Amer. J. Kidney.* **45**:626-637, 2005.

62. Walker RJ, Weggery S, Bedford JJ et al: Lithium induced reduction in urinary concentrating ability and urinary Aquaporin 2 (AQP2) excretion in healthy volunteers. *Kidney Internat.* **67**:291-4, 2005.

63. Bedford JJ, Weggery, S, Ellis G, et al: Lithium induced Diabetes Insipidus: Renal effects of Amiloride. Clinical J Amer Soc Nephrol.doi:10 2215/CJN 01640408 July 2 2008

64. Stuart CA, Neelan FA Lebovitz HE: Disordered Control of Thirst in Hypothalamic-Pituitary Sarcoidosis. *NEJM.* **303**:1078-1082, 1980.

65. Palevsky Paul M, Bhagrath Ravinder, Greenberg Arthur: Hypernatraemia in Hospitalised Patients. *Ann Intern. Med.* **124(2)**:197-203, 1996.

66. Snyder Neil A, Feigal David W, Arieff Allen I: Hypernatraemia in Elderly Patients. *Annals of Intern. Med.* **107**:309-319, 1987.

67. MacDonald NJ, McConnell KN, Stephen MR, Dennigan MG: A Hypernatraemic dehydration in patients in a large hospital for the mentally handicapped. **BMJ.299**:1426-1429, 1989.

68. Sterns RH: Hypernatraemia in the Intensive Care Unit: Instant quality—Just add water. *Crit. Care Med.* **27**:1041-1042, 1999.

69. Richardson DW, Robinson AG: Desmopressin. *Ann. Int. Med.* **103**:228-239, 1985.

70. Barlow, ED, de Wardener, HE: Compulsive Water Drinking. *QJM.* **28**:235-258, 1959.

71. Talbot N, Richie R, Crawford J: Metabolic Homeostasis: Normal Limits of total Body tolerance for Water. p18. *Harvard Univ. Press* 1959.

72. Adrogue Horacio J; Madias Nicolaos E: Hyponatraemia. *New J. Eng. Med.* **342(21)**:1581-1589, 2000.

73. Kumar Sumit, Berl Tomas: Sodium. *The Lancet.* **352**:220, 1998.

74. Ellison DH, Berl T: The syndrome of Inappropriate Antidiuresis. *New Engl J Med.* **356**:2064-2072, 2007.

75. Schrier RW: Pathogenesis of sodium and water in high output and low output Cardiac failure. Nephrotic Syndrome, Cirrhosis and Pregnancy (First of Two Parts. *New Engl J Med.* **319**:1065-1071, 1988.

76. Schrier Robert W: Water and Sodium Retention in Edematous Disorders: Role of Vasopressin and Aldosterone. *Amer. J. Med.* **119(7A)**:S47-S53, 2006.

77. Oren Ron M: Hyponatraemia in Congestive Heart Failure. *Amer. J. Cardiology* **95**:2B-7B, 2005.

78. Fraser Cosmo L, Arieff Allen I: Epidemiology, Pathophysiology and Management of Hyponatraemic Encephalopathy. *Amer. J. Med.* **102**:67-77, 1997.

79. Forfia PR, Mathai FC, Fisher MR et al: Hyponatraemia predicts right heart failure and poor survival in pulmonary arterial hypertension. *Amer. J. Respiratory & Critical Care Medicine.* **177**:1364-9, 2008.

80. Robertson JIS: Salt, volume and hypertension: Causation or correlation. *Kidney International.* **32**:590-602, 1987.

81. Atkinson AB, Davies DL, Leckie B et al: Hyponatraemic Hypertensive syndrome with renal-artery occlusion corrected by Captopril. *Lancet.* **2**:606-608, 1979.

82. Sekkarie Mohamed, Olutade Babatunde, Peterson Phillip: Multiple Manifestations of Renovascular Hypertension. *Amer. J. Kidney Diseases.* **23(6)**:866-868, 1994.

83. McAreavey D, Brown JJ, Cumming AM et al: Inverse relation of exchangeable sodium and blood pressure in hypertensive patients with renal artery stenosis. *J. Hypertension.* **1**:297-302, 1983.

84. Fichman MP, Vorherr H, Kleeman CR, Telfer N: Diuretic-induced Hyponatraemia. *Ann. Int. Med.* **75**:853-863, 1971.

85. Sonnenblick Moshe, Friedlander Yechiel, Rosin Arnold J: Diuretic-induced Severe Hyponatraemia—Review and Analysis of 129 Reported Patients. *Chest.* **103(2)**:601-606, 1993.

86. Ayus J. Carlos, Arieff Allen I: Chronic Hyponatraemic Encephalopathy in Postmenopausal Women. *JAMA.* **281(24)**:2299, 1999.

87. Friedman E, Shadel M, Halkin H, Farfel Z: Thiazide-induced Hyponatraemia. *Ann. Int. Med.* **110**:24-30, 1989.

88. Liamis G, Haralampos M, Elisaf M: A Review of Drug-Induced Hyponatraemia. *Amer. J. Kidney Dis.* **52**:144-153, 2008.

89. Berl, T; Schrier, RW: Disorders of Water Metabolism. *In textbook:* Renal & Electrolyte disorders. p45. Ed. R.W. Schrier. 6th Ed.2003 Lippincott, Williams and Wilkins.

90. Schindel A, Tobin G, Klutke C. Hyponatraemia associated with Desmopressin for the treatment of nocturnal polyuria. *Urology.* **60**:344, 2002.

91. Stratton JF, Stronge J, Boylan PC: Hyponatraemia and non-electrolyte solutions in labouring primigravida. *European J. Of Obstetrics, Gynaecology & Reproductive Biology.* **59(2)**:145-151, 1995.

92. Feeney, J G. Water Intoxication and Oxytocin. *BMJ.* **285**:243, 1982.

93. Schwartz RH, Jones RWA: Transplacental Hyponatraemia due to Oxytocin. *BMJ.* **1**:152-153 1978.

94. Smith NJ, Espir MLE, Baylis PH: Raised plasma arginine vasopressin concentration in carbamazepine-induced water intoxication. *BMJ.* **2**:804, 1977.

95. Bissram M, Scott FD, Liu L Rosner MH: Risk factors for symptomatic hyponatraemia in the role of pre-existing asymptomatic hyponatraemia. *Int. Med. J.* **33**:149-55, 2007.

96. Fabian TJ, Amico JA et al: Paroxetine-Induced hyponatraemia in older adults: a 12-week prospective study. *Arch. Intern. Med.* **164(3)**:327-332, 2004.

97. Wilkinson TJ, Begg E, Winter A: Incidence and risk factors for hyponatraemia following treatment with fluoxetine or Paroxetine in elderly people. *Brit. J. Clin. Pharmacol.* **47**:211-217, 1999.

98.   Jacob S, Spinler SA: Hyponatraemia associated with selective serotonin—reuptakeinhibitorsinolderadults. *Annals of Pharmacotherapy.* **40**:1618-22, 2006.

99.   Liu BA, Mittman N, Knowles SR, Shear NH: Hyponatraemia and the syndrome of inappropriate secretion of Antidiuretic hormone associated with the use of selective serotonin reuptake inhibitors: A review of spontaneous reports. *Canadian Medical Association Journal—JAMC.* **155**:519-527, 1996.

100. Holmes SB, Banerjee AK, Alexander WD: Hyponatraemia and seizures after ecstasy use. *Post Grad. Med. J.* **75**:32-33, 1999.

101. Cherney D, Davids MR, Halperin ML: Acute Hyponatraemia and "Ecstasy": Insights from a quantitative and integrative analysis. *QJM.* **95**:475-483, 2002.

102. Chung HM, Kluge R, Schrier RW, AndersonJ: Postoperative hyponatraemia. A prospective study. *Arch. Intern. Med.* **146(2)**:333-336, 1986.

103. Arieff AI: Hyponatraemia, convulsions, respiratory arrest, and permanent brain damage after elective surgery in healthy women. *New Eng. J. Med.* **314**:1529-1535, 1986.

104. Lane N, Allen K. Hyponatraemia after orthopaedic surgery. *BMJ.* **318**:1363, 1999.

105. Ayus J. Carlos, Wheeler James M, Arieff Allen I: Postoperative Hyponatraemia Encephalopathy in Menstruant Women. *Annals of Intern. Med.* **117(11)**:891, 1992.

106. Steele A, Gowrishankar M, Abrahamson S, et al: Postoperative Hyponatraemia despite Near-Isotonic Saline Infusion: A Phenomenon of Desalination. *Annals of Intern. Med.* **126**:20-25, 1997.

107. Arieff Allen I, Ayus J. Carlos, Fraser Cosmo L: Hyponatraemia and death or permanent brain damage in healthy children. *BMJ.* **304**:1218, 1992.

108. Kirby Robert R: Perioperative Fluid Therapy and Postoperative Pulmonary Edema—Cause-Effect Relationship? *Chest.* **115(5)**:1224-1226, 1999.

109. Choong K, Kho ME et al: Hypotonic versus isotonic saline in hospitalized children: a systematic review. *Archives Dis. Childhood.* **91**:828-835, 2006.

110. Way C, Dhamrait R, Wade A, Walker I: Perioperative fluid therapy in children: a survey of current prescribing practice. *Brit J Anaesthesia.* **97(3)**:371-379, 2006.

111. Editorial. Four and a Fifth and All That. Brit J Anaesthesia. **97(3)**:274-277, 2006.

112. Halberthal Michael, Halperin Mitchell L, Bohn Desmond: Acute hyponatraemia in children admitted to hospital: retrospective analysis of factors contributing to its development and resolution. *BMJ.* **322**:780-782, 2001.

113. Jackson J, Bolte RG: Risks of intravenous administration of hypotonic fluids for paediatric patients in ED and prehospital settings: let's remove the handle from the pump. *Amer. J. Med.* **18(3)**:269-270, 2000.

114. Taylor D, Durward A: Pouring salt on troubled waters. *Arch. Dis. Child.* **89**:411-414, 2004.

115. Carlos AJ, Arieff AI: Glycine-Induced Hypo-osmolar Hyponatraemia. *Arch. Intern. Med.* **157**:223-226, 1997.

116. Gonzales R, Brensilver JM, Rovinsky JJ: Post-hysteroscopic Hyponatraemia. *Am. J. Kidney Dis.* **23**:735-738, 1994.

117. Hew-Butler T, Jordaane E, Stuemfle KJ, et al: Exercise Associated Hyponatraemia. *J. Clin. Endocrinol & Metab.* **93**:2072-8, 2008.

118. Speedy Dale B, Rogers Ian R et al: Exercise-Induced Hyponatraemia in Ultra Distance Triathletes Is Caused by Inappropriate Fluid Retension. *Clin. J. Sport Med.* **10(4)**:272-278, 2000.

119. Almond C, Shin Andrew Y et al: Hyponatraemia among Runners in the Boston Marathon. *New Eng. J. Med.* **352(5)**:1550-1556, 2005.

120. Hew-Butler T, Ayus JC, Kipps C, et al: Statement of the Second International Exercise-Associated Hyponatraemia Consensus Development Conference, New Zealand. *Clin. J. Sport Med.* **18**:111-117, 2008.

121. Davis D, Videen JS; Marino A et al: Exercise-associated hyponatraemia in marathon runners: a two-year experience. *Journ. Emer. Med.* **21(1)**:47-57, 2001.

122. Ayus JC, Varon J, Arieff AI: Hyponatraemia, Cerebral Edema and Noncardiogenic Pulmonary Edema in Marathon Runners. *Annals Intern. Med.* **132(9)**:711-714, 2000.

123. Siegel AJ: Exercise-associated **hyponatraemia:** role of cytokines. *Amer. J. Med.* **119(7 Suppl 1)**:S74-S78, 2006.

124. Noakes TD, Sharwood K, Speedy D et al: Three independent biological mechanisms cause exercise-associated **hyponatraemia:** evidence from 2,135 weighed competitive athletic performances. *Proceedings of the National Academy of Sciences of the United States of America.* **102(51)**:18550-18555, 2005.

125. Siegel AJ, Verbalis JG, Clement S et al: Hyponatraemia in Marathon Runners due to inappropriate arginine vasopressin secretion. *American Journal of Medicine.* **120**, 2007.

126. Noakes TD: Over consumption of fluids by athletes. *BMJ.* **327**:113, 2003.

127. Montain SJ, Cheuvront SN, Sawka MN: Exercise associated hyponatraemia: Quantitative analysis to understand the etiology. *Brit. J. Sports Med.* **40**:98-105, 2006.

128. Gardener JW: Death by Water Intoxication. *Military Medicine.* **167**:432-434, 2002.

129. Garigan TP, Ristedt DE: Death from hyponatraemia as a result of acute water intoxication in an army basic trainee. *Military Medicine.* **164**:234-8, 1999.

130. Levine BJ, Thompson PD: Marathon Maladies. *NEJM.* **352**:1516-1518, 2005.

131. Noakes TD: Sports drinks: Prevention of "Voluntary Dehydration" and Development of Exercise-Associated Hyponatraemia. *Med. Sci. Sports Exerc.* **38(1)**:193, 2006.

132. Ayus JC, Arieff AI: Pulmonary Complications of Hyponatraemia Encephalopathy: Non-cardiogenic Pulmonary edema and Hypercapnic Respiratory Failure. *CHEST.* **107(2)**:517-521, 1995.

133. Frizzell RT, Lang GH, Lowance DG, Lathan RS: Hyponatraemia and Ultra Marathon Running. *JAMA.* **255**:772-774, 1986.

134. Levine S, McManus BM; Blackbourne BD, Roberts William C: Fatal Water Intoxication, Schizophrenia and Diuretic Therapy for Systemic Hypertension. *Amer. J. Med.* **82**:153-155, 1987.

135. Singh S, Padi MH, Bullard H and Freeman H: Water Intoxication in Psychiatric Patients. *Brit. J. Psychiatry.* **146**:127-131, 1985.

136. Goldman MB, Robertson GL et al: Psychotic Exacerbations and Enhanced Vasopressin Secretion in Schizophrenic Patients with Hyponatraemia and Polydipsia. *Arch. Gen. Psych.* **54(5)**:443-449, 1997.

137. Cheng C, Zikos D, Skopicki HA; Peterson D et al: Long-Term Neurologic Outcome in Psychogenic Water Drinkers with Severe Symptomatic Hyponatraemia: The Effect of Rapid Correction. *Amer. J. Med.* **88**:561, 1990.

138. Goldman MB, Luchins Daniel J, Robertson GL: Mechanisms of Altered Water Metabolism in Psychotic Patients with Polydipsia and Hyponatraemia. *New Eng. J. Med.* **318(7)**:397-403, 1988.

139. Demanet JC, Bonnyns M, Bleiberg H: Coma Due to Water Intoxication in Beer Drinkers. *The Lancet.* 2:1115-1117, 1971.

140. Sanghvi SR, Kellerman PS, Nanovic L: Beer Potomania: An unusual cause of Hyponatraemia at High Risk of Complications from Rapid Correction. *Amer. J. Kidney Dis.* **50**:673-680, 2007.

141. Kelly J, Wassif W, Mitchard J, Gardner WN: Severe hyponatraemia secondary to beer potomania complicated by central pontine myelinosis. *Internation. J. Clin. Practice.* **52**:585-587.1998

142. Leens C, Mukendi R, Foret F et al: Central and extrapontine myelinosis in a patient in spite of careful correction of hyponatraemia. *Clin. Nephrology.* **56**:490, 2001.

143. Committee on Nutrition. American Academy of Pediatrics—Report 1957. *Pediat.* **19**:339.

144. Oelkers W: Hyponatraemia and Inappropriate Secretion of Vasopressin (Antidiuretic Hormone) In Patients with Hypopituitarism. *New Eng. J. Med.* **321**:492-496, 1989.

145. Hanna FWF, Scanlon MF: Hyponatraemia, Hypothyroidism and Role of Arginine-Vasopressin. *The Lancet.* **350**:755, 1997.

146. Kubota H, Tanabe Y, Takanashi J, Kohno Y: Episodic hyponatraemia in mitochondrial encephalomyopathy, lactic acidosis and stroke-like episodes (MELAS). *J. Child Neurology.* **20**:116-20, 2005.

147. Miller AC: Hyponatraemia in legionnaire's Disease. *BMJ.* **284**:558, 1982.

148. Thomas TH, Morgan DB, Swaminathan R et al: Severe Hyponatraemia: A study of 17 patients. *The Lancet.* **1**:621-623, 1978.

149. Kennedy PGE, Mitchell DM, Hoffbrand BI: Severe hyponatraemia in hospital inpatients. *BMJ.* **2**:1251-53, 1978.

150. Ross Hill A, Uribarri J, Mann J, Berl T: Altered Water Metabolism in Tuberculosis: Role of Vasopressin. *Amer J. Med.* **88**:357-363, 1990.

151. Ayus JC; Achinger SG; Arief A. Brain volume regulation in hyponatremai: role of sex, age, vasopressin and hypoxia. Am J Physiol Renal Physiol.295: F619-F 624.2008

152. Vitting Kevin E; Gardenswartz Mark H, Zabetakis PM et al: Frequency of Hyponatraemia and Nonosmolar Vasopressin Release in the Acquired Immunodeficiency Syndrome. *JAMA.* **263(7)**:973 -978, 1990.

153. Rose DR, Post TW: Physiological Approach to Acid-Base and Electrolyte Disorders. p704. McGraw-Hill 2001.

154. Harrigan MR: Cerebral Salt Wasting Syndrome Critical Care Clinics 2001. **17**:125-136, 2001.

155. Singh S, Bohn D et al: Cerebral Salt wasting: Truths, fallacies, theories and challenges. *Critical Care Medicine.* **30**:2575-2579, 2002.

156. Berendes E, Walter M et al: Secretion of brain natriuretic peptide in patients with aneurismal subarachnoid haemorrhage. *Lancet.* **349**:245-249, 197.

157. Gutierrez OM, Lin HY: Refractory hyponatraemia. *Kidney Internat.* **71**:79-82, 2007.

158. Upadhyay Ashish, Jaber Bertrand L, Madias Nicolaos E: Incidence and prevalence of Hyponatraemia. *Amer. J. Med.* **119(7A)**:S30-S35, 2006.

159. Hirshberg Boaz, Ben-Yehuda Arie: The Syndrome of Inappropriate Antidiuretic Hormone Secretion in the Elderly. *Amer. J. Med.* **103**:270-273, 1997.

160. Anderson Robert J, Chung Hsiao-Min, Kluge R, Schrier RW et al: Hyponatraemia: A Prospective Analysis of Its Epidemiology and the Pathogenic Role of Vasopressin. *Annals of Intern. Med.* **102**:164-168, 1985.

161. Hoorn EJ, Lindemans J, Zietse R: Development of severe hyponatraemia in hospitalized patients: treatment-related risk factors and inadequate management. *Nephrol. Dial. Transplant.* **21(1)**:70-76, 2006.

162. Torres JM, Cardenas O, Vasquez A, Schlossberg D: Streptococcus pneumoniae Bacteraemia in a Community Hospital. *CHEST.* **113**:387-90, 1998.

163. Bartter Frederic C, Schwartz William B: The Syndrome of Inappropriate Secretion of Antidiuretic Hormone. *Amer. J. Med.* **42**:790-805, 1967.

164. Musch W, Hedeshi A, Decaux G. Low Sodium Excretion in SIADH Patients with Low Diuresis. Nephron Physiology **96** 11-18 2004

165. Verbalis JG. Whole- Body Volume Regulation and Escape from Antidiuresis. Amer J med **119** S21-S29 2006

166. Robertson Gary L: Regulation of Arginine Vasopressin in the Syndrome of Inappropriate Antidiuresis. *Amer. J. Med.* **119(7A)**:S36-S42, 2006.

167. Gietlman Stephen E, Feldman Brian J: Rosenthal, Stephen M: Nephrogenic Syndrome of Inappropriate Antidiuresis: A Novel Disorder in Water Balance in Paediatric Patients. *Amer. J. Med.* **119(7A)**:S54-S58, 2006.

168. Cohen CD; Keuneke C; Sciermann; et al. Hyponatremia as a complication of colonoscopy. Lancet **357**: 282-283 2001.

169. Nagler J, Poppers D, Turetz M: Severe hyponatraemia and seizure following a Polyethylene glycol based bowel preparation for colonoscopy. *J. Clin. Gastroent.* **40**:558-559, 2006.

170. Lewis M, Rugg-Gunn F, Don C, Woods W: Bowel preparation at home in elderly people: patients should be warned not to drink too much or too little fluid. *BMJ.* **314**:7073, 1997.

171. Frizelle F, Colls B: Hyponatraemia and seizures after bowel preparation: report of three cases. *Diseases of Colon and Rectum.* **48**:393-396, 2005.

172. Clemens D et al: Hyponatraemia as a complication of colonoscopy. *Lancet.* **357**:282-283, 2001.

173. Fong M: Fluid deficits and hypotension during colonoscopy. *Anaesth Intensive Care.* **34**:305-306, 2006.

174. Sanders G, Mercer SJ, Saeb-Parsey K et al: Randomised clinical trial of intravenous fluid replacement during bowel preparation for surgery. *Brit. J. Surgery.* **88**:1363-1365, 2001.

175. Shapira I, Isakov A, Almog C: Hyponatremia as a result of preparation for abdominal ultrasound examination Clin Ultrasound **16** 61-62 1988

176. Arieff Allen I: Influence of hypoxia and Sex on Hyponatraemic Encephalopathy. *Amer. J. Med.* **119(7 Suppl 1)**:S59-S64, 2006.

177. Arieff Allen I, Llach Francisco, Massry Shaul G: Neurological Manifestations and Morbidity of Hyponatraemia: Correlation with Brain Water and Electrolytes. *Medicine.* **55(2)**:121, 1976.

178. Ayus J. Carlos, Krothapalli Radha K, Arieff Allen I: Treatment of Symptomatic Hyponatraemia and Its Relation to Brain Damage. *New Eng. J. Med.* **317(19)**:1190, 1987.

179. Ayus JC, Armstrong D, Arieff AI: Hyponatraemia with hypoxia: Effects on brain adaption, perfusion and histology in rodents. *Kidney Internat.* **69**:1319-1325, 2006

180. Knochel J: Hypoxia is the cause of brain damage in hyponatraemia. *JAMA.* **281**:2342-2343, 1999.

181. Arieff AI: Management of hyponatraemia. *BMJ.* **307**:305-308, 1993.

182. Kokko JP: Symptomatic hyponatraemia with hypoxia is a medical emergency. *Kidney International.* **69**:1291-1293, 2006.

183. Achinger S, Moritz M, Ayus J: Dysnatraemias: why are patients still dying. *Southern Med. J.* **99**:353-362, 2006.

184. Fraser CL, Arieff AJ: Fatal Central Diabetes mellitus and Insipidus resulting from untreated hyponatraemia: A new syndrome. *Ann. Int. Med.* **112**:113-119, 1990.

185. Decaux G: Is Asymptomatic Hyponatraemia really asymptomatic? *Am. J. Med.* **119**:S7-S82, 2006.

186. Chung HM; Kluger R; Schrier RW, Anderson RJ: Clinical Assessment of Extracellular Fluid Volume in Hyponatraemia. *Amer. J. Med.* **83**:905-908, 1980.

187. Musch W, Thimpont J, Vandervelde D et al: Combined fractional excretion of sodium and Urea better predicts response to saline in hyponatraemia than do usual clinical and biochemical parameters. *Amer. J. Med.* **99**:348-355, 1995.

188. Musch W, Decaux G Treating the syndrome of inappropriate ADH secretion with isotonic saline. QJM **91** 749-753 1998

189. Brown W: Osmotic Demyelination Disorders: Central Pontine and Extrapontine Myelinosis. *Current Opinion in Neurology.* **13**:691-697, 2000.

190. Ashrafian H, Davey P: A review of the causes of central pontine myelinosis: yet another apoptotic illness. *European J. Neurology.* **8**:103-109, 2001.

191. Murase T, Sugimura Y, Takefuji S et al: Mechanism and Therapy of Osmotic Demyelination. *Amer. J. Med.* **119(7A)**:69-73, 2006.

192. Brown W, Caruso J: Extrapontine myelinosis with involvement of the Hippocampus in three children with severe hypernatraemia. *J. Child Neurol.* **14**:428-433, 1999.

193. Lilje C, Heinen F, Laubenberger J et al. Benign course of central pontine myelinosis in a patient with anorexia nervosa. *Paediatric Neurology.* **27**:132-135, 2002.

194. Kilinc M, Benli U S, Can U. Osmotic myelinosis in a normonatraemic patient. *Acta Neurologica Belgica.* **102**:87-89, 2002.

195. Casey E, Evans A, Krentz A et al: Central Pontine Myelinosis and an unusual complication of diabetes. *Diabetes Care.* **22**:998-1000, 1999.

196. Shintani M, Yamashita M, Nakan A et al: Central pontine and extrapontine myelinosis associated with type 2 diabetic patient with hypokalaemia. *Diabetes Research & Clinical Practice.* **68**:75-80, 2005.

197. Karp BI, Laureno R: Pontine and Extrapontine Myelinosis: A neurological Disorder following rapid correction of Hyponatraemia. *Medicine.* **72**:359-373, 1993.

198. Lohr James W: Osmotic Demyelination Syndrome Following Correction of Hyponatraemia: Association With Hypokalaemia. *Amer. J. Med.* **96**:408, 1994.

199. Laureno Robert, Karp Barbara I; Myelinolysis after Correction of Hyponatraemia. *Annals of Intern. Med.* **126(1)**:57-61, 1997.

200. Endo Y, Oda M, Hara J: Central pontine myelinosis. *Acta Neuropathol.* **53**:145-153, 1981.

201. Tien Robert, Arieff Allen I, Kucharczk W, Kucharczk J: Hyponatraemic Encephalopathy: Is Central Pontine Myelinolysis a Component? *Amer. J. Med.* **92**:513-521, 1992.

202. Lampal C, Yazdi K: Central Pontine Myelinosis. *European Neurology.* **47**:3-10, 2002.

203. Adams DH, Gunson B, Honigsberger L et al: Neurological complications following liver transplantation. *The Lancet.* **329**:949-951.

204. Uchino A, Yuzuriha T, Murakami M al: Magnetic resonance imaging of sequelae of central pontine myelinosis in chronic alcohol abusers. *Neuroradiol.* **45**:877-880, 2003.

205. Kleinschmidt-Demasters BK, Anderson CA, Rubinstein D: Asymptomatic Pontine Lesions found by Magnetic Resonance Imaging: are they central pontine myelinosis? *J. Neurol. Sci.* **149**:27-35, 1997.

206. Berl T Editorial. Treating Hyponatraemia: What is all the controversy about? *Annals of Intern. Med.* **113(6)**:417, 1990.

207. Sterns Richard H: Severe Symptomatic Hyponatraemia: Treatment and Outcome. *Annals of Intern. Med.* **107**:656-664, 1987.

208. Sterns RH, Thomas DJ, Herndon RM: Brain Dehydration and Neurological Deterioration after rapid correction of hyponatraemia. *Kidney Int.* **35**:69-75, 1989.

209. Abbott R, Silber E, Felber J, et al: Osmotic Demyelination syndrome. BMJ **331**:829-830 2005

210. Sterns Richard H, Riggs Jack E, Schochet, Sydney S: Osmotic Demyelination Syndrome Following Correction of Hyponatraemia. *New Eng. J. Med.* **314(24)**:1535-1542, 1986.

211. Narins RG: Therapy of Hyponatraemia. Does Haste Make Waste. *NEJM.* **314**:1573-1574, 1986.

212. Sterns Richard H: The Treatment of Hyponatraemia: First, Do No Harm. *Amer. J. Med.* **88**:557-560, 1990.

213. Berl Tomas: Treating Hyponatraemia: Damned if we do and damned if we don't. *Kidney International.* **17**:1006-1018, 1990.

214. Pirzada N, Ali I: Central Pontine Myelinosis. *Mayo Clin. Proc.* **76**:559-562, 2001.

215. Ruzek KA, Campeau NG, Miller GM: Early diagnosis of Central Pontine Myelinosis with Diffusion—Weighted imaging. *Amer. J. Neuroradiol.* **25**:210-213, 2004.

216. Ayus JC, Krothapilli RK, Arieff AI: Changing Concepts in Treatment of Severe Symptomatic Hyponatraemia. *Amer. J. Med.* **78**:897, 1985.

217. Ayus J. Carlos, Olivero Juan J, Frommer J. Pedro: Rapid Correction of Severe Hyponatraemia with Intravenous Hypertonic Saline Solution. Amer. J. Med. 72:43, 1982.

218. Laureno R, Karp BI: Pontine and Extrapontine Myelinosis following rapid correction of hyponatraemia. *Lancet.* p1439-1441, 1988.

219. Goldszmidt MA: DDAVP to prevent rapid correction in hyponatraemia. *Clinical Nephrology.* **53**:226-229, 2000.

220. Soupart A, Ngassa M, Decaux G: Therapeutic re-lowering of the serum sodium in a patient after excessive correction of hyponatraemia. *Clinical Nephrology.* **51**:383-386, 1999.

221. Soupart A, Penninckx R, Crenier L et al: Prevention of brain Demyelination in rats after excessive correction of chronic hyponatraemia by serum sodium lowering. *Kidney International.* **45**:193-200, 1994.

222. Perianayagam A, Sterns RH, Silver SM et al: DDAVP is effective in preventing and reversing inadvertent overcorrection of Hyponatraemia. *Clin. J. Amer. Soc. Nephrol.* **3**:331-336, 2008.

223. Worthley LIG, Thomas PD: Treatment of hyponatraemic seizures with intravenous 29.2% saline. *BMJ.* **292**:168-170, 1986.

224. Sarnaik A, Meert K, Hackbarth R, Fleischmann L: Management of hyponatraemic seizures in children with hypertonic saline: a safe and effective strategy. *Crit. Care Med.* **19**:758-762.

225. Hew-Butler T, Noakes TD, Siegel AJ: Practical Management of Exercise-Associated Hyponatraemic Encephalopathy: The Sodium Paradox of Non-osmotic Vasopressin Secretion. *Clin. J. Sports Med.* **18**:350-354. 2008.

226. Kempski Oliver: Hypertonic saline and stroke: *Crit. Care Med.* **33(1)**:259. 2005.

227. Stocchetti Nino: Salt saves the hot brain? *Intensive. Care Med.* **29**:1409-1410, 2003.

228. Kolsen-Petersen JA, Nielsen JO, Tonnesen E: Acid base and electrolyte changes after hypertonic saline (7.5%) infusion: a randomised controlled clinical trial. *Scand. J. Clin. & Lab. Investigation.* **65(1)**:13-22, 2005.

229. Prough Donald S, Zornow Mark H: Hypertonic maintenance fluids for patients with cerebral edema: Does the evidence support a "phase II" trial. *Crit. Care Med.* **26(3)**:421-422, 1998.

230. Kamat Pradip, Vats Atul et al: Use of hypertonic saline for the treatment of altered mental status associated with diabetic Ketoacidosis. *Pediatric Crit. Care.* **4(2)**:239-242, 2003.

231. Battison Claire, Andrews Peter JD et al: Randomised, controlled trial on the effect of a 20% mannitol solution and a 7.5% saline/6% dextran solution on increased intracranial pressure after brain injury. *Crit Care Med.* **33(1)**:196-202, 2005.

232. Bentsen G, Breivik H, Lundar T et al: Hypertonic saline (7.2%) in 6% hydroxyethyl starch reduces intracranial pressure and improves haemodynamics in a placebo-controlled study involving stable patients with subarachnoid haemorrhage. *Crit. Care Med.* **34**:2912-2917, 2006.

233. Bhardwaj Anish, Ulatowski John A: Hypertonic saline solutions in brain injury. *Curr. Opin. Crit. Care.* **10(2)**:126-131, 2004.

234. Editorial Levine J: Hypertonic Saline for the treatment of intracranial hypertension: Worth its salt. *Crit. Care Med.* **34**:3037-3039, 2006.

235. Kamel KS, Bear RA: Treatment of Hyponatraemia: A Quantitative Analysis. *Am. J. Kid. Dis.* **21**:439-443, 1993.

236. Forrest JN, Cox M, Hong C et al: Superiority of Demeclocyline over Lithium in the treatment of chronic syndrome of inappropriate secretion of Antidiuretic hormone. *New Engl J Med.* **298**:173-177, 1978.

237. Miller PD, Linas SL, Schrier RW: Plasma Demeclocyline and Nephrotoxicity. *JAMA.* **243**:2513-2515, 1980.

238. Decaux G, Waterlot Y, Genette F, Mockel J: Treatment of the syndrome of inappropriate secretion of Antidiuretic hormone with frusemide. *New Engl J Med.* **304**:329-330, 1981.

239. Palm C, Pistrosch ;F Herbrig K; Gross P: Vasopressin Antagonists as Aquaretic gents for the Treatment of Hyponatraemia. *Amer. J. Med.* **119(7A)**:S87-S92, 2006.

240. Goldsmith Steven R: Is There a Cardiovascular Rationale for the Use of Combined Vasopressin V_{1a}/V_2 Receptor Antagonists? *Amer. J. Med.* **119(7A)**:S93-S96, 2006.

241. Gheorghiade Mihai, Gottlieb Stephen S; Udelson J: Vasopressin V2 Receptor Blockade with *Tolvaptan* versus Fluid Restriction in the Treatment of Hyponatraemia. *Amer. J. Cardiology.* 1064-1067, 2006

242. Schrier R, Gross P et al: Tolvaptan, a selective oral vasopressin, V_2-receptor antagonist, for hypernatraemia. *New Engl J Med.* **355**:2099-2112, 2006.

CARDIOVASCULAR INTEGRITY, HYPOVOLAEMIA, SODIUM DISORDERS, Heart failure and Shock. Part 1.

Not all that is measured is important
not all that is important can be measured Albert Einstein

The function of the circulation depends on a pump, a system of blood vessels of various sizes and the fluid within. (Fig 1)

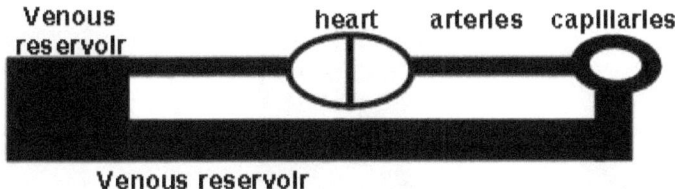

Figure 1: Model of Circulation

Disordered function results from :

- Defective pump (heart) including obstruction to its output.
- Inadequate filling of blood vessels.
- Metarteriole or capillary constriction or bypass causing tissue hypoxia.

Inadequate filling of blood vessels, causing circulatory failure is due to:

- Increase in vascular capacity (vascular dilatation)
- Hypovolaemia—Low intravascular volume.
- Low cardiac output (CO) from cardiac dysfunction.

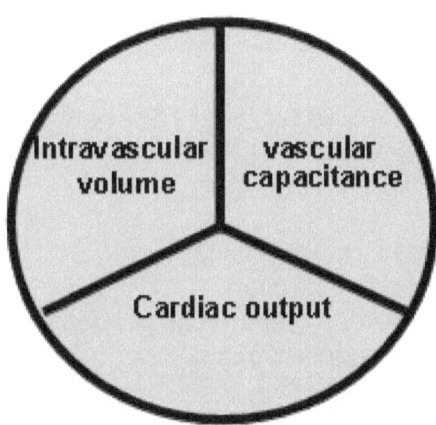

Figure 2: Determinants of circulatory sufficiency.

Vascular capacity comprises both venous (65% circulatory volume) and arterial blood volume (~700 mL) sides of the circulation. Filling of venous capacity determines cardiac filling, (preload). Underfilling of venous capacity is due to hypovolaemia or an increase in capacity for the same volume. (Figure 3) Increase in venous capacity occurs in sepsis, fever, from the effects of drugs, sympathetic dysfunction, for example, spinal cord transection or high spinal block.

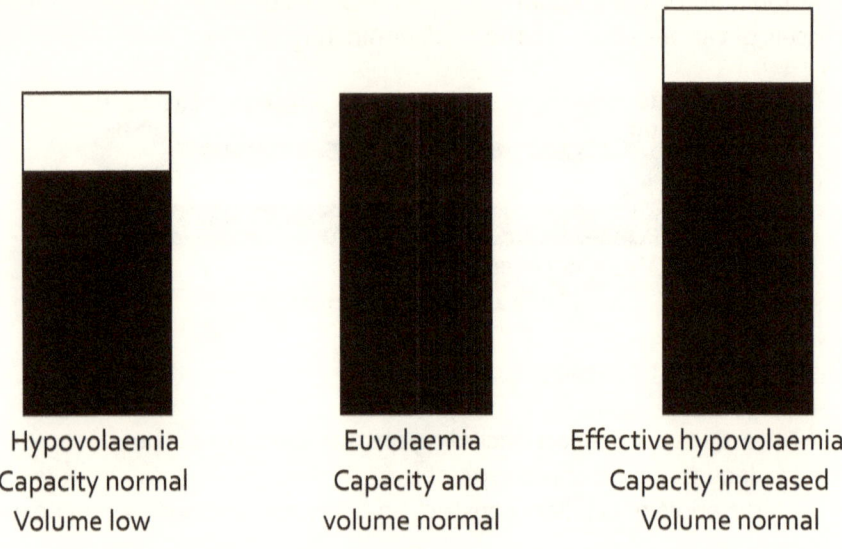

Hypovolaemia	Euvolaemia	Effective hypovolaemia
Capacity normal	Capacity and	Capacity increased
Volume low	volume normal	Volume normal

Figure 3: *Model of venous capacity in relation to volume.*

Decrease in cardiac filling, in the absence of hypovolaemia, may also result from obstruction to venous return: from high intrapleural pressure, positive pressure ventilation, pericardial fluid or tension pneumothorax. Increasing volume improves cardiac filling.

The term effective hypovolaemia is used to include hypovolaemia itself, an increase in venous capacity for a normal volume or both. Impaired cardiac output results from:

- Decrease in preload (cardiac filling).
- Intrinsic malfunction of the heart.
- Obstruction to cardiac output e.g. pulmonary embolism, aortic dissection or severe vasoconstriction.

Arterial filling is a useful term which relates cardiac output to arterial rather than venous capacity. Effective arterial blood volume depends on matching of cardiac output to arterial capacity. The arterial system may be underfilled because cardiac output is low or arterial capacity increased from dilatation of the arterial side of the circulation. [5-7] Arterial dilatation occurs in pregnancy, [5-7] liver cirrhosis, [5-7] conditions of high cardiac output failure, [4-6] as in thiamine deficiency, sepsis and arteriovenous fistulae. [5,6] Sodium and water retention are common to these conditions (Table 1).

The arterial system is highly sensitive because it contains only 0.5-0.7L of the vascular volume. Arterial dilatation or low cardiac output under fills the arterial capacity. Arterial over-filling suppresses these responses and stimulates secretion of natriuretic peptides which cause natriuresis.

	Total Blood Volume	Venous Return	Arterial filling	Pathophysiology
Volume Loss	↓	↓	↓	↓ CO
Congestive Heart Failure	↑	↑	↓	↓ CO
High Output Cardiac Failure	↑	↑	↓	Vascular Dilatation
Sepsis	N	N or ↓	↓	↓ CO, third space loss, Vascular dilatation
Pregnancy	↑	↑	↓	Vascular dilatation
Cirrhosis	↑	↓ or N	↓	Vascular dilatation
AV Fistulae	↑	↑	↓	Arterial dilatation and AV bypass

Table 1: *Changes in total blood volume, venous return, effective arterial volume and pathophysiology of several disease states. (N=normal), CO=cardiac output)*

Intravascular volume, vascular capacity and cardiac output are integrated by a monitoring and response system.

MONITORING SYSTEM

The circulation has a monitoring system which responds in order to achieve optimum venous and arterial filling.

Low pressure High volume receptors.

70% of intravascular fluid is present in veins. High volume low pressure receptors, which monitor stretch, are present in veins, pulmonary vessels, atria, ventricles and portal circulation. Underfilling stimulates the Renin Angiotensin Aldosterone System (RAAS), Sympathetic Nervous System (SNS) and Arginine Vasopressin (AVP,ADH) secretion. On the other hand atrial or ventricular distension decreases stimulation of these systems and releases natriuretic peptides-atrial (ANP) and brain (BNP).

High pressure low volume receptors.

Monitor pressure in the aortic arch, carotid sinus and renal afferent arterioles. Decrease in pressure stimulates the SNS, RAAS, and AVP secretion. Sensors, which monitor filling of the arterial system –low cardiac output or peripheral arterial dilatation, are the most important for maintaining optimum vascular filling. [5-7]

Monitors of sodium status.

Macula densa, part of renal juxtaglomerular system, are specialised cells in distal tubules in contact with renal afferent arterioles. They monitor Na^+ and Cl^- delivery to distal nephrons. Gastrointestinal sensors may monitor sodium content in food.

RESPONSE (EFFECTOR SYSTEM).

Maintenance of optimal vascular filling, in response to the monitoring system, is achieved by stimulation and integration of:

- Sympathetic nervous system (SNS).
- Renin angiotensin aldosterone System (RAAS).
- ADH (Vasopressin) secretion.
- ANP and prostaglandin secretion.
- Renal control of sodium.
- Redistribution of blood flow.
- Fluid shifts between interstitial and vascular compartments.

Sympathetic Nervous System (SNS).

High pressure baroreceptors in the ventricle, carotid artery, aortic arch and renal afferent arterioles react immediately to low pressure to increase sympathetic discharge from hypothalamus and medulla. This increases cardiac output, peripheral vascular resistance and ADH secretion. Catecholamines and sympathetic nerve fibres stimulate renin secretion from juxtaglomerular (JGA) cells and increase Na^+ reabsorption.

Renin Angiotensin System (RAAS) (figure 4).

The JGA (juxtaglomerular apparatus) consists of highly differentiated cells of Macula densa, which sense NaCl delivery to distal nephrons; and juxtaglomerular cells in afferent arterioles which monitor arteriolar pressure. The juxta- glomerular cells synthesise renin from pro-renin, a circulating precursor protein, which is stored in secretory granules. Renin is secreted from juxtaglomerular granular cells of afferent arterioles in response to:

- Decrease in blood pressure in afferent arterioles.
- Increase in catecholamine and SNS stimulation.
- Decrease in glomerular filtration rate.
- Decrease in NaCl delivery to distal nephrons, sensed by macula densa cells.

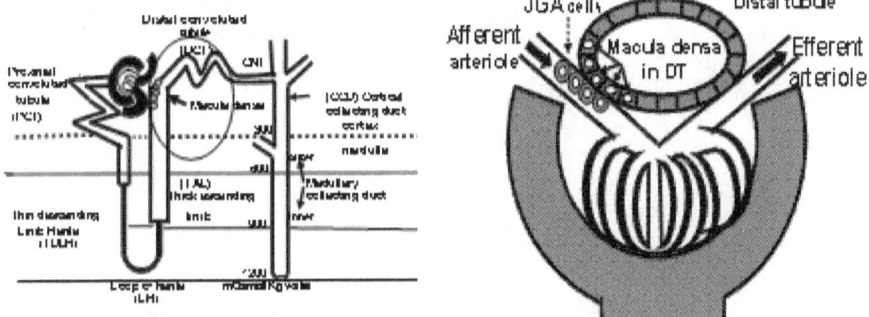

Figure 4: Renin is secreted by juxtaglomerular cells of afferent arterioles from circulating prorennin in response to sympathetic nervous system stimulation, decrease in afferent arteriolar pressure or glomerular filtration rate and stimulation by macula densa. The Macula densa, specialised cells in distal tubules in contact with afferent arterioles, monitor NaCl delivery to distal nephrons.

Renin acts on angiotensinogen, an α globulin produced by liver, to produce Angiotensin 1 (A_1). A_1 is also synthesised by the kidney. A_1 is converted to angiotensin 2 (A_2) by angiotensin converting enzyme (ACE) in pulmonary capillary endothelial cells and other tissues. A_2 acts on 2 principal receptors: AT_1 and AT_2. The AT_2 receptor is important in decreasing uncontrolled growth of normal tissue, in promoting apoptosis and stimulating bradykinin and nitric oxide synthesis. The AT_1 receptor mediates:

* Vasoconstriction of peripheral arterioles.
* Stimulation of aldosterone secretion.
* Stimulation of thirst by acting on the hypothalamic thirst centre and salt intake from a salt-sensing system
* Constriction of afferent arterioles and mesangial cells: this decreases GFR, the effective area for filtration, and thus sodium and water filtration.
* Reduction of medullary blood flow and enhancement of Na^+ reabsorption in ascending loops of Henle.
* Enhancement of proximal and distal tubule Na^+:H^+ exchange and basolateral membrane Na^+:HCO_3^- co-transporters which increases $NaHCO_3$ reabsorption.
* SNS stimulation and catecholamine release.
* AT_1 receptors promote endothelial dysfunction, vascular remodelling, oxidative stress and atherosclerosis.

Components of the effector system and their interaction in matching blood volume to vascular capacity are summarised in figure 5.

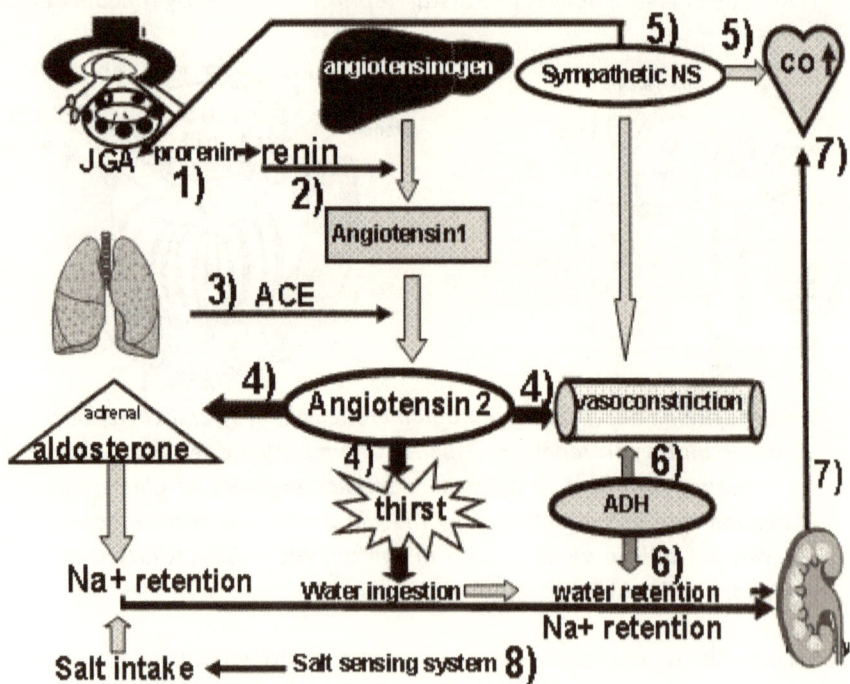

Figure 5: *Interaction of the Renin Angiotensin Aldosterone system (RAAS), Sympathetic Nervous system (SNS) and ADH in regulating cardiac output, sodium and water retention. (Produced using Servier medical art) Numbers refer to text*

1) Renin is produced by JGA from circulating prorenin.,
2) Converts angiotensinogen, produced by the liver to Angiotensin 1.
3) ACE converts A_1 to A_2 in lung capillaries by angiotensin converting enzyme (ACE) and chymostatin-sensitive generating enzyme (CAGE).
4) A_2 stimulates aldosterone secretion, thirst and vasoconstriction.
5) Sympathetic nervous system (SNS) stimulates renin secretion, causes vasoconstriction and increases cardiac contractility.
6) Secretion of ADH is stimulated by hypovolaemia, causes vascular constriction, water reabsorption by collecting ducts and Na^+ reabsorption.
7) Cardiac output increases from sympathetic, catecholamine stimulation and increase in preload from sodium, water retention and vasoconstriction.
8) Salt intake is stimulated by a salt-sensing system.

Antidiuretic Hormone (ADH) Arginine Vasopressin

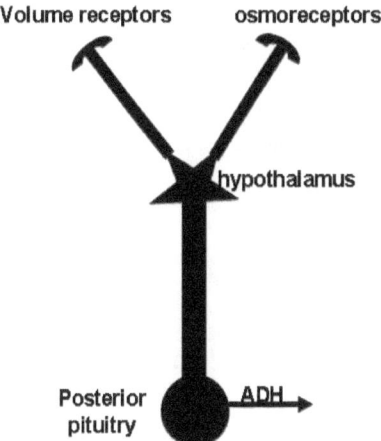

ADH is secreted by cells of paraventricular and supraoptic nuclei of hypothalamus in response to 1 % change in plasma osmolality or 10% decrease in blood volume. Baroreceptors, unloading of arterial capacity, angiotensin 2 and the SNS trigger release of AVP. Decrease in cardiac output, rather than fall in mean arterial pressure, is the main stimulus for non osmotic release of ADH in hypovolaemia and heart failure.

Figure 6: Model of ADH (AVP) Production.

AVP causes vasoconstriction of blood vessels by acting on V_{1R} receptors; myocardial hypertrophy; water reabsorption by acting on V_2 receptors of collecting ducts; and sodium reabsorption by acting on Na:Cl transporters in the DCT and collecting ducts. ADH increases GFR by efferent arteriolar constriction and thus the filtration fraction. This increases sodium reabsorption by proximal tubules. GFR is selectively preserved because AVP acts on efferent but not afferent arterioles compared to adrenaline and n,adrenaline.

Natriuretic Peptides. [8]

Natriuretic peptides inhibit renin secretion, increase GFR and Na^+ excretion, decrease medullary urea and solute concentration and move fluid from vascular into medullary interstitial space. Natriuretic peptides suppress RAAS, SNS and endothelin to modulate vasoconstrictive responses and increase excretion of sodium. They also have anti-fibrotic effects on the heart. [8] ANP is secreted in short bursts; BNP activation is regulated by gene expression and responds in a more sustained way to heart failure. Natriuretic peptides are important markers of cardiac failure. [8]

Prostaglandins

Prostaglandins modulate vasoconstriction: they counteract the effect of A2 on vasoconstriction and sodium retention and preserve GFR during hypovolaemia by dilatation of afferent arterioles. Inhibition may decrease GFR sufficiently to cause renal failure in states of low cardiac output. A_2 stimulates synthesis of E2 and E1 prostaglandins in a feedback system.

LOCAL CONTROL OF BLOOD FLOW AND REDISTRIBUTION. [4]

Blood flow to tissues is regulated to supply tissue requirements. [4] This is achieved within seconds of change in flow or pressure by local vasodilatation or constriction of arterioles, metarterioles and precapillary sphincters. Factors responsible are:

Autoregulation. [4]

An increase in arterial pressure, which normally increases blood flow, evokes reflex smooth muscle contraction to oppose it, called stretch activated muscle contraction. This restores normal flow.

Chemical Mediators. [4]

Adenosine, low pO_2, high pCO_2, H^+, cytokines in sepsis and other mediators cause marked vasodilatation and control flow to tissues. K_{ATP} channels, which are stimulated by adenosine, low cellular ATP levels, lactate, H^+ and other mediators are important in vasodilation due to sepsis. Ca^{2+} causes vasoconstriction.

Renal mechanisms.

Macula densa receptors sense high flow of Na^+ and fluid passing down distal tubules which activate reflex vasoconstriction of afferent arterioles and decrease GFR.

Blood is diverted from viscera, muscle, skin and extremities to maintain brain, cardiac and lung perfusion if cardiac output decreases.

Locally Produced Tissue Mediators. [9-12]

Several tissues, including kidney, heart and blood vessels produce angiotensin 2, aldosterone and other mediators locally rather than systemically (paracrine action). A_2 is synthesised in cardiac myocytes, fibroblasts and vascular smooth muscle, catalysed by renin and cathepsin D, and in a second stage by chymase rather than ACE. Tissue ACE and A_2, produced locally, modulate regulation of blood pressure, cardiovascular responses, repair, plaque structure and metabolism. Local action on angiotensin 1 receptors (AT_1) mediate vasoconstriction, aldosterone and ADH release, sodium and water retention and SNS stimulation. Intrarenal dopamine provides a counterregulatory system which controls sodium balance by acting on dopamine receptors to cause natriuresis during high sodium intake. Dopamine antagonises AT1 receptors which decrease NHE_3 (Na^+:H^+ exchanger) abundance and activity. [9] During a low sodium diet RAAS is upregulated to produce A_2 which increases sodium reabsorption in proximal tubules by acting on AT_1 receptors. During high sodium intake or volume expansion dopamine antagonises AT1 receptors to decrease Na^+ reabsorption. An enteral hormonal system activates local dopamine secretion during sodium intake. [9]

All components of the RAAS are present in kidney. [10] Renal tubules and interstitium contain 1000 fold more angiotensin 2 than plasma and also produces aldosterone, ACE_2, other angiotensins locally renin and AT_2 receptors. Action on AT_2, rather than A_1 receptors, counteracts several of these responses and inhibits renin secretion. [9]

The renal medulla is a major site of nitric oxide (NO) and endothelin 1 (ET1) synthesis. [11] ET1, acting locally, increases blood flow and inhibits Na^+ and water reabsorption in the medulla, and Cl^- reabsorption in thick ascending limbs, loops of Henle. NO controls sodium excretion by modulating renal blood flow, GFR, and by direct tubular action. Natriuretic peptides are also produced locally by kidney: for example, urodilatin is secreted into distal nephrons and acts on medullary collecting ducts (CD) to promote natriuresis.

Thus local and global production of Angiotensin 2 and other mediators regulate blood pressure, sodium reabsorption and cardiovascular responses. Muscle hypertrophy, fibrosis and vascular remodelling are important detrimental effects. The contribution of local production of mediators is uncertain.

Fluid shifts between interstitial and vascular compartments

The extracellular fluid compartment has two main roles:

- Providing cells with an optimum supportive environment.
- Defence of vascular volume.

Interstitiium consists of collagen and elastin fibres with spaces between filled by proteoglycans (sugar coated protein molecules), which combine with water to form a gel, and act like a sponge to entrap interstitial fluid. Interstitial fluid contains 60% (4-5g/kg body weight) and plasma volume 40% total body albumin. Interstitiium has traditionally been considered to play a passive role in fluid balance: changes in interstitial hydrostatic and colloid osmotic pressure counteract changes in capillary filtration—a form of autoregulation. However interstitial matrix is dynamic: connective tissue cells can contract collagen gel by influencing the tension of fibre networks. (Chapter 2)

The capillary exchange network in interstitium has the largest cross sectional area of the vascular system. A dynamic equilibrium exists between vascular and interstitial compartments. The sum of forces shift fluid into interstitiium at the arterial end and back again at the venous end of capillaries. Precapillary sphincters control blood flow through capillary networks but blood can bypass tissues by direct movement from arteriole to venule. (chapter1).The balance normally favours fluid movement into interstitium at approximately 2.0 mL/minute. Fluid returns to large veins by lymphatics. Reduction in capillary pressure decreases filtration. [4] Normal fluid movement reverses in severe haemorrhage or saline deficiency. Plasma refill increases considerably in severe blood loss: [13, 14] albumin moves from interstitiium to vascular space and synthesis increases.

Volunteers bled 10-20% of blood volume increased plasma refill to 90mL-120 mL/minute from interstitium within minutes in the first 2 hours; and then at 40-60mL/minute for 6-10 hours. [13] This was complete and blood volume normal at 30-40 hours: the increase in plasma volume from interstitial fluid approximately equalled the volume of blood lost. Serum albumin did not decrease. Plasma refill increased up to 1000mL/hour in young males presenting with profound shock from bleeding. [14]

Oedema also occurs in injured tissues, depending on severity, due to a systemic inflammatory response from release of cytokines. [15]The leak from capillaries to interstitium increases in septic shock and postoperative patients. Transcapillary leak of albumin, normally 5% per hour, increases by over 300% and constitutes a third space loss of fluid. [16]

Renal conservation or excretion of Sodium (chapter 3)

Until recently salt was often unavailable and highly valued. [17-20] Food eaten by man in the past often consisted of vegetables, leaves and fruit containing high potassium concentration with accompanying organic anions rather than chloride. [18] The Paleolithic diet contained considerably more K^+ than Na^+ [18] and often only ~30mmol Na^+ from a mixed diet and 6-7mmol from a vegetable diet. [18] Breast milk contains only 5-6mmol Na^+/L. Na^+. was vital in evolution because of man's predisposition to hypovolaemia from childbirth, trauma and gastroenteritis. [20]

Approximately 20,000-25,000 mmol of Na^+ are filtered each day, compared to 700mmol of K^+. 1% decrease in Na^+ reabsorption leads to loss of the equivalent of 1.5L of saline but only 7.0 mmol loss of potassium. Thus man has evolved with extremely efficient mechanisms to reabsorb Na^+.

60-70% of Na^+ is reabsorbed in proximal tubules, 25% in ascending limbs loops of Henle, 5% in distal convoluted tubules and 5% in collecting ducts. Normally 99% of filtered sodium is reabsorbed –filtration fraction < 1% ($FeNa^+$<1%). Cellular mechanisms involved are discussed in chapter 3. Several renal mechanisms defend Na^+ homeostasis and optimise vascular filling.

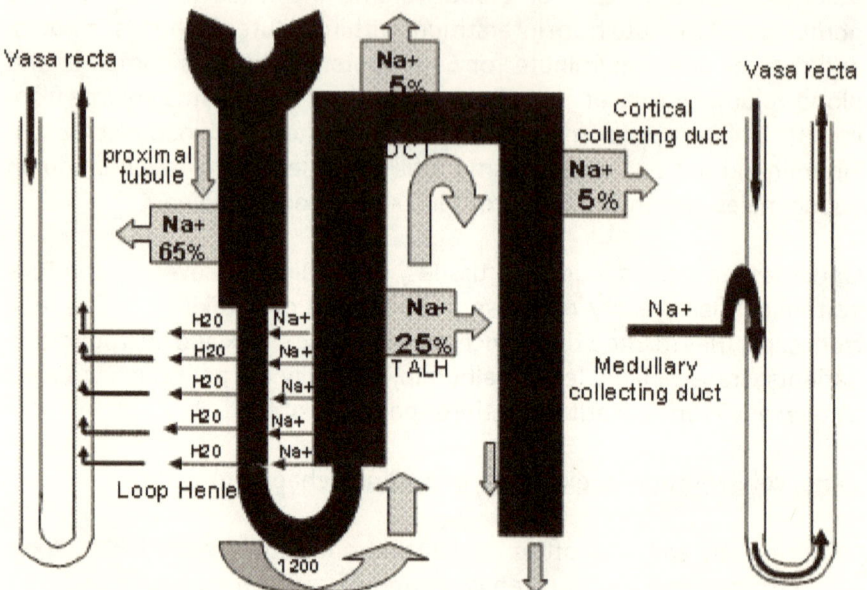

Figure 7: Model of reabsorption of sodium and its recycling into the descending loop of Henle and descending vasa recta. Grey boxes show amount of Na+ reabsorbed in different parts of the nephron. Na+ in vasa recta moves in direction of medulla while water moves to cortex. Urea is transported from medullary collecting ducts and recycles to descending limbs of loops of Henle.Thus Na+ and urea are concentrated in medulla.

- <u>Extrarenal mechanisms</u>: SNS, RAAS,AVP, and natriuretic peptides.
- <u>Local renal tissue mediators</u>: renin, angiotensin 2, dopamine, aldosterone, natriuretic peptides, nitric oxide, endothelin 1, prostaglandins.
- <u>Haemodynamic factors.</u>

Resistance of afferent and efferent arterioles, which are influenced by mediator and haemodynamic factors, determine per i- tubular capillary hydrostatic pressure, oncotic pressure, and reabsorption.

Sodium depletion decreases capillary hydrostatic pressure by lowering both afferent and efferent arteriolar pressure. This promotes Na+ reabsorption by decreasing Na+ filtration and increasing peritubular oncotic pressure. The opposite occurs during volume expansion and gives rise to pressure natriuresis.

A2 increases Na^+ reabsorption in proximal tubules while dopamine decreases reabsorption by acting on $Na:H^+$ (NHE3) exchangers. Decreased flow and sodium chloride delivery to Macula densa stimulates renin release, increases aldosterone secretion, thus increasing sodium reabsorption in distal nephrons.

Aldosterone, A2 and ADH increase Na^+ reabsorption in exchange for K^+ and H^+ in distal nephrons and A_2 stimulate Na^+ reabsorption with bicarbonate in proximal tubules. Local A_2, ADH, thromboxane and other mediators, cause afferent arteriolar constriction and decrease sodium filtration.

To summarise (figure 8):

Blood volume, vascular capacity and cardiac output determine optimum blood supply to tissues. These are monitored by high and low pressure volume sensors which stimulate responses from the SNS, RAAS, hypothalamus and local mediators. Na^+ retention or excretion maintains optimum arterial filling.

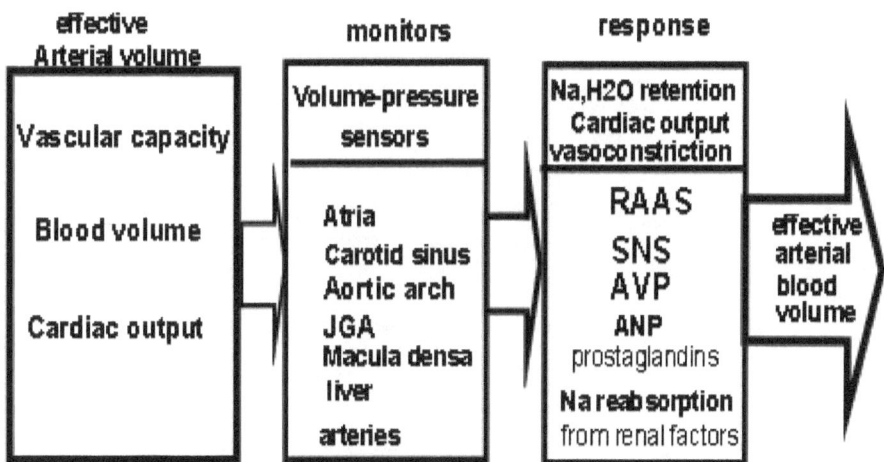

Fig 8: *Determinants of arterial filling, monitoring and response systems.*
SNS =sympathetic nervous system; ANP =atrial natriuretic peptide; RAAS = Renin-aldosterone angiotensin2 system; AVP=Arginine vasopressin.

Arterial underfilling, either from vascular dilatation or decrease in cardiac output, is probably the most important stimulus defending the circulation [21] (Figure 9). Arterial underfilling occurs from:

- Effective hypovolaemia
- Primary cardiac disorders causing low CO.
- Arterial dilatation.
- Combination of the above.

A combination of these factors causes arterial underfilling in:

SEPSIS: causes both arterial and venous vascular dilatation; cardiac dysfunction; and fluid loss from vascular to interstitial space (third space losses). [22] Cardiac output is initially normal or higher than normal, despite cardiac dysfunction, but falls subsequently.

ANAPHYLAXIS: causes venous and arterial dilatation, cardiac dysfunction and interstitial fluid loss due to increased capillary permeability.

ADDISON'S DISEASE: vascular dilatation occurs from lack of cortisol and renal sodium loss from inadequate aldosterone secretion.

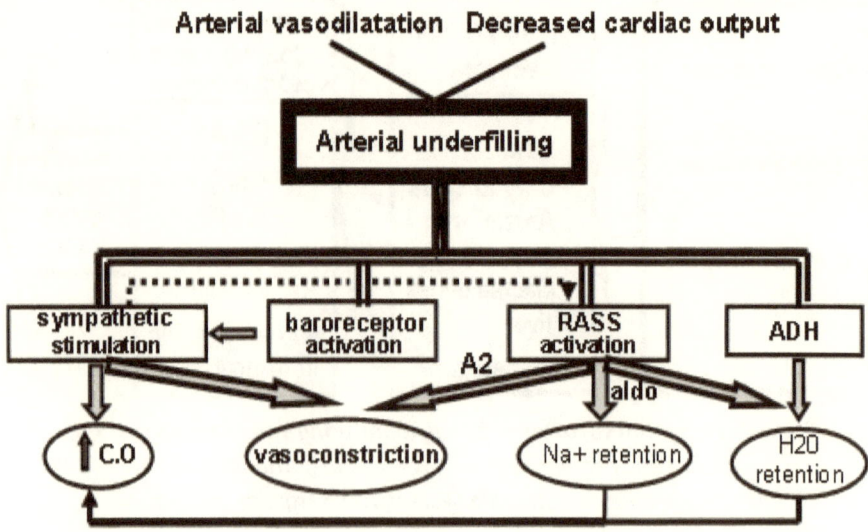

Figure 9: Role of arterial underfilling in activating systems to maintain cardiac output and blood pressure.(aldo=aldosterone; CO=cardiac output;A2 =angiotensin 2; RAAS =Renin angiotensin aldosterone system).

DISORDERS CAUSING LOW CARDIAC OUTPUT

EFFECTIVE HYPOVOLAEMIA.

Effective hypovolaemia is present when the venous compartment is underfilled sufficiently to decrease venous return and lower cardiac output. There are 3 main causes:

Hypovolaemia.

Increase in capacity of the venous system.

Obstruction to venous return.

INCREASE IN VENOUS CAPACITY (65-70% of blood is contained in systemic veins) occurs from:

* Sympathetic system failure: from cervical cord transection, peripheral neuropathy (eg.Guillain Barre syndrome, porphyria) high spinal anaesthesia, cerebral disorders, drugs, poisons and general anaesthesia.
* Sepsis.
* Anaphylaxis and Angioedema.

OBSTRUCTION TO VENOUS RETURN

* Increased intrathoracic or pericardial pressure.
* Intermittent positive pressure ventilation.
* Pneumothorax.
* Pericardial effusion.

These conditions require high venous pressure to maintain cardiac filling. This may be achieved by saline infusion.

The term effective hypovolaemia covers hypovolaemia and an increase in venous capacity or obstruction to venous return.

HYPOVOLAEMIA is due to loss of one or a combination of:

• Blood.
• Colloid.
• Saline.

Losses may be <u>overt</u> or <u>concealed</u>.

<u>BLOOD AND COLLOID LOSSES</u>

Common causes of blood and colloid losses are shown in table 2 but will not be discussed further.

BLOOD LOSSES

OVERT LOSSES: - external loss of blood.

COVERT LOSSES.

<u>Retroperitoneal or intraperitoneal</u> haemorrhage e.g. ectopic pregnancy, aneurysm rupture, hemothorax, retroperitoneal haemorrhage from anticoagulation or trauma.

<u>Fractures</u>—blood, colloid and saline.

<u>Pulmonary haemorrhage.</u>

<u>Blood in gastrointestinal tract.</u>

COLLOID LOSSES:

Burns, pancreatitis.

Table 2. Common causes of blood and colloid losses.

<u>SALINE DEPLETION</u>

Most sodium is lost as hypotonic or isotonic fluids. Hypovolaemia or low cardiac output stimulate thirst and water intake which usually result in additional free water. This is initially excreted to maintain normal serum tonicity. Thus sodium losses are initially accompanied by water in a ratio similar to ECF.

However, when hypovolaemia is sufficiently severe, free water is retained and results in hyponatraemia. This occurs when more than 3L of saline are lost or > 1000 mL of blood in average young males. This may occur earlier if nausea, stress or pain is present.

Sodium depletion plus an isosmotic equivalent of water is called saline depletion or excess. Plasma sodium is normal. The anion accompanying Na⁺ depends on acid-base balance.

Abnormal plasma sodium implies that a coexisting (free) water abnormality is also present:

* Raised plasma sodium implies a free water deficit.
* Low plasma Na⁺ (if it reflects tonicity) implies water excess.
* (Free) water gains or losses have only a slight effect on the ECV (extracellular volume).

COVERT LOSSES. (Third space losses)

Peritoneal cavity—peritonitis, ascites, pancreatitis.
Gastrointestinal tract from obstruction.
Interstitial space: sepsis, anaphylaxis, trauma, operation.
Capillary leak syndrome.
Muscle—rhabdomyolysis.
Bone fracture.

EXTERNAL LOSSES

Gastrointestinal: Diarrhoea, vomiting, ileostomies, fistulae.

Renal: Diuretics, Hereditary tubular disorders, post-obstructive diuresis, renal failure, renal tubulointerstitial disease.
Diabetic Ketoacidosis or hyperglycaemia.
Cerebral salt wasting.
Hypoaldostereonism.
Alkalosis.

Skin Burns, Sweating, Exfoliative dermatitis.

Table 3. Causes of saline depletion.

Inadequate intake of sodium by itself rarely causes severe sodium depletion in those with normal renal function as is often implied: the ability to limit urine sodium excretion to 5- 20 mmol a day suggests that it would take several weeks to cause loss of 1-2 litres of saline. However plasma volume increases by as much as 10% in those taking high sodium containing "Western" diets compared to those taking low sodium or Paleolithic diets. [23, 24] Osmotically inactive sodium may be sequestered in interstitial space and bone on high sodium diet [23, 24] and may have been an important buffer for salt losses in pregnancy, trauma and gastrointestinal disease when salt was scarce. [20] Increase in Na^+ excretion, greater than sodium intake, occurs in the early days of low Na^+ intake. [24] Decrease in food intake, as a result of illness, may initially result in losses of sodium equivalent to 1-2L of saline but is not sufficient to cause symptomatic hypovolaemia. Effective hypovolaemia in those presenting to the Emergency department with fever or infection is usually due to one or a combination of venous dilatation, arterial dilatation and capillary leak, due to cytokines and other factors, rather than decreased intake as is often implied.

External Losses of Saline (chapters 3, 12,- 15 for more detail).

Diarrhoeal Disorders.

The severity of sodium and potassium losses in diarrhoeal disorders are related to the site of bowel affected; organism involved; severity of water and electrolyte losses, which determines Na^+ exchange for K^+ in colon; rapidity of development; and composition of diet.

Cholera, a small intestinal disease characterised by enormous transfer of water, Na^+ and Cl^- into the lumen of small bowel, leads to diarrhoeal stools with much lower concentrations of K^+ and higher concentrations of Na^+ than occurs in other diarrhoeal disorders. Less severe diarrhoea, malabsorption, colonic disorders, such as inflammatory colitis, laxative abuse and villous adenoma, which allow time for Na^+/K^+ exchange in colon, result in severe potassium deficiency as well as sodium depletion. Stool K^+ losses from non cholera diarrhoea in children are higher, but variable: potassium 27-60mmol/ℓ, mean 44.0mmol/L.

Small intestinal fluid has high Na^+ but low K^+ concentration (<10 mmol/L) and relatively high Mg^{2+} concentration (5 mmol/L.) Ileostomy losses cause sodium depletion and often magnesium depletion but severe potassium depletion is uncommon. Laxative use may not be volunteered. The clue to diagnosis is in low urinary potassium and hyperchloraemic acidosis.

Vomiting.

Vomiting causes loss of isotonic fluid containing approximately 150mmol/L Cl^-, 60 mmol/L Na^+ and 2-10mmol K^+. Loss of Na^+ leads to hypovolaemia and Cl^- loss in excess of Na^+ to alkalosis. Hypovolaemia stimulates the SNS, RAAS and ADH secretion. Initially HCO_3^- is excreted with sodium in distal tubules because it is a poorly reabsorbable anion. Urine initially contains high Na^+ concentration despite Na^+ depletion, but Cl^- is low from the outset.

Efficiency of Na^+ conservation increases when hypovolaemia increases in severity: reabsorption of $NaHCO_3^-$ increases in proximal tubules and maintains alkalosis; stimulation of Na^+ reabsorption in distal tubules, in exchange for K^+, increases losses of K^+ in urine. Hypovolaemia from Na^+ depletion, metabolic alkalosis and hypokalaemia result. Hypokalaemia is due to loss of K^+ in urine and not from loss in vomitus.

Renal causes

Loop diuretics.

Frusemide, Torsemide and Bumetanide decrease action of Na^+K^+2Cl (NKCC2) cotransporters in thick ascending limbs loops of Henle. This increases urine Na^+ excretion because the capacity of principal cells to reabsorb the large load of Na^+ delivered to them is exceeded. Hypovolaemia due to Na^+ depletion increases aldosterone secretion. This and increased Na^+ delivery to principal cells of distal tubules increases K^+ secretion in exchange for luminal Na^+ reabsorption. Chloride lost in urine and hypovolaemia stimulate bicarbonate reabsorption to accompany Na^+ in proximal tubules and results in metabolic alkalosis. Calcium excretion also increases because its reabsorption in thick ascending limbs is linked to Na^+ reabsorption. Saline depletion, metabolic alkalosis, hypokalaemia and hypercalciuria result.

Thiazides and Indapamide.

Thiazide diuretics and indapamide decrease function of Na^+Cl^- transporters (NCC) in distal convoluted tubules (DCT) and cortical collecting ducts (CCD). This increases Na^+ delivery to distal nephrons. Thiazide diuretics are less potent and cause less Na^+ loss than loop diuretics because the DCT normally reabsorbs only 5% of filtered sodium. Hypokalaemia develops from exchange of Na^+ for K^+ in CD and leads to urinary K^+ loss. There are two other differences: Ca^{2+} excretion decreases and maximal urinary dilution, which occurs in the DCT from absorption of Na^+, decreases.

Bartters and Gitelmans Syndrome.

These are hereditary syndromes due to mutations which cause dysfunction of Na^+: K^+ $2Cl^-$ cotransporters in thick ascending limbs loops of Henle (TAL) and Na^+Cl^- transporters of distal convoluted tubules respectively. For ease of recall the effects of Bartters syndrome resembles the action of loop diuretics because of interference with function of $Na^+K^+2Cl^-$ cotransporters; while Gitelmans syndrome resembles the action of thiazide diuretics because both decrease function of Na^+Cl^- transporters in DCT.

Diabetic Ketoacidosis and Non-Ketotic Hyperglycaemia (chapter 14)

Osmotic diuresis, secondary to glycosuria and ketonuria, cause urine losses of Na^+, K^+ and water. Increased delivery of Na^+ to principal cells and aldosterone secretion, secondary to volume depletion, increase K^+ loss in exchange for Na^+ in distal tubules. Na^+ and K^+ are also excreted with hydroxybutyrate, a poorly absorbed anion.

Plasma K^+ may be normal or high on presentation from the effects of volume depletion, hypertonicity, insulinopenia, cell necrosis, glycogen depletion and hyperchloraemic acidosis, which are present to a varying extent. Diabetic Ketoacidosis and Hyperosmolar states cause hypovolaemia from Na^+ depletion, K^+ depletion and both hyperchloraemic and anion gap acidosis. Severe hypokalaemia may develop following rehydration, insulin treatment, reformation of glycogen and correction of acidosis.

Acquired renal tubular disorders (chapter 15).

Chronic pyelonephritis.

Obstructive uropathy.

AIDS.

Interstitial nephritis from drugs, medullary cystic disease, autoimmune disease and Sickle cell disease.

Renal transplantation.

These conditions lead to highly variable losses of sodium. Losses are especially high in conditions which involve distal nephrons such as in medullary cystic disease, medullary sponge kidney and chronic interstitial renal disease. They cause natriuresis, with or without, renal tubular acidosis. Na^+ depletion usually only occurs if food contains inadequate Na^+.

Renal Failure.

Patients develop either Na^+ excess or depletion depending on dietary sodium and the speed of dietary change -which influences adaption. [25] Sodium wasting in chronic renal failure is due to damage to remaining nephrons which limit their capacity to reabsorb Na^+. Osmotic diuresis in remaining functioning nephrons obligates Na^+ excretion and delivery of Na^+ to fewer nephrons exceeds their capacity for distal reabsorption. [25]

However patients with chronic renal failure can reduce urinary sodium excretion provided Na^+ restriction or loss develops slowly. Adaptive natriuresis, to a previous high Na^+ diet, takes time to turn off; and negative Na^+ balance or even hypovolaemia can develop before adaption occurs. Na^+ conservation is efficient in both diseases of the medulla and cortex provided sufficient time permits adaption. [25]

Non-Reabsorbable Anions.

Chloride is the only readily reabsorbed anion in distal tubules. Anions such as HCO_3^-, SO_4^{2-}, penicillinate⁻, and ßhydroxybutyrate⁻ are poorly reabsorbed. These anions must be excreted with cations. Distal Na^+ and K^+ excretion increase when anions other than Cl^- reach distal tubules: Na^+:K^+ exchange results in excretion of poorly absorbed anions with potassium or sodium.

Renal artery stenosis.

High pressure in afferent arterioles increases filtration of Na^+, called pressure natriuresis, and increases sodium loss.

Hypoaldostereonism and Pseudohypoaldostereonism.

Hypoaldostereonism decreases function of sodium channels, potassium channels and Na^+:K^+ pumps in distal tubules. This decreases sodium reabsorption and electrogenic K^+ secretion in exchange for Na^+.

Pseudohypoaldostereonism is due to conditions in which aldosterone secretion is normal but function defective. Increase in sodium excretion results from defective aldosterone receptors or function of Na^+ channels (EnaC). Sodium depletion, hyperkalaemia and hyperchloraemic acidosis result.

Hyporeninaemic hypoaldostereonism due to defective renin secretion by the juxtaglomerular cells is the most common cause of hypoaldostereonism. It is associated with diabetes and tubulointerstitial disease. Mild to moderate renal failure is required for its clinical expression. Na^+ depletion commonly occurs but hyperkalemia, with or without renal tubular acidosis, is the most common presentation.

Addison's disease.

This causes effective hypovolaemia due to both aldosterone and cortisol deficiency. Cortisol deficiency decreases vascular responsiveness to sympathetic stimulation and catecholamines and hypoaldostereonism increase renal losses of Na^+ and decrease excretion of K^+. Severe hypotension and shock may result from severe sodium depletion in combination with decreased vascular responsiveness. Lack of cortisol decreases GFR and decreases suppression of ADH secretion which can lead to hyponatraemia. Patients treated with cortisol alone may continue to lose sodium because of under-treatment with fludrocortisone. [26]

Cerebral Salt Wasting Syndromes. [27-29]

Cerebral salt wasting is a highly controversial condition due to excessive urine Na^+ and Cl^- losses in the absence of a physiological stimulus to excretion and in association with a cerebral condition. Hyponatraemia may or may not be present. Subarachnoid haemorrhage, brain trauma, brain tumours and chronic meningitis are common causes. [27-29].The diagnosis should not be made unless the following are met. [27, 28]

• Deficiency of sodium and hypovolaemia are absent.
• Causes of Na^+ loss, such as hypoaldostereonism, are excluded.
• Urinary sodium loss due to intrinsic renal disease is excluded.
• The response to correction of sodium depletion is beneficial.

When hyponatraemia is present differentiation from the syndrome of inappropriate ADH secretion, which is commonly present in cerebral conditions, is difficult but important, because water restriction in cerebral salt wasting is detrimental. Urinary Na$^+$ concentration is raised in both conditions. There are several caveats in making the diagnosis. [28]

- The sodium deficit must exceed 2 mmol/kg body weight - approximately the amount that occurs in normal subjects who markedly reduce sodium intake. [28]
- Administering infusions of saline to prevent cerebral vasoconstriction from subarachnoid haemorrhage may increase urinary sodium excretion despite normovolaemia.
- Capacity of the circulation decreases from marked increase in catecholamine secretion, for example from subarachnoid haemorrhage. Adrenergic surges cause natriuresis. [28]
- Diagnosis of sodium depletion is difficult to establish. [28]

The pathogenesis has not been established but includes cerebral secretion of atrial natriuretic peptides; [27-29] decrease in vascular capacity due to vasoconstriction causing natriuresis, followed by normalisation of vascular capacity; [28] pressure natriuresis when systemic blood pressure increases, followed by resolution; [28] direct neural effects of the sympathetic nervous system; [27] and abnormal function of Na$^+$: K$^+$ pumps. [27, 29]

The main emphasis in treatment is to ensure that positive sodium balance is achieved by correcting sodium depletion. However treatment with saline can decrease serum Na$^+$ further if inappropriate ADH secretion, rather than cerebral salt wasting, is present by a process of "desalination". Thus serum sodium should be monitored if normal saline is given.

Musch et al [30] showed that intravascular infusion of 2 L saline over 24 hours was safe in differentiating sodium depletion from inappropriate ADH secretion: serum sodium fell in the latter but only by 2-4 mmol/L, which was safe, but serum sodium increased if saline depletion was present. Both cerebral salt wasting and inappropriate ADH secretion may coexist and make diagnosis more difficult.

LOSSES FROM SKIN.

Burns. [31-34]

Losses of colloid, saline and red cells result from increased capillary permeability. Losses are greatest in the first eight hours and progressively decrease. Capillary integrity is restored during the second 24 hours. [31]

Various formulas have been used to calculate saline, colloid and red cell requirements. [31] These have usually included 2000mL of glucose in water for insensible water loss; normal saline or lactated ringers of 1.0 - 4.0mL per kg per percent of burn; sufficient isotonic fluid to maintain urine output above 30mL/hour; and additional colloid. [31] Decrease in saline and colloid infusion was recommended in the subsequent 24 hours. Red cell replacement was deferred until capillary permeability normalised, and colloids were deferred by some until the second 24 hours post burn. [31]

A volume of crystalloid of approximately 4mL/kg/percent of burn given initially was found to be effective and well tolerated. Subsequently satisfactory resuscitation was achieved using only Ringers Lactate, 2mL/kg/percent of burn without colloid until the second 24 hours. [32, 33] Blood transfusion was restricted unless haemoglobin decreased below 70g/L. [33] Transfusion increases infection and mortality: infection increases 13% for each unit transfused. [34]

Automated fluid infusion, based on urinary output or Doppler ultrasound measurement of renal perfusion, safely allows fluid restriction because this has a closer correlation with renal cortical perfusion than urine output. This approach decreases complications such as oedema and compartmental syndromes. [32, 33] Modern treatment of fluid therapy is to restrict use of saline, without compromising renal function, and to avoid blood transfusion unless haemoglobin decreases below 70g/L. [33]

Environment and exercise causing sodium chloride losses.

Sodium and chloride concentration of sweat, 10-60mmol/L (mean 28.5mmol/L) [35] are approximately equal and vary with rate of flow and acclimatisation. [35] However Na^+ concentration is greater than 50mmol/L in some adults. This causes Na^+ depletion and predisposes to metabolic alkalosis because the ratio of Cl^- to Na^+ is higher in sweat than extracellular fluid. Increase in renal tubular Na^+: K^+ exchange, secondary to Na^+ depletion and increased aldosterone secretion, lead to hypokalaemia and metabolic alkalosis.

Sweating increases when environmental temperature and humidity increase. High humidity decreases (free) water losses from both lungs and skin. Thus heat dissipation is mainly dependent on sweating. Patients may present with severe muscle cramps, hypotension and tetany from severe metabolic alkalosis. This decreases ionised calcium. [Personal observations]

Cystic Fibrosis:

Cystic fibrosis is due to a genetic disorder of the cystic fibrosis transmembrane conductance regulator (CFTR) gene which controls function of cAMP regulated chloride channels. The higher NaCl concentration of sweat, 90-100mmol/L, mean chloride 96mmol/L, [35] increases risk of sodium depletion, metabolic alkalosis and hypokalaemia.

Cystic fibrosis may present for the first time in adults with recurrent episodes of sodium depletion and hypokalaemic metabolic alkalosis, sometimes causing tetany. Common abnormalities are bronchiectasis, especially of upper lobes; malabsorption from pancreatic insufficiency; recurrent pancreatitis; liver cirrhosis; and infertility in males due to failure of the epididymis and vas deferens to develop.

THIRD SPACE LOSSES.

Third space losses occur into the peritoneal cavity from peritonitis; ascites; pancreatitis; into the intestine in acute intestinal obstruction or inflammation; into muscle in rhabdomyolysis and compartment syndromes; around bone fractures; and into interstitium in sepsis, anaphylaxis, trauma, haemorrhage and the capillary leak syndrome. These involve predominantly saline but colloid loss may be substantial in inflammatory conditions such as pancreatitis and peritonitis.

Rhabdomyolysis. [36]

Rhabdomyolysis results from trauma, especially compartment syndromes; infection; seizures; coma; drugs such as alcohol, lipid lowering agents and illicit drugs; hyperpyrexia and genetic diseases. Hypovolaemia develops as fluid is sequestered in muscle. Hyperkalaemia, hyperphosphataemia, hyperuricaemia and anion gap acidosis result from necrosed muscle and hypocalcaemia may occur from calcium entry into ischaemic muscle. Volume depletion, renal vasoconstriction and myoglobin predispose to renal failure. Surprisingly the $FeNa^+$ is usually <1%.

Large volumes of isotonic sodium containing fluid are given to correct volume depletion and maintain a high urine flow rate. Use of bicarbonate is controversial: it prevents the nephrotoxicity of myoglobin and decreases hyperchloraemic acidosis from saline administration but may cause or worsen hypocalcaemia.

Haemorrhage and operations.

Operation and traumatic haemorrhage were traditionally considered to cause considerable interstitial losses of fluid in addition to blood. This was considered to lead to extracellular volume contraction and led to aggressive saline replacement in excess of overt losses. In a systematic review of trials, in which extracellular volume was measured Brandstrup et al [37] challenged this view and concluded that previous methodology was flawed. Aggressive saline infusion in excess of need increased the frequency of complications. Therefore the best evidence is that covert losses of interstitial fluid are not substantial in most trauma and as a result of operations.

Capillary Leak. [38, 39]

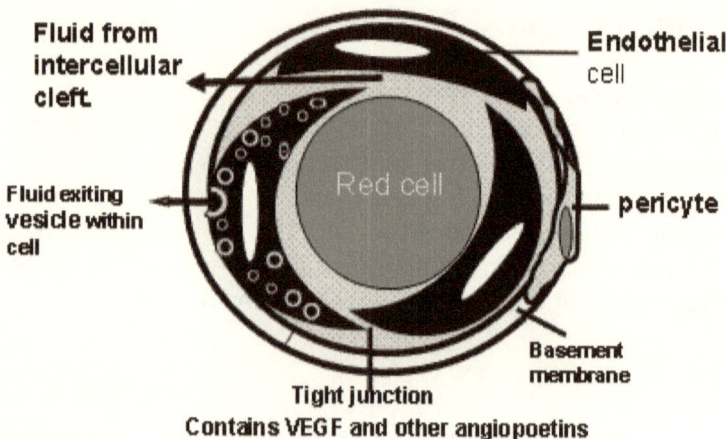

Figure.10. Model of capillary showing fluid exiting from intercellular cleft and from vesicle in endothelial cell.

The normal barrier to endothelial permeability includes endothelial cells, coated by a glycocalyx, (not shown), basement membrane, and pericytes. Endothelial cells contain cytoplasmic vesicles which are involved in the transcellular passage of plasma proteins. Normally small molecules, such as water and solutes, move between endothelial cell clefts (paracellular) and only to a limited extent through cells by vesicles (transcellular).The junction between cells contain several proteins which influence endothelial permeability. Sepsis; several viral infections, for example Dengue fever, [39] drugs and toxins, anaphylaxis, angioedema and rare endocrine disorders cause widespread increase in capillary permeability. This causes vascular loss of saline and plasma into interstitiium and hypovolaemia.

Ovarian Hyperstimulation syndrome.

This syndrome has become important since βHCG and gonadotrophic releasing hormones were used to enhance fertility. Normally a tightly coordinated cycle, controlled by hormones and other mediators, results in the release of a single mature oocyte from thousands of primordial oocytes. Ovarian Hyperstimulation from gonadotrophic treatment results in luteinisation of multiple follicles and marked enlargement of individual follicles. This results in large ovaries containing cysts: Grade 1 - 5X5 cm, longitudinal axis,; and grade 3, above 12X12 cm. Ovarian cysts leak several mediators, including VEGF (vascular endothelial growth factor) which increase vascular permeability. There are 2 main manifestations:

Ovarian enlargement with cysts which are liable to rupture.

Leakage of ovarian mediators into the peritoneal cavity and vascular space.

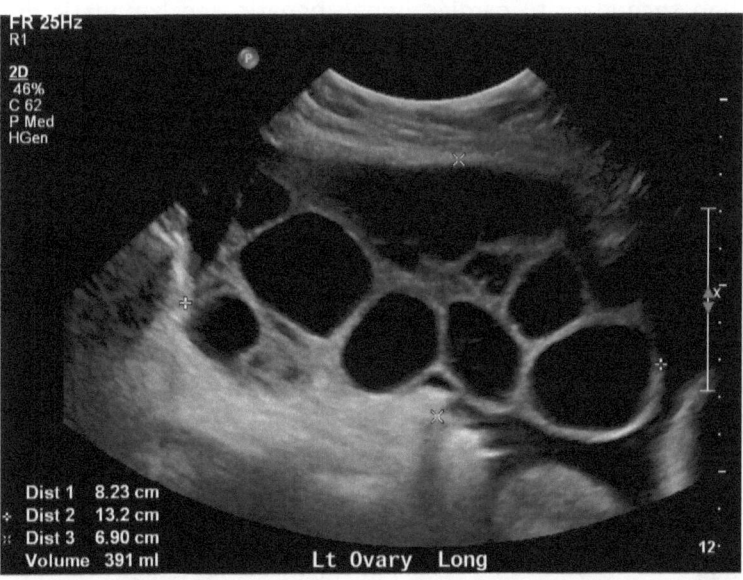

Figure 11. Ultrasound of Left ovary measuring 13 cm in longitudinal axis.

This results in ascites, occasionally pericardial and pleural fluid collections, hypovolaemia, renal failure, raised haematocrit, and predisposes to thrombosis of veins and less commonly arteries. Renal failure predisposes to hyperkalaemia and hyponatraemia. Ascites is often prominent because of leakage of mediators from cysts directly into the peritoneal cavity;

and pain may be severe because the acute onset limits the capacity for abdominal distension. Respiratory symptoms are due to restriction, atelectasis, secondary to ascites, and pulmonary oedema from vascular leakage. Weight, abdominal girth, serum creatinine, electrolytes, haematocrit, fluid balance, blood pressure, SO_2, respiratory rate and abdominal symptoms should be monitored closely.

Conservative treatment, while awaiting spontaneous resolution in 9-14 days, is indicated. However judicious saline or albumin infusion (40-50 gm over several hours) may be indicated to prevent renal failure; anticoagulation to prevent vascular thrombosis; and paracentesis (under ultrasonic guidance is essential) if indicated.

Idiopathic Systemic capillary leak syndrome. [38]

This rare condition is characterised by unexplained episodic capillary hyperpermeability. There should be no evidence of salt and water retention secondary to cardiac, renal, hepatic and lymphatic disease; drugs causing sodium retention; anaphylaxis and angioedema; and severe sepsis. Fluid and protein shift rapidly from intravascular to interstitial space and results in diffuse oedema, hypovolaemia, hypoalbuminaemia, shock and renal failure. Renal failure is due to hypovolaemia combined with rhabdomyolysis.

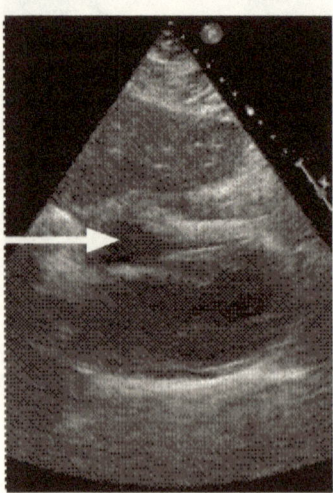 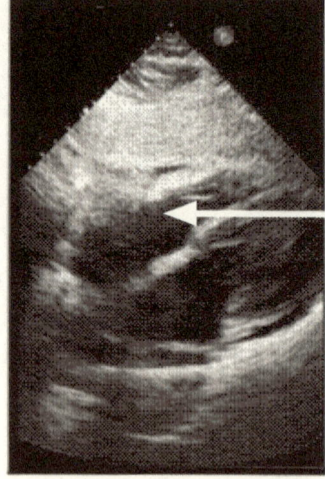

Figure 12. Echocardiogram showing very small right atrium outlined by arrows during hypovolaemic shock on left and 3 months later following recovery on right: note marked increase in size.

Sudden onset of the Systemic Capillary leak syndrome: haemoglobin 200g/L, CPK>50.000U/L, renal failure, generalised oedema, Monoclonal gammopathy. Pulseless Electrical Arrest developed and was followed by flash pulmonary oedema during recovery.

Marked haemoconcentration, leucocytosis, hypoalbuminaemia, raised CPK and neutrocytosis are common. Rhabdomyolysis is due to hypotension and pressure of interstitial fluid in muscle.

Monoclonal gammopathy occurs in approximately 80 %.

There are 2 phases: severe hypovolaemia and shock due to loss of plasma volume into the interstitiium; followed in 1-3 days by return of fluid to the circulation and often flash pulmonary oedema. Therefore fluid given in the first phase is detrimental when capillary permeability normalises and causes a dilemma in initial treatment. Attacks are often preceded by malaise, myalgia and fatigue. The median age is 45 years. Intravenous immunoglobulin at high dose and theophylline-in prevention has been reported to be beneficial in case reports. [38]

CLINICAL SIGNS OF HYPOVOLAEMIA AND INTERSTITIAL FLUID DEPLETION.

Hypovolaemia due to blood loss.

The American College of Surgeons and several others have proposed a relation between the amount of blood loss and clinical signs. This is shown in the following table.

	Blood loss	% Blood Loss	Pulse	BP	Pulse Pressure	UO	RR
Class I	500-750	10-15	<100	N	N	>30	N
Class II	750-1500	15-30	>100	N	↓	20-30	20-30
Class III	1500-2000	30-40	>120	↓	↓	5-15	30-40
Class IV	>2000	>40	>140	↓	↓	0	>35

Table 4: Relation between blood loss and physical signs. Modified from Advanced Life Support, American College of Surgeons 2004.[15] UO = urine output mL/hour, RR=respiratory rate. Blood loss applies to a 70 kg adult with a blood volume of 5L (7% body weight) comprising 3L plasma and 2L red cells.

Blood loss of 500-750mL causes few clinical manifestations in adults. More severe blood loss causes tachycardia, hypotension, decrease in urine output, and increase in respiratory rate due to decreased lung compliance, vasoconstriction of skin, anxiety and agitation, followed by confusion. Vasoconstriction of skin causes pallor, peripheral cyanosis, decreased temperature and prolonged capillary refill. A narrow pulse pressure, due to increase in diastolic blood pressure from catecholamines, indicates that clinically significant blood loss has occurred. [15]

A high respiratory rate [40] leads to alkalosis and decrease in tissue perfusion which causes lactic acidosis and raised anion gap. Oliguria indicates severe blood loss is present. Disseminated intrascular coagulation occurs in severe haemorrhagic shock. [40]

Poor correlation exists between blood volume and blood pressure until blood loss is appreciable. [41] Supine hypotension may be absent until losses exceed 1500-2000mL. [15] Indeed, in traumatic haemorrhage, hypertension may occur until over 25-30% of blood is lost. [41] Most subjects with systolic blood pressure less than 100mmHg have lost 30% of blood volume. [41]

The pulse rate usually increases more often than BP decreases from moderate and severe (Class II, III) blood loss but is unreliable and shows poor correlation with amount of blood lost [41]. Paradoxically, when blood loss is severe, bradycardia occurs in animals [41, 42] and man. [41-45] Inappropriate bradycardia is more common when supine hypotension is present:

In one study pulse rate < 100 beats per minute (bpm) occurred in 35% of patients presenting with systolic blood pressure of < 90 mmHg compared to only 1.8-3.1 % in those without hypotension. Indeed the pulse rate was negatively correlated with blood pressure (BP). [45] In patients, in whom severe hypovolaemia was induced by negative pressure to the lower extremities, tachycardia and normal BP suddenly gave way to bradycardia and hypotension. Syncope occurred as hypovolaemia worsened. [42]

In 20 consecutive patients with mean blood loss of 2.3 L, equivalent to 36% of their estimated blood volume, mean BP was 81:55 mmHg and pulse rate only 73 bpm. This rapidly reversed following infusion of n. saline. [43]

It has been suggested that an initial phase of blood loss results in vasoconstriction and tachycardia but when greater loss develops sympathetic inhibition and vagal stimulation commonly occur. [42] In one study a blood pressure of less than 100 mmHg indicated occurrence of blood loss > 35%.

Combination of systolic blood pressure (SBP) and pulse was found to be a better predictor of acute blood loss than either alone or measurement of central venous pressure. A shock index (SBP/pulse) of greater than 1.0 predicted a loss of blood of at least 20-30% of blood volume [41] and a shock index of 1.38 a loss of over 40% of blood volume.

Thus in evaluating blood loss the combination of both pulse rate and blood pressure are better than either alone. Severe hypotension suggests blood loss of at least 1500mL.

Absence of both hypotension and tachycardia [46-48] occur in some subjects, leading to under estimation of blood loss. Patients may appear deceptively stable. [47] Blood pressure may suddenly fall precipitously [41,46] or organ failure develop later because of inadequate early resuscitation. [47] Controlled observations were carried out in volunteers who were bled 450-1000mL. The data on orthostatic change in pulse rate are shown in table 5.

Author	n	Age (years)	increase in standing pulse beats/min	Sensitivity	Specificity
Loss	450-500 mL				
Witting[49]	292 44	< 65 (Mean 37) ≥ 65 (Mean 68)	≥ 20	43% 25%	91% 100%
Knopp[50]	56	17-55	≥ 30	57%	
Baraff[51]	200		≥ 20	9%	98%
Loss	1000	mL			
Knopp[50]	44	17-55	≥ 30*	98%	98%
Green[52]	25	-	≥ 25	100%	100%

Table 5: Sensitivity and specificity of increase in pulse from supine to standing in studies of phlebotomy of 450-500 mL and 1 L. n= number * Pulse ≥ 30 beats per minute or severe symptoms.

Baraff and Schriger [51] measured blood pressure and pulse in 100 healthy blood donors and 100 healthy elderly ambulatory subjects following phlebotomy of 450 mL blood, excluding those with prior orthostatic hypotension. There was no significant variation of orthostatic blood pressure or pulse with age. Increase in orthostatic pulse rate was the most sensitive sign following phlebotomy.

Knopp et al [50] bled 100 subjects aged 17-55 years: 500 mL in 56 subjects followed by an additional 500 mL for a total of approximately 1000 mL in 44 subjects. In those bled 1000 mL measured blood volume decreased from 9.7-29.6% (mean 22.7%) and correlated with an increase in pulse on standing and presence of severe symptoms, whereas 500 mL loss could not be distinguished from controls. 43 of 44 subjects with 1000 mL loss developed severe symptoms and an increase in standing pulse of ≥ 30 bpm.

Green and Metheney [52] phlebotomised 1000mL of blood from 25 volunteers. The standing pulse rate exceeded supine by 25 beats per minute or over in all cases and a mean decrease in systolic blood pressure of 10mmHg and increase in diastolic blood pressure occurred on standing.

Shenkin [53] *et al* bled 18 volunteers: cardiac output and stroke volume showed minimal change following phlebotomy of 500 mL (n=18) but cardiac output decreased following 1000 mL blood loss (n=17). In these cases the subjects were either unable to tolerate standing or showed orthostatic tachycardia. However the supine pulse rate was usually normal and bradycardia occurred in 9 of 11 subjects.

Based on his observations and experience he considered manifestations of blood loss followed 3 stages:

First stage   500 mL   - minimum symptoms.

Second stage   1000 mL   - symptoms present and pulse rate increases
                                on standing.

Third stage   1500 mL   - symptoms while supine. Vasovagal effects
                                of bradycardia, hypotension, pallor,
                                sweating, hyperpnoea, restlessness, nausea
                                and faintness developed. [53]

Nine studies of blood loss of 450 and 1000 mLs showed that the most useful signs were either postural dizziness, sufficiently severe to prevent standing, or standing pulse increment of ≥ 30 bpm. Supine hypotension and supine tachycardia were frequently absent, even following blood losses of 1000 mL [54]. Capillary refill time was not useful. [54]

Postural changes, without phlebotomy, were reviewed from 25 studies in young and elderly subjects: the mean pulse rate on standing increased by 10.9 bpm (8.9-12.8); the systolic blood pressure decreased by a mean of 3.5 mmHg and diastolic blood pressure increased by a mean of 5.2 mmHg. [54]

Loss of approximately 500 mL blood is usually asymptomatic, causes no consistent signs, and subjects can resume normal activities. The standing pulse rate and blood pressure show minimal differences to controls. The above data suggest:

*   Loss of 1000 mL usually shows no consistent changes in supine blood pressure or pulse and on standing systolic blood pressure does not consistently decrease. However the standing pulse rate increases in nearly all cases. [54]

*   When blood losses exceed 1000 mL bradycardia and supine hypotension are common. Signs should be measured supine after two minutes and one minute after standing. Sitting decreases the sensitivity of orthostatic signs. [50, 54] Counting the pulse for 30 rather than 15 seconds is more accurate. [54] There are several caveats which should be considered in interpretation of this data.

Female subjects, who have lower blood volumes, were not separated from male subjects: manifestations probably occur with lesser of blood loss in women.

Medications such as β blockers and vasodilators may decrease cardiovascular responses to hypovolaemia while diuretics and vasodilators may lead to hypovolaemia or an increase in vascular capacity prior to blood or saline loss.

The impact of blood or saline losses is also probably related to their rate of loss which influences adaptation.

Either tachycardia or bradycardia, from vasovagal stimulation, can be due to anxiety, pain or other factors.

Given the above, the inexact correlation between the quantity of blood loss and physical signs, crystalloid or blood should be rapidly given until urine output is ≥ 0.5 mL/kg (≥ 30-50 mL/minute). The American College of Surgeons[15] recommend the 3-1 rule: 3L saline for each estimated 1L blood loss. A transient response suggests the need for blood supplementation and absence of an adequate response suggests occurrence of ongoing haemorrhage.

HYPOVOLAEMIA DUE TO SODIUM DEPLETION

Sodium depletion causes symptoms due to:

Decreased interstitial fluid.

Hypovolaemia.

The distinction between salt depletion and water depletion in animals was first made by Kerpel-Froinius in 1935[55] and confirmed by Elkinton et al. [56] The differences in man were emphasised by Nadal, Pedersen and Maddocks, [55] Marriot [57] and McCance. [58, 59] McCance emphasised the difficulty of producing sodium depletion: this failed to occur despite the absence of sodium in the diet for 7 days.

Sodium depletion, equivalent to 3-7L of saline, produced in volunteers[55, 58, 59] caused severe fatigue, profound apathy, nausea, anorexia, hypogeusia, muscle cramps, fainting and hypotension of varying severity. Thirst was not prominent provided water was allowed. There were no changes in BP, pulse or serum sodium from 10 % decrease of ECV.

McCance [59] reported normal BP, despite a decrease of 30 % in the ECV of his subjects, whereas Nadal et al reported hypotension and fainting. This was probably due to the speed of development of sodium depletion, which was slower in McCance's subjects.

Urine output varied from normal to oliguria and water loads were excreted after a delay. Hyponatraemia only developed after a loss of approximately 3L saline. Losses beyond this caused 'sacrifice' of osmolality for defence of ECV. [58] However, slow rather than rapid development of sodium depletion, allows adaption of the circulation to occur, decreases severity and delays onset of hyponatraemia. [60] On restoration of sodium intake weight loss initially increased, due to excretion of free water. [58]

In the same way, patients with adrenal insufficiency maintained with cortisone alone, may gradually become depleted of body sodium while maintaining normal plasma sodium by gradual contraction of their extracellular and plasma volume: acute salt depletion due to gastrointestinal fluid losses causes severe hyponatraemia. [59, 61]

Development of water excess and hyponatraemia depend on both the rate of development and extent of sodium depletion.

Dehydration from free water alone compared to sodium loss is completely different; and circulatory insufficiency does not occur from water loss alone. [55-59]

Several authors [55-59, 62] have emphasised the marked differences between sodium and free water depletion. Burnell et al [62] added considerable conceptual clarity to the problem of descriptions and definitions of sodium and water disorders: these were based on the principle that sodium disorders are solely extracellular volume disorders and water disorders osmolality disorders—hyponatraemia and hypernatraemia indicate relative excess and deficiency of free water regardless of sodium status.

They introduced the term saline deficiency and excess—sodium with an isosmotic equivalent of water (with the anionic composition dependent on acid base status) to emphasize the volume aspect of sodium disorders.

Mixed disorders are those in which both saline deficiency and (free) water deficiency are present. In a patient with hypernatraemia saline deficiency may be more severe than (free) water deficiency suggested by serum sodium.

In addition to hypovolaemia, signs of enophthalmos and skin inelasticity are important signs of sodium depletion but may be absent in water depletion. [63-67] Zvi Laron and Crawford [68] in rats and Zvi Laron [63] in infants quantified the degree of skin elasticity in the two syndromes and demonstrated the much greater skin inelasticity from sodium depletion.

These signs lack prominence and are frequently absent in (free) water depletion. [63-67, 69, 70 personal observations]

Normal skin turgor is related to interstitial fluid surrounding collagen or elastic fibres. [63, 71] Skin inelasticity is a sign of saline and not free water depletion.

Mucous membranes are parched in free water depletion. Contrary to some accounts mucous membranes may be either dry or moist in severe saline depletion. [72] Hyperactivity, hyperreflexia, rigidity and less commonly opisthotonos occur in free water depletion or hypernatraemic dehydration, [55, 64-67] neurological signs are prominent [64, 66] and seizures may occur. [64, 70] Severe circulatory failure is uncommon in free water depletion, [70, 56] compared to severe sodium depletion in which peripheral pulses may be absent and peripheral cyanosis present. [55-58, 68].

Free water depletion is physiologically unlikely to cause manifestations of hypovolaemia: in a 70 kg adult a loss of 7L of water without salt decreases plasma volume by only approximately 400 mL, an amount insufficient to cause symptoms of hypovolaemia. (Chapter 2)

Published literature on the relation between extent of dehydration and loss of skin turgor, enophthalmos and other signs is confounded by failure to separate (free) water depletion from saline depletion. [73] Several publications have attempted to establish the sensitivity and specificity of the signs of "dehydration". McGee et al [54] reviewed 13 studies from a Medline search on dehydration which met predetermined criteria. None were of high quality. Unfortunately these low quality observational studies failed to separate free water depletion from sodium depletion and several were methodologically flawed. Steiner et al [74] reviewed 13 studies from 1,561 potential publications on dehydration. They found signs of dehydration were of limited usefulness but capillary refill time, skin turgor, respiratory pattern and the combination were the best. However these studies also failed to separate free water depletion from sodium depletion.

MacKenzie et al [75] evaluated 102 children with gastroenteritis who were thought to be at least 5% 'dehydrated'. Although he failed to separate sodium depletion from free water depletion serum sodium ≥ 152mmol/L was only present in 4 children and therefore most did not have free water depletion. 26% had greater than 5% "dehydration" based on gain in body weight and the mean true dehydration was 3.4%. Despite the serious limitations of this study decrease in peripheral perfusion and skin turgor, high serum urea, low pH and deep breathing achieved statistical significance as signs of mild to moderate dehydration.

I assessed 270 consecutive, mainly demand breast feeding infants, with diarrhoea and recorded signs of sodium depletion and free water depletion on admission. [72, 76]

Electrolytes were done in 80 cases and showed hypernatraemia in only four. All infants considered to have severe sodium depletion gained between 8-20% of their admission body weight 24-72 hours following admission. Eleven received brief 24-48 hour balance studies. All infants with severe sodium depletion showed skin inelasticity, enophthalmos, inactivity and apathy, including a minimal response to arterial puncture. The veins were so collapsed that cut down was required to administer fluids in the majority. Surprisingly the mucous membranes were often moist and tear secretion maintained. The first urine passed was of low specific gravity and osmolality and low Na^+ concentration (<5 mmol/L) suggesting that renal function was normal. Marked polyuria occurred within a short time of saline infusion, so that hypoosmolality was corrected before full volume restoration.

I conclude that skin inelasticity, enophthalmos and inactivity are signs of sodium depletion. (Figures 13-15) These signs and hypovolaemia are absent in water depletion without sodium depletion. Free water depletion causes irritability, agitation and other neurological signs. Mucous membranes are dry or parched. Mucous membranes may be moist (figure 13) and urine output maintained in severe sodium depletion. However the speed of development of sodium depletion and retention of free water, which supports ECV, probably plays an important role in circulatory signs, urine output and osmolality.

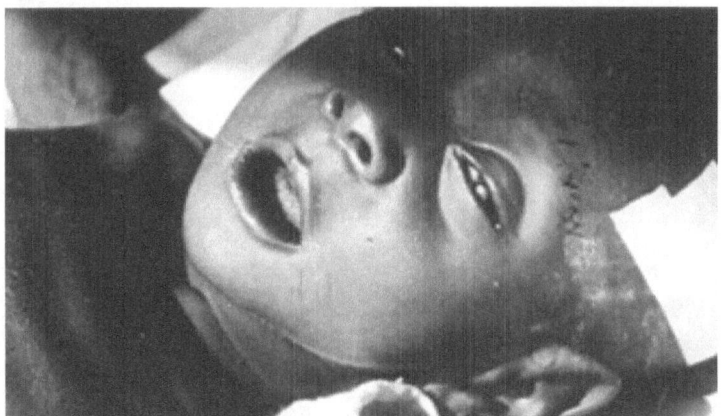

Figure 13. Severe enophthalmos and tear secretion from L. eye in infant with severe Na^+ depletion. Serum Na^+ =111, K+=1.8.mmol/L.

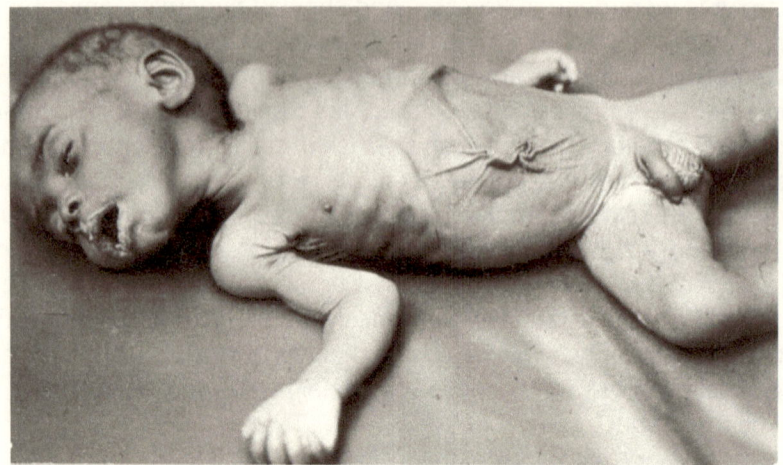

Figure 14:Severe saline depletion in an 8 month old infant from diarrhoea and vomiting. Serum Na⁺ 113 mmol/L K⁺ 1.6 mmol/L. NOTE: Semi comatose state, severe skin inelasticity, sunken abdomen. Following saline and potassium repletion the gain in weight was approximately 20% of admission weight.

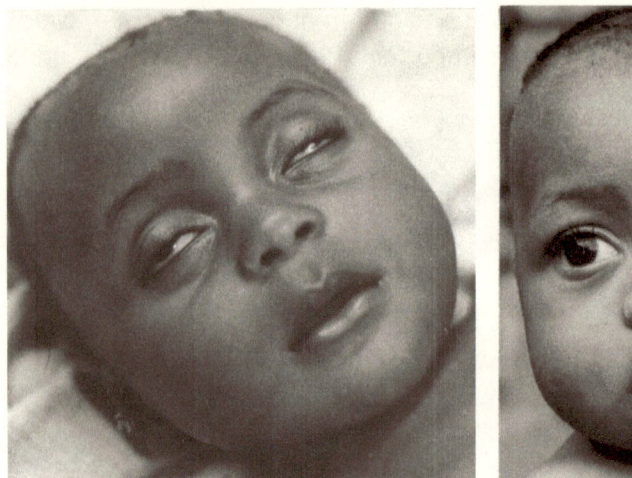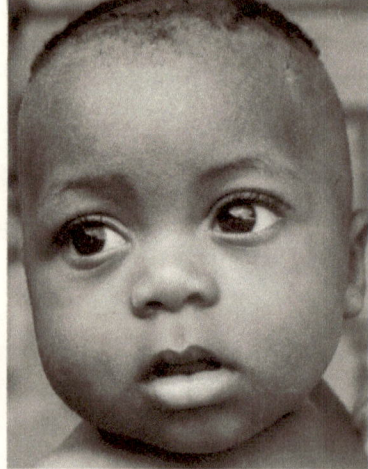

Figure 15:Severe sodium and potassium depletion in an infant before and after correction serum Na 114 mmol/L. K 1.7 mmol/L NOTE: Semi closed sunken eyes (sleeping with the eyes open sign)

During cholera [77, 78] fluid losses occur rapidly; infants present in shock and renal failure with much smaller losses of fluid than do those with less fulminant diarrhoea. Venoconstriction and redistribution of blood flow is probably more efficient when fluid losses occur more slowly. Water excess also allows hyponatraemia to buffer a low interstitial and plasma volume.

Studies in adults to determine the reliability of signs of dehydration are flawed because of failure to separate (free) water from sodium depletion. [79-81] One of the few methodologically sound studies assessed the usefulness of clinical signs in differentiating normovolaemia from hypovolaemia in patients with hyponatraemia: clinical assessment was of limited sensitivity and specificity; the concentration of sodium in a spot sample of urine was considerably better. [82] Capillary refill was not found to be useful to detect mild-moderate hypovolaemia based on orthostatic signs or frank hypotension. [83]

There are no reliable quantitative data on the relation between cardiovascular manifestations and extent of saline depletion. In young volunteers who were depleted of salt but with normal access to water signs were absent and water was normally excreted (hyponatraemia did not occur) until at least 3L of saline was lost. Losses of up to 30% extracellular fluid are tolerated if they occur slowly. [58] In six normal human volunteers decrease in extracellular volume of 10% resulted in minimal changes in blood pressure or serum sodium, although GFR was slightly decreased, and renin and aldosterone increased. [55]

If the data on blood loss is extrapolated and 1L blood is considered to be equivalent to 3L of saline, orthostatic tachycardia would be expected from losses of over 3L saline and supine hypotension from losses of approximately 4-5L.

In conclusion, although controlled observations are not available, sodium depletion should be suspected when a cause is present. Severity is suggested by lying or orthostatic tachycardia (figure 16), hypotension, oliguria, hyponatraemia, a raised serum creatinine and other laboratory tests.

The concentration of sodium in a spot urine sample is superior to clinical signs in separating hypovolaemia from normovolaemic patients with hyponatraemia. [82] My observations suggest that orthostatic tachycardia is considerably more sensitive than orthostatic hypotension in the diagnosis of severe sodium depletion. The following case illustrates this.

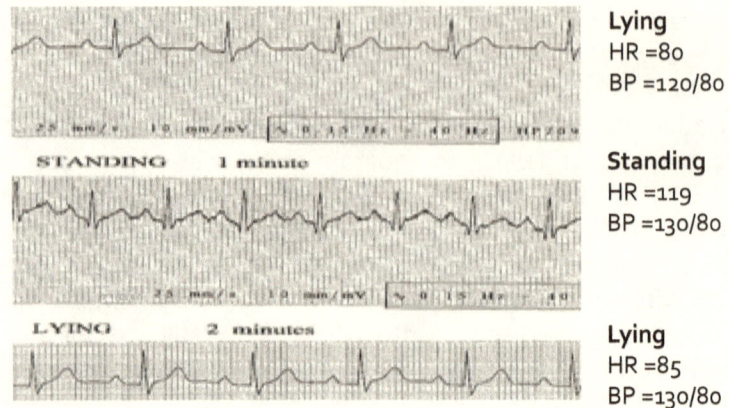

Lying
HR =80
BP =120/80

Standing
HR =119
BP =130/80

Lying
HR =85
BP =130/80

Figure 16: ECG showing orthostatic tachycardia in a

young man with chronic sodium depletion due to Gitelman Syndrome. HR=heart rate; BP=blood pressure. Orthostatic tachycardia was demonstrated on 10 occasions during a year but orthostatic hypotension never developed. Serum renin and aldosterone levels were markedly increased on all occasions. The first tracing shows the BP and heart rate lying, the second standing and the third lying following standing. Note there is no change in BP but the pulse increases from 80 bpm to 119 bpm on standing.

Laboratory Tests

Serum creatinine, urea creatinine ratio, serum electrolytes and urine electrolytes aid in diagnosis.

<u>Serum creatinine</u>: is usually raised to a slight or moderate extent from hypovolaemia, elevated to a greater extent in renal failure and lower than normal when unsuppressed ADH secretion is the main cause of hyponatraemia. Serum creatinine uncommonly rises above 300 μmol/L during volume depletion or cardiac failure unless there is pre-existing renal dysfunction.

The urea creatinine ratio is the ratio of urea to creatinine. It is raised above 60, if both are measured in mmol/L, in low cardiac output states from both volume depletion and cardiac failure. Ratios above 100 are usually due to low cardiac output. The ratio is usually ≤ 60 in renal failure from intrinsic renal disease.

Hyponatraemia develops when hypovolaemia is sufficiently severe to limit free water excretion; but also occurs from low cardiac output from primary cardiac disease; and from unsuppressed ADH secretion. Thus, if intrinsic cardiac disease is excluded, hyponatraemia is evidence for hypovolaemia.

Serum uric acid is usually very low from hyponatraemia due to unsuppressed ADH secretion, compared to hypovolaemia.

Urine electrolytes chapter 12, 15). Low urine Na^+ and/or Cl^- occur in severe Na^+ depletion, other causes of hypovolaemia and low cardiac output from heart disease. Both are usually increased if hyponatraemia is due to unsuppressed ADH secretion. Urine Na^+ decreases within minutes of the onset of haemorrhage.[20] Low urine sodium separated hypovolaemia from normovolaemia in one study. [82]

Urine osmolality does not give useful information additional to urine Na^+ and Cl^- measurement: it can be low or high in severe sodium depletion. [72, 76]

There is no laboratory test, clinical sign or gold standard which is diagnostic for saline deficiency.

Therefore diagnosis of saline depletion is based on several bits of information.

- Evidence for a cause of sodium depletion or for ineffective arterial filling: external or internal losses of sodium containing fluids, expansion of the venous capacitance bed or vascular dilatation from sepsis.
- Exclusion of a cardiac cause of low cardiac output or hypotension.
- Orthostatic or supine hypotension and/or tachycardia which is otherwise unexplained.
- Oliguria, raised urea/creatinine ratio, slight to moderately raised serum creatinine in the absence of previous renal dysfunction.
- Acute loss of weight (within one week).
- Impaired skin turgor.
- Unexplained raised haemoglobin or haematocrit—especially useful if a previous record is available.
- Hyponatraemia provided cardiac failure and other causes of ADH secretion are excluded.
- Low urine Na^+ or Cl^-: serum Cl^- is a more useful guide to Na^+ deficiency during alkalosis.

There is limited useful information on the correlation of the signs and extent of sodium (saline) deficiency. Thus, treatment has to be based on the response to saline infusion: urine output, increase in blood pressure, resolution of hyponatraemia, improvement in serum creatinine, symptomatic improvement and absence of heart failure.

However, the extent of saline deficiency can be estimated (very approximately) by several rules of thumb.

- The signs given for blood loss can be used for saline depletion by multiplying 1L blood loss by 3.0-4.0 (i.e. 1L blood loss ≡ 3L-4L saline loss).
- In normal male subjects hyponatraemia (decreased excretion of free water) usually does not occur until approximately > 3L saline are lost.
- Orthostatic hypotension and tachycardia suggest that between 3-5L saline have been lost. However orthostatic hypotension is common in the elderly, [54, 84-86] is highly variable [86] and may also result from the effects of vasodilators or other drugs.
- <u>Supine</u> hypotension and tachycardia, when a cause of fluid loss is present, suggests loss of 5-7L of saline in an average sized male.

However the size of the subject, gender (females have lower interstitial and plasma volume per weight than males), existing comorbidity and the effects of medications such as diuretics, β blockers and vasodilators influence physical signs.

The elderly and those with underlying heart disease are more likely to develop heart failure but are also more likely to develop complications of slow correction of volume depletion, [15, 84] arteries narrowed from atherosclerosis predispose to cardiac infarction and stroke; irreversible renal failure; and the complications of sepsis are likely to be higher.

Adequate venous return is crucial if diastolic dysfunction or atrial fibrillation is present, as is the case in many elderly subjects. Cardiac dysfunction may also result from inadequate flow in narrowed coronary arteries.

Patients with low ejection fraction are more dependent on adequate cardiac filling. Those with chronic hypovolaemia from diuretics or underfilled vascular beds from vasodilators are especially vulnerable to additional blood loss, saline losses or arterial dilatation from sepsis. These patients <u>need the same or greater initial rapid volume repletion</u> as normal subjects.

They may need more careful or frequent monitoring or the use of bolus infusions but this should not prevent rapid volume resuscitation. (Chapter 11)

CARDIAC FAILURE [87-90]

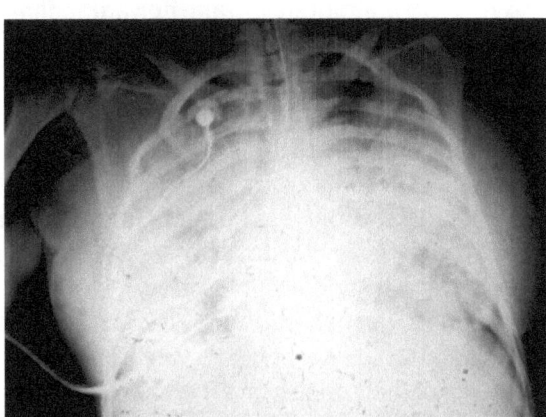

Figure 17. Acute cardiogenic pulmonary oedema.

The heart, like other pumps, may fail because of inadequate filling (effective hypovolaemia) or defective function.

Defective function may be due <u>to loss of muscle or abnormal muscle; obstruction to flow; or faulty valves.</u>

The cardiac ventricles may fail independently. Additional volume loading may be appropriate in right ventricular failure from right ventricular infarction, pulmonary embolism or other causes of right heart failure. Heart failure leads to low cardiac output (CO) and compensatory responses similar to those described for arterial underfilling. <u>Arterial underfilling,</u> either from a <u>low CO or arterial dilatation,</u> is considered to be the main activating mechanism [87] which leads to stimulation of the following :[87-90]

<u>Sympathetic nervous system (SNS)</u>—causing vasoconstriction, tachycardia, increased cardiac contractility and stimulation of the RAAS (renin angiotensin aldosterone system) and ADH secretion.

<u>RAAS</u>: Angiotensin II (A_2) causes vasoconstriction, stimulates aldosterone secretion, ADH secretion and thirst.

ADH,(AVP): causes vasoconstriction by acting on V_1r receptors; water retention by acting on V_2 receptors; Na^+ reabsorption and stimulation of the SNS, A_2, endothelin and ACTH secretion.

Plasma levels of AVP (ADH), angiotensin II and nor-adrenaline are increased In heart failure.[89] Sodium retention results from actions of aldosterone, ADH, renal afferent and efferent arteriolar constriction and increased proximal tubule Na^+ reabsorption despite the presence of an increase in blood volume. [87, 91] This is due to the following:

* Low glomerular filtration rate results from low cardiac output, renal afferent arteriolar constriction and decrease in glomerular surface area from mesangial contraction. [87]
* Efferent arteriolar constriction causes an increased filtration fraction. This increases oncotic pressure in peritubular capillaries surrounding proximal tubules and increases sodium reabsorption.
* Angiotensin II increases proximal tubule $NaHCO_3$ reabsorption by stimulating $Na^+:H^+$ exchangers.
* Aldosterone stimulates Na^+ reabsorption in exchange for K^+ by distal tubule principal cells.
* ADH stimulates water reabsorption by collecting duct principal cells and Na^+ reabsorption by distal convoluted tubules and collecting ducts.
* Aldosterone and angiotensin II are released locally by the left ventricle. Neuro-hormonal activation occurs in the early stages of heart failure before symptoms are apparent. [89]

These variables act together to increase:

Preload: from sodium, water retention and venous constriction.

Blood pressure: by arteriolar constriction.

Cardiac output: Increased contractility and tachycardia stimulated by catecholamines and the sympathetic nervous.

These have detrimental effects in the short and long term.

• Arteriolar vasoconstriction increases cardiac work and may decrease cardiac output.
• Sodium, water retention and increase in preload may lead to excessive cardiac dilatation, increase in work of the heart and decrease in stroke volume by the Starling mechanism. Increase

in left ventricular filling pressure leads to increase in pulmonary capillary venous pressure, pulmonary artery capillary pressure and pulmonary congestion.

- Tachycardia, from sympathetic stimulation, decreases time for cardiac filling—especially important if atrial fibrillation and diastolic dysfunction are present.
- ADH(AVP) secretion increases free water reabsorption, predisposes to hyponatraemia and causes severe vascular constriction. [89, 92, 93]

Natriuretic peptides, NO (Nitric Oxide) [95] and prostaglandins [87] oppose these mechanisms, but are relatively ineffective in counteracting them. Natriuretic peptides, produced systemically and locally in response to stretch, include ANP (atrial natriuretic peptide), BNP (brain natriuretic peptide), produced mainly in the myocardium, and C type peptide produced mainly in vascular endothelium. [94] The main actions of ANP and BNP are to promote natriuresis, increase GFR, less importantly inhibit RAAS and reduce sympathetic vascular tone.

Prostacyclin and prostaglandin E attenuate renal afferent arteriolar vasoconstriction. Non-steroidal inflammatory drugs, which inhibit their production, may impair this, decrease GFR and causes renal failure. [87] Endothelin, a potent vasoconstrictor is increased in some patients with heart failure. [87] Stimulation of the SNS, RAAS aldosterone and perhaps nitric oxide [95] have long term deleterious effects in enhancing cardiac remodelling: alteration in size, shape and function of the left ventricle. [90] Remodelling of the left ventricle increases ventricular dilatation and sphericity and contributes to mitral regurgitation. [89] Left ventricular fibrosis and hypertrophy contribute to subendocardial ischaemia and predispose to arrhythmia and remodelling. Increase in left ventricle stiffness decreases cardiac filling for a particular pressure (diastolic dysfunction). Elevated filling pressure causes tachycardia, vasoconstriction, fluid retention, interstitial oedema and fibrosis. [89]

Administration of β blockers, ACE inhibitors and aldosterone antagonists (eg spironolactone 25mg) are given to decrease remodelling. β Blockers and spironolactone decrease mortality in heart failure. Diuretics have not been shown to do so.

Acute heart failure, as in myocardial infarction, may cause either :

- Raised pulmonary capillary wedge pressure which predisposes to pulmonary oedema.
- Decrease in cardiac output.

These underlie the clinical symptoms and signs of acute heart failure.[96] (Table 6) The earliest change due to raised PCWP is redistribution of blood flow to upper lobes followed by fluid extravasation to the perivascular space and interstitium. Chest imaging shows decreased clarity of medium sized pulmonary arteries and a perihilar haze.[96] Increase in oedema results in periacinar rosettes which coalesce to form frank pulmonary oedema. Clinical criteria predict the correct subset in approximately 80% of cases of myocardial infarction. Compensation, such as peripheral vasoconstriction and thickened vascular walls, cause a disparity between clinical and haemodynamic manifestations. Hypoperfusion increase mortality ten times; hypoperfusion and congestion together have the worst mortality. [96]

Normal, Dry and Warm			Wet and Warm		
PCWP	Normal	<18mmHg	PCWP	High	>18mmHg
CI	Normal	>2.7L/min/m²	CI	>2.7L/min/m²	Normal
Dry but Cold			Wet and Cold		
PCWP	Normal	<18mmHg	PCWP	High	>20mmHg
CI	Low	<2.7L/min/m²	CI	Low	<2.7L/min/m²

Table 6: Presentation subsets of myocardial infarction. [96] PCWP = pulmonary capillary wedge pressure C1 = Cardiac Index. Wet = pulmonary oedema, Cold = low cardiac output. Modified from Forrester J S et al. [96]

RIGHT VENTRICULAR FAILURE

Heart failure may involve the right ventricle alone. The function of the right ventricle (RV) is very different to the left ventricle because the RV is thin walled, has low muscle mass and moves blood through a low pressure, low impedance system with much less oxygen demand. Management and recovery of LV and RV failure are different. RV failure is characterised by low cardiac output, hypotension, raised jugular venous pressure and liver congestion but peripheral oedema may be absent, [97] Figure 18.

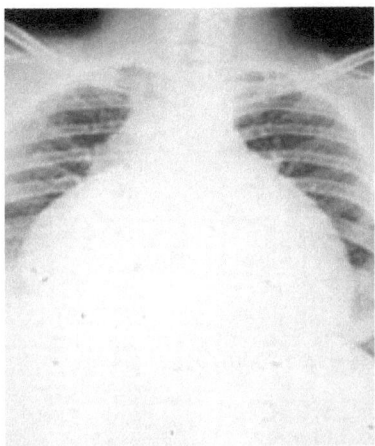 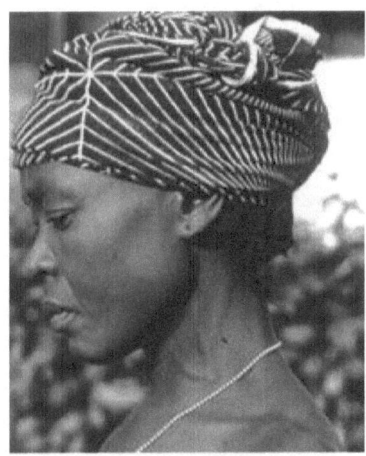

Figure.18 Severe right heart failure due to endomyocardial fibrosis of the right ventricle. The patient had minimal dyspnoea, absent peripheral oedema, absent pulmonary venous congestion on imaging but severe venous congestion (approximately 40 cm water above the right atrium.

In acute pulmonary embolism the right ventricle has limited capacity to increase contractility, dilates, and may decrease left ventricular volume. [97] Chronic pulmonary hypertension may be primary or secondary to hypoxaemia, chronic pulmonary embolism, vasculitis or congestive cardiac failure.

Treatment with prostaglandins, oral Bosentan or phosphodiesterase inhibitors, such as Sildenafil, is partly effective in treatment of primary and secondary pulmonary hypertension from vasculitis. Oxygen is effective in pulmonary hypertension due to hypoxaemia. There is no evidence that diuretics improve outcome in (predominant) right ventricular failure. Underloading in acute pulmonary hypertension may be detrimental.

RV infarction, accompanying anterior myocardial infarction, is associated with a higher mortality than left ventricular infarction alone and should be considered for early reperfusion. However RV ischaemia is more common than RV infarction and usually recovers completely. Common causes of right sided heart failure are shown in table 7.

Pulmonary embolism.

Right ventricular infarction.

Acute Respiratory Distress Syndrome (ARDS).

Decompensated chronic pulmonary hypertension.

Cardiomyopathy involving right ventricle e.g. endomyocardial fibrosis.

Sepsis: both right and left ventricular dysfunction.

Table 7: Common causes of right ventricular failure.

Diastolic Dysfunction. [98-101]

Diastolic dysfunction causes congestive cardiac failure despite a normal ejection fraction. Ventricular relaxation is abnormal. Thus elevated ventricular pressure for a given ventricular volume is abnormal. This leads to pulmonary congestion, dyspnoea and oedema similar to systolic dysfunction.

Diastolic dysfunction is common in the elderly, especially women, those with hypertension, obesity and diabetes. Flash pulmonary oedema develops due to surges of hypertension [100], ischaemic episodes, sudden onset of rapid atrial fibrillation and other tachyarrhythmias, and rapidly improves when these factors are corrected. Rapid heart rates and loss of atrial contraction allow less time for filling of a "stiff" ventricle.

Diagnosis is initially suspected following an episode of congestive cardiac failure when the ejection fraction is found to be normal; and is confirmed by a combination of several echocardiographic criteria [98, 99] Natriuretic peptides are elevated.

Diagnosis of Heart Failure:

Several papers have reported the correlation between clinical, imaging and laboratory manifestations with congestive cardiac failure. In a systematic review of 22 studies [102] from 815 citations the following were considered useful in predicting the presence or absence of heart failure in patients presenting to the Emergency Department (Table 8).

Positive Likelihood Ratio		Negative Likelihood Ratio	
Chest imaging pulmonary vein distension	12.0	Absent cardiomegaly	0.33
Third heart sound	11.0	Absence RALES	0.51
Increase in Jugular venous pressure	5.8	Absent JVD	0.66
Past history of heart failure	5.8	No past history	0.45
Atrial fibrillation on ECG	3.8	Normal ECG	0.64
Paroxysmal nocturnal dyspnoea	2.6	No dyspnoea	0.48

Table 8: Prediction of signs and symptoms in patients presenting to an Emergency Department. Modified from reference 102.

Low serum BNP was the best test but added little to the above. [102] A combination of manifestations rather than individual symptoms and signs were highly predictive.

In another systematic review of 1254 papers jugular venous pressure and imaging signs of pulmonary venous hypertension were 'very helpful' for diagnosing left-sided heart failure but their absence could not exclude an increase in filling pressure.[103] Dyspnoea, orthopnoea, decrease in systolic or pulse pressure and third heart sound were 'somewhat useful'.

In a prospective cross sectional study of 71 randomly selected patients admitted with acute dyspnoea the sensitivity of overall clinical assessment was 81% for the diagnosis of congestive cardiac failure but the specificity was only 47%.This increased to 92% following chest imaging and electrocardiography. [104]

A third heart sound is highly specific but is only heard in a minority of those with heart failure [102, 105,] and carries a worse prognosis [105]. An auscultated third heart sound, compared to phonocardiography, has low sensitivity but high specificity for detecting abnormal ventricular function. [111]

The problem with these studies is the lack of an independent gold standard for diagnosis of heart failure, especially diastolic dysfunction, in which the ejection fraction may be normal; and that the poor predictive value of clinical signs may be due to the lack of skills of auscultation and estimation of JVP by clinicians. [106-111]

Clinical estimation of jugular venous pressure (JVP) has been compared to central venous pressure (CVP) measurement by catheter. [112] The predictiveness of clinical examination, which is controversial, is discussed in chapter. 11

Both internal and external jugular venous pressure (JVP) estimation correlate well with raised or normal CVP. [112] The presence of raised jugular venous pressure and third heart sound also correlates with severity and outcome. [106, 114] The hepatojugular reflux is useful and valid in evaluating dyspnoeic patients. [113]

Clinical, imaging and laboratory manifestations have also been related to abnormal pulmonary capillary wedge pressures (PCWP) and ejection fraction. In a prospective study of 50 consecutive patients, with pulmonary capillary wedge pressure >22mmHg, raised jugular venous pressure and pulmonary oedema were both absent in 40% (18/43) but when present were 100% specific [115]. In 52 consecutive patients with a mean ejection fraction of 19% both clinical and radiological signs of congestion could not be relied on for identifying patients with PCWP ≥30mmHg. [116]

In conclusion clinical signs and imaging together are predictive for the diagnosis when congestive cardiac failure is decompensated and is clinically apparent to independent blinded assessors. However they are not reliable for identifying functional abnormalities such as a low cardiac output or increased PCWP.

An important question is whether measurement of more sensitive markers of heart failure such as natriuretic peptides can guide therapy and improve outcomes.

Natriuretic Peptides

Natriuretic peptides, secreted in response to atrial or ventricular stretch, are elevated early in heart failure [117] and are more predictive than physical signs for diagnosis. [118] BNP (Brain Natriuretic Peptide) is predictive for separating pulmonary from cardiac causes of dyspnoea which may be difficult when both conditions coexist.[117] BNP is elevated in diastolic dysfunction and acute coronary syndromes, but is also elevated in pulmonary hypertension, pulmonary embolism and critically ill patients. [119] Natriuretic peptides have been compared with clinical manifestations for guiding therapy of chronic heart failure. In a randomised study of class 2 and 3 heart failure an improved outcome-hospitalisation or heart failure associated death, occurred in those whose treatment was guided by BNP compared to clinical guidelines. [120] Serum troponin levels are also increased in heart failure without ischaemia. [119]

Treatment of Systolic Dysfunction.

* Treat volume excess with diuretics and preload with nitrates.
* Decrease vasoconstriction and remodelling by ACE inhibitors or ACE Receptor Blockers
* Administer β blockers—when volume excess has resolved.
* Administer anti-aldosterone drugs in low dose: spironolactone, 25mg, or eprelenone 50 mg.

Both ACE inhibitors and β blockers are started in low doses and gradually increased. Long acting are probably better than short acting beta blockers. Renal function, serum potassium, blood pressure and weight should be monitored: (**start low, go slow**).

To aid memory ABCD: A= ACE, aspirin aldosterone antagonists),B= β blockers, C=cholesterol reduction, D-diuretics and diet.

Nitrates and morphine decrease preload and nitrates dilate coronary arteries. Morphine also decreases anxiety, slows and regularises breathing and probably decreases catecholamine secretion. ACE inhibitors inhibit RAAS, decrease vasoconstriction and improve cardiac output.

When fluid excess and raised venous pressure has been effectively treated and cardiac output improves measures are taken to decrease left ventricular remodelling and muscle hypertrophy: β blockers and spironolactone (25mg) in addition to continuing ACE inhibitors and β blockers should be given. ACE inhibitors and β blockers are gradually increased to maximum tolerated doses. Loop diuretics should be decreased and subsequently discontinued If oedema and pulmonary hypertension resolve and improvement is sufficient.

Diastolic Dysfunction. [98-101]

There is inadequate evidence to inform practice. Treatment recommended is similar to that of systolic dysfunction and is based on optimising physiological variables. Special emphasis is given to slowing heart rate, especially in atrial fibrillation, to allow adequate filling of a ventricle which relaxes poorly; and early treatment to decrease remodelling as a result of hypertension. Several randomised trials are underway with the intention to change physiological logic to good evidence.

The advantages and disadvantages of drugs for use in both systolic and diastolic dysfunction are shown in Table 9.

Diuretics. [121-125] (chapter 14).

Diuretics are considered the standard of care for treating volume overload in decompensated heart failure.[121] They relieve congestion, decrease intracardiac pressure and improve cardiac performance. However their efficacy is based on few trials of limited quality and contradictory results.[121]

In acute decompensated heart failure a bolus of intravenous furosemide, 20-100mg; Torsemide, 10-100mg, or Bumetanide, 0.5-4mg, are recommended. [121] A bolus peaks in 1-2 hours and lasts for six hours. [121] Their action is decreased in the presence of renal dysfunction (dependent on GFR) and poor intestinal absorption especially in congestive cardiac failure.

Renal dysfunction decreases effectiveness but prolongs action. [122] They are less effective when non-steroidal anti-inflammatory drugs, including aspirin and thiazolidenediones, are used.

More importantly loop diuretics such as furosemide [121] act over 2-4 hours. Sodium loss is followed by avid sodium retention in the following 20 hours. Thus an increase in frequency rather than higher single dose should be given or salt restricted in order to increase sodium excretion.[122] There are several actual and theoretical risks in using diuretics.

Metabolic problems.

- Thiazide diuretics predispose to hyponatraemia because they act on distal convoluted tubules, where further dilution of tubular fluid occurs, and are less effective than loop diuretics. Furosemide is a more potent and less commonly causes hyponatraemia unless cardiac output is severely decreased. Hypokalaemia and hypomagnesaemia promote cardiac arrhythmias and calcium loss from loop diuretics may cause secondary hyperparathyroidism. [121,122]
- Potassium losses from loop or thiazide diuretics can be decreased by addition of a K+ sparing diuretic, such as spironolactone, enalrepone or amiloride. However, K+ sparing diuretics predispose to hyperkalaemia, which is especially dangerous if renal dysfunction is present in those with underlying heart disease or diabetes.
- Thiazide diuretics may increase glucose intolerance.
- Decrease in cardiac output commonly results and may cause hypotension, fatigue, depression, renal dysfunction [123,125] and impotence. Decreased recovery of renal function and an increase in mortality occur when diuretics are used in critically ill patients. [125]
- In diastolic dysfunction a sudden drop in diastolic filling and peripheral vasoconstriction may worsen cardiac output.
- RAAS activation [121,123] results from decrease in cardiac output or hypotension: increase in renin, nor epinephrine and AVP has been shown following intravenous furosemide [121]. Ventricular remodelling may be increase and RAAS activation may cause further systemic vasoconstriction. [123,124]

Consider whether <u>diuretics should be decreased or stopped when volume excess has been corrected</u> because of these risks and the absence of evidence that diuretic use decreases mortality or myocardial remodelling in the long term.

CLASS	BENEFICIAL ACTIONS	IMPORTANT ADVERSE EFFECTS
Diuretics	↓ filling pressure.	Decrease CO.
	Improve pulmonary congestion.	Increase vasoconstriction.
	↓ peripheral oedema.	Activate RAAS.
		Increase remodelling.
Spironolactone Eprelenone	↓ Remodelling. Limited diuresis.	Contributes to ↑serum K⁺.
ACE inhibitors and ARB	↓ vasoconstriction and BP.	May ↑ renal failure and hyperkalaemia.
	May improve CO.	
	↑ speed of ventricular relaxation. ↓ diastolic pressure.	
	↓ remodelling and LVH.	
β blockers	Slow heart rate. ↓ remodelling.	↓ contractility. Slow diastolic relaxation.
	↓ ischaemia and arrhythmias.	
Ca²⁺ Channel Blockers	↓ VC and ↓ BP.	↓ diastolic relaxation.
Non-Dehydroperidine	Slow HR.	↓ contractility.
Dehydroperidine	↑ HR.	↓ contractility.
Nitrates	↑ local NO.	Headache.
	↓ Preload.	↓ Preload.
Morphine	↓ Preload.	Constipation, nausea.
	↓ Anxiety pain.	Hypotension.
	↓ Catecholamines and Hypertension.	Respiratory depression.

Table 10: Drugs used for treatment of heart failure (excluding drug side effect). CO = Cardiac Output. VC = Vasoconstriction. BP = Blood Pressure. HR = Heart Rate. ARB = Angiotensin Receptor Blockers. Remodelling = Muscle hypertrophy and fibrosis.

Further unloading of the heart by diuretics and vasodilators is undertaken in patients who deteriorate. As <u>end stage heart failure</u> approaches management becomes a balancing act—a trade off between the distress of breathlessness and suffocation from pulmonary congestion; and weakness, depression, hyponatraemia, dizziness and renal failure from low CO due to drugs used to relieve pulmonary congestion. The extent of underloading (table 12) must be made in collaboration with the patient.

The therapeutic ratio of drug treatment narrows with progression so that a small change in drugs such as diuretics may tip the balance to pulmonary oedema on the one hand or renal failure and hypotension on the other. Rarely reduction of BP may worsen pulmonary congestion—if coronary perfusion is reduced through narrowed coronary arteries. Diuretics, which decrease venous return (preload) and increase heart rate secondary to hypovolaemia, may decrease filling in diastolic dysfunction.

- **Standing Blood** pressure—and complaints of dizziness on standing or walking.

- **Evidence of inadequate** CO—increasing serum creatinine, hyponatraemia, weakness, depression.

- **Neck veins**—with the exception of predominantly right heart failure it is safe to underload to a normal JVP.

- **Evidence of pulmonary congestion**—the most sensitive indication is the history of dyspnoea, effort intolerance and orthopnea. However the usefulness of measuring natriuretic peptides are being investigated.

- **Change in body weight**.

Table 11. Clinical variables used in the decision on whether further cardiac unloading is indicated.

Other end stage measures are teaching patients to breathe efficiently: slow regular breathing and coordinated diaphragm and chest breathing. <u>Morphine</u> may also regularise and improve the efficiency of ventilation, facilitates sleep and improve Quality of Life in those with end stage heart failure. Other aspects of the treatment of heart failure such as arrhythmia control, treatment of aggravating factors, the causes of heart failure and rehabilitation are not discussed.

Hyponatraemia and diuretic resistance are important problems as heart failure progresses. This is usually asymptomatic and does not need urgent treatment. If symptoms such as confusion and seizures occur urgent correction of serum Na+ should be carried out (with furosemide if heart failure is present or likely to occur) (chapter 4). Other approaches to hyponatraemia are:

- Water restriction—this is difficult and works slowly (often only an increase of1-2mmol/L serum Na+ per day).
- ADH receptor blockers (viptans). [121,126]
- However always consider whether underloading is excessive. In some patients left ventricular failure changes to predominant right ventricular failure with time and a high venous pressure may be required to sustain cardiac output.

Diuretic resistance [121,122] in heart failure may be due to:

- Decreased absorption.
- Decreased response due to decreasing effectiveness as sodium depletion develops.
- Increase in sodium reabsorption occurs from hypertrophy of cells of the distal medullary nephrons.
- Development of renal failure.

The approach should be to increase the number of times loop diuretics are given in order to decrease avid reabsorption of sodium which follows the first dose; and to increase the dose in renal failure.

Thiazides and or spironolactone can be given to block sodium reabsorption in distal convoluted tubules.

Manifestations of a low CO are standing hypotension, fatigue, dizziness, oliguria, rising serum creatinine and hyponatraemia. Measurement of BP must be done standing because a normal supine BP may be irrelevant if the standing BP is low.

In ongoing assessment always consider:

- Is pulmonary congestion present?
- Is fluid retention, weight gain or peripheral oedema present?
- Is venous pressure elevated or low?

- Is cardiac output low, high or normal?
- Is standing blood pressure low or high and if low is it symptomatic?
- Are aggravating factors present? Is their treatment optimum?
- Are risk factors for vascular complications optimally managed?
- Is treatment of arrhythmias optimum?
- If adequacy of underloading is uncertain measure BNP.

REFERENCES:

General Reading:

1.   Scrier RW, Gurevich AK, Abraham WT. Renal Sodium Excretion, Edematous Disease and diuretic use. P64-114 in Renal & Electrolyte disorders. Ed R.W. Schrier. 6th Ed. 2003 Lippincott, Williams and Wilkins.
2.   Brenner RM, Miller JA, Tobe SW, Skorecki KL: Control of extracellular fluid volume and pathogenesis of oedema formation. P817-872 in The Kidney 5th Ed. Ed. Brenner BM, 1996.
3.   Rose BD, Post TW: Regulation of the effective circulatory volume in Clinical Physiology of Acid Base and Electrolyte disorders 5th Ed.2001 Eds. Rose BD and Post TW. McGraw-Hill
4.   Textbook of Medical Physiology. p195-203. 11th Edition.2006. Eds. Guyton AC, Hall JE, Elsevier Saunders.

Specific References:

5.   Schrier RW: Pathogenesis of sodium and water in high output and low output Cardiac failure. Nephrotic Syndrome, Cirrhosis and Pregnancy (First of Two Parts. *NEJM.* **319**:1065-1071, 1988.
6.   Schrier RW: Pathogenesis of sodium and water in high output and low output Cardiac failure. Nephrotic Syndrome, Cirrhosis and Pregnancy (Second of Two Parts. *NEJM.* **319**:1127-1134, 1988.
7.   Schrier RW, Fassett RG, O'Hara M, Yves Martin P: Pathophysiology of renal fluid retention. *Kidney Int.* **54**(Suppl 67):S127-132, 1998.
8.   Silver MA: The Natriuretic Peptide System: Kidney & Cardiovascular Effects. *Current Opinion in Nephrology and Hypertension.* **15**:14-21, 2006.
9.   Wang X, Armando I, Upadhyay K et al. The regulation of proximal tubular salt transport in hypertension: an update.Current Opinion Nephrol Hypert.**18**:412-42.2009.

10. Siragy HM: Angiotensin II compartmentalization within the kidney: effects of salt diet and blood pressure alteration. *Current Opinion in Nephrology and Hypertension.* **15**:50-53, 2006.

11. Pollock JS, Pollock DM. Endothelin and NOS/1 nitric oxide signaling and regulation of sodium homeostasis. Current Opinion Nephrol Hypertens:**17** 70-75 2008

12. Kumar R, Singh VP, Baker KM: The intracellular renin-angiotensin system—implications in cardiovascular remodeling. *Current Opinion in Nephrology and Hypertension.* **17**:168-173, 2008.

13. Moore FD: The effects of haemorrhage on body composition. *NEJM.* **273**:567-577, 1965.

14. Carey LC, Lowery BD, Cloutier CT: Haemorrhagic Shock. *Current problems in surgery.* **62** 3-48, January 1971. Year Book Medical Publishers.

15. Advanced Trauma Life Support. 7th Ed. 2004. Amer. College of Surgeons.

16. Fleck A, Raines G, Hawker F. et al: Increased vascular permeability: A major cause of Hypoalbuminaemia in Disease and Injury. *Lancet.* 781-783, 1985.

17. Kurlansky M. Salt A World History, Vintage 2003.

18. Eaton SB, Konner M: Paleolithic Nutrition. New Engl J Med **312**:283-289, 1985.

19. Chevalier RL: The moth and the aspen tree: Sodium in early post natal development. *Kidney Int.* **59**:1617-1625, 2001.

20. Hollenberg NK: Set point for Sodium Homeostasis: Surfeit, deficit and their implication. *Kidney Int.* **17**:423-429, 1980.

21. Schrier RW: Volume regulation in health and Disease: A unifying Hypothesis. *Ann. Int. Med.* **113**:155-159, 1990.

22. Parillo JE: Pathogenic Mechanisms of Septic Shock. *NEJM.* **328**:141-1477, 1993.

23. Humphreys MH: Salt intake and body fluid volumes: Have we learned all there is to know? *Amer. J. Kidney Dis.* **37**:648-652, 2001.

24. Heer M, Baisch F, Kropp J. et al: High dietary sodium chloride consumption may not induce body fluid retention in humans. *Amer. J. Physiol. Renal Physiol.* **278**:F585-595, 2000.

25. Danovitch GM, Bourgoigne J, Bricke RNS: Reversibility of "salt losing" tendency of Chronic Renal Failure. *NEJM.* **296**:14-19, 1977.

26. Smith SJ, Markandu ND Macgregor GA et al: Evidence that patients with Addison's disease are undertreated with Fludrocortisone. *The Lancet.* 11-14, 1984.

27. Harrigan MR: Cerebral Salt Wasting Syndrome. *Critical Care Clinics.* **17**:125-136, 2001.

28. Singh S, Bohn D, et al: Cerebral Salt Wasting: Truths, fallacies, theories and challenges. *Critical Care Medicine.* **30**:2575-2579, 2002.

29. Berendes E, Walter M, et al: Secretion of Brain Natriuretic peptide in patients with aneurismal subarachnoid haemorrhage. *The Lancet.* **349**:245-249, 1997.

30. Musch W,Decaux G Treating the syndrome of inappropriate ADH secretion with isotonic saline.QJM **91** 749-753 1998

31. Pruitt BA: Fluid and electrolyte Replacement in the Burned Patient. *Surgical Clinics of N. America.* **58**:1291-1311, 1978.

32. Loyd, JR: Thermal Trauma: Therapeutic Achievements and Investigative Horizons. *Surg. Clin. N. America.* **57**:p121-134, 1971.

33. Nicholas N: Advances in burn care. *Current Opinion in Critical Care.* **13**:405-410, 2007.

34. Palmieri T, Caruso DM, Daniel M et al: Effect of blood transfusion on outcome after major burn injury: A multicentre study. *Crit. Care Med.* **34**:1602-1607, 2006.

35. Canciani M, Forno S, Mastela G: Borderline Sweat Test: Criteria for Cystic Fibrosis Diagnosis. *Scandinavian J. Gastroenterology.* **143**(Suppl):p19-27, 1988.

36. Bosch X, Poch E, Grau JM.Rhabdomyolysis and Acute Kidney Injury. New Engl J medicine.361:62-72.2009

37. Brandstrup B, Svensen C, Engquist A. Hemhorrhage and operation cause a contraction of the extracellular space needing replacement. A systematic review. Surgery.**139**:413-432 2006

38. Kirk MD, Greipp PR. Narrative Review: The Systemic Capillary Leak Syndrome. Annals Intern Med. **153**:90-98.2010

39. Wills BA, Dung NM, Loan HT et al.Comparison of Three Fluid Solutions for Resuscitation in Dengue Shock Syndrome. New Engl J Med.**353**:877-889.2005

40. Moss GS, Saletta JD: Traumatic Shock in Man. *New Eng J Med.* **290**:724-726, 1974.

41. Burri C, Henkemeyer H, Passler HH, Allgower M: Evaluation of Acute Blood Loss by Means of Simple Haemodynamic Parameters. *Progr. Surg.* **11**:109-127, 1973.

42. Sanders JS, Ferguson DW: Profound Sympathoinhibition Complicating Hypovolaemia in Humans. *Ann. Int. Med.* **111**:439-441, 1989.

43. Sander-Jensen K, Secher NH, Bie P, et al: Vagal slowing of the heart during haemorrhage: Observation from 20 consecutive hypotensive patients, *BMJ.* **292**:364-366, 1986.

44. Demetrios D, Chan L, Bhasin P et al: Relative Bradycardia in Patients with Traumatic Hypotension. *Journal of Trauma.* **45**:534-539, 1998.

45. Thompson D, Adams SL, Barrett J: Relating Bradycardia in Patients with Isolated Penetrating Abdominal Trauma and Isolated Extremity Trauma. *Ann. Emerg. Med.* **19**:268-275, 1990.

46. Wo, CCJ, Shoemaker WC, et al: Unreliability of blood pressure and heart rate to evaluate cardiac output in emergency resuscitation and critical illness. *Critical Care Medicine.* **21**:218-223, 1993.

47. Abou Khali B, Scalea TM, Appel PL et al: Haemodynamic responses to shock in young trauma patients: Need for invasive monitoring. *Crit. Care Med.* **22**:633-639, 1994.

48. Emergency Medicine. p226-227. Ed Tintinalli JE, Sixth edition. 2004 McGraw-Hill,

49. Witting MD, Wears RL, Sergio Li: Defining the Positive Tilt Test: A Study of healthy Adults with Moderate Acute Blood Loss. *Ann. Emerg. Med.* **23**:1320-1323, 1994.

50. Knopp R, Claypool R, Leonardi D, California F: Use of the tilt Test in measuring Acute Blood Loss. *Ann. Emerg. Med.* **9**:72-75, 1980.

51. Baraff LI, Schriger DL: Orthostatic Vital Signs : Variation with age, specificity and sensitivity in detecting a 450mL blood loss. *Am. J. Emerg. Med.* **10**:99-103, 1992.

52. Green DM, Metheny D: The estimation of acute blood loss by the tilt test. *Surg. Gynecol/Obstet.* **84**:1045-1050, 1947.

53. Shenkin HA, Cheney RH, Govons SR et al: On the diagnosis of haemorrhage in man. *Am. J. Med. Sci.* **208**:421-436, 1944.

54. McGee S, Abernethy WB, Simel DL: Is this patient Hypovolaemic. *JAMA.* **281**:1022-1029, 1999.

55. Nadal JW, Pedersen S, Maddock WG: Comparison between dehydration from sodium loss and water deprivation. *J. Clin. Invest.* **20**:691-703, 1941.

56. Elkinton JR, Danowski TS, Winkler AW: Haemodynamic changes in salt depletion and in dehydration. *J. Clin. Invest.* **25**:264-266, 1946.

57. Marriot H: Water and salt depletion. *Brit. Med. J.* **245**:328; 285, 1947.

58. McCance RA: Experimental sodium chloride deficiency in man. *Proc. Roy. Soc.* Series B **119**:245, 1936,

59. McCance RA: Medical problems in mineral metabolism. III Experimental Human Salt Deficiency. *Lancet.* **230**:823-830, 1936.

60. Cizek LJ, Huang KC: Water diuresis in the salt depleted dog. *Amer. J. Physiol.* **167**:413, 1951.

61. Lipsett MB, Pearson OH: Sodium depletion in adrenelectomised humans. *J. Clin. Invest.* **37**:1394, 1958.

62. Burnell JM, Paton RP, Scribner BH: The problem of sodium and water needs of patients. *J. Chronic Dis.* **11**:189, 1960.

63.   Laron Z: Skin Turgor as a Quantitative Index of Dehydration in Children. *Pediat.* **19**:816 1957.

64.   Finberg L, Harrison HE: Hypernatraemia in infants. *Pediat.* **16**:1, 1955.

65.   Weil WB, Wallace WM: Hypertonic dehydration in infancy. *Pediat.* **17**:171, 1956.

66.   McCaulay D, Blackhall MI: Hypernatraemic dehydration in infantile gastroenteritis. *Arch. Dis. Child.* **36**:543, 1961.

67.   Ahmed I, Augusto-Odutola TB: Hypernatraemia in diarrhoeal infants in Lagos. *Arch. Dis. Child.* **45**:97, 1970.

68.   Laron Z, Crawford JD: Skin turgor as a Quantitative index of dehydration in Rats. *Pediat.* **9**:810, 1957.

69.   Black DAK, McCance RA, Young WF: A study of dehydration by means of balance experiments. *J. Physiol.* **102**:406, 1944.

70.   Bruck E, Abal G, Aceto T: Pathogenesis and pathophysiology of Hypertonic Dehydration. *Amer. J. Dis. Child.* **115**:122, 1968.

71.   Dorrington KL: Skin Turgor: Do we understand the clinical signs? *Lancet* 1. *264-265* 1981.

72.   Kingston M: Biochemical disturbances in Breast fed infants with gastroenteritis and dehydration. *J. Pediat.* **82**:1073-1081, 1973.

73.   Mange K, Matsuura D, et al: Language Guiding Therapy : The Case of Dehydration versus Volume Depletion. *Ann. Int. Med.* **127**:848-853, 1997.

74.   Steiner MJ, De Walt DH, Byerley JS: Is this child dehydrated? *JAMA.* **291**:2746-2754, 2004.

75.   Mackenzie A, Barnes G, Shann F: Clinical signs of Dehydration in children. *Lancet.* 605-607, 1989.

76.   Kingston M: Electrolyte and fluid disturbances in Liberian Children. A thesis submitted for the Degree of Doctor of Medicine. University of London. 1974.

77.   Mahalanabis P: Water and electrolyte losses due to cholera in infants. *Pediat.* **45**:374, 1970.

78.   Griffiths LFC: Electrolyte Replacement in Pediatric Cholera. *Lancet.* **1**:1197, 1967.

79.   Gross CR, Lindquist RD, Wooley AC et al. Clinical Indicators of Dehydration Severity In Elderly Patients. *J. of Emergency Medicine.* **10**:267-274, 1992.

80.   Levitt MA, Lopez B, Lieberman HE, Sutton M: Evaluation of the tilt test in an Adult Emergency Medicine Population. *Ann. Emerg. Med.* **21**:713-718, 1992.

81.   Eaton D, Bannister P, Hulley GP, Connolly MJ: Axillary sweating in clinical assessment of dehydration in ill elderly patients. *BMJ.* **308**:1271, 1994.

82.   Chung HM, Kluge, Schrier RW, Anderson RJ: Clinical Assessment of Extracellular Fluid Volume in Hyponatraemia. *Amer. J. Med.* **83**:905-908, 1987.

83.   Schriger DL, Baraff LJ: Capillary Refill—Is it a useful predictor of hypovolaemic states? *Ann. Emerg. Med.* **20**:601-605, 1991.

84.   Lipsitz LA: Orthostatic Hypotension in the Elderly. *New Eng J Med.* **321**:952-957, 1989.

85.   Raiha I, Luutonen S, Piha J, et al: Prevalence, Predisposing factors and Prognostic importance of Postural Hypotension. *Arch. Int. Med.* **155**:930-935, 1995.

86.   Ooi WL, Barrett S, Hossain M et al: Patterns of orthostatic blood pressure change and their clinical correlates in a frail, elderly population. *JAMA.* **277**:1299-1304, 1997.

87.   Schrier RW, Abraham WT: Hormones and Haemodynamics in heart failure. *NEJM.* **341**:577-585, 1999.

88.   Chen HH, Schier RW: Pathophysiology of Volume Overload in Acute heart failure syndromes. *Amer. J. Med.* **119**(12A):S11-S16, 2006.

89.   Chatterjee K: Neurohormonal activation in Congestive Heart Failure and the Role of Vasopressin. *Am. J. Cardiol.* **95**(Suppl):8B-13B, 2005.

90.   Jessup M, Brozena S: Heart Failure. *NEJM.* **348**:2007-2018, 2003.

91.   Cannon PJ: The Kidney in heart Failure. *NEJM.* **296**:26-32, 1977.

92.   Szatalowicz VL, Arnold PE, Chaimovitz C et al: Radioimmunoassay of plasma Arginine Vasopressin in Hyponatraemic Patients with Congestive Heart Failure. *NEJM.* **305**:263-266, 1981.

93.   Riegger GAJ, Liebau G, Kochsiek K: Antidiuretic Hormone in Congestive Heart Failure. *Amer. J. Med.* **72**:49-52, 1982.

94.   Onwuanyi A, Taylor M: Acute Decompensated Heart Failure: Pathophysiology and Treatment. *Amer. J. Cardiol.* **99**(Suppl):25D-30D, 2007.

95.   Lapu-Bula R, Ofili E: From Hypertension to Heart Failure: Role of nitric oxide-mediated Endothelial Dysfunction and Emerging Insights from Myocardial Contrast Echocardiography. *Amer. J. Cardiol.* **99**(Suppl):7D-14D, 2007.

96.   Forrester JS, Diamond G, Chatterjee K et al: Medical Therapy of Acute Myocardial Infarction by application of Haemodynamic Subsets. *New Eng J Med.* **295**:1356-1362, 1976.

97.   Woods J, Monteiro P, Rhodes A: Right ventricular dysfunction. *Current Opinion in Critical Care.* **13**:532-540, 2007.

98.   Chinnaiyan KM, Alexander D, Madden SM, McCullough PA: Curriculum in Cardiology: Integrated diagnosis and management of diastolic heart failure. *Amer. Heart J.* **153**:189-200, 2007.

99. Kitzman DW, Little WC, Brubaker PH. Pathophysiological Characterization of Isolated Diastolic Heart Failure in comparison to Systolic Heart Failure. JAMA :**288**:2144-2150 2002

100. Little WC, Brucks S: Therapy for Diastolic Heart Failure. *Progress in Cardiovasc. Dis.* **47**:380-388, 2005.

101. Massie BM, Fabi RM: Clinical Trials in Diastolic Heart Failure. *Prog. Cardiovasc. Dis.* **47**:389-395, 2005.

102. Wang C, Fitzgerald JM, Mark DM et al: Does this Dyspnoeic Patient in the Emergency Department have Congestive Heart Failure. *JAMA.* **294**:1944-1956, 2005.

103. Badgett RG, Lucey CR, Mulrow CD: Can the Clinical Examination Diagnose Left-Sided Heart Failure in Adults. *JAMA.* **277**:1712-1719, 1997.

104. Gillespie ND, McNeill G, Prigle T et al: Gross sectional study of contribution of clinical assessment and simple cardiac investigations to diagnosis of left ventricular systolic dysfunction in patients admitted with acute dyspnoea. *BMJ.* **314**:936-940, 1997.

105. Drazner MH, Rame JE, Stephenson LW, Dries DL: Prognostic importance of elevated jugular venous pressure and a third heart sound I Patients with Heart Failure. *New Eng J Med.* **345**:574-81, 2001.

106. Perloff JK: The Jugular Venous Pulse and Third Heart Sound in Patients with Heart Failure. *New Eng J Med.* **345**:612-614, 2001.

107. Mangione S, Nieman LZ: Cardiac Auscultatory Skills of Internal Medicine and Family Practice Trainees. *JAMA.* **278**:717-722, 1997.

108. March SK, Bedynek JL, Chezner MA: Teaching Cardiac Auscultation : Effectiveness of a Patient-Centered Teaching Conference on Improving Cardiac Auscultatory Skills. *Mayo Clin. Proc.* **80**:1443-1448, 2005.

109. St Clair EW, Oddone EZ, Waugh RA, Corey R: Assessing Housestaff Diagnostic Skills using a Cardiology Patient Simulator. *Ann. Int. Med.* **117**:751-756, 1992.

110. Vukanovic-Criley JM, Criley S, Warde CM et al: Competency in Cardiac Examination Skills in Medical Students, Trainees, Physicians and Faculty. *Arch. Int. Med.* **166**:610-616, 2006.

111. Marcus G, Vessey J, Jordan MV et al: Relationship between Accurate Auscultation of a Clinically Useful Third Heart Sound and Level of Experience. *Arch. Int. Med.* **166**:617-622, 2006.

112. Vinayak AG, Levitt J, Gehlbach B, et al: usefulness of the External Jugular Vein Examination in Detecting Abnormal Central Venous Pressure in critically ill patients. *Arch. Int. Med.* **166**:2132-2137, 2006.

113. Marantz PR, Kaplan MC, Alderman MH: Clinical Diagnosis of Congestive Heart Failure in Patients with Acute Dyspnoea. *Chest.* **97**:766-81, 1990.

114. Drazner MH, Rame JE, Dries DL: Third heart sound and elevated jugular venous pressure as markers of the subsequent development of heart

Failure in patients with Asymptomatic Left Ventricular Dysfunction. *Amer. J. Med.* **114**:431-437, 2003.

115. Stephenson LW, Perloff JK: The Limited Reliability of Physical Signs for estimating Haemodynamics in Chronic Heart Failure. *JAMA.* **261**:884-888, 1989.

116. Chakko S, Woska D, Martinez H et al: Clinical, Radiographic and Haemodynamic Correlations in Chronic Congestive Heart Failure : Conflicting results may lead to inappropriate care. *Amer. J. Med.* **90**:353-359, 1991.

117. Davis M, Espiner E, Richards G et al: Plasma brain natriuretic peptide in assessment of acute dyspnoea. *Lancet.* **343**:440-44, 1994.

118. Maisel AS, Krishnaswamy P, Nowak RM et al: Rapid measurement of B-type Natriuretic Peptide in the Emergency Diagnosis of Heart Failure. *New Eng J Med.* **347**:161-167, 2002.

119. Braunwald E: Biomarkers in Heart Failure. *New Eng J Med.* **358**:2148-2159, 2008.

120. Jourdain P, Jondeau G, Funk F et al Plasma Brain Natriuretic Peptide-Guided Therapy to Improve Outcome in Heart Failure. The STARS-BNP Multicenter Study. J Amer Coll Cardiology **49**:1733-9.2007

121. Cleland JGF, Coletta A, Witte K: Practical Applications of Intravenous Diuretic Therapy in Decompensated Heart Failure. *Amer. J. Med.* **119**(12A):S26-S36, 2006.

122. Brater DC: Diuretic Therapy. *New Eng J Med.* **339**:387-395, 1998.

123. Hill JA, Yancy CW, Abraham WT: Beyond Diuretics: Management of volume overload in Acute Heart Failure Syndromes. *Amer. J. Med.* **119**:S37-S44, 2006.

124. Francis GS, Siegel RM, Goldsmith SR, et al: Acute Vasoconstrictor Response to Intravenous Furosemide in Patients with Chronic congestive heart Failure. *Ann. Int. Med.* **103**:1-5, 1985.

125. Mehta RL, Pascual MT, Soroko S, Chertow GM: Diuretics, Mortality and non-recovery of Renal Function in Acute Renal Failure. *JAMA.* **288**:2547-2553, 2002.

126. Goldsmith SR: Current Treatments and Novel Pharmacologic Treatments for Hyponatraemia in Congestive Heart Failure. *Amer. J. Cardiol.* **95**(Suppl):14B-23B, 2005.

Part 2. SHOCK [1-7]

"A momentary pause in the act of death" John Collins Warren [1]

Shock is widespread inadequate tissue perfusion sufficiently severe to cause cellular hypoxia and lactic acidosis.

The determinants of systemic oxygen delivery (DO_2) are cardiac output (CO) L/minute; haemoglobin (HB) g/L ; and o_2 saturation (So_2).[1,2]

$$DO_2 = CO \times (HB \times 1.34) \times SO_2$$

1gm HB binds 1.34mL oxygen, 150g binds 200mLO_2

Therefore **DO2 = 5 x 200 x 98%.**

Therefore at rest approximately 1000mLo_2/minute is delivered when the CO is 5L/minute. Tissues need approximately 200mL-250mL oxygen/minute but cannot abstract oxygen beyond SO_2 of 20%. Thus effective oxygen delivery is 750-800mL/minute.

Cardiac output decreases to one third of normal before inadequate oxygen delivery occurs at rest. However tissue oxygen uptake (VO_2) depends on metabolic demand. This increases in sepsis. If delivery of oxygen (DO_2) decreases below demand oxygen extraction increases until it is maximal: VO_2 is independent of DO_2 over a wide range(5).If DO_2 decreases below this—to a critical level, tissue oxygen uptake (VO_2),which is supply dependent, is inadequate to sustain oxidative glycolysis. [1,2,5]

Glycolysis occurs in three stages:

1. Anaerobic production of 2 moles of pyruvate from 1 mole of glucose in the cytosol.
2. Mitochondrial conversion of pyruvate to AcCoA, CO_2 and hydrogen in the Tricarboxylic Acid Cycle (TCA)—provided o_2 is available.
3. Transfer of hydrogen H (hydrogen atom), H+[(proton); H [without an electron] and electrons, liberated from the breakdown of pyruvate, to the electron chain for synthesis of ATP.

Only Stage 1, conversion to pyruvate, proceeds without oxygen.

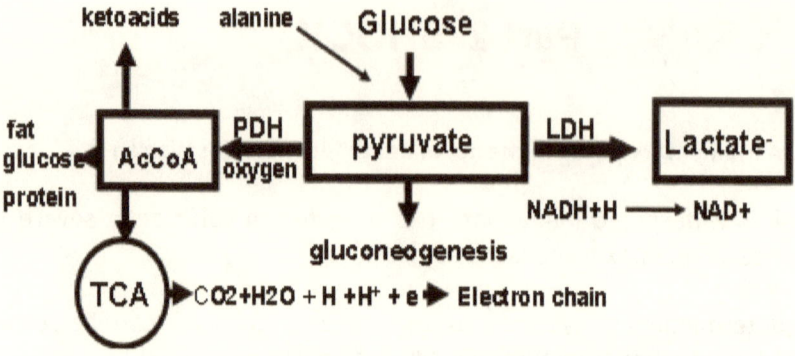

Figure 1: Simplified model of glucose metabolism. (TCA=tricarboxylicacid cycle; PDH=pyruvate dehydrogenase; LDH=lactic dehydrogenase) see text below.

Pyruvate is transported to mitochondria if oxygen is available and converted to acetyl coenzyme A (AcCoA), the pivotal substance in aerobic glycolysis.

AcCoA has three fates: metabolism in the Krebs (tricarboxylic acid cycle); conversion to ketoacids; and synthesis of fat, glucose and protein. Acetyl CoA is broken down to Co_2 and hydrogen atoms (H) in the TCA cycle. Hydrogen is the main source of energy which is used to transform ADP to ATP (chapter 6).

NADH and FADH accumulate in the absence of oxygen. Absence of (oxidised) NAD^+ and FAD prevents transfer of H, H^+ and e^- to the electron chain. Aerobic glycolysis ceases and pyruvate accumulates. The lactate: pyruvate ratio is proportional to the $NADH/NAD^+$ ratio in the cytosol. An increase in NADH (reduced NAD), compared to NAD^+ (oxidised NAD), increases the <u>redox</u> state (<u>red</u>uction-<u>ox</u>idation) which increases pyruvate conversion to lactate⁻ by mass action. [8]

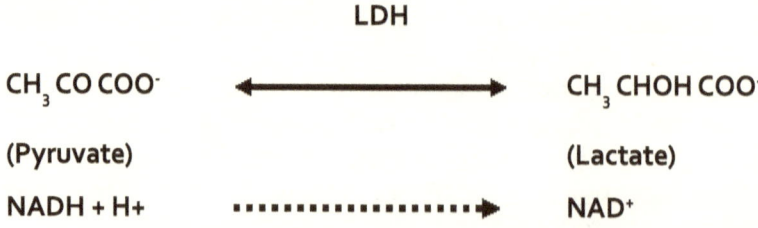

In the process NADH + H$^+$ is converted to NAD$^+$, as shown, which allows anaerobic glycolysis to continue. Normallly the ratio is 10-1 in favour of lactate.

Note that it is <u>lactate⁻ not lactic acid</u> which is formed.

Only 2 moles of ATP are produced from anaerobic glycolysis per mole of glucose compared to 36 moles from aerobic glycolysis. However the small amount of ATP generated is used for vital cellular metabolic work; and the NAD$^+$ generated enables anaerobic glycolysis to continue. *(P = inorganic phosphate)*

$$\text{Glucose} + 2\,\text{ADP} + 2\text{P} \longrightarrow 2\,\text{lactate}^- + 2\,\text{ATP} + 2\,\text{H}_2\text{O}$$

Each time a molecule of ATP is hydrolysed a proton (H$^+$) is released which would lead to increasing cellular acidosis.

$$\text{ATP} + \text{H}_2\text{O} \longrightarrow \text{ADP} + \text{P} + \text{H}^+$$

However H$^+$ ions released react with lactate to form lactic acid.

$$\text{H}^+ + \text{CH}_3\,\text{CHOH COO}^- \longrightarrow \text{CH}_3\,\text{CHOH COOH}$$

(lactate)   **(lactic acid)**

Lactic acid diffuses out of cells to extracellular fluid. Lactic acid is a strong acid. Buffering by $NaHCO_3$ limits the acidosis that would otherwise occur but at the expense of decreasing extracellular bicarbonate (buffer base).

$$\text{CH}_3\text{CHOH COOH} + \text{NaHCO}_3 \rightleftharpoons \text{CH}_3\text{CHOH COO}^-\text{Na}^+ + \text{H}_2\text{CO}_3 \longrightarrow \text{CO}_2 + \text{H}_2\text{O}$$

(Lactic Acid)   **(Na$^+$ lactate)**

Lactate is converted to pyruvate if oxygen availability improves. This is oxidised to CO_2 and H_2O by the reverse of the process described and $NaHCO_3$ (buffer base) is restored.

Between 1000-1500mmol of lactate are produced daily (15-20 mmol/kg/day) by muscle, skin, renal medulla, intestine and brain. Lactate is used as a fuel by myocardium, brain, kidney, and if sufficiently raised, skeletal muscle, and can be converted to glucose in liver and kidney (Cori cycle).

Filtered lactate is efficiently reabsorbed by transporters in proximal tubules and only appears in urine when the blood level reaches 6-7mmol/L.

The normal blood or plasma lactate is 0.7-2.5 mmol/L but depends on the specific laboratory reference range. Lactate production provides the following advantages: [9]

- Provision of a fuel during shock. Lactate, produced by inadequately perfused tissues, such as skeletal muscle, can be used by relatively well perfused and more vital organs, such as brain and myocardium, to which blood is preferentially delivered (autoregulation). This is converted to glucose and glycogen in the liver.
- Provision of a small amount of ATP for local use.
- Decrease in NADH accumulation, increase in NAD^+ and a decrease in cellular H^+ from local conversion of lactate to lactic acid. This allows anaerobic glycolysis to continue.

There is no evidence that lactate itself is harmful: it is infused as Ringers lactate; and during extreme exercise plasma lactate may increase above 20mmol/L. Hyperlactataemia in shock is a beneficial adaption to hypoxia: production by muscle provides fuel utilised by brain and heart. However lactic acidosis is a marker of disease severity in shock: levels >10mmol/L carry a poor prognosis. [10]

Although hypoxia, from inadequate tissue perfusion, is the most common underlying cause, metabolic factors associated with the inflammatory response, catecholamine secretion, liver dysfunction, which decreases lactate metabolism, and increased glycolysis play a role in sepsis. Increase in production, rather than hypoxia, may be the most important mechanism of lactate production in septic patients. [10-12]

When oxygen supply and ATP production decrease further key metabolic processes, such as operation of membrane pumps, are affected. [1,8] Muscle Na^+:K^+ ATPase activity correlates with lactic acid levels in sepsis. [11,12] This leads to cellular depolarisation (increased intracellular Na^+ and decreased K^+), calcium influx and apoptosis—the end result in all forms of shock.

In septic (distributive) shock, compared to hypovolaemic and cardiogenic shock, DO_2 and VO_2 are both initially increased. [1,5] Inadequate tissue perfusion in septic shock may be due to one or a combination of abnormalities of the microcirculation, cellular dysfunction from cytokines, the effects of catecholamines or mitochondrial dysfunction.

The components of the circulation which may fail and lead to inadequate tissue perfusion are:

- Vascular capacity. ⎤ Which determine preload and arterial filling?
- Intravascular volume. ⎦
- Cardiac function; or obstruction to pulmonary arteries or aorta.
- Precapillary arterioles—resistance part of circulation.
- Capillary exchange network.

The main causes of shock are:
- Severe hypovolaemia.
- Cardiogenic dysfunction.
- Sepsis.

Less common causes are:

- Severe vascular dilatation (venous and arteriolar) from sympathetic failure as in spinal cord transection, high spinal anaesthetic, effects of poisons (carbon monoxide, cyanide), general anaesthesia and severe brain damage.
- Obstruction to venous return—severe pneumothorax, pericardial effusion or constriction.
- Severe vascular constriction (precapillary arterioles) from phaeochromocytoma and amphetamines.
- Anaphylaxis: This decreases sympathetic vascular resistance causing vasodilatation; increases vascular capacity; increases leak of fluid from capillaries; myocardial depression; and bronchospasm.
- Addisonian Crisis: due to a combination of hypovolaemia and cortisol deficiency: cortisol deficiency decreases vascular constriction and glomerular filtration rate (GFR).
- Mitochondrial dysfunction: mitochondrial disorders, carbon monoxide, cyanide, medication, such as metformin.

The three most common causes of shock, cardiogenic, hypovolaemic and sepsis often pass through three stages: compensated, decompensated and irreversible, and have many similarities. Haemhorrhage and cardiogenic shock are initially characterised by vasoconstriction; septic shock by vasodilation. However decompensation in all forms of shock can lead to vasodilation.

HYPOVOLAEMIC SHOCK[1-4,13]

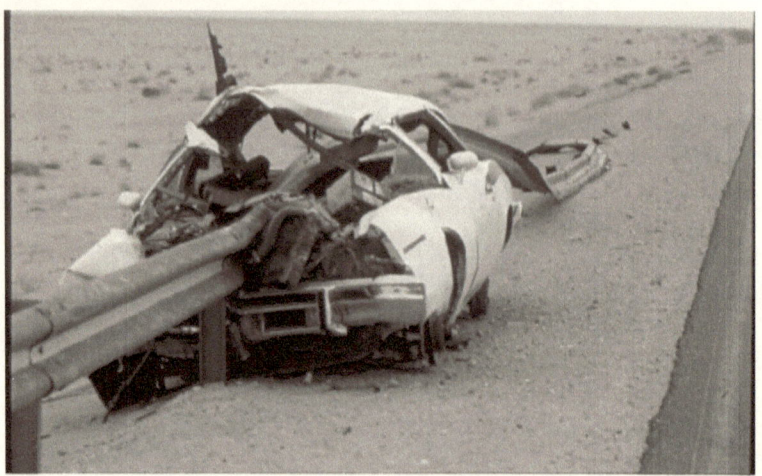

This may be due to overt or hidden losses of <u>blood, colloid or saline</u>

Rapid reversal with appropriate fluids and termination of blood or fluid loss should be carried out before irreversible shock occurs. The following compensate for severe hypovolaemia:

- Vasoconstriction of precapillary arterioles, from stimulation of α adrenergic receptors by circulating catecholamines, sympathetic nerves and direct vasoconstriction by angiotensin 2 and arginine vasopressin (AVP, ADH) acting on VI_R receptors.
- Decrease in vascular capacity (predominantly venous) by venoconstriction.
- Redistribution of blood flow to vital organs. Cerebral and cardiac perfusion are independent of blood pressure above a minimal level. Cerebral autoregulation maintains flow up to a mean blood pressure of 50-60mmHg in normal subjects.
- Increase in cardiac contractility and tachycardia from stimulation of β1 receptors by catecholamines and Sympathetic Nervous System (SNS).
- Vascular refill from interstitial fluid and albumin. Plasma compartment refill can reach 1 L/hour and albumin 1g/hour in severe shock. [6]
- Increase in plasma cortisol from ACTH stimulation.
- Marked sodium and water reabsorption—within minutes of a decrease in cardiac output.

There are several detrimental effects of the compensatory response:

- Increase in pressure in precapillary arterioles increases cardiac work.
- Restriction of blood flow and precapillary arteriovenous shunting leads to ischaemia of skin, muscle, splanchnic organs and kidney. This leads to cellular dysfunction, lactic acidosis and eventually irreversible ischaemic damage.
- Blood flow to kidneys is diverted from cortex to medulla.
- Mitochondrial failure leads to anaerobic glycolysis and lactic acidosis.

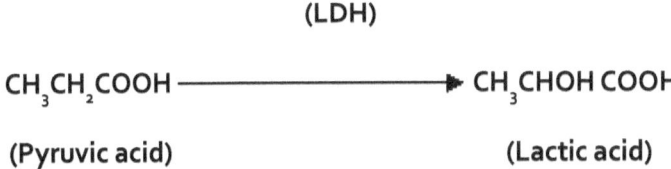

(LDH)

$$CH_3CH_2COOH \longrightarrow CH_3CHOH\,COOH$$

(Pyruvic acid)   **(Lactic acid)**

When shock progresses:

- Increase in capillary permeability causes loss of both saline and albumin from vascular to interstitial space.
- The microvasculature becomes plugged because of endothelial swelling, platelets, leucocyte aggregates and red cells with decreased deformability.
- Consumptive coagulopathy occurs from disseminated intravascular coagulation (DIC). [14]
- Vasoconstriction may eventually lead to vasodilation and <u>irreversibility</u>.

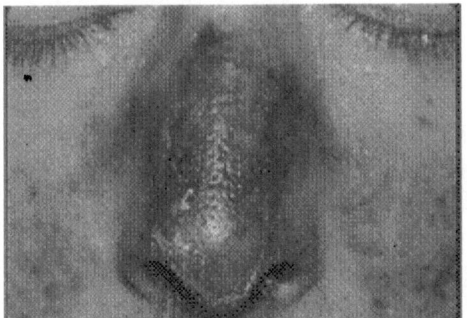 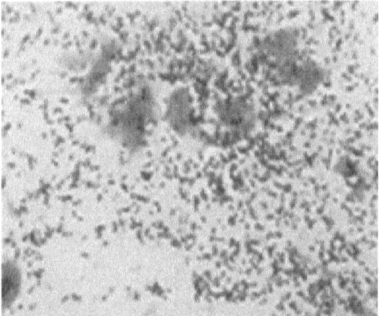

<u>Disseminatedintravascular coagulation due to Pneumococcaemia in in a patient with asplenia. Grams smear of skin showing large numbers of pneumococci</u>

CLINICAL MANIFESTATIONS [1-4, 7, 13]

Tachycardia.

This may be attenuated from the effects of drugs such as β blockers. Bradycardia, probably vagally mediated, is common in severe haemorrhage and bradycardia may occur in myocardial infarction.

Hypotension.

Hypotension is a late manifestation of shock in both sepsis and hypovolaemia, discussed in part 1.

Shock index—pulse rate / systolic blood pressure may be more reliable than either heart rate or systolic blood pressure alone [7]. An abnormal index (>0.9) indicates that severe circulatory failure is present but has poor sensitivity.

Pulse Pressure.

A narrow pulse pressure suggests that significant blood has been lost [2] or hypovolaemia is present but this does not occur in neurogenic shock. [2]

Extremities.

Cold, pale and blue extremities, slow capillary refill, and diaphoresis indicate inadequate skin perfusion. The core temperature may decrease or increase during sepsis. An exception is neurogenic shock due to sympathetic paralysis: the skin may be warm and red despite hypotension.

Respiratory Rate.

Increase in lung water causes stiff uncompliant lungs. The respiratory rate increases but may decrease in narcotic overdose. Tachypnoea, due to stiff lungs, and respiratory alkalosis are common [2]. Metabolic acidosis, due to lactic acid, causes Kussmaul type breathing—regular deep hyperventilation. The characteristic arterial blood gas profile is primary (anion gap) metabolic acidosis from lactic acid combined with acute primary respiratory alkalosis from hyperventilation.

Oliguria.

Urine output (< 30mL/hour) is the most important indicator of inadequate tissue perfusion and an important target for treatment [2]. The glomerular filtration (GFR) decreases, but to a lesser extent than renal plasma flow, due to increases in resistance in both afferent and efferent glomerular arterioles. The filtration fraction increases and blood is redistributed from renal cortex to medulla.

Splanchnic Organ Ischaemia.

This predisposes to erosive gastritis, pancreatitis and bacteraemia from compromised barrier function of the intestine (translocation). Centrilobular hepatic necrosis (shock liver) causes liver enzyme elevation and liver cell necrosis.

Confusion.

Confusion is an ominous sign which usually indicates that brain perfusion is inadequate or brain injury or severe metabolic encephalopathy is present.

Cardiac Arrhythmia and Ischaemia. Angina, ST segment depression or elevation, and arrhythmias occur secondary to inadequate myocardial perfusion or to a cardiac cause of shock.

Laboratory Tests.

Blood gas shows an anion gap lactic acidosis (base deficit) combined with respiratory alkalosis from hyperventilation. Hypoxaemia suggests lung trauma, pulmonary oedema or sepsis is present. Marked elevation of serum C reactive protein (CRP) occurs in sepsis but also occurs in severe trauma without sepsis and other inflammatory conditions.

Haemoglobin and haematocrit are unreliable signs of blood loss but decrease as haemodilution develops.

Liver enzymes may reach high levels from ischaemia.

An increase in serum troponin correlates with severity of shock and does not necessarily indicate that an acute coronary event has occurred.

Disseminated Intravascular Coagulation.

Thrombocytopaenia, raised prothrombin time, partial thromboplastin time and low serum fibrinogen occur in severe sepsis, but also in severe hypovolaemic shock. [14]

Hypocalcaemia and Hypophosphataemia of uncertain cause, are very common in critically ill patients (chapters 9, 10)

The most reliable signs of shock, and useful in guiding therapy, are urine output, heart rate, mean arterial pressure and the shock index. However these indicators perform less well than more invasive investigations: measurement of cardiac output, central venous oxygen saturation and central venous pressure, especially their response to fluid challenge.

TREATMENT.

The optimum approach is to:

* Identify shock in the early phase before decompensation occurs.
* Rapidly identify and treat the cause.
* Rapidly infuse fluids in non cardiogenic shock to maintain urine output, blood pressure, cardiac output and decrease lactic acidosis (discussed at the end of the section). Fluids should be given in the ratio of 3L crystalloid to 1L colloid.
* Treat associated conditions or complications.

> **CARDIOGENIC SHOCK:** [1, 15-18]

CO = SV x HR (CO = cardiac output, HR = heart rate, SV=stroke volume)

SV is determined by Preload, Afterload and Cardiac Contractility.

Preload depends on left ventricular end diastolic volume (LVEDV). Shortening or contraction of muscle depends on its stretch up to a certain (maximum) point. However the relationship between LVEDV and LVEDP (left ventricular end diastolic pressure) also depends on compliance of the ventricle: a stiff ventricle requires a higher filling pressure to achieve the same filling as a less stiff ventricle. The optimum Pulmonary Capillary Wedge Pressure (PCWP) varies with ventricular compliance. Thus a normal maximum central venous pressure (CVP) or PCWP may not rule out a further response to a fluid load: [1, 2, 7] a higher than normal venous return may be needed to overcome the high intrathoracic pressure of pneumothorax, intermittent positive pressure ventilation or raised intrapericardial pressure from pericardial effusion. The implementation of IPPV, when hypovolaemia is present, decreases CO.

Afterload is the resistance against which the left ventricle ejects blood: it is mainly determined by Systemic Vascular Resistance (SVR), but other factors, including aortic wall compliance, are involved.[1] Loss of atrial contraction due to atrial fibrillation or a very fast heart rate, decreases SV because there is inadequate time for ventricular filling, especially if diastolic dysfunction is present.

Venous return to the left ventricle may also decrease from impingement of the interventricular septum into the left ventricle from right ventricular overload in pulmonary embolism.

The cardiogenic index is usually <2.2L/min/m^2, pulmonary wedge pressure >15mmHg and AV O$_2$ difference increases in cardiogenic shock. [15]

Cardiogenic shock occurs from:

- Disorder of cardiac function from loss of muscle or disordered muscle function.
- Obstruction to output: pulmonary embolus, aortic dissection.
- Severe valvular dysfunction—ruptured chordae, papillary muscle infarction.
- Arrhythmias.

Myocardial infarction is the most common cause. Shock occurs when 40% or more of the left ventricle is involved.

Signs of heart failure may resemble those of hypovolaemic shock described previously. The following aid in separating cardiogenic from hypovolaemic shock (chapter 11):

- Raised jugular venous pressure.
- Presence of pulmonary oedema—by clinical signs or imaging.
- S3 gallop.
- ECG or other evidence for a cardiac cause.

An elevated jugular venous pressure, without pulmonary oedema, occurs from right ventricular infarction, tension pneumothorax, pericardial fluid or constriction, pulmonary embolism, pulmonary hypertension and superior vena cava obstruction.

A normal chest x-ray in the presence of cardiogenic shock, severe hypoxaemia and or jugular venous distension should suggest the diagnosis of severe pulmonary embolism.

The function of the right ventricle (RV) is very different from the left ventricle (LV): the RV is thin walled with one sixth the mass of the LV and moves blood volume through a low pressure, low impedance system, with less oxygen demand. [16, 17] RV infarction is uncommon because of this, compared to RV ischaemia, and has a high rate of recovery without loss of function.

Management and recovery of LV and RV failure are therefore different. [16, 17]

Right ventricular infarction, accompanying anterior myocardial infarction, is associated with higher mortality than left ventricular infarction alone; should be diagnosed by using right-sided precordial leads in the presence of inferior wall ischaemia; and should be considered for early reperfusion. [18]

TREATMENT.

Treatment of cardiogenic shock is not discussed further. Fluid infusion, discussed later, has a limited role in right ventricular infarction and perhaps pulmonary embolism. The role of catecholamines and vasodilators are also discussed at the end of this chapter. Afterload reduction is especially important in acute mitral regurgitation. Vasodilators may however be detrimental in aortic stenosis because lowering diastolic blood pressure has a small effect on CO while decreasing coronary perfusion. Inotropic drugs may exacerbate obstruction to ventricular ejection in eccentric aortic stenosis or hypertrophic obstructive cardiomyopathy. [1]

SEPTIC SHOCK ('DISTRIBUTIVE' SHOCK

This is due to infection or toxin production by micro-organisms. Anaphylaxis, severe allergic reactions, inflammatory conditions, such as pancreatitis, cyanide and carbon monoxide poisoning, metformin toxicity and some mitochondrial disorders produce a similar state.

Sepsis is due to gram positive and gram negative bacteria; fungal infections in up to 15%; but organisms may not be isolated. The response to infection is initiated by Toll-like receptors (innate immunity) which recognise molecules on immune and other cells. These release mediators such as NFkb and a cascade of proinflammatory cytokines; activate complement and the coagulation cascade; and promote development of adhesion molecules on endothelial cells.

Vasoconstriction is the normal response to inadequate tissue perfusion in cardiogenic and hypovolaemic shock. However, sepsis causes vasodilatory shock with hypotension due to failure of vascular smooth to contract in response to activation of the Sympathetic nervous system (SNS); Renin angiotensin aldosterone system(RAAS); and secretion of vasopressin(AVP,ADH).[19]

The following is a very simplified account of the mechanism of smooth muscle contraction and dilatation. [19]

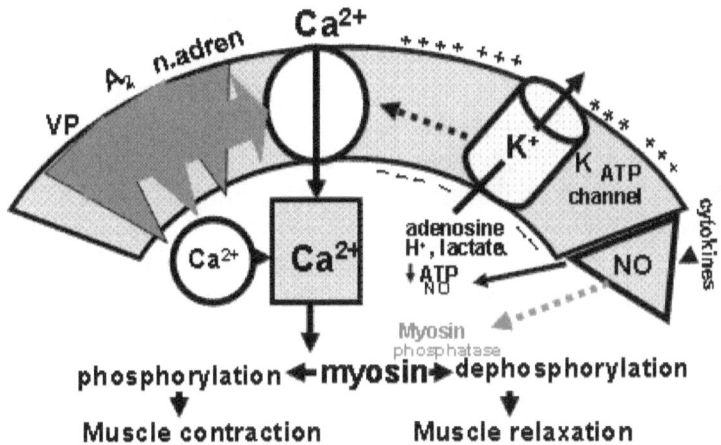

Figure 2: Simplified model of mechanisms of vasoconstriction and vasodilation in vascular smooth muscle cells.

The membrane, which is negative on the inside, has voltage gated calcium (Ca^{2+}) and K $_{ATP}$ channels and receptors for vasopressin VP, angiotensin II (A$_2$) and n adrenaline (n.adren.). Phosphorylation of myosin results in muscle contraction and dephosphorylation in muscle relaxation.

Phosphorylation is stimulated by Ca²⁺ entry into cells and from intracellular stores stimulated by vasopressin (VP), A2 and n,adrenaline. Opening of K$_{ATP}$ channels hyperpolarises inner cell membranes (become more negative as K⁺ leaves cells) which closes voltage gated Ca²⁺ channels and thus inhibits phosphorylation of myosin. K$_{ATP}$ channels are opened by adenosine, lactate, H⁺, NO(Nitric oxide) and decreased availability of ATP, all of which increase in sepsis or inadequate oxygen availability. (NO) synthesis is increased in sepsis and causes muscle relaxation by 2 mechanisms: stimulation of myosin phosphatase and opening of K$_{ATP}$ channels.

- <u>Contraction</u> of smooth muscle occurs in response to phosphorylation of myosin. This is initiated by Ca²⁺ entry into cells from voltage gated Ca²⁺ channels and release from cell stores. Ca²⁺ activates a kinase which phosphorylates myosin.
- <u>Vasodilation</u> is produced by dephosphorylation of myosin, due to stimulation of myosin phosphatase, following a cascade initiated by nitric oxide (NO).Vasodilation is also produced by hyperpolarisation of cell membranes (inner cell membrane becomes more negative) induced by efflux of K⁺ via K⁺$_{ATP}$ channels. This closes voltage gated Ca²⁺ channels which inhibit phosphorylation and muscle contraction.
- Normal tone results from a balance between these mechanisms.
- Angiotensin 2, nor adrenaline and vasopressin (VP) lock into receptors on smooth muscle cell membranes and stimulate Ca²⁺ entry into cells via voltage gated Ca²⁺ channels iIn hypovolaemic and cardiogenic shock. This results in vasoconstriction.
- Vasodilation In septic shock is produced by increase in synthesis of nitric oxide and other vasodilators and activation of K⁺$_{ATP}$ channels: efflux of K⁺ hyperpolarises the cell membrane which closes voltage gated Ca²⁺ channels. A decrease in cell ATP and increase of H⁺, adenosine and lactate activate K⁺$_{ATP}$ channels.[19,20]

<u>Vascular permeability</u>

Interstitial fluid leaks between endothelial cells due to disruption of cell junctions from the effect of cytokines and other inflammatory mediators. Endothelial damage during sepsis causes microthrombus formation and consumptive coagulopathy. Generation of reactive oxygen radicals may contribute to endothelial damage.

Two phases of septic shock have been described: an initial <u>warm phase,</u> superseded after a highly variable interval, by a <u>cold, often irreversible phase.</u> Septic shock is initially characterised by:

- Early increase in cardiac output (CO) above normal levels, decrease in ejection fraction (EF) and ventricular compliance (increased cardiac stiffness).
- Decrease in cardiac filling pressure—effective hypovolaemia, due to vascular dilatation, described above, and capillary loss of fluid into tissues from an increase in permeability.
- Maldistribution of blood flow and capillary arterio-venous bypass which decreases blood flow in the microcirculation.
- Increase in lactate production due to stimulation of Na^+:K^+ pumps by catecholamines and other ligands involved in the inflammatory process, especially in muscle,.
- An increase in central venous oxygen saturation (cVO_2) due to decreased oxygen extraction by tissues.
- Renal sodium and water reabsorption are normal in early sepsis suggesting that intervention at an early stage may prevent irreversible renal failure. [21]

Thus, although cardiac output is elevated, myocardial contractility is decreased; blood flow is maldistributed; arterial underfilling (effective hypovolaemia) develops from vascular dilatation; and fluid loss into the third space. The Systemic Inflammatory Response Syndrome (SIRS) is characterised by two or more of the following:

- * Tachycardia (≥ 90/minute).
- * Tachypnoea (respiratory rate > 20/minute; decreased pO_2 or pCO_2 < 32 mmHg).
- * Hyperthermia > 38° C or hypothermia < 36° C.
- * Neutrophil count :> 12,000 or < 4000 or 20% bands.

A cold phase develops if treatment is delayed or ineffective. This is characterised by hypotension (systolic BP <90mmHg), lactic acidosis, oliguria, low arteriovenous oxygen saturation difference (increased S_cVO_2), suggesting inadequate tissue oxygen utilisation, multiple organ dysfunction and disseminated intravascular coagulation. (Table 1)

Cardiac Dysfunction. [15-22]

Systolic and diastolic dysfunction occurs and resolves in 7-10 days if the patient survives. Decrease in cardiac contractility occurs in 60% of patients with sepsis and is partly corrected by dobutamine. The lowest LVEF (left ventricular ejection fraction) in patients with previous normal cardiac function was 31% in one study. [22] Serum Troponin levels increase and are a marker of severity. [23] Sodium and calcium accumulate in myocytes.

Critical Illness Related Corticosteroid Insufficiency.

Some experts consider that relative corticosteroid deficiency occurs due to a combination of adrenal insufficiency and tissue resistance to corticosteroids; and should be suspected in hypotensive patients who respond poorly to fluids and vasopressors. [24]

Lung	Adult respiratory distress syndrome. **(ARDS)** Hypoxaemia, pulmonary oedema, infiltrates.
Kidney	Urine output ≤ 0.5 ml/kg/hour but occasionally greater (non-oliguric renal failure). Increasing serum creatinine. Acute renal failure in 19% with moderate sepsis, 23% with severe sepsis and 51% of patients with septic shock. [21]
Liver	Elevation of liver enzymes and bilirubin.
Gastrointestinal Tract	Mucosal damage and translocation of micro-organisms into the blood stream.
Disseminated intravascular	**coagulation**

Table.1 MODS (Multiple Organ Dysfunction Syndrome)

TREATMENT:

Goal directed therapy of hypoperfusion, [1, 2, 25-28] following the seminal study by Rivers et al, [25] and early antibiotic therapy [25, 26, 28] are standard practice in treatment of severe sepsis.

Detailed guidelines for treatment of severe sepsis have been formulated by Critical Care and Infectious disease experts representing 11 international organisations. [26] The main points from the "Surviving Sepsis Campaign" guidelines for the management of severe sepsis in adults are: [26]

Rapid initial resuscitation to specific goals.

* CVP 8-12mmHg.
* MAP ≥65mmHg.
* Urine output >0.5mL/kg/hour.
* Central venous (CV SO_2) or mixed venous SO_2 ≥ 70%.

If CV SO_2 >70% is not achieved following fluid resuscitation to a CVP of 8-12mmHg, packed cells are infused to achieve a haematocrit ≥ 30% and or dobutamine is administered up to 20µg/kg/min. Increasing oxygen delivery to supranormal levels is not beneficial. [26, 29 -31]

* Two or more blood cultures should be taken. Intravenous antibiotics, active against the most likely pathogens, should be started within the first hour after cultures. This should be reassessed after 48 hours with the goal to change to narrow spectrum antibiotics to decrease development of resistance and super infection. A combination of antibiotics is appropriate for neutropenic sepsis. However blood cultures are negative in many cases and treatment may have to be guided by clinical judgement, including the likely source of infection, and response.
* Other measures may be indicated in sepsis: abscess drainage, debridement of infected tissue, removal of an infected device and surgical treatment of gastrointestinal perforation. However the risks of an intervention must be balanced by the potential benefit.
* Fluid Therapy.

Administrations of Colloids or Crystalloids have no major outcome differences. A fluid challenge may be given as 500-1000mL of crystalloid or 300-500mL of colloid over 30 minutes and repeated based on response. (I emphasise however that 500mL colloid is equivalent to 1.5 L rather than 1L of crystalloid).

* Vasopressor and Inotropic therapy. An arterial catheter should be placed to facilitate accurate blood pressure measurements.

Vasopressors should be used when a fluid challenge fails to restore blood pressure or organ perfusion. Either norepinephrine or dopamine is the first choice. Dobutamine is the preferred inotrope for improving low cardiac output in the presence of adequate left ventricular filling pressure. Both a vasoconstrictor and dobutamine may be used together.

Low dose dopamine should not be used as a renal protective agent.

Vasopressin may be considered in refractory shock despite absence of adequate evidence for its effectiveness.

* <u>Corticosteroids</u>.

Hydrocortisone, 200-300mg/day for seven days, in three divided doses, or by continuous infusion are recommended for those who fail therapy with fluid and require vasodepressor support. Higher doses of corticosteroid are ineffective or harmful. More recent guidelines suggest administration of hydrocortisone 200mg/day in four divided doses or by continuous infusion of 240mg/day for >7 days. [26] Glucocorticoid should be weaned and not stopped abruptly. [26]

   * <u>Recombinant Human Activated Protein C</u> is recommended for those at high risk of death.
   * <u>Red Cell Transfusions</u> should only be given if the haemoglobin level drops below 70g/L to a target of 70-90 g/L unless severe cardiac disease or acute haemorrhage suggest otherwise.
   * Mechanical <u>Ventilation</u> for Adult Respiratory Distress Syndrome (ARDS):

Low tidal volumes (~6mL/kg predicted body weight) are used as a goal to maintain end inspiratory plateau pressures less than <30cmH$_2$o. Permissive hypercapnia may be used.

A minimum amount of positive end-expiration pressure should be set to prevent lung collapse at end expiration. The prone position should be considered if experience in this technique is available. A semirecumbent position, to decrease ventilator-acquired pneumonia, and a weaning protocol should be used if appropriate. Neuromuscular blockers should be avoided if possible. A longer duration of mechanical ventilation increases mortality from renal failure. [32] Interruption of sedation—drug infusions shortens the duration of mechanical ventilation. [33]

For ARDS methyl prednisolone, 1mg/kg/day for 14 days, is recommended by the American College of Critical Care Medicine. [24]

   * <u>Glucose Control</u>.

Serum glucose should be maintained below 8.3mmol/L, preferably by continuous infusion.

Sodium bicarbonate infusion should not be given.

Stress ulcer and deep vein prophylaxis should be given to all patients.

* Enteral Nutrition.

Parenteral nutrition increases mortality. Early enteral nutrition improves outcome and should be used in preference to parenteral nutrition. [37]

Since these guidelines were published two randomised double blind trials found that administration of both intensive insulin [34] and hydrocortisone [35] were ineffective in critically ill patients. Intensive insulin, compared to conventional insulin therapy, in critically ill medical patients showed a similar mortality but an increase in severe hypoglycaemia and other adverse events in the intensively treated group. In the Corticut trial [35] there was no advantage to patients given hydrocortisone, 200mg day for five days, and then tapered over six days compared to placebo. Moreover the corticotrophin stimulation test is unreliable in critically ill patients. [36]

Trials of Novel Drugs are being undertaken but their usefulness is uncertain. These are designed to counteract the immune reaction, cytokine related vasodilatation and vascular hyporesponsiveness in Septic Shock—for example NO scavengers such as Polyoxethylene [38] and K^+_{ATP} channel blockers. [20]

FLUID THERAPY IN SHOCK

The most important issues in fluid therapy of shock are the timing, quantity and composition of fluids used; and the use and timing of vasoactive drugs following initial correction of hypovolaemia.

There is consensus that effective hypovolaemia should be corrected early and rapidly with the exception of ongoing blood loss in trauma: In penetrating torso injuries delay in aggressive fluid therapy, until operative intervention is available, improves outcome. [39] Other forms of trauma may also not benefit from early rapid volume replacement until haemorrhage is controlled. [40]

Rapid infusion of fluid to achieve specific goals in severe sepsis is based on only 2 randomised trials in human subjects [25, 27]. Although these trials had limitations, it is physiologically plausible that early effective treatment to decrease irreversible changes in the microcirculation should be undertaken. In septic shock this has been endorsed by several Societies and Associations.[26] Early and rapid fluid infusion is probably crucial in improving outcome in septic shock.[42,43] Implementation of standard guidelines for treatment of septic shock in an Emergency Department led to more vigorous administration of fluids and a lower 28 day mortality. [44] The elderly and those with cardiac disease are often administrated fluids at a slower rate than are younger patients (personal observations). This is theoretically unsound for several reasons. The elderly:

* Have limited physiological reserve.
* Less ability to increase cardiac output in response to injury. [13]
* A high frequency of increased myocardial stiffness [13] and atrial fibrillation, which increases the need for adequate preload, are often on medications which cause hypovolaemia and compromise appropriate cardiovascular responses. [13]
* Stroke, myocardial infarction and multi-organ dysfunction are theoretically much more likely to occur during hypotension in those with narrowed arteries.
* A high frequency of comorbidity increases risk of complications.

In the absence of randomised controlled studies the elderly should receive at least as rapid and adequate fluid therapy as younger subjects. Subjects with underlying cardiac disease, especially with diastolic dysfunction or atrial fibrillation, are especially dependent on an adequate preload.

Hypotension (BP <100mmHg) in non-trauma patients before hospitalisation [42] and in the Emergency Department [43] carries a higher mortality than patients with normotension.

<u>Although early and adequate correction of hypovolaemia is physiologically sound, an over liberal administration of fluids may have adverse effects.</u>

Infusion of fluids and sympathomimetic drugs to achieve supra-physiological goals fail to improve outcome in septic shock and do not improve organ dysfunction or mortality. [1, 29-31]

Once acute respiratory distress syndrome develops a restrictive rather than liberal fluid therapy improves lung function and ventilator free days, although mortality is similar. [45] An increase in crystalloid infusion after colonic resection leads to an increase in gastrointestinal fluid and oedema and decreased recovery of function. [46-48] A liberal, compared to a restricted use of fluids post operatively, which led to a positive cumulative fluid balance, resulted in more complications and longer length of stay. [46, 47] In studies of intraabdominal surgery post operative complications were reduced and length of stay decreased. [49] However other studies have come to different conclusions. [50]It has been emphasised, however, that a restrictive fluid policy may have been governed by specific goals. [51]

In conclusion <u>sufficient fluid should be given rapidly to maintain adequate blood pressure and urine output but fluids in excess of this may be detrimental.</u>

CARDIOGENIC SHOCK OR HYPOTENSION.

Fluids are clearly contraindicated when cardiogenic pulmonary oedema is present. [15]

Right ventricular infarction decreases diastolic compliance and systolic function of the right ventricle. This results in a volume sensitive, rather than pressure sensitive state, compared to the left ventricle. [1] Diagnosis is suggested by the <u>triad of clear lung fields, elevated jugular venous pressure and inferior wall infarction.</u> The venous pressure may decrease rather than increase on inspiration. Right ventricular (RV) infarction is confirmed by ST segment elevation or the presence of Q waves in right precordial leads. [52]

Fluid loading may also be considered for improving cardiac output in acute massive pulmonary embolism before diagnosis is established and thrombolysis administered. [54] However fluid loading may worsen haemodynamic status, as in many animal models: fluid loading may cause the interventricular septum to bulge into the left ventricle and decrease CO; and worsen right ventricular ischaemia or oxygen demand. [1]In one observational study, however, infusion of 500mL of dextran over 20 minutes to patients with acute circulatory failure (cardiac index <2.5L/min/m²) increased right atrial pressure and cardiac index from 1.6 to 2.0L//m²/min. [54]

Volume loading with normal saline improves cardiac output and hypotension in RV failure. However Dobutamine may be more effective than volume loading. [53]

COMPOSITION OF FLUID USED.

Sodium bicarbonate for treatment of lactic acidosis is of no proven benefit and is theoretically unsound because it generates CO_2 production and has other harmful effects (chapter 6).

$NaHCO_3$ + lactic acid $\longrightarrow$ Na Lactate + H_2CO_3 $\longrightarrow$ CO_2 + H_2O

Carbicarb, a mixture of Na_2Co_3 and $NaHCo_3$ is similar but does not generate net Co_2. However there is no evidence for benefit.

Crystalloid, colloid or blood can be used to increase the volume of the vascular space and improve cardiac output or delivery of oxygen (DO_2).

Colloids contain particles sufficiently large to exert an oncotic pressure. Thus colloids initially increase vascular filling to a greater extent than crystalloids. Saline administration distributes to the plasma volume and interstitial fluid in a ratio of approximately 1:3. Thus theoretically 3 times the amount of crystalloid should be given, compared to colloid, to increase plasma volume to the same extent. [55] Theoretically 1L normal saline distributes as 250mL in the vascular and 750mL in the interstitial space (normal ratio of interstitial—vascular space 3-1). [55,56] It is therefore surprising that Guidelines for shock recommend giving either 500 mL colloid or 1000 mL saline for fluid challenge.

Only 21% of normal saline infused in critically ill septic patients remained in the plasma volume at the end of the infusion. However neither saline nor colloid improved oxygen delivery, perhaps because hypovolaemia was absent. [56]In another study only 194 mL of each litre of Ringers lactate infused remained in the vascular compartment and this decreased in the next hour. 1 gram albumin increased plasma volume by ~18mL and 25g by 465 ± 47mL. Albumin infusion doubled the ECV: equal amounts remained in plasma volume and interstitial volume although there was wide variability. There was a suggestion that intracellular fluid participated in shift of fluid into ECV. [57]

Although 90% of albumin remains in the vascular space for two hours, equilibrium with the interstitial space leads to a 75% decrease from the vascular space within two days. This is highly variable, however, and is probably higher in sepsis or ischaemia because capillary permeability is increased. Thus colloids may leak into the interstitial space and increase interstitial oedema.

Protagonists for the use of colloids, rather than crystalloids, argue that colloid infusion increases plasma volume with less expansion of interstitial fluid than occurs with crystalloid infusion; and that leakage of fluid into interstitial space is less. On the other hand leakage of albumin may make subsequent mobilisation of fluid more difficult and a normal interstitial fluid volume may be important in itself.

The vigorous debate on the advantages of colloid versus crystalloid continues although a meta-analysis [58] and recent randomised trials have failed to establish a significant advantage for albumin over crystalloid administration.[59, 60] It is possible that albumin may be more effective than crystalloid in specific subgroups of patients. A subgroup, involving patients with traumatic brain injury from the SAFE study, [61] showed a trend for mortality reduction. Even patients with hypoalbuminemia do no better with albumin compared to colloid infusion. [62]

Albumin administration in some critically ill patients may improve organ function. [63] Mortality and renal impairment are decreased in patients with liver cirrhosis and peritonitis who are given albumin. [64] However correction of hypovolaemia may have been responsible because albumin was used alone and was not compared with an equivalent volume of crystalloid.

Colloids other than albumin have not been shown to be superior to crystalloids in volume repletion; are more expensive; and cause complications, although these are uncommon (Table 1). An increase in oncotic pressure resulting from artificial colloids may decrease the glomerular filtration rate. [65] A recent randomised double blind trial comparing HES (hydroxy ethyl starch) with Ringers solution showed more adverse effects from HES including an increase in renal failure and coagulopathy. [34]

Saline has the disadvantage, not shared by Ringer lactate or similar solutions, of causing hyperchloraemic acidosis [66] (chapter 7). This is due to increase in Cl^- (or decrease in HCo_3^-) compared to the plasma concentration or decrease in SID (strong ion difference) compared to plasma}. Whether this is detrimental is uncertain. Other solutions such as Hartmans have the disadvantage of being hypotonic.

Crystalloid solutions may also increase tissue oedema, especially if given to excess. Whether this is detrimental is controversial. Tissue oedema in wounds and lung may also occur from albumin infusion, due to an increase in capillary permeability and has the disadvantage that subsequent mobilisation of fluid may be slower than occurs with interstitial fluid alone. If total crystalloid volume is controlled to avoid volume overload there may be no difference in pulmonary function between using crystalloid and colloid [55]. Oncotic pressure may be a minor determinant of fluid translocation [55]. Interestingly subjects with <u>Hereditary Analbuminemia</u> (complete absence of albumin) do not usually develop oedema. [67]

Synthetic colloids are made from carbohydrates, dextran or animal collagen—gelatines. They contain molecules of varying molecular weight which govern their duration in the circulation. Colloids remain in the blood stream for longer than crystalloids and increase oncotic pressure which expands plasma volume. Duration of action depends on clearance from the circulation, which is related to their permeability through capillary membranes, degradation and renal excretion.

Specific colloids have important differences and some of these properties may have an advantage in specific situations. Colloids differ in the size and weight of molecules; their contribution to oncotic pressure; half life; and side effects. There are claims that some colloids improve the microcirculation, [68-70] inflammation, [68-70] haemodynamic stability and fluid shift out of capillaries compared to crystalloids. [68, 71] The main colloids and some of their properties are shown in Table 2.

Plasma expansion was better preserved with 6% dextran 70 than with 5% albumin, 6% HES and 3.5% gelatin in an animal model with trauma. A considerable increase in capillary permeability limited duration of plasma volume expansion. [72] Colloids, other than albumin, have a higher frequency of anaphylactoid reactions, [73] coagulopathy, [74] and renal failure than albumin.

<u>Hydroxy ethyl Starch (HES)</u> is a modification of amylopectin and is hypertonic compared to albumin. 46% percent of an administered dose is excreted within two day.1L increases plasma volume by approximately 790mL. [55] Coagulopathy and anaphylactoid reactions occur, but are rare. Renal function may decrease. [34, 75, 76] In a randomised double blind trial comparing crystalloid with HES the mortality was the same but renal failure and coagulopathy were more common from use of HES. [34] Pentastarch is similar to HES but is cleared more rapidly.

<u>Dextrans</u> [55] are mixtures of glucose polymers produced by Leuconostoc mesenteroides, a bacterium grown on a sucrose medium. Dextran 70 (average MW 70,000) is usually used as a 6% solution in normal saline and Dextran 40 (average MW 40,000) is available as a 10% solution in

either saline or dextrose water. Dextran 70, results in more effective and prolonged volume expansion because of its higher MW. Infusion increases the plasma volume to a similar extent (average 790mL) as does 6% HES. It is claimed that Dextran, especially Dextran 40, improves peripheral blood flow in the microcirculation. Dextran infusion may cause anaphylaxis, bleeding and renal failure.

Gelatins: These are produced by modification of collagen. The low molecular weight results in rapid renal excretion. The most important complication is anaphylactoid reactions associated with histamine release. Coagulopathy occurs less commonly compared to Dextran and HES. [74] Gelatin is less effective than both albumin and dextran in its water pulling capacity. [72, 77]

COLLOID	Na	Cℓ	Complications
5% albumin	130-160	130-160	Hypocalcaemia, mild acidosis
(250-500mL)			? Pulmonary oedema
			Anaphylaxis less common than other colloids
6%Hetastarch(HES) (500mL)	154	154	Coagulopathy—decrease in factor VIII and VWf (von Willebrand's factor)
			Anaphylaxis, renal failure
10% Pentastarch	154	154	Similar to above
6% Dextran 70	154 or 0	154 or 0	Renal failure, anaphylaxis, coagulopathy
10% Dextran 40 (500mL)	154	120	Anaphylaxis, coagulopathy

Table 2: Commonly used colloids and their complications. (Na, Cl in mmol/L.)

In conclusion: at present albumin cannot be justified for either expanding volume or correcting hypoalbuminemia other than for use during paracentesis in cirrhotic patients with bacterial peritonitis. Other colloids have not been shown to be better than crystalloids or albumin for volume correction. In view of this, their cost and potential complications, they should not be considered for first line therapy.

Blood.

The current fashion is to avoid blood transfusion unless anaemia is severe. [78, 79] Evidence of cardiac ischaemia and subtle cognitive dysfunction only occurred when the haemoglobin fell to 50-60g/L (5-6g/dL) in healthy volunteers and surgical patients.[80] Cardiovascular compensation was adequate to a haemoglobin level of 5g/dL (50g/L) In healthy volunteers. [81]

A randomised controlled trial showed that a restrictive red cell transfusion strategy was as good as and possibly superior to a liberal transfusion strategy. A threshold for red cell transfusion of 70g/L (7g/dL), maintaining haemoglobin between 70-90g/L (7-9g/dL), was used. [82]

Blood transfusions compromise immunity, increase infections, [83] may compromise the microcirculation and have serious complications. Concerns have been expressed that a restricted transfusion policy may be inappropriate in those with severe coronary artery disease, aortic stenosis or in the very old. In a retrospective study mortality was increased in patients with cardiovascular disease who declined a blood transfusion. [84] However in another retrospective study of elderly (>65 years of age) subjects with myocardial infarction mortality was higher in patients who received a blood transfusion. [85] A combination of three large randomised trials of 24,111 patients with acute coronary syndromes showed an increase in mortality of nearly four times in those receiving blood transfusion. [86]

Thus, evidence at present, suggests that blood transfusions are rarely beneficial above haemoglobin of 100g/L (10g/dL) or haematocrit >30% but benefit exceeds risks when haemoglobin falls below (70g/L). [87]

Hypertonic Saline:

Hypertonic saline has been suggested for the treatment of hypovolaemia associated with trauma: [88, 89] brain trauma with raised intracranial pressure;[90-92]in sepsis;[93] and in diabetic ketoacidosis with altered mental state.[94] Apart from logistical advantages, in expanding the plasma volume with a smaller quantity of fluid, its place in the treatment of shock has not been established. Rapid development of hypernatraemia and osmotic demyelination is a potential hazard.

Vasoactive Drugs. [95-110]

The purpose of using vasoactive drug therapy is to improve tissue perfusion. Severe vasoconstriction is characteristic of hypovolaemic, cardiogenic and obstructive shock whereas septic shock is characterised by vasodilation, myocardial depression and altered distribution of blood flow. [1, 2] There are inadequate trials to guide therapy. A Cochrane review concluded that studies were unsatisfactory and that current available evidence was not suited to inform clinical practice for circulatory shock. [98] This is therefore based on expert opinion. There seems to be general consensus that:

Hypovolaemia should be corrected before vasoconstrictive drugs are used.

Adrenaline (epinephrine) should not be used as a first line vasopressor [95, 96] except in anaphylaxis.

N-adrenaline (n-epinephrine) is the preferred vasoconstrictor. [95, 96]

Dobutamine is preferred to increase cardiac output. [96]

Raising MAP from 65mmHg to >85mmHg or the use of dobutamine to boost cardiac output is not beneficial. [97]

The effect of catecholamines result from actions on alpha (α), beta (β) and dopamine receptors. The action on each of these receptors is dose dependent. (Table 3).

It is important to start low and go slow and titrate to clinical response. A large vein or CV line should be used.

N-adrenaline (nor epinephrine) is recommended as the initial catecholamine for septic shock. [99,100] It has a dose dependent effect on both α and β adrenergic receptors and maintains a higher cardiac index than AVP. Decrease in cardiac output, increase in organ ischaemia and arrhythmias are important adverse effects. N adrenaline does not cause deterioration and may improve renal function [96,100] when used for shock and is considered the catecholamine of choice for renal protection in critically ill patients. [101]

Adrenaline (epinephrine) has potent α and β effects. It is the vasoactive drug of choice for anaphylaxis but is not used in septic shock because of its detrimental effect on regional circulation and its effect in increasing lactic acidosis. [96]

DRUG	USUAL IV DOSE	Effects of Receptors			CLINICAL USE
		α	β_1	Dopamine	
Dopamine	1-2 µg/kg/min°	+	+	+++	Vasodilatation
	2-10 µg/kg/min	+	+	+++	Inotropism
	10-30 µg/kg/min	++	++	+++	Vasoconstriction
Dobutamine	2-10µg/kg/min	+	+++	0	Cardiogenic shock, pulmonary embolism
n.Adrenaline	2-40 µg/min	+++	++	0	Hypotension
Adrenaline	0.5-1 mg (1:10,000)	+	++	0	Cardiac arrest Anaphylaxis
	1-200 µg/min	++	+++	0	
Isoprenaline	2-10 µg/min	0	+++	0	Bradycardiac, Torsades, heart block
AVP (ADH)	01-.04ug/min	Vi receptor			

Table 3: *Commonly used vasoactive drugs, action on receptors and clinical use. Dose recommendations vary and change with time.*

Vasopressin (ADH) [AVP]:

Occupancy of Vir AVP receptors by vasopressin increases Ca^{2+} entry into smooth muscle cells and releases Ca^{2+} from stores. This causes vasoconstriction by phosphorylating myosin. Vasopressin also inactivates K^+_{ATP} channels which normally cause vasodilation. Vasoconstriction therefore results. The degree of vasoconstriction in response to AVP depends on plasma levels. Vasopressin is secreted in considerably greater amounts in shock, 9-189 pmol/L, than in response to increase in osmolality,

0.9-6.5 pmol/L. Vasopressin in high concentration decreases considerably when shock worsens. This and vascular resistance to A_2 and noradrenaline provide the rationale for its use.

AVP predominantly constricts the splanchnic circulation, muscles, skin, and glomerular efferent arterioles. It increases filtration pressure and GFR in comparison to n-adrenaline which constricts afferent rather than efferent arterioles, decreases filtration pressure and may prolong the course of renal failure. [21]

Vasopressin is a potent vasopressor [21,102] which may have a place in haemorrhagic shock unresponsive to other agents; [103] and for uncontrolled haemorrhagic shock to decrease bleeding below the diaphragm while increasing perfusion above. [104] It has also been used in septic shock. [105] Vasopressin infusion increases blood pressure and urine output and decreases the dose of n-adrenaline required to maintain blood pressure. However its place in both septic and haemorrhagic shock has not been established. [105] AVP does not have an inotropic effect, as does n-adrenaline, decreases cardiac output and constricts coronary arteries. [21]

There was no difference in outcome in a recent randomised double blind trial, comparing vasopressin with n-adrenaline. [106] However AVP and n, adrenaline in combination resulted in fewer side effects than n, adrenaline alone. [107]

Dopamine:

There is a variable interaction on receptors (Table 2) which depends on dose. At low dose (<5.0 µg/kg/min dopamine causes vasodilation in mesenteric and renal beds; at doses of 5-10 µg/kg/min β receptors are activated resulting in positive inotropic effects; and at high doses (10-20 µg/kg/min) systemic vasoconstriction results from activation of α adrenergic receptors. In a multicenter randomised trial, comparing dopamine with n, adrenaline for treatment of shock there was no difference in mortality but dopamine therapy was associated with more adverse events. [108]

Dobutamine is considered the preferred drug for inotropic support in septic shock, [95, 96,109] pulmonary embolism and cardiogenic shock. [109] It increases stroke volume for a particular LVEDV. However elevation of oxygen delivery by dobutamine, to specific target levels, is ineffective and possibly detrimental in critically ill patients. [101] Dobutamine improves the percent of small vessels which are continuously perfused in septic shock. [110]

REFERENCES

1. Intensive Care Medicine. Eds. Rippe JM, Irwin RS, Fink MP, Cerra FB. 3rd Edition 1996.

2. Rivers EP, Otero RM, Nguyen HB: Approach to the patient in shock. p219-225 Emergency Medicine. Ed. Tintinalli JD, Kelen GD, Stapczynski JS. 6th Edition 2004.

3. Textbook of Adult Emergency Medicine. p 23-32 Eds. Cameron P, Jelinek G, Kelly AM et al. 2 edition 2004 Elsevier.

4. Jimenez EJ: Shock in Critical Care. p359-376 in Critical Care. Eds Civetta JM, Taylor RW, Kirby RR. 1997. Lippincott Raven.

5. Vincent JL, De Backer D: Oxygen transport—the oxygen delivery controversy. *Int. Care Med.* **30**:1990-1996, 2004.

6. Carey LC, Lowery BD, Cloutier CT: Haemorrhagic Shock. *Current Problems in Surgery.* p1-47. 1971. Year Book Medical Publishers Inc.

7. Dabrowski GP, Steinberg SM, Ferrara JF, Flint LM: A critical assessment of end points of shock resuscitation. *Surg. Clin. N. Amer.* **80**:825-844, 2000.

8. Somero G: Protons, osmolytes and fitness of the internal milieu for protein function. *Amer. J. Physiol.* **20**:197-213, 1986

9. Gutierrez G, Wulf ME: Lactic Acidosis in Sepsis: Another Commentary. *Critic. Care Med.* **33**:2420-2422, 2005.

10. Kellum JA: Lactate and pHi; our continued search for markers of tissue distress. *Crit. Care Med.* **26**:1783-1784, 1998.

11. Levy B: Lactate and Shock State: The Metabolic View. *Crit. Care Med.* **12**:315-321, 2006.

12. Levy B, Gibot S, Franck P et al: Relation between muscle $Na^+ H^+$ ATPase activity and raised lactate concentration in septic shock: a prospective study. *Lancet.* **365**:871-875, 2005.

13. Advanced Trauma Life Support. 7th Ed. 2004. *Amer. College Surgeons.*

14. Attar H, Hanashiro P, Hansberger A et al: Intravascular Coagulation—Reality or Myth. *Surgery.* **68**:27-33, 1970.

15. Califf RM, Bengston JR: Cardiogenic Shock. *NEJM.* **330**:1724-1730, 1994.

16. Goldstein JA: Right versus left ventricular shock: A tale of two ventricles. *J. Amer. Coll. Cardiol.* **41**:1280-1282, 2003.

17. Yen AD, Parillo JE: The golden hour of right ventricular ischaemia. *Crit. Care Med.* **36**:2194-2195, 2008.

18. Hamon M, Agostini D, Lepage O et al. Prognostic impact of right ventricular involvement in patients with acute myocardial infarction. *Crit. Care. Med.* **36**:2023-2033, 2008.

19. Landry DW, Oliver JA. The Pathogenesis of Vasodilatory Shock. NEJM **345** 588-592 2001

20. Lange M, Morelli A, Westphal M: Inhibition of potassium channels in critical illness. *Current Opinion in Anesthesiology.* **27**:105-110, 2008.

21. Schrier RW, Wang W: Acute Renal Failure and Sepsis. *New Engl J Med.* **351**:159-168, 2004.

22. Charron C, Belliard G, Page B, Jardin F: Actual incidence of global left ventricular hypokinesia in adult septic shock. *Crit. Care Med.* **36**:1701

23. Fernandez CJ, Akaminic N, Knobel E: Cardiac Troponin: A new serum marker of myocardial injury in sepsis. *Int. Care Med.* **25**:1165-1168, 1999.

24. Marik PE, Pastores SM, Annane D et al. Recommendation for the diagnosis and management of corticosteroid insufficiency in critically ill adult patients: Consensus statements from an internal taskforce by the American College of Critical Care Medicine. *Crit. Care Med.* **36**:1937-1949, 2008.

25. Rivers E, Nguyen B, Havstad S et al: Early goal directed therapy in the treatment of severe sepsis and septic shock. *New Engl J Med.* **345**:1368-1377, 2001.

26. Delinger RP, Carlet JM, Masur H et al: Surviving sepsis campaign guidelines for management of severe sepsis and septic shock. *Crit. Care Med.* **32**:858-873, 2004.

27. Oleivera CF, Oleivera DS, Gottschald AF, Moura JD et al. ACCM/PALS haemodynamic support guidelines for paediatric septic shock: an outcome comparison with and without monitoring central venous oxygen saturation. Intensive Care Medicine DOI 10.1007/s 00134-008-1085-9.2008

28. Vandack H, Sarasin F, Pugin J: Prompt antibiotic administration and goal-directed therapy haemodynamic support in patients with severe sepsis and septic shock. *Current Opinion in Crit. Care.* **13**:586-591, 2007.

29. Hayes MA, Timmins AC, Yau EH et al: Elevation of Systemic Oxygen Delivery in the Treatment of Critically Ill Patients. *New Engl J Med.* **330**:1717-1722, 1994.

30. Shoemaker WC, Appel PL, Kram HB et al: Prospective trial of supranormal values of survivors as therapeutic goals in high-risk surgical patients. *Chest.* **94**:1176-1186, 1989.

31. Gattinoni L, Brazzi L, Pelosi P et al: A trial of goal-oriented haemodynamic therapy in critically ill patients. *New Engl J Med.* **333**:1025-1032, 1995.

32. Neveu H, Kleinknecht D, Loirat Ph et al: Prognostic factors in acute renal failure due to sepsis. Results of a prospective multicentre study. *Nephrol Dial. Transplant.* **11**:293-299, 1996.

33. Kress JP, Pohlman HS, O'Connor MF, Hall JB. Daily interruptions of sedative infusions in critically ill patients undergoing mechanical ventilation. *New Engl J Med* **342** 1471-1477 2000

34. Brunkkorst FM, Engel C, Bloos F et al: Intensive insulin therapy and Pentastarch Resuscitation in Severe Sepsis. New Eng J Med.**358**:125-9 2008

35. Sprung CL, Annane D, Keh D et al: Hydrocortisone therapy for patients with septic shock. *New Engl J Med.* **358**:111-124, 2008.

36. Hamrahian AH, Oseni TS Arafah BM. Measurements of serum free cortisol in critically ill patients.NEJM **350** 1629-1638 2004

37. Marik PE: Death by TPN....the final chapter? *Crit Care Med.* **36**:1964-1965, 2008.

38. Djukom C: Polyoxethylene: A breakthrough in the fight against distributive shock? *Crit Care Med.* **36**:2189-2190, 2008.

39. Bickell WH, Wall JM, Pepe PE et al: Immediate versus delayed fluid resuscitation for hypotensive patients with penetrating torso injuries. *New Engl J Med.* **331**:1105-1109, 1994.

40. Bickell WH, Stern S: Fluid replacement for hypotensive injury victims: How, When and What Risks? *Current Opinion in Anesthesiology.* **11**:177-180, 1998.

41. Peters MJ, BrierlyJ. Back to the basics in septic shock. Intensive Care Medicine **34** 991-993 2008

42. Jones AE, Stiell IG, Nesbitt LP et al: Non-Traumatic out of hospital hypotension predicts in hospital mortality. *Ann. Emerg. Med.* **43**:106-13, 2004.

43. Jones AE, Yiannibas V, Johnson C, Kline JA: Emergency Department hypotension predicts sudden unexpected in-hospital mortality. Chest. **130**:941-6 2006.

44. Micek ST, Roubinian N, Heuring T et al: Before and after study of a standardized hospital order set for the management of septic shock. *Crit. Care Med.* **34**:2707-2713, 2006.

45. Wiedeman HP, Wheeler AP, Bernard GR et al: Comparison of two fluid-management strategies in acute lung injury. *New. Engl. J Med.* **354**:2564-2575, 2006.

46. Lobo DN, Bostock KA, Neal KR et al: Effect of salt and water balance on recovery of gastrointestinal function after elective colonic resection: a randomised controlled trial. *Lancet.* **359**:1812-1818, 2002.

47. Brandstrup B, Tonnesen H, Beier-Holgersen R et al: Effects of intravenous fluid restriction on postoperative complications: comparison of two perioperative fluid regiments: a randomised assessor-blinded multicenter trial. *Ann. Surg.* **238**:641-648, 2003.

48. Weinstein PD, Doerfler ME: Systemic Complications of Fluid Resuscitation. *Critical Care Clinics.* **8**:439-448, 1992.

49. Nisanevich V, Felsenstein I, Almogy G et al: Effect of intraoperative fluid management on outcome after intra-abdominal surgery. *Anaesthesiology.* **103**:25-32, 2005.

50. Holte K, Klarskov B, Christensen DS et al: Liberal versus restrictive fluid administration to improve recovery after laparoscopic cholecystectomy: a randomised double-blind study. *Ann. Surg.* **240**:892-899, 2004.

51. Bagshaw SM, Bellomor: The influence of volume management on outcome. *Current Opinion in Crit. Care.* **73**:541-548, 2007.

52. Kinch JW, Ryan TJ: Right Ventricular Infarction. *New Engl J Med.* **330**:1211-1217.

53. Ferrario M, Poli A, Previtali M et al: Haemodynamics of volume loading compared with dobutamine in severe right ventricular infarction. *Amer. J. Cardiol.* **74**:329-333, 1994.

54. Mercat A, Diel JL, Meyer G et al: Haemodynamic effects of fluid loading in acute massive pulmonary embolism. *Crit. Care Med.* **27**:540-544, 1999.

55. Griffel MI, Kaufman BS: Pharmacology of Colloids and Crystalloids. *Critic. Care Clinics.* **8**:235-253, 1992.

56. Ernest D, Belzberg AS, Dodek P: Distribution of normal saline and 5% albumin infusions in septic patients. *Crit. Care Med.* **27**:46-50, 1999.

57. Hauser J, Shoemaker WC, Turpin I et al: Oxygen transport responses to colloids and crystalloids in critically ill surgical patients. *Surg. Gynaecol. Obstet.* **150**:811, 1980.

58. Cochrane Group Albumin Reviewers. Human albumin administration in critically ill patients: systematic review of randomised controlled trials. *BMJ.* **317**:235-240, 1998.

59. Finfer S, Bellomo R, Boyce N et al: A comparison of albumin and saline for fluid resuscitation in the intensive care unit. *N. Engl. J. Med.* **350**:2247-2256, 2004.

60. Roberts I, Alderson P, Bunn F et al: Colloids versus crystalloids for fluid resuscitation in critically ill patients. *Cochrane Database Syst Rev.* CD000567, 2004.

61. The SAFE Study Investigators. Saline or albumin for fluid resuscitation in patients with traumatic brain injury. *New Engl J Med.* **357**:874-884, 2007.

62. Saline versus albumin fluid evaluation study investigators. Effect of baseline serum albumin concentration on outcome of resuscitation with albumin or saline in patients in intensive care units: analysis of data from the saline versus albumin fluid evaluation (SAFE) study. *BMJ.* **353**:1044-1046, 2006.

63. Dubois MJ, Carlos OJ, Melot C et al: "Albumin administration improves organ function in critically ill hypoalbuminaemic patients: a prospective randomised controlled, pilot study. *Crit. Care Med.* **34**:2536-2540, 2006.

64. Sort P, Navasa M, Arroyo V et al: Effects of intravenous albumin on renal impairment and mortality in patients with cirrhosis and spontaneous bacterial peritonitis. *New Engl J Med.* **341**:403-409, 1999.

65. Thomas G, Balk EM, Jaber BL. Effect of Insulin Therapy and Pentastarch Resuscitation on Acute Kidney Injury in Severe Sepsis. Commentary. Amer J Kidney Diseases. **52** 13-17 2008.

66. Acidosis is a predictable consequence of intraoperative infusion of 0.9% saline. *Amer. Soc. Anaes.* **90**:1247-1249, 1999.

67. Baldo-Enzi G, Baiocchi MR, Vignag et al: Analbuminaemia: a natural model of metabolic compensatory systems. *J. Inher. Metab. Dis.* **10**:317-322, 1987.

68. Traylor R, Pearl R: Crystalloid versus colloid versus colloid: All colloids are not created equal. *Anaesthesia and Analgesia.* **83**:209-212, 1996.

69. Boldt J: The holy grail of volume resuscitation in the septic patient is...... *Crit. Care Med.* **34**:248-251, 2006.

70. Hoffman JN, Volmar B, Laschke MW et al: Hydroxyethyl starch (130kD), but not crystalloid volume support, improves microcirculation during normotensive endotoxaemia. *Anaesthesiol.* **97**:460-470, 2002.

71. Funk W, Baldinger V: Microcirculatory perfusion during volume therapy. *Anaesthesiol.* **82**:975-982, 1995.

72. Persson J, Grande PO: Plasma volume expansion and transcapillary fluid exchange in skeletal muscle of albumin, Dextran, gelatin, hydroxyethyl starch, and saline after trauma in the cat. *Crit. Care Med.* **34**:2456-2462, 2006.

73. Boldt J: The Good, the Bad and the Ugly: should we completely banish human albumin from our Intensive Care Units. *Anaesthesia and Analgesia.* **91**:887-895, 2000.

74. De Jonge E, Levi M: Effects of different plasma substitutes on blood coagulation: A comparative review. *Crit. Care Med.* **29**:1261-1267, 2001.

75. Cittanova ML, Leblanc I, Egendre C Mouquet C et al: Effect of hydroxyethyl starch in brain-dead kidney donors on renal function in kidney transplant recipients. *Lancet.* **348**:1620-1622, 1996.

76. Schortgen F, Lacherade JC, Bruneel F et al: Effects of hydroxyethyl starch and gelatin on renal function in severe sepsis: a multicenter randomised study. *Lancet.* **357**:911-916, 2001.

77. Silva MR: Transcapillary fluid exchange. *Crit. Care Med.* **34**:2506-2507, 2006.

78. Harvey K: Blood avoidance for the critically ill: Another blow to liberalism? *Crit. Care Med.* **34**:2013-2014, 2006.

79. Carson JL, Noveck H, Berlin JA, Gould SA: Mortality and morbidity in patients with very low postoperative Hb levels who decline blood transfusion. *Transfusion.* **42**:812-818, 2002.

80. Weiskopf RB, Kramer JH, Viele M Neumann M et al: Acute severe isovolaemic anaemia impairs cognitive function and memory in humans. *Anaesthesiology.* **92**:1646-1652, 2000.

81. Weiskopf RB, Kramer JH, Viele M, Feiner J, Kelly S et al: Human cardiovascular and metabolic response to acute, severe isovolaemic anaemia. *JAMA.* **279**:217-221, 1998.
82. Hebert PC, Wells G, Blajchman MA Marshall J et al: A Multicenter Randomized, Controlled Clinical Trial of Transfusion Requirements in Critical Care. *NEJM.* **340**:409-417, 1999.
83. Agrawal N, Murphy JG, Cayten CG, Stahl WM: Blood transfusion increases the risk of infection after trauma. *Arch Surg.* **128**:171-177, 1993.
84. Carson JL, Duff A, Poses RM Berlin JA et al: Effects of anaemia and cardiovascular disease on surgical mortality and morbidity. *Lancet.* **348**:1055-1060, 1996.
85. Wu WC, Rathore SS, Wang Y et al: Blood transfusion in elderly patients with acute myocardial infarction. *New Engl J Med.* **345**:1230-1236, 2001.
86. Rao SV, Jollis JG, Harrington RA, Granger CB et al: Relationship of blood transfusion and clinical outcomes in patients with acute coronary syndromes. *JAMA.* **292**:1555-1562, 2004.
87. Hebert PC, Fergusson DA: Do transfusions get to the heart of the matter? *JAMA.* **292**:1610-1612, 2004.
88. Cooper DJ, Myles PS, McDermott FT: Prehospital hypertonic saline resuscitation of patients with hypotension and severe traumatic brain injury. *JAMA.* **291**:1350-1357, 2004.
89. Vassar MJ, Fischer RP, O'Brien PE et al: A multicenter trial for resuscitation of injured patients with 7.5% sodium chloride: the effect of added Dextran 70. The multicenter Group for the Study of Hypertonic Saline in Trauma Patients. *Arch. Surg.* **128**:1003-1011, 1993.
90. Battison Claire, Andrews Peter JD et al: Randomised, controlled trial on the effect of a 20% mannitol solution and a 7.5% saline/6% Dextran solution on increased intracranial pressure after brain injury. *Crit Care Med.* **33(1)**:196-202, 2005.
91. Bhardwaj Anish, Ulatowski John A: Hypertonic saline solutions in brain injury. *Curr. Opin. Crit. Care.* **10(2)**:126-131, 2004.
92. Cooper DJ, Myles PS, McDermott FT et al: Prehospital hypertonic saline resuscitation of patients with hypotension and severe traumatic brain injury. *JAMA.* **291**:1350-1357, 2004.
93. Oliviera RP, Weingartner R, Ribas EO: Acute haemodynamic effects of a hypertonic saline/Dextran solution in stable patients with severe sepsis. *Int. Care Med.* **28**:1574-1581, 2002.
94. Kamat Pradip, Vats Atul et al: Use of hypertonic saline for the treatment of altered mental status associated with diabetic Ketoacidosis. *Pediatric Crit. Care.* **4(2)**:239-242, 2003.

95. Beale RJ, Hollenberg S, Vincent JL, Parillo JE: Vasopressor and inotropic support in septic shock: An evidence-based review. *Crit. Care Med.* **32**(Suppl):S455-465, 2004.

96. Holmes CL: Vasoactive drugs in the intensive care unit. *Current Opinion in Crit. Care.* **11**:413-417, 2005.

97. Hayes MA, Timmins AC, Yau EHS et al: Elevation of systemic oxygen delivery in the treatment of critically ill patients. *New Engl J Med.* **330**:1717-1722, 1994.

98. Mullner M, Urbanek B, Havel C et al: Vasopressors for shock. The Cochrane Database of Systematic Reviews. **2** *Accession.*12732600, 2008.

99. Bourgoin A, Leone M, Delman A et al: Increasing mean arterial pressure in patients with septic shock : effects on oxygen variables and renal function. *Crit. Care Med.* **33**:780-786, 2005.

100. Albanese J, Leone M, Garnier F et al: Renal effects of norepinephrine in septic and non-septic patients. *Chest.* **126**:534-539, 2004.

101. Bellomo R, Bonventre J, Macias W, Pinsky M: Management of early acute renal failure: focus on post injury prevention. *Curr. Opinion in Critical Care.* **11**:542-547, 2005.

102. Holmes CL Walley KR: Vasopressin in the ICU. *Curr. Opin. Crit. Care.* **10**:442-448, 2004.

103. Dunser MW, Lindner KH, Volker W: Vasopressin. Multitalented hormone among shock hormones? *Critical Care Med.* **34**:562-564, 2006.

104. Stadlbauer KH, Wenzel V, Krismer AC et al: Vasopressin during uncontrolled haemorrhagic shock: Less bleeding below the diaphragm, more perfusion above. *Anaesth. Analg.* **101**:830-832, 2005.

105. Russel JA: Vasopressin in vasodilatory and septic shock. *Current Opinion in Crit. Care.* **13**:383-391, 2007.

106. Russell JA, Walley KR, Singer J et al: Vasopressin versus Norepinephrine Infusion in Patients with Septic Shock. *New Engl J Med.* **358**:877-887, 2008

107. Dunser MW, Mayr AJ, Ulmer H et al: Arginine Vasopressin in Advanced Vasodilatory Shock: A Prospective Randomized Controlled Study. *Circulation.* **107**:2313-2319, 2003.

108. De Backer D, Biston B, Devriendt J et al: Comparison of Dopamine and Norepinephrine in the Treatment of Shock. New Eng J Med **362**:779-789 2010

109. Cuthbertson BH, Hunter J, Webster NR: Inotropic agents in the critically ill. *Brit. J. Hosp. Med.* **56**:386-390, 1996.

110. De Backer D, Creuter J, Dubois MJ et al: The effects of dobutamine on microcirculatory alterations in patients with septic shock are independent of its systemic effects. *Crit. Care Med.* **34**:403-408, 2006.

ACID-BASE DISORDERS [1-14] PART 1.

"The great masses of the people will more easily fall victims to a great lie than to a small one"—Adolf Hitler.

Approximate normal values: $[H^+]$ = H^+ concentration.

Arterial blood pH	7.40 units.
Arterial blood $[H^+]$	40 nmol/L (0.000040 mmol/L).
Arterial blood pCo_2	40 mm/Hg.
Intracellular H^+	80-100 nmol/L.
Serum HCo_3^-	24 mmol/L Total Co_2 22-27 mmol/L.

H^+ (hydrogen ion) is a proton—a hydrogen atom without an electron. H^+ are not free in solution, react with water to form hydronium ions (H_3O^+), but can be considered as H^+ in practice. The concentration of free H^+ $[H^+]$ is only one millionth or less than the concentration of commonly measured electrolytes such as Na^+, K^+, Cl^- and Mg^{2+}. This unwieldy number, for example the normal $[H^+]$ of .000040 mmol/L, can be made manageable by multiplying by 1 million to give the concentration in nmol/L. Thus normal $[H^+]$ of arterial blood is 40nmol/L.

Despite the extremely low H^+ concentration, regulation is vital because H^+ binds to negatively charged molecules, such as proteins, causing alteration of their structure, shape and function [15]. In addition small cellular biosynthetic molecular intermediates are ionised and trapped within cells at <u>neutral</u> pH. Neutrality exists when H^+ =OH^- and varies with body and cellular temperature: pH is neutral at pH 7.0 at 25 degrees Celsius but neutral at pH 6.8 at 37 degrees Celsius. Neutral intracellular pH is defended by buffers, mainly proteins with imidazole groups, when temperature changes (Alphastat hypothesis). Thus a neutral pH is vital for trapping cellular intermediates to maintain optimum cellular function.

The range of pH compatible with life is greater than for other ions, varying from ~10 nmol/L (pH 8.0) to nearly 160 nmol/L (pH 6.8).

Hydrogen ions are present in aqueous solutions. The property of water to ionise, although slight, represents an inexhaustible supply of H^+ and OH^- ions. At 25°C 1L of pure water dissociates into 0.0000001 mol/L H^+ and 0.0000001 mol/L OH^- and has neutral P^H 7.0. The product $[H^+]$ $[OH^-]$ is 10^{-14}.

$$H_2O \longleftrightarrow OH^- + H^+.$$

The number 0.0000001 can be written as 1×10^{-7} which is 1 with the decimal point moved 7 places to the left. pH is the negative exponent (-7) of [H+] in moles changed to a positive number. Thus 0.0000001 mole [H+] which=10^{-7}, equals pH of 7.0.

H+, as in HCl (hydrochloric acid) added to water, combines with free OH- to form HOH (H_2O) and causes a proportionate decrease in OH-. Although the product of H+ and OH- remains the same at 10^{-14} the solution is acid because H+ is now greater than OH-. When NaOH is added to water OH- combines with H+ ions to form water leaving a greater concentration of OH- than H+. However the product [H+] [OH-] remains 10^{-14}.

By convention acid–base characteristics of a solution is based on hydrogen ion concentration [H+] rather than hydroxyl ion concentration [OH-].

Thus H+ > OH- is an acid solution and H+ < OH+ is an alkaline solution.

		Exponent	pH
H+0.00000001 mol/L (10^{-8})	and OH-10^{-6}	-8	8 alkaline
H+ 0.0000001 mol/L (10^{-7})	and OH-10^{-7}	-7	7 neutral
H+0.000001 mol/L (10^{-6})	and OH-10^{-8}	-6	6 acid

In each case the product [H+] [OH-] is 10^{-14}.

An acid is a substance which can donate (H+) to another substance; a base accepts a proton (H+)(Bronsted-Lowry model).The strength of acids or bases depends on their dissociation.

HCl is a strong acid because its disosciation to H+ and Cl- is nearly complete. K (dissociation constant) =~1.0. H_2CO_3 is weaker because less dissociates to form H+. Dissociation of a weak acid is as follows:

$$HA \longleftrightarrow H^+ + A^-$$

The reaction continues until the speed of the reaction of HA to H+ + A- equals the reverse reaction of H+ + A- to HA. A constant relationship or equilibrium occurs between the products on one side of a reaction and those on the other side.- law of mass action.

Thus at equilibrium K (constant): = [H+][A-]/HA

K, the measure of dissociation, increases as dissociation of HA to $[H^+] + [A^-]$ increases. Strong acids such as HCl have a K of ≈1.0 because their dissociation is almost complete. A buffer is most effective when the weak acid HA equals $[A^-]$, the conjugate base of the weak acid; alternatively when pH and pK are equal. The degree of dissociation also depends on the prevailing $[H^+]$ (pH) of a solution. For example: the ratio of HPO_4^{-2} to $H_2PO_4^-$ varies as follows:

	Ratio		HPO_4^{-2}	$H_2PO_4^-$
pH7.4	$[H^+]$ 40	in extracellular fluid	4	1
pH7.1	[H+] 80	in intracellular fluid	2	1
pH5.8	[H+]>1000	in urine	1	10

Use of the pH scale mystifies clinicians who try to interpret acid base problems. Advocates argue that low $[H^+]$ concentration in mmol/L is cumbersome—easily remedied by converting to nmol/L; and that $[H^+]$ measured by a potentiometer is proportional to the logarithm of $[H^+]$ concentration. However several other chemical measurements are extrapolated from non linear relationships, including logarithmic scales, and are reported in nmol or picomol concentrations.

Use of the pH scale requires an understanding of logarithms (an unnecessary use of clinician's time); access to logarithmic tables, which are usually inaccessible; and distorts the conceptual clarity of acid base data:

- For example a strong acid has a high K, which is easy to understand, but a low pK!!
- A pH change from 7.0 to 8.0 represents a 10 fold change in $[H^+]$.
- A change of pH of 0.3 from a pH of 7.4 is a decrease in $[H^+]$ of 20 nmol/L for a pH of 7.7; but an increase in 40 nmol/L for a pH of 7.1-despite a similar magnitude of pH change of 0.3 in both cases.

It should be a "simple" matter for laboratories, reporting blood gas measurements, to convert pH to $[H^+]$ (or to report both) for users of their data.

The following is a practical conversion guide for those who prefer to think in terms of $[H^+]$. pH and $[H^+]$ are inversely related: higher pH represents a lower $[H^+]$. The exponent of the H^+ in mol/L is used as the pH when the H^+ is a multiple of 10.

$$pH = \log \frac{1}{[H_+]} = -\log [H^+]$$

Note that the exponent, for example 6, 7 and 8 in 10^{-6}, 10^{-7}, 10^{-8}, which represents the number of zeros before 1, indicates p^H with the negative sign changed (negative logarithm to base 10). Thus:

H^+ mol/L		pH	nmol/L (H^+ X 10^9)
0.00000001	10^{-8}	8	10
0.0000001	10^{-7}	7	100
0.000001	10^{-6}	6	1000
0.00000004	4×10^{-8}	7.4	40

Fortunately, the normal H^+ of 40 nmol/L (.000000040 mol/L), is equivalent to pH of 7.40 which is easy to remember. Over a wide range of pH, 7.28-7.45, a change of [H^+] of 1 nmol/L corresponds to a pH deviation of 0.01 units [16]. An additional bit of useful information is that the log of 2.0 is 0.3: thus H^+ ion doubles or halves for each change in pH of 0.3 unit.

Given this the H^+ or pH can be derived if one of these are known.

pH		nmol/L	
7.40	(Normal)	H^+40	4×10^{-8}
7.70	increase by 0.3 from 7.4	H^+20	(half 40)
8.0	increase by 0.3 from 7.7	H^+10	(half 20), $H^+ = 10^{-8}$ mol/L
7.1	decrease by 0.3 from 7.4	H^+80	(double 40)
6.8	decrease by 0.3 from 7.1	H^+160	(double 80)
6.0		H^+1000	$H^+ = 10^{-6}$ mol/L
6.9	increase by 0.9 from 6.0	H^+125	(1000 x ½ x ½ x ½)
7.2	increase by 0.3 from 6.9	H^+62.5	(½ x 125)
7.0		H^+100	(10^{-7}) mol/L
7.3	increase of 0.3 from 7.0	H^+50	(½ x 100)
7.6	increase of 0.3 from 7.3	H^+25	(½ x 50)
7.5	increase by 0.3 from 7.2	H^+31.2	(½ x 62.5)
7.8	increase of 0.3 from 7.5	H^+ ~ 15	(½ x 31.25)

Table 1: Change of pH corresponding to change of H^+.

Despite the small quantity of total body H^+ ions ~ 3000 nmol, approximately 70, 000, 000 nmol of H^+ are generated daily. H^+ ions are generated in the body from 3 main sources:

* Complete oxidation of carbohydrate, fat and neutral amino acids generates CO_2—a volatile acid.

$$CO_2 + H_2O \longleftrightarrow H_2CO_3 \longleftrightarrow H^+ + HCO_3^-$$

* Incomplete oxidation of carbohydrate or fat generates lactic or keto acids.

Glucose → Pyruvic acid → Oxidation in Krebs cycle to $CO_2 + H_2O$

↘ Anaerobic metabolism to lactate.

Fatty Acids → Acetyl CoA → incomplete oxidation to Ketoacids (→ Ketoanions⁻ + H^+).

↘ Oxidation → $CO_2 + H_2O$.

Both lactic and keto acids however undergo further oxidation to HCO_3^-. This regenerates HCO_3^- consumed in their buffering.

Thus they only cause acidosis in the interval before complete oxidation or excretion by the kidney with cations.

* Metabolism of Aminoacids.

Metabolism of some dietary amino acids produces HCl, H_2SO4 or H_3PO4 (hydrochloric, sulphuric, phosphoric acid) with 'fixed anions' which require renal excretion.

Aminoacids with more carboxyl (COOH) than amino (NH_3) groups give rise to net HCO_3^- which requires excretion.

H^+ GENERATED FROM METABOLIC PRODUCTION OF CO_2.

H^+ ions are continuously generated from metabolism: ~ 10,000 - 15,000 mmol of CO_2 daily. Although not an acid CO_2 combines with water to form carbonic acid, which dissociates into H^+ and HCO_3^-.

$$H_2O + CO_2 \longleftrightarrow H_2CO_3 \longleftrightarrow H^+ + HCO_3$$

Ventilation eliminates this source of hydrogen ions as CO_2, (which is therefore called volatile acid). Decrease in alveolar respiration increases pCO_2 and thus H^+ ions—called respiratory acidosis: the higher the pCO_2 the higher the quantity of carbonic acid (H_2CO_3) which disosciates to H^+. Fortuitously, if the plasma HCO_3 is normal, 24 mmol/L, the [H^+] doubles or halves for each doubling or halving of pCO_2 in the absence of buffering.

DIETARY SOURCES OF H^+ AND HCO_3^-.

Amino acids have NH_3 and COOH groups. Metabolism of COOH gives rise to HCO_3^- and metabolism of amino groups to H^+. Metabolism of aminoacids, with equal numbers of carboxyl and amino groups, has no effect on acid –base balance because HCO_3^- formed from carboxyl groups consumes H^+ released from NH_3 groups in formation of urea. H^+ ions associated with anions such as sulphate, (SO_4^{2-}), phosphate and Cl^- in excess of sodium, which form strong acids, (fixed acids), must be excreted by kidneys as NH_4Cl or $NH_4SO_4^{2-}$. Anionic aminoacids with more carboxyl than amino groups form HCO_3^- on metabolism. This is excreted by kidneys or combines with H^+ in formation of urea.

Metabolism of Protein which produce H+ from aminoacids.

Metabolism of sulphur-containing aminoacids (methionine, cystine) produces H_2SO_4; phosphorylated aminoacids produce H_3PO_4 and metabolism of arginine and lysine produce HCl.These are 'fixed' anions associated with H^+–fixed because they must be excreted with a cation.

Methionine, cysteine → urea+CO_2+ H_2O + H_2SO_4 (~20-40mmol/day)
Arginine and Lysine → urea + CO_2 + H_2O + H^+Cl^-
Organic phosphates → HPO_4^{2-}, $H_2PO_4^-$, H_3PO_4
Strong anions SO_4^{2-} and Cl^- from meat sources require NH_4^+ or other cation for excretion. HPO_4^{2-} can be excreted as NaH_2PO_4 in acid urine and therefore does not obligate excretion of NH_4^+.

Metabolism of Dietary Protein which produce HCO3-

Carboxyl groups in amino acids from vegetables, fruit, leaves and dietary sources of citrate, succinate and malate lead to net HCO_3^- ion production. Despite the large amount of HCO_3^- produced alkalosis is prevented by formation of H^+ ions in synthesis of urea: H^+ produced in formation of urea reacts with HCO_3^- to produce carbonic acid which is eliminated as CO_2. This is important because alkaline urine promotes calcium precipitation which is potentially harmful. [17, 18]

$$NH_4^+ + CO_2 \longrightarrow 2H^+ + urea + H_2O$$

$$2HCO_3^- + 2H^+ \longrightarrow 2H_2CO_3 \longleftrightarrow CO_2 + H_2O.$$

Combining equations: $2NH_4^+ + 2HCO_3^- \longrightarrow urea + 3H_2O + CO_2$

Therefore food intake results in either:

- Net H^+ production, associated with SO_4^{2-} and Cl^-, especially if meat is consumed.
- Net HCO_3^- production predominantly from vegetables and fruit.

However metabolism of the majority of aminoacids generates urea, glucose, CO_2 and water and does not generate net H^+ or HCO_3^-.

Thus the main H^+ load in non-vegetarian diets is the need to excrete 'fixed' sulphuric and HCl acids. A normal meat intake of 100 g leads, on average, to 70 mmol H^+: 40 mmol from $H_2SO_4^{2-}$, ~30mmol from HCl, and $H_2PO_4^-$. The latter can be excreted as titratable acid whereas SO_4^{-2} and Cl^- require excretion with NH_4^+. [9] On the other hand consumption of a "vegetarian" diet may lead to net production of bicarbonate which is eliminated in formation of urea or excreted as HCo_3^-.

The liver plays a key role in acid-base balance.

Urea and glutamine are synthesised by anatomically discrete populations of cells in liver. [19-24] Thus liver orchestrates the balance between:

- Removal of HCO_3^- derived from carboxyl amino acids by producing urea. HCO_3^- resulting from metabolism of carboxylated aminoacids combines with H^+ which is formed in synthesis of urea.
- Synthesis of glutamine for production of NH_4^+ by kidney in order to excrete SO_4^{2-} and Cl^- as NH_4Cl. [19-24]

During acidosis ureagenesis is inhibited and liver produces glutamine from amino acids. This is transported to the kidney for NH_4^+ synthesis and enables excretion of Cl^- and other anions associated with H^+.

Glutamine $\longrightarrow$ $3CO_2 + 2NH_4^+ + 2HCO_3^-$ [21]

However proteolysis increases loss of aminoacids.

During alkalosis ureagenesis increases and HCO_3^- is eliminated in formation of urea.

Given the low concentration of H^+ ions, (in nanomol/L) in plasma and interstitial fluid, and daily production of H^+ ions in mmol amounts (70,000,000 nmol) an efficient buffering process is essential in the period before the kidney can correct acid-base disturbances. This is achieved by:

Immediate buffering in body fluids (within seconds)

Ventilation to change pCO_2 (minutes—hours)

Renal excretion of hydrogen ions / retention of bicarbonate: (hours-

days) (in Stewart-Fencl's model the excretion or retention of Cl^-)

BUFFERING IN THE BODY FLUIDS.

Buffers minimise changes of $[H^+]$ when acid or base are added.

Buffers act rapidly to temporarily remove or add H^+ in order to maintain $[H^+]$ as near normal as possible.

A buffer is a substance which can reversibly bind to or release hydrogen ions and thus limit the free H^+ concentration $[H^+]$ (p^H) which would otherwise result from addition of strong acid or base.

Buffer + H^+ $\longleftrightarrow$ H Buffer

Addition of strong acids, such as HCl, or strong bases, such as NaOH, which completely disosciate, increase or decrease H^+ ion considerably. For example 1mmol HCl added to water decreases the pH to 3.0. However combination with $NaHCO_3$ leads to formation of the weaker acid, carbonic acid. In addition carbonic acid dissociates to CO_2 and H_2O which further limits the increase in H^+ that would otherwise occur and therefore increases the power of this buffer system.

$$HCl + NaHCO_3 \longleftrightarrow Na\,Cl + H_2CO_3 \longleftrightarrow CO_2 + H_2O$$

Buffers do not eliminate H^+ ions but partly neutralise them until permanently removed. $NaHCO_3$ is consumed in buffering HCl but must ultimately be regenerated by the kidney. The buffer systems of the body are:

- Bicarbonate: (mainly ECF) $HCO_3^- $-$H_2CO_3$-$CO_2$ system
- Protein buffer system : $Protein^- + H+ \longleftrightarrow HProtein$ (mainly in cells)
- Haemoglobin buffer system: $Hb- + H+ \longleftrightarrow HbH$
  in red cells
- Phosphate buffer system: $HPO_4^{2-} + H^+ \longleftrightarrow H_2PO_4^-$
  in cells, acidification of urine, 8% in the ECF.
- Bone buffer system—contains large stores of carbonate⁻, phosphate⁻ and Na^+ which buffer H^+ ions.

$HCO_3^- - H_2CO_3 - CO_2$ BUFFER SYSTEM.

Consists of a relatively weak acid, H_2CO_3, and $NaHCO_3$.

On addition of strong acid, for example lactic acid:

$$Lactic\ acid + NaHCO_3 \longleftrightarrow Na\ lactate + H_2CO_3 \longrightarrow CO_2 + H_2o$$

$(H^+ lactate^-)$

The dissociation of H_2CO_3 to CO_2, which is eliminated by lungs, decreases concentration of H_2CO_3 and increases the power of this buffer system.

If a strong base such as NaOH is added:

$$NaOH + H_2CO_3 \longleftrightarrow Na\,HCO_3 + H_2O$$

The weak base $NaHCO_3$ replaces the strong base NaOH.

PROTEIN BUFFER SYSTEM.

Imidazole groups of proteins are the major contributors to intracellular buffering. Protein is composed of carboxyl groups—COOH and at least one amino group (NH_2) and are amphoteric: In buffering they act as acids or bases in cells and plasma. The free carboxyl group acts like an acid by releasing H^+ when the $[H^+]$ decreases and the NH_2 group accepts H^+ when $[H^+]$ increases. The negative charges of protein in plasma can take up or release H^+ and contribute to buffering in plasma and cells.

$$
\begin{array}{ccccc}
\text{R} & & \text{R} & & \text{R} \\
| & +H^+ & | & & | \\
NH_3-C\text{-}COOH & \longleftarrow & NH_2-C-COOH & \longrightarrow & NH_2\text{-}C\text{-}Coo^- + H+ \\
| & & | & & | \\
\text{H} & & \text{H} & & \text{H}
\end{array}
$$

PHOSPHATE BUFFER SYSTEM.

This is relatively unimportant in buffering extracellular fluid because its concentration is low but is important in cells, where phosphate is the main anion, and in urine where change of HPO_4^{2-} to $H_2PO_4^-$ enables titratable acid excretion.

$$Na_2HPO_4^- + HCl \longleftrightarrow NaH_2PO_4^- + NaCl$$

A strong acid HCl is replaced by a weak acid NaH_2PO_4.

HAEMOGLOBIN BUFFER SYSTEM. (figure 1)

Haemoglobin has charged side chains which can bind H^+. CO_2 produced in tissues diffuses freely into red cells and forms H_2CO_3, catalysed by carbonic anhydrase, which increases the speed of reaction 5000 times. H_2CO_3 dissociates into HCO_3^- and H^+. HCO_3^- is exchanged with Cl^- present in plasma (chloride shift) while haemoglobin takes up H^+ resulting from the reaction. This enables transport of the majority of CO_2 as bicarbonate.

$$Hb^- + H^+ \longleftrightarrow HHb$$

When haemoglobin releases oxygen and takes up CO_2, reduced haemoglobin accepts H^+ ions more avidly: deoxygenated haemoglobin takes up 0.7mol H^+ for each mole O_2 released which offsets acidosis resulting from CO_2 carriage. If the respiratory quotient is 0.7 (0.7 mol CO_2 produced for each 1.0 mol O_2 consumed) $[H^+]$ (pH) does not change and buffering is complete.

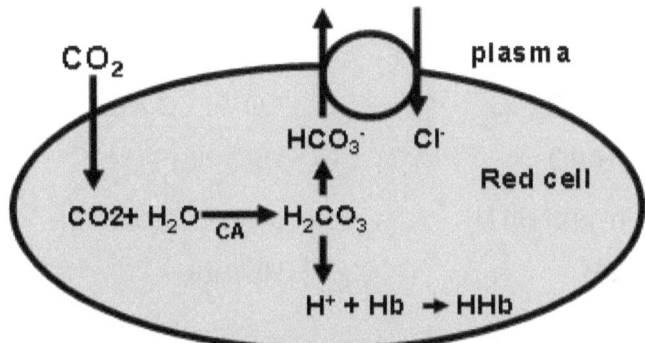

Figure 1: *Model of red cell bicarbonate: chloride exchange in buffering of H^+. CA = carbonic anhydrase. Hb = haemoglobin.*

BONE BUFFERING.

Bone carries out considerable buffering, especially in chronic acidosis of renal failure. H^+ exchanges with Na^+ and Ca^{2+} in bone in acute acidosis but mainly Ca^{2+} in chronic acidosis. This can cause osteomalacia, nephrocalcinosis and urolithiasis.

TOTAL BODY BUFFERING.

Buffering in plasma is immediate; interstitial buffering takes minutes; and complete cellular buffering takes several hours.

Approximately 50% of buffering of acid is carried out by E.C.F. and 50% by cells, but bone and cellular buffering increase with time. To maintain electroneutrality, Cl⁻ or other anion must enter cells, or cations, such as K^+, leave cells in exchange for H^+. The concerted action of several acid-base transporters in cell membranes defends cells against changes in pH: $Na:H^+$: antiporters; H^+ pumps and $Cl^-:HCO_3^-$ exchangers. Cellular pH and buffering may be more important than extracellular but is difficult to measure.

ISOHYDRIC PRINCIPLE.

All buffer systems are in equilibrium because H^+ ions are common to all. Therefore measurement of one system reflects the H^+ concentration (pH) in all the others. However cellular H^+ concentration is higher than extracellular concentration (figure 2).

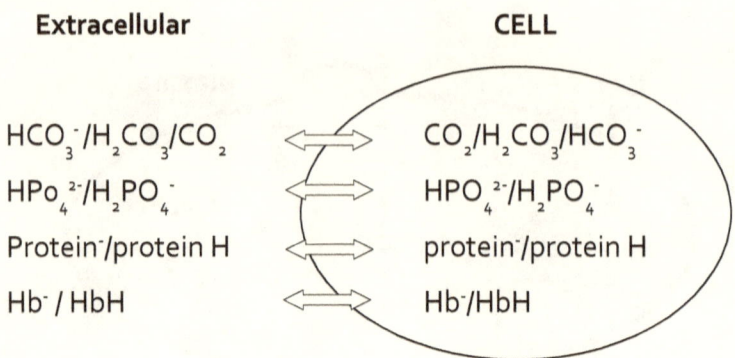

Figure 2: Buffer systems in cell and extracellular fluid. These are in equilibrium so that measurement in one buffer system reflects H^+ concentration in others. (= isohydric principle).

In acid-base homeostasis all approaches should satisfy the following:

- Electroneutrality: sum of cations = sum of anions.
- Dissociation equilibria of acids and bases.
- Conservation of mass. The total concentration of a substance must be accounted for by the sum of disosciated plus undisosciated forms.

Assessment of acid-base status is traditionally based on the HCO_3 H_2CO_3 - CO_2 system because:

- Serum HCO_3^- and arterial pCO_2 are easy to measure.
- Both CO_2, produced by metabolism, and H_2CO_3, which is converted to CO_2, are eliminated by lungs as CO_2. Changes in arterial pCO_2 compensate for changes in H^+.
- HCO_3^- excreted or produced by kidney provides the non respiratory compensation for H^+ ion (pH) changes.

Although cellular ($[H^+]$) pH may be more important than extracellular pH ($[H^+]$), changes in cellular pH, which are difficult to measure, are reflected by extracellular pH ($[H^+]$).

Acid base balance thus depends on two key variables:

- pCO_2 – respiratory component.
- HCO_3^- - metabolic component (or Cl^- rather than HCO_3^-)in the Stewart Fencl approach-discussed later.

HCO_3^- METABOLIC COMPONENT. [25-27]

Arterial pH of blood is 7.40 (H^+ 40nmol/L) which is slightly alkalaemic. Venous blood pH is less alkalaemic because CO_2 produced by tissues contributes to $[H^+]$.

Total plasma CO_2: (measured in venous blood with electrolytes) Normal range (22-27 mmol/L).

A measure of HCO_3^- plus dissolved CO_2. Plasma total CO_2 varies with pCO_2. It is increased by high pCO_2 and decreased by low pCO_2. In the range of pCO_2 40-100 mmHg bicarbonate rises by approximately 1 mmol/L for every 10-15 mm Hg increase of pCO_2. Moreover pCO_2 reflects CO_2 produced locally: thus exercise and tourniquet should be avoided in blood sampling.

Standard bicarbonate (normal 24-25mmol/L).

To make plasma total CO_2 more representative of the metabolic component of acid-base balance—to exclude the effect of pCO_2, blood is equilibrated with a normal pCO_2 of 40mmHg at 38°C, to give standard bicarbonate. However this does not take buffering by haemoglobin and albumin into account. This has led to measurement of:

Whole Buffer Base. (40-42 mEq/L.).

The sum of the concentration of all blood buffers: HCO_3^-, haemoglobin and albumin. It is the amount of acid or base that must be added to 1L of blood at 38° C while keeping pCO_2 constant at 40mmHg. It is the same as the strong ion difference (SID). Strong ion difference (SID), is the sum of cations minus (Cl⁻ + strong organic acids). Whole buffer base is estimated from standard HCO_3^- by multiplying the deviation of standard HCO_3^- from a mean of 22.9 by 1.2, a correction factor derived from pH, PCO_2 and haemoglobin, using the normogram established empirically by Siggard-Andersen.

Base Excess.   positive value (>5) = excess base.
                   negative value (<5) = excess fixed acid.

The extent to which whole buffer base deviates from normal: the quantity of strong acid or base required to restore pH to 7.40 in blood equilibrated under standard conditions of pCO_2 40mmHg and 38°C.

A negative base excess (< -5.0 mmol/L) is similar to a low plasma bicarbonate and indicates that an acidosis is present.

Standard Base Excess.

However the whole blood buffer base does not truly reflect extracellular acid-base status because haemoglobin is absent in interstitial fluid. This was modified by assigning a value for haemoglobin of 50g/L instead of 150g/L (ratio of plasma to interstitial fluid =1:3). This is called Standard Base Excess.

In essence:

Total plasma CO_2 = plasma HCO_3^- + contribution from dissolved CO_2.

Standard bicarbonate = Plasma total CO_2 minus dissolved CO_2.

Whole buffer base: = contribution of plasma HCO_3^-, blood and albumin. Also equals SID. (Strong ion difference)

Standard buffer base = whole buffer base but using haemoglobin of 50g/L rather than 150g/L.

Base excess or standard base excess = deviation of buffer base, or Standard buffer base respectively from normal:

Minus >5mmol/L = acidosis.

Plus >5mmol/L = alkalosis.

A good account of the various measures of the bicarbonate component of acid base balance is given in references 25-27.

The following diagram shows the interrelations of the HCO_3^- - H_2CO_3 – CO_2 system and rationalises the quantitative aspects of H^+ concentration in blood.

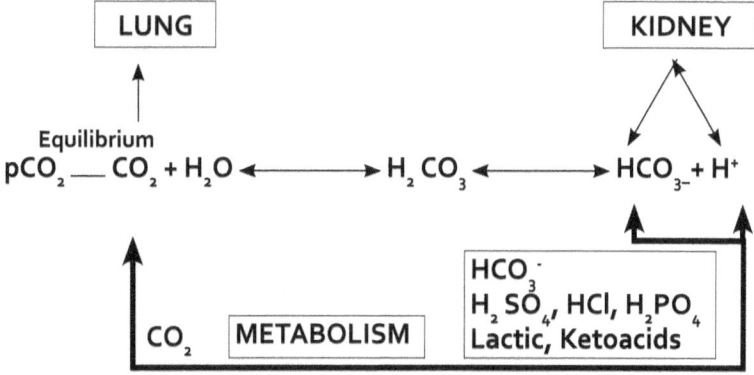

Figure 3: Interrelations of HCo_3^- - H_2CO_3 – pCO_2 system of buffering.

Metabolism gives rise to:

- CO_2 *from complete oxidation of fatty acids or glucose.*
- *Lactic or keto-acids from incomplete oxidation of fatty acids and glucose.*
- *Sulphate, chloride and phosphate associated with H^+ from food.*
- HCO_3^- *from aminoacids with COOH groups greater than NH_3 groups.*

CO_2 is excreted in ventilation and thus decreases H_2CO_3 - H^+ ions of strong acids react with $NaHCO_3$ and form $H_2CO_3^-$ which dissociates to CO_2 + H_2O.

H^+ ions increase the ratio of H_2CO_3 / HCO_3^-.

$$H + HCO_{3-} \rightleftharpoons H_2CO_3 \rightleftharpoons CO_2 + H_2O$$

K_1 is the extent to which H_2CO_3 disosciates to HCO_3^- + H^+

$$H_2CO_3^- = K_1 (HCO_3^- + H^+)$$

Rearranging the equation:

$$H^+ = K_1 H_2CO_3/HCO_3^-$$

H_2CO_3 dissociates into CO_2 + H_2O, but occurs too rapidly to measure [1, 10, 28]. Solubility of CO_2 in plasma is .03.

Therefore $\quad [H^+] = K_2 [.03\ pCO_2] / [HCO_3^-]$ [1, 10, 28]

K_2 is the amount that H_2CO_3 disosciates to form CO_2 -approximately. 0008%. [28]

Therefore $[H+] = .0008 \times .03 / HCO_3^-$ mmol/L

$$= .000024 \, pCO_2 / [HCO_3^-] \text{ mmol.}$$

To convert this to manageable numbers this is multiplied by 1 million (10^6) to give [H$^+$] in nmol/L rather than mmol/L.Therefore:

$$[H^+] \text{ nmol/L} = 24 \, pCO_2 / HCO_3^- \qquad \text{(approximately)}$$

The ratio of pCO_2 to HCO_3^-, not the amount of either, governs [H$^+$] or pH. This key equation shows that if plasma HCO_3^- is kept constant, at 24 mmol/L, [H$^+$] doubles or halves as the pCO_2 doubles or halves. Alternatively, if pCO_2 is kept constant, and HCO_3^- doubles or halves [H$^+$] will halve or double.

The constant 24 is easy to remember because the numerical value, fortuitously, is the same as normal plasma bicarbonate ~ 24mmol/L. pCO_2 must be the numerator because the [H$^+$] will increase with a rise in pCO_2 and decrease when HCO_3^- (the denominator) is increased.

When plasma HCO_3^- is 24mmol/L (normal) and pCO_2 is normal (40 mmHg).

$$H^+ \text{ 4onmol/l} = pCO_2 \text{ 40mmHg} = P^H \text{ 7.40}$$

Figure 3 also illustrates that CO_2 is eliminated by lungs, while H$^+$ associated with H_2SO_4 from food, lactic and ketoacids, derived from incomplete oxidation of glucose and fatty acids, are excreted.

Each H$^+$ excreted by the kidney generates HCO_3^- which is reabsorbed. Thus the kidneys role can be considered as excretion of H$^+$ or reabsorption of HCO_3^-.

Each net gain or loss of HCo_3^- must be accompanied by an equivalent loss or gain of Cl$^-$ or be accompanied by a cation to maintain electroneutrality. In excretion of acid, H_2PO_4 or NH_4Cl is excreted, while $NaHCO_3^-$ (or other cation / HCO_3^-) is reabsorbed.

Buffering limits change in [H$^+$] pH.

The effectiveness of buffering is shown in the following example:

If the HCO_3^- is 24mmol/L, pCO2 40mmHg, K=24.

$$H^+ = \frac{24 \times pCO_2}{HCO_3^-} = \frac{24 \times 40L}{24} = 40nmol/L$$

If 12mmol of HCl (12 million nmol H$^+$) is added to IL of plasma 12mmol of HCO_3^- is consumed.

12mmol HCl + 12mmol $NaHCO_3$ ⟶ 12 mmol NaCl + 12mmol H_2CO_3 ⟶ CO_2 + H_2O.

The normal $NaHCO_3$ of 24 mmol/L decreases to 12 mmol/L.

The [H$^+$] is now $= \dfrac{24 \times 40}{12} = 80nmol/L$ (pH 7.1).

99.99% of H+ has been immediately buffered. Subsequently cellular buffering ($\approx$50%) contributes so that HCO_3^- in each litre of plasma will only decrease to 18mmol/L. This results in [H$^+$] of 53nmol/L) pH~7.28).

On the other hand if 12 mmol of HCl were added to 3L water rather than plasma the [H$^+$] would increase to 12,000,000 /3 = 4,000,000 nmol/L.

Two further systems compensate to limit acid base change and to restore buffer base.

* Respiratory compensation.
* Regeneration of HCO_3^- lost in buffering.

RESPIRATORY COMPENSATION SYSTEM.

Respiratory compensation for metabolic acidosis or alkalosis takes minutes to hours to be fully effective because H$^+$ and HCO_3^- pass slowly into cells compared to CO_2. Medullary chemoreceptors respond to cerebrospinal fluid (CSF)[H$^+$] rather than blood pH. If pCO$_2$ increases rapid diffusion of CO$_2$ into cells stimulates both central and peripheral chemoreceptors. During metabolic acidosis CO$_2$ decreases, secondary to peripheral chemoreceptor stimulation, and rapidly moves into cerebrospinal fluid (CSF), while H$^+$ ions, which are impermeable, take time to move into CSF.[28]. Paradoxically CSF initially becomes alkaline. Full respiratory stimulation (compensation) takes time to develop but persists for longer. [28] Respiratory compensation for metabolic acidosis is ultimately greater than for metabolic alkalosis, presumably because hypoventilation, in response to metabolic alkalosis, decreases pO_2, which is potentially harmful.

pCO_2 normally decreases between 1-1.5mmHg (average 1.2mmHg) for each mmol decrease in HCO_3^- during metabolic acidosis. The pCO_2 response to acidosis also approximates the last 2 digits of the pH to a pCO_2 of 15mmHg. For example the appropriate pCO_2 compensation for arterial blood pH of 7.20 should be 20 mmHg.

During metabolic alkalosis pCO_2 approximately increases by 0.5mmHg for each1 mmol increase of plasma HCO_3^- above normal but rarely rises above a pCO_2 of 50 mmHg. [28]

The combination of buffering in interstitial fluids, cells and lungs restores $[H^+]$ towards normal. For example in buffering lactic acid:

$$H^+ \text{ lactate}^- + NaHCO_3^- \leftrightarrow Na^+ \text{ lactate}^- + H_2CO_3 \leftrightarrow CO_2 + H_2O$$

However buffering reduces bicarbonate and other buffers. Plasma HCO_3^- of 2.4 mmol/L has 1/10 the buffering capacity of an HCO_3^- of 24 mmol/L. Further reduction in plasma HCO_3^- of only1.2 mmol/L doubles the arterial blood $[H^+]$ if respiration and buffering remain the same. Increase in respiration due to metabolic acidosis is detrimental because work of breathing and pulmonary oxygen consumption increase disproportionately. Restoration of serum HCO_3^- and other buffers must be carried out by kidneys to produce new HCO_3^- (or excrete H^+ and Cl^- ions).

RENAL COMPENSATORY SYSTEM

The kidneys excrete net H^+ ion or HCO_3^- (or excrete or reabsorb Cl^-) to compensate for acidosis or alkalosis of both respiratory and metabolic origin. This takes hours—days because of time taken to synthesise ammonium to accompany Cl^-.

For each Cl^- excreted without cation one HCO_3^- is reabsorbed and vice versa. Both H^+ and HCO_3^- are generated from H_2O and CO_2 in tubule cells.

Thus if H^+ is secreted into the tubular lumen HCO_3^- is reabsorbed into blood. Either HCO_3^- or H^+ is excreted, depending on acid base balance. Plasma bicarbonate, which has been consumed in buffering H^+, is regenerated by the kidney and H^+ excreted. Thus the buffering process in blood is reversed.

The role of the kidney in acid base balance can be thought of as either net H^+ excretion and HCO_3^- reabsorption or net H^+ reabsorption and HCO_3^- excretion. If HCO_3^- is reabsorbed, without a cation, Cl^- must be excreted; if HCO_3^- is excreted without a cation Cl^- must be reabsorbed to balance electrical charges. Therefore the role of the kidney in acid-base balance can also be considered to be the excretion or reabsorption of Cl^- without a strong cation (strong cations = Na^+, K^+, Ca^{2+}, Mg^{2+}) Given that HCO_3^- can be synthesised, but Cl^- cannot, chloride excretion with NH_4^+ is the mechanism for changing the metabolic component of acid-base balance. The kidney has 2 main roles in the acid base balance:

- To reclaim (reabsorb) the large amount of filtered HCO_3^- ~ (3000 mmol/day at a GFR of 100 ml/min). This will not generate new HCO_3^-.
- To generate new HCO_3^- or excrete Cl^-; or to excrete HCO_3^- efficiently if there is excess.

In generating new HCO_3^- proximal tubules also play an important role in synthesising NH_4^+ and HCO_3^- from glutamine produced by liver.

Simplistically, HCO_3^- is exchanged for Cl^-, probably in distal tubules. NH_4Cl is then eliminated in urine and HCO_3^- reabsorbed.

Although the traditional approach focuses on HCO_3^- regeneration and reabsorption it is conceptually easier to view NH_4^+ synthesis as the means to excrete Cl^- without Na^+, thus increasing the extracellular Na^+: Cl^- ratio and the strong ion difference (SID). An explanation of this approach follows later. During alkalosis HCO_3^- is excreted in exchange for Cl^- which is reabsorbed.

Cellular mechanisms. [2, 9, 10, 11, 13-14, 19-24, 29-37]

Proximal tubules reabsorb ~ 90% of filtered HCO_3^- and in addition synthesise NH_4^+ and HCO_3^- from glutamine for use in generation of new HCO_3^- (secretion of H^+ and Cl^-) by distal tubules.

Reabsorption of filtered bicarbonate does not produce additional HCO_3^-: it only reclaims HCO_3^- filtered. This action is therefore called reclamation and should be distinguished from regeneration in which HCo_3^-, in excess of that filtered, is reabsorbed and increases total body bicarbonate. Proximal tubules do not simply reabsorb $NaHCO_3$ directly: they do this by indirectly converting HCO_3^- to CO_2 in tubule lumens and reform HCO_3^- in tubule cells as shown in fig 4.

The net result is reabsorption of filtered $NaHCO_3$ by this indirect process. Most HCO_3^- reclamation is due to transcellular coupling of $Na^+:H^+$ exchangers (NHE-3) and $H^+:ATPase$ pumps with basolateral $Na^+: HCO_3$ (NBC) cotransporters.

Proximal tubules also plays a key role in production of new HCO_3^- by synthesising $NH_4^+ + HCO_3^-$ for excretion of NH_4^+ by distal tubules—called regeneration). This occurs as follows:

Glutamine is synthesised by cells in a specific anatomic location in the liver. Synthesis increases during metabolic acidosis and decreases during alkalosis.[19-21]Glutamine is absorbed into proximal tubule cells by specific (SNAT3) transporters. [21-23] Glutamine is converted to NH_4^+ and HCO_3^- in proximal tubule cells.

$$Glutamine \longrightarrow NH_4^+ + HCO_3^-$$

NH_4^+ is secreted into the lumen by taking the place of H^+ on NHE-3 ($Na^+:$ H^+) exchangers. [22-24]

NH_4^+ is reabsorbed into cells in the ascending loop of Henle by replacing K^+ on $Na^+ :K^+ :2Cl^-$ cotransporters or is reabsorbed by the paracellular route due to the positive lumen potential created by K^+ secretion. NH_4^+ is transported out of cells, enters the interstitial part of the medulla and is concentrated there. [21-24].NH_4^+ dissociates into NH_3 and H^+ in the medulla.

$$NH_4^+ \longleftrightarrow NH_3 + H^+$$

NH_4^+ is also recycled by counter current exchange, from the TALH into descending loops of Henle This concentrates NH_4^+ in the medulla. [22, 23, 31, 32]

85% of filtered $HCO_3^-$is reabsorbed in proximal tubules; 10% in loops of Henle and approximately 5-10% by distal convoluted tubules and collecting ducts. There is normally a threshold for HCO_3^- reabsorption which maintains serum HCO_3^- at normal levels, ~ 24 mmol/L.

When the threshold is exceeded, as a result of high dietary base intake, $HCo_3^-$is not reabsorbed beyond the Tm (Tm = maximum HCO_3 reabsorption). This threshold is increased by sodium depletion, raised pCO_2, aldosterone, angiotensin II [24] and severe K^+ deficiency. The Tm HCO_3^- is decreased by volume expansion and low pCO_2.

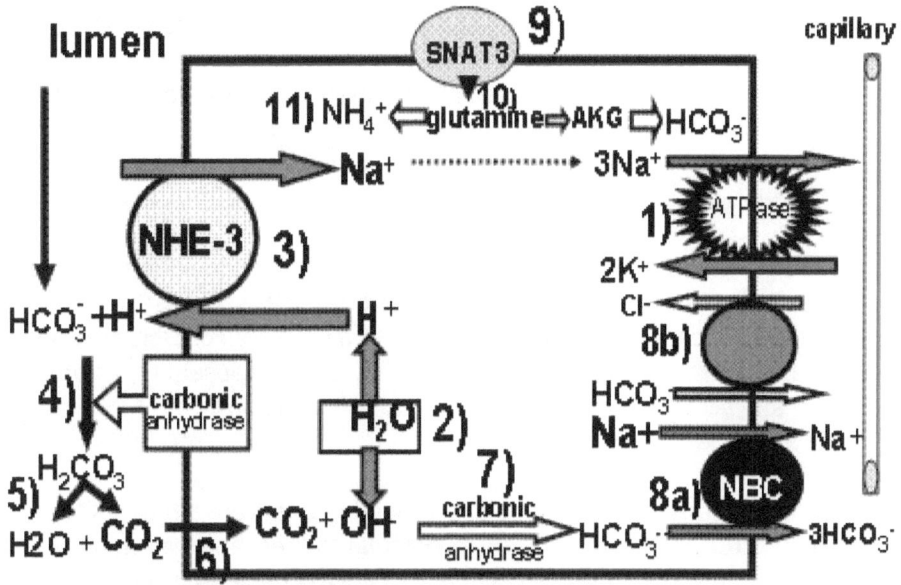

Figure 4: Simplified model of role of proximal tubule cell in acid base balance. Numbers correspond to numbers in the text below.

AKG = α ketoglutarate. Oval clear Circle = Na⁺:H⁺ exchanger (NHE-3). Oval black circle is Na⁺:3HCO₃ transporter (NBC) and grey circle Cl⁻:HCO₃⁻ exchanger. Serrated oval circle = Na⁺:K⁺ pump.

1. $Na^+:K^+$ pumps generate negative intracellular potential and low intracellular Na^+.
2. H^+ ions are generated from dissociation of water.
3. H^+ is exchanged for Na^+ by Na^+: H^+ exchangers,(NHE3) and enters the lumen).
4. H^+ ions in lumen react with filtered HCO_3^- to form H_2CO_3 accelerated 500 times by carbonic anhydrase, on the brush border of tubular cell.
5. Luminal H_2CO_3 rapidly dissociates into CO_2 and H_2O.
6. CO_2, which is lipid soluble, rapidly diffuses into tubule cell.
7. CO_2 reacts with the OH^- remaining from dissociation of water. The reaction is accelerated by intracellular carbonic anhydrase.
8. HCO_3^- is reabsorbed with Na^+ on $Na^+:3HCO_3^-$ exchangers (NBC) (8a); or transported by HCO_3^-: Cl^- exchangers (8b) through basolateral membrane into interstitial fluid and circulation. NBC is up regulated in response to metabolic acidosis and potassium depletion.

9. Glutamine is absorbed into proximal tubule cells by specific (SNAT 3) transporters [21-23]
10. Glutamine is converted to NH_4^+ and HCo_3 via α ketoglutarate in proximal tubule cells. Glutamine $NH_4^+ + HCO_3^-$
11. NH_4^+ is secreted into the lumen by taking the place of H^+ on NHE-3 (Na^+: H^+) exchangers

Fine tuning of acid-base balance is carried out by collecting ducts of distal tubules. Two types of cell α (A for acid secretion) and β (B for base secretion) secrete acid or base into tubular lumens. [33-35] α Cells are concentrated and active in outer medullary collecting ducts; [35] β cells are absent here but are present and act in cortical collecting ducts. [33] Non α non β cells function in either way. [32, 34]

Terminal portions of inner medullary collecting ducts are a major site for net acid secretion. [35] There are three postulated mechanisms for entry of NH_4^+ or NH_3 into the lumen of collecting ducts to enable excretion. [21-23]

1. NH_3, which dissociates from NH_4^+ in the medulla, enters the tubular lumen by non-ionic diffusion and is fixed by H^+ secreted by H: ATPase pumps, to form NH_4^+, which is not lipid soluble, and cannot diffuse back.
2. NH_4^+ enters collecting duct cells by replacing K^+ on either basolateral Na^+: K^+ pumps, Na^+ K^+ $2Cl^-$ cotransporters or NH_4^+ transporters-RhBG.
3. NH_4^+ moves from cell to lumen by NH_4^+ transporters. (RhCG) [19, 21, 23]

During potassium deficiency NH_4^+ can take the place of K^+ on basolateral Na^+: K^+ pumps or Na^+ K^+ $2Cl^-$ cotransporters which decreases K^+ entry into cells. [32] This increases urine NH_4^+ (Cl^-) excretion and causes metabolic alkalosis. NH_4^+ synthesis also increases in proximal tubules. [32]

During hyperkalaemia less NH_4^+ is synthesised in proximal tubules and less NH_4^+ enters α intercalated cells in place of K^+. α cells secrete H^+, which acidifies tubular fluid, and secrete NH_4^+ into tubular fluid. Cl^- is secreted into the lumen to maintain electro neutrality$^+$. H^+ is secreted by:

* Proton pumps (H^+ ATPase).
* H^+: K^+ pumps: increase K^+ reabsorption in exchange for H^+ secretion when deficiency occurs. [36]

Cellular mechanisms in the distal Tubule. [11, 13, 14, 36, 37] (figure 5)

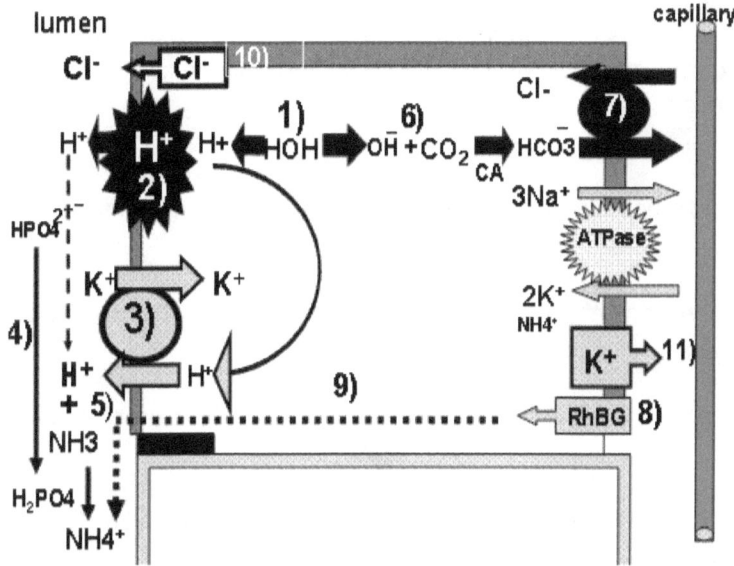

Figure 5. α intercalated cell (Numbers correspond to text below.)

1. H^+ and OH^- ions are generated from dissociation of H_2O
2. H^+ is secreted by proton (H^+ ATPase) pumps or
3. in exchange for K^+ on $H^+:K^+$ ATPase exchangers.
4. H^+ either combines with HPO_4^{2-} to form $H_2PO_4^-$
5. or with NH_3 to form NH_4.
   (NH_3 diffuses into the tubule lumen from the medulla and combines with H^+ to form NH_4^+. Formation of non lipid NH_4^+ prevents its back leak into the cell).
6. CO_2 in cell combines with OH^-, remaining from dissociation of H_2O, to form HCo_3^- catalysed by carbonic anhydrase.: $CO_2 + OH^- = HCO_3^-$
7. HCo_3^- exits cells on $Cl^-:HCo_3^-$ exchangers.
8. NH_4^+ enters cells by NH_4^+ transporters, (RhBG), or by substituting for K^+ on $Na^+:K^+$ pumps or basolateral $Na^+:K^+:2Cl^-$ transporters.
9. NH_4^+ enters the tubular lumen by NH_4^+ transporters.
10. Cl^- enters tubular lumen to accompany NH_4^+ via Cl^- channels.
11. K^+ exits cell via basolateral K^+ channels

α cells are responsible for excreting NH_4Cl or $H_2PO_4^-$ with another cation; β cells are responsible for excreting $NaHCO_3^-$ in urine and reabsorbing Cl^-. Operation of $Cl^-:HCo_3^-$ exchangers are linked to excretion of NH_4Cl. The principal method of acid excretion is achieved by excretion of NH_4Cl rather than $H_2Po_4^-$.Combination of H^+ ions with HPO_4^{2-} or NH_3 fixes H^+ ions, prevents their leak back into cells, and lowers H^+ concentration.

This decreases the luminal-cellular H⁺ gradient and enables excretion of large amounts of H⁺ in maximally acid urine. (pH 4.4.) The net effect is to excrete NH_4Cl and NaH_2PO_4. Synthesis and excretion of NH_4^+ is summarised. fig 6:

Synthesis of glutamine by liver increases during acidosis.

Glutamine enters proximal tubule cells by SNAT3 transporters.

Glutamine is converted to $NH_4^+ + HCO_3^-$ in renal proximal tubules.

NH_4^+ is secreted into lumen by substituting for H⁺ on Na⁺: H⁺ (NHE) transporters.

NH_4^+ moves into TAL cells by replacing K⁺ on the Na⁺: K⁺ 2Cl⁻ cotransporters of the TAL; or enters medulla through cells.

NH_4^+ is recycled and concentrated in the medulla by countercurrent exchange.

NH_4^+ dissociates to NH_3: $NH_4^+ \longleftrightarrow NH_3 + H^+$

NH_3 diffuses into lumen; or NH_4^+ is transported into α cells by RhBG NH_4^+ transporters or by substituting for K⁺ on Na⁺:K⁺ pumps.

NH_3 combines with H⁺, secreted by α cells, in tubular lumen in collecting ducts to form NH_4^+ which is excreted with Cl⁻. Alternatively NH_4^+ is secreted directly into the lumen by RhBC transporters.

Figure 6: Model of synthesis and excretion of ammonium (CD= collecting duct)

Metabolic acidosis. [21-24]

A proton [H⁺] sensing system stimulates several transporters during metabolic acidosis. [21]

- Liver increases glutamine synthesis. Glutamine transporters (SNAT 3) are up regulated and increase entry of glutamine into proximal tubule cells for NH_4^+ synthesis.
- $NaHCo_3$ reabsorption increases in renal proximal tubules from stimulation of Na^+:H^+ exchangers (NHE-3) and basolateral Na^+: $3HCO_3^-$ cotransporters.
- Metabolic acidosis increases NH_4^+ reabsorbed by Na^+ K^+ $2Cl$ cotransporters in the TALH. This is transported into the medulla and increases medullary NH_4^+. The increase facilitates NH_3 entry into the lumen of the CD [23]. Ammonium transporters (RhBG, RhCG) increase in metabolic acidosis [22,23] and increase cellular uptake and secretion of NH_4^+ into the lumen.

Urine H^+ secretion depends on:

1. Production of negative voltage in the lumen of principal cells by Na^+ reabsorption without Cl^-.
2. Secretion of H^+ by H^+: ATPase or H^+: K^+ pumps.
3. Aldosterone and angiotensin2 secretion. Aldosterone secretion drives Na^+ reabsorption by sodium channels (ENaC), stimulates Na^+:K^+ ATPase pumps, H^+ :ATPase and H^+:K^+ ATPase pumps. Angiotensin 2, produced both locally and systemically, increases proximal and distal tubule acid secretion and HCO_3^- reabsorption. [24]
4. High medullary concentration of NH_3 and its diffusion into the lumen to combine with and trap H^+.
5. A relatively H^+ leak proof luminal membrane to prevent back leak of secreted H^+.
6. Cytosolic carbonic anhydrase to convert OH^- remaining from dissociation of water to HCO_3^-.Rate of H^+ secretion is $\propto$ to:

- pCO_2—raised pCO_2 increases H^+ secretion and therefore HCO_3^- reabsorption.
- Mineralocorticoids—increases HCO_3^- reabsorption and H^+ secretion.
- K^+ status—hypokalaemia increases K^+ reabsorption by stimulating H^+: K^+ pumps and thus HCO_3^- reabsorption. A high plasma K^+ decreases HCO_3^- reabsorption by decreasing K^+ reabsorption and H^+ secretion by

$H^+:K^+$ pumps. NH_4^+ synthesis increases in proximal tubules during K^+ deficiency, from increase in aldosterone secretion and raised pCO_2, and decreases from low nephron mass and hyperkalaemia.

During alkalosis or diet high in potential HCO_3^- β intercalated cells act in the opposite manner, by secreting HCO_3^- plus cation into tubular lumens and reabsorbing H^+ with Cl^- from basolateral membranes into blood. The structure of β intercalated cells is the same as α intercalated cells but a mirror image in polarity and function. Cl^-: HCO_3^- exchange operates in tandem with basolateral chloride channels.[78] The anion exchanger, Pendrin, is probably the most important HCO_3^- exchanger and has an important role in Cl^- conservation.[21]

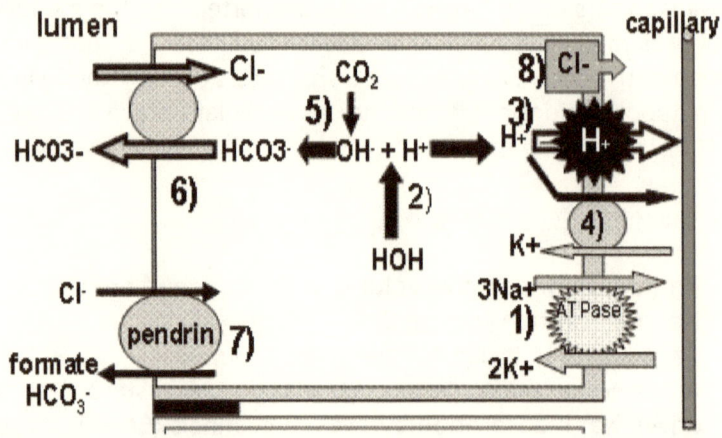

Fig 7 β intercalated cell. Structure and function are the mirror image of α intercalated cells. HCl is transported into the circulation and HCo_3^- secreted into lumen in exchange for Cl^- which is reabsorbed.

1. *Na^+: K^+ pumps create Na^+ and negative potential gradients.*
2. *H^+ and OH^- ions are generated from dissociation of H_2O*
3. *H^+ transported via basolateral membranes by H^+:ATPase pumps*
4. *or $H^{+:}K^+$ pumps*
5. *CO_2 combines with OH^-, from dissociation of H_2O, to form HCO_3^-*
6. *Cl^- is transported into the cell from the lumen in exchange for HCO_3^- by $Cl:HCO_3^-$ transporters or*
7. *by anion exchangers (pendrin)*
8. *Cl^- exits through chloride channels in basolateral membranes.*

TO SUMMARISE: (figure 8).

An increase or decrease of H^+ is immediately buffered by:

* Extracellular HCo_3^- H_2CO_3 - CO_2 system followed by
* Haemoglobin in red cells.
* Protein and phosphate buffer systems in cells.
* Buffering by bone.

<u>All Buffering Systems are in equilibrium.</u> H^+ and OH^- ions are common to all, thus the CO_2 - H_2CO_3 - HCO_3^- system reflects the acid base balance despite the higher cellular $[H^+]$ than plasma $[H^+]$.

Three main organs are involved in acid-based balance: <u>LUNGS, LIVER AND KIDNEY.(figure 8)</u>

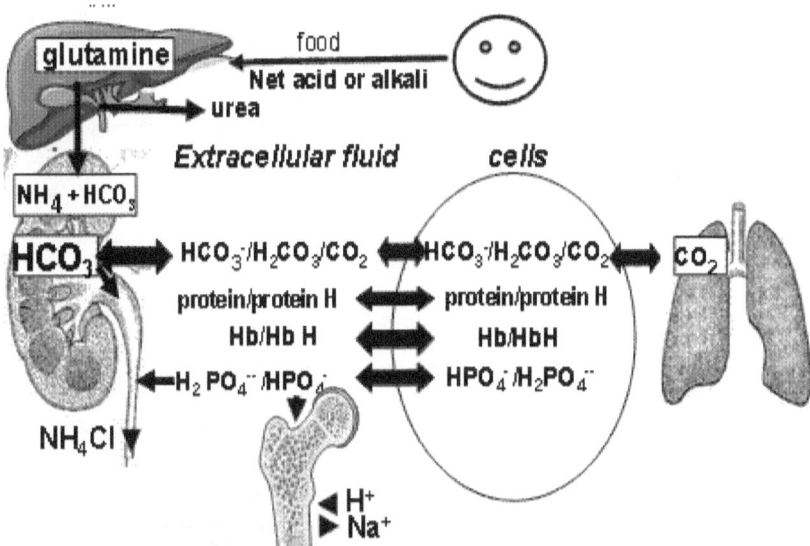

Figure 8: *Acid-Base balance and organs involved. (produced using Servier medical art)Extracellular buffers interact with cellular buffers, lungs; kidney and bone. Food intake results in net acid or alkali. The liver increases glutamine synthesis during net acid diet or acidosis. Glutamine is converted to NH_4^+ + HCO_3^- by renal proximal tubules. This enables excretion of Cl^- with NH_4^+ and retention of HCO_3^-. If net alkali diet is ingested the liver converts COOH groups to urea and the kidney excretes excess HCO_3^-. Bone participates in buffering acid by exchanging H^+ for sodium and Ca $^{2+}$.Lungs increase ventilation and CO_2 excretion during acidosis and retain CO_2 during alkalosis.*

<u>LUNGS</u> increase ventilation in response to metabolic acidosis to decrease pCO_2, $H_2CO_3^-$ and H^+ ions. To a lesser extent hypoventilation compensates for alkalosis.

<u>LIVER (figures 8 and 9)</u> produces CO_2 from complete oxidation of fuels and ketoacids and lactic acid from incomplete oxidation. It oxidises lactic acid produced by other tissues; produces SO_4^{2-}, Cl^- and $H_2PO_4^+$, associated with H^+, from metabolism of amino acids containing strong anions; net HCO_3^- from metabolism of aminoacids with more COOH than NH_3 groups; and urea or glutamine from aminoacids with equal numbers of NH_3 and COOH groups.

<u>Liver responds to acidosis by:</u>

- Synthesis of glutamine for production of NH_4^+ + HCO_3^- by proximal tubules.

<u>Liver responds to alkalosis or an "alkaline diet:</u> (vegetables, fruit):

- By metabolising amino-acids with net COOH groups: these combine with H^+ during synthesis of urea.

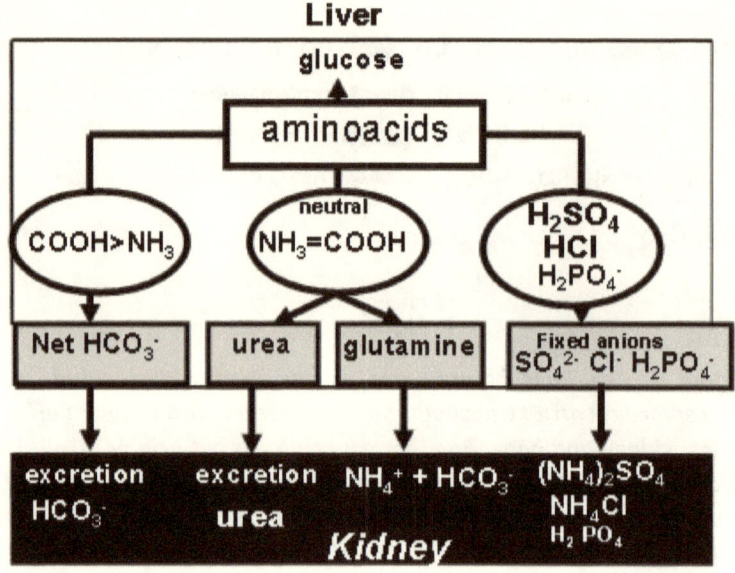

Figure 9. Metabolism of aminoacids by liver and interaction with kidney.

SO_4^{2-}, Cl^- and $H_2PO_4^+$, associated with H^+, results from metabolism of amino acids containing strong anions. Net HCO_3^- is produced from metabolism of aminoacids with more COOH than NH_3 groups. Urea or glutamine results from aminoacids with equal numbers of NH_3 and

COOH groups. Glutamine is transported to the kidneys for production of $NH_4^+ + HCO_3^-$.

The KIDNEY has three major roles in acid-base balance.

Reclamation (reabsorption) of filtered HCO3-.

by proximal tubules is achieved by the indirect process of converting filtered HCO_3^- into H_2CO_3 by combination with secreted H^+ ions, catalysed by carbonic anhydrase. H_2CO_3 rapidly dissociates into H_2O and CO_2. CO_2 is rapidly absorbed into cells and is reconverted into HCO_3^- and H^+ catalysed by cytosolic carbonic anhydrase. HCO_3^- is reabsorbed into the circulation through basolateral membranes by $Na^+:3HCO_3^-$ transporters or $HCO_3^-:Cl^-$ exchangers. H^+ ions are secreted into the proximal tubule lumen by exchange with Na^+.

Synthesis of new HCO3-: is achieved in distal tubules by:

* Excretion of titratable acid: HPO_4^{2-} combines with H^+ secreted by H^+ ATPase pumps to form $H_2PO_4^-$ to increase H^+ excretion.
* Excretion of NH_4Cl: the most important mechanism. NH_4^+ is synthesised and secreted into the lumen by proximal tubular cells; reabsorbed in the medullary TALH; and transported out of cells to accumulate by counter current exchange in medullary interstitium. NH_4^+ is transported into α intercalated cells in medullary collecting ducts and secreted into the lumen. Alternatively NH_3, which dissociates from NH_4^+, diffuses from medulla to collecting duct lumens, followed by combination with H^+, secreted by H^+ ATPase pumps, to form NH_4^+. Cl^- is secreted into the lumen by Cl^- channels to be excreted as NH_4Cl.

During K^+ deficiency synthesis of NH_4^+ is increased; more NH_4^+ takes the place of K^+ on $Na^+:K^+$ pumps or transporters; and more H^+ is transported into the lumen in exchange for K^+ by $H^+:K^+$ pumps rather than H^+ ATPase pumps. [32]

The normal Western diet requires excretion of approximately 70 mmol H^+ derived from non-volatile acids. Normally 30 -40 mmol H^+ are titrated with HPO_4^{2-} to form $H_2PO_4^-$ and 30 mmol excreted as NH_4Cl.

Net Acid Excretion: = titratable acid as $H_2PO_4^-$ + NH_4Cl minus free HCO_3^-.

It is equivalent to net HCO_3^- generated and requires both adequate NH_4^+ generation from glutamine by proximal tubules and H^+ secretion by distal tubules.

NH_4^+ is the most important method of H^+ excretion and is capable of reaching 300 mmol during severe acidosis compared to 80 mmol for titratable acid.

Conceptually the most important reason for NH_4^+ production and excretion is to excrete Cl^- without Na^+ thus increasing the SID (strong ion difference) predominantly (Na^+ minus Cl^-).

NET BASE EXCRETION.

The kidney has an enormous capacity to excrete HCO_3^-. This was important in Paleolithic times when vegetarian diets gave rise to base rather than acid. An intake of up to 140 g sodium bicarbonate daily in human volunteers for three weeks led to an increase of plasma total CO_2 to only 35-40mEq/L and a blood pH increase of less than 0.1 unit from the initial value. [38] This is achieved by decreasing reclamation of bicarbonate above a Tm max of 24.0mmol/L and increasing HCO_3^- excretion by cortical medullary ducts.

Citrate excretion, which increases in alkaline urine or when alkalosis is present, is a further defence against precipitation of Ca^{2+} with phosphate. [17, 18] This is especially important when the diet is largely vegetarian as occurred in the past (Paleolithic nutrition).

Citrate is also a significant component of total base excretion because it is converted to bicarbonate. [17, 18]

Metabolism of Keto acids and Lactate

A further defence against acid base changes is that an increase in lactate and ketoacids occurs during metabolic alkalosis. [39]

Thus depending on whether the diet has an alkaline or acid load—or disordered acid-base balance:

•   Liver synthesises glutamine in response to acidosis. Aminoacids with more COOH than NH_3 groups are converted to urea and H^+ in response to alkalosis. H^+ combines with HCO_3^- to form CO_2 and H_2O.

- If glutamine is converted to NH_4^+ and HCO_3^- in the kidney, NH_4^+ can be reabsorbed into the circulation for metabolism in liver or is secreted into the tubular lumen with Cl^- which generates HCO_3^-.

"Genetic economy" leads to utilisation of the same chemical reaction for several functions:

$$CO_2 + H_2O \longleftrightarrow H_2CO_3 \longleftrightarrow H^+ + HCO_3^-$$

- Buffering in plasma :

  $Na\,HCO_3 + H^+\,Cl^- \longleftrightarrow Na\,Cl + H_2CO_3 \longleftrightarrow CO_2 + H_2O.$

- Buffering by red cells.

- Proximal tubule reclamation of HCO_3^-.

- Distal tubule secretion of H^+ or reabsorption of HCO_3^- ions—the generation or loss of new HCO_3^-.

HCO_3^-, which buffers H^+ and is consumed in the process, is regenerated by a similar reaction in the kidney. When net HCO_3^- excretion is required the same reaction occurs in β cells and H^+ is reabsorbed instead of HCO_3^-.

α cells (A for acid) excrete acid. β Intercalated cells (B for base) excrete HCO_3^-. HCO_3^- regeneration is tightly linked to H^+ excretion and vice versa so that net H^+ excretion = net HCO_3^- regeneration (new HCO_3^-).

HCO_3^- and Cl^-, unaccompanied by non-NH_4^+ cations, are reciprocally related so that excretion of Cl^- without cation must be accompanied by HCO_3^- reabsorption to satisfy electroneutrality—and vice versa.

HCO_3^- regeneration (new HCO_3^-) is linked to Cl^- excretion. Cl^- excretion increases the strong ion difference (SID).

The renal component of acid base homeostasis given here is a very simplified account of a highly complex and controversial subject. The section on the Stewart-Fencl approach [40] which follows can be omitted for those who are content to use the traditional approach.

Analysis of acid-base disorders by the Stewart-Fencl model is conceptually clearer but offers minimal or no practical advantages [41] provided albumin, which has 12 negative charges, is considered in calculation of the anion gap. The main differences are that Cl⁻ rather than HCO_3^- is considered the important independent metabolic variable in acid-base balance and the Stewart approach uses a more comprehensive (and complicated) method to analyse the anion gap. Whether this changes diagnosis, prognosis or management is controversial. In a recent review of 943 critically ill patients, analysis using the Stewart approach, showed no advantage over the traditional approach using standard bicarbonate or base excess—provided albumin was corrected if abnormal.[41]Others also consider that there is no advantage for the Stewart Fencl method. [42]

Stewart's/Fencl approach to acid-base haemostasis. [25, 40-45]

Both Stewart-Fencl and traditional approaches to Acid-Base disorders consider:

* pCO_2, the respiratory component, in the same way.
*   However Cl⁻ rather than HCO_3^- is the focus of the metabolic component in the Stewart Fencl approach: HCO_3^- merely fills the gap between strong cations and anions. NH_4^+ is synthesised by the kidney to enable the excretion of Cl⁻ rather than reabsorption of HCo_3^-, which secondarily follows to maintain electroneutrality.

The Stewart model does not change assessment of acid-base disorders because changes in Cl⁻ and HCO_3^- are reciprocally related. To satisfy electroneutrality HCO_3^- must be reabsorbed when Cl⁻ is excreted for acid –base purposes; and when Cl⁻ is reabsorbed without a cation HCO_3^- must be excreted. Cl⁻ and HCO_3^- are the predominant anions which exchange for acid-base purposes and are the main anions in extracellular fluid.

Cl⁻ is the main actor because it cannot be synthesised and must be retained or eliminated, whereas H⁺ and HCO_3^- can be produced from an inexhaustible supply of H_2O and CO_2:

H⁺ and OH⁻ dissociate from water and HCO_3^- is formed from CO_2 and H_2O. Thus H⁺, OH⁻ and HCO_3^- can be produced as required in response to acid base disturbances.

$$H_2O \longleftrightarrow OH^- + H^+$$

$$CO_2 + H_2O \longrightarrow H_2CO_3 \longrightarrow HCO_3^- + H^+$$

Stewart emphasised that:

* The laws of electroneutrality, dissociation equilibria and mass conservation must be satisfied. For example a single ion by itself cannot be added– an ion of the same charge must be exchanged or ion of opposite charge added at the same time.
* Intercompartmental acid-base balance is based on differentiating independent from dependent variables. Independent variables are pCO_2 and strong ions, those which are nearly completely dissociated: Na^+, K^+, Ca^{2+}, Mg^{2+} Cl^-, SO_4^{2-} and organic anions.
* Contrary to the traditional approach HCO_3^- is not an independent variable. It cannot be changed independently but only indirectly from a change in an independent variable. It is therefore a dependent variable.
* Changes in acid-base balance only occur from changes in independent variables—each of which can be changed independently of the others.
* Acid-base balance is analysed between any two compartments rather than in the body as a whole. For acid base change to occur in two compartments independent variables must assume different values in each compartment.

Strong ions cannot be created or destroyed to satisfy electroneutrality but H^+, OH^- can be generated from disosciation of water. This provides an inexhaustible supply of H^+ and OH^- ions and HCO_3^- generated from OH^- and CO_2.

Strong ions have a powerful effect on dissociation of water: in a solution containing strong ions $[H^+]$ is determined by the difference between positively charged and negatively charged strong ions. For example if net negative strong ions (anions) increase H^+ increases in response; if net positive strong ions (cations) increase H^+ decreases.

Independent variables are:

* pCO_2 – as in the traditional approach.
* SID – strong ion difference.

SID is the difference between the sum of all strong cations and strong anions: those which are (nearly) completely disosciated in solution.

Normally: $Na^+ + K^+ + Ca^{2+} + Mg^{2+} = Cl^-, + SO_4^{2-}$ + organic anions.

Anions associated with lactic and ketoacids are considered <u>strong ions</u> because they are highly dissociated and are therefore included with Cl^- in SID.

<u>SID (strong ion difference) = Na^++ K^+ +Ca^{2+}+Mg^{2+} minus (Cl +SO_4 + organic anions).</u>

<u>The SID is positive in extracellular fluid because strong cations exceed strong anions.</u> SID is normally +40-42 and is the same numerically as base excess. When SID is positive free OH^- ions are greater than H^+ ions.

<u>Dependent variables are</u>:

<u>HCO_3^-, OH^-, CO_3^{2-}, H^+, charges on albumin$^-$ and phosphate$^-$.</u>

(Note: CO_2 dissolved in water produces CO_2, H_2CO_3, HCO_3^-, CO_3^{2-}.

Dependent variables, shown above, only change in response to changes in independent variables and do not primarily change acid-base balance. They increase or decrease in response to changes in independent variables such as pCO_2 or strong ions. They change to fill the gap between strong anions and cations to satisfy electroneutrality. SID must be balanced by charges on dependent variables to satisfy electroneutrality.

This includes <u>charges</u> on albumin (not concentration), phosphate and organic ions.

As SID become more positive, H^+ decreases, as one of the dependent variables, to maintain electroneutrality. This results in alkalosis. When SID becomes less positive H^+ increases and acidosis results.

<u>All dependent variables change simultaneously when an independent variable changes.</u>

Dependent variables include <u>charges</u> on albumin (not concentration), phosphate and organic ions.

H^+, OH^-, CO_3^{2-} are present in minute amounts. Therefore dependent variables which contribute significant amounts of negative charges are HCO_3^- albumin and phosphate.

HCO_3^- is normally 24 mmol/L. Non-volatile weak acids are albumin (~ 12 negative charges)[46] and phosphate.

Thus SID, the difference in strong ions, must = weak anions.= HCO_3^- + albumin (approximately 12 negative charges) + Phosphate⁻, to satisfy electroneutrality.

Volatile weak acids albumin and phosphate are called A(tot) In the Stewart model.

Thus dependant variables are also equal to HCO_3^- + A(tot).

PLASMA-CELLULAR COMPARTMENTAL INTERACTION.

In plasma electro-neutrality must be satisfied:

$Na^+ + K^+ + Ca^{2+} + Mg^{2+} + H^+ = OH^- + Cl^- + HCO_3^- + albumin^{x-1} + P^{y-1} + OA$

(x and y= number of charges. P = phosphate; OA=organic acids).

Strong ion difference (SID) is $Na^+ + K^+ + Ca^{2+} + Mg^{2+}$ minus Cl^-.

SID can be calculated, as above from strong cations minus Cl + strong organic anions, called SIDa (SID apparent).

Weak anions called SIDe are HCO_3^- + Atot (=albumin and phosphate).

To satisfy electroneutrality the difference in strong ions must be balanced by negative charges on anions, essentially HCO_3^- and A(tot).

Therefore: SIDa = SIDe.

Or rearranging the above equation: SIDa – SIDe = 0.

Therefore net positive strong ions (cations minus Cl⁻) should equal the sum of weak anions. If they do not, SIDa does not = SIDe, a strong ion gap called SIG is present: SIG is the amount by which SIDa minus SIDe does not equal zero.

SIG is theoretically zero but has a normal range of 0 to -2 mEq/L although other values have been suggested. A positive SIG indicates that unmeasured cations are present and a negative SIG, a more common event, indicates that <u>unmeasured anions are present.</u> SIG greater than -2 suggests that abnormal <u>unmeasured anions</u> such as SO_4^{2-}, keto anions, lactate, citrate, cellular organic acids and other anions are present.

In analysing acid-base changes between plasma and cells <u>CO_2,</u> which is <u>lipid soluble,</u> rapidly diffuses across biological membranes, so that it's concentration inside and outside of cells is equal. It therefore <u>cannot change intercompartmental acid-base balance.</u>

H^+ and OH^- are present in very small nanomolar amounts. Albumin does not cross cell membranes and phosphate is not regulated for acid-base purposes. Na^+ is primarily regulated to maintain euvolaemia and Ca^{2+} Mg^{2+} and K^+ are tightly regulated for reasons other than for acid-base balance.

Thus Cl- is the predominant ion which influences plasma-cellular pH changes.

This contrasts with the traditional approach which emphasises H^+ exchange with Na^+ and K^+ by H^+ pumps and HCO_3^- or OH^- exchange with Cl^-, by $Na^+{:}3HCO_3^-$ transporters or Cl^-/HCO_3^- exchangers.

In the Stewart approach renal excretion of H^+ ions, which can be readily produced from dissociation of water, is not relevant. <u>The purpose of renal ammoniagenesis is excretion of Cl^- without Na^+ or K^+ which increases the SID.</u> Regulation of acid base balance requires a change in:

<u>pCO_2</u> (respiratory component as in the traditional approach).

<u>SID</u> – (metabolic component) essentially <u>Cl^- not HCO_3^-</u> is the focus of metabolic acid- base balance: Cl^- excretion or reabsorption by the kidney.

Primary metabolic acidosis.

This is due to a decrease in either SID (becomes less positive) or less commonly an increase in albumin or phosphate (Atot).Hyperalbuminemia, resulting from haemoconcentration, contributes to the acidosis in cholera and a raised phosphate to the acidosis of renal failure.

The main causes of metabolic acidosis however are a decrease in SID either from cation loss or an increase in Cl^- (hyperchloraemic acidosis) or strong organic acids (lactic acid and keto acids). Decrease in SID produces an electrochemical force which results in an increase in free {H^+].The causes of metabolic acidosis are therefore a decrease in SID or increase in [Atot] (table 2).

- Loss of cations > chloride, e.g. diarrhoea.
- Decrease in Cl⁻ excretion – renal tubular acidosis.
- Generation of organic anions – lactate and ketoanions.
- Addition of exogenous organic anions – poisons.
- Increase in plasma albumin containing negative charges (weak acid).
- Increase in inorganic anions – SO_4^{2-}, HPO_4^{2-}.

Table 2: Causes of metabolic acidosis by Stewart/Fencl approach to Acid- Base disorders.

Primary metabolic alkalosis is due to:

- An increase in SID – loss of strong anions greater than cations, usually Cl⁻ (diuretics, vomiting, chloride diarrhoea) or gain of strong cations (predominantly Na⁺) greater than anions.
- Decrease in A(tot) :albumin and phosphate.

The normal concentration of plasma phosphate is approximately 1.8 meq/L; therefore a decrease has a negligible effect. However decrease in serum albumin, which has approximately 12 negative charges, [46] causes mild metabolic alkalosis. However severe metabolic alkalosis is due to Cl⁻ depletion—conceptually sounder than an increase in plasma HCO_3^-.

Other Changes to SID.

Increase or decrease in extracellular volume, contrary to some accounts, does not change SID and does not cause acid base changes because the ratio of negative to positive ions remains the same. A change in water balance (free water changes), although not altering the ratio of cations to anions, dilutes or concentrates SID—decreases or increases the concentration of strong ions and causes a slight acidosis or alkalosis: a decrease in free water (causing hypernatraemia) increases the SID and causes mild contraction alkalosis; increase in free water (hyponatraemia) decreases the SID and causes mild acidosis.

Acidosis due to treatment with saline causes a more severe acidosis due to infusion of excess Cl⁻ compared to cations, not from volume expansion as some allege,—thus decreasing SID and causing hyperchloraemic acidosis: the SID of normal plasma is 40-42 mEq/L; that of saline is zero. Alternatively NaCl without HCO_3^- is infused into extracellular fluid with HCO_3^- concentration of 24 mmol/L.

The Stewart approach gives similar analytic results, compared to the traditional approach, but may improve conceptual clarity. For example: gastric secretion of HCl is achieved by proton pump secretion of H^+ which accompanies Cl^- from NaCl. The HCO_3^-, required to accompany Na^+ transfer out of cells is produced from H_2O and CO_2 in oxynctic cells catalysed by carbonic anhydrase. HCl is secreted into the stomach and $NaHCO_3$ reabsorbed into the circulation-the so called post prandial alkaline tide.

In essence NaCl has changed to $NaHCO_3$ which is reabsorbed and HCl is secreted into the stomach:

$NaCl = Na + Cl^-$. $H^+ + Cl^- = HCl$. $H_2O + CO_2 = HCO_3^- + H^+$

$HCO_3 + Na^+ = NaHCO_3^-$. HCl is secreted into stomach; $NaHCO_3$ is reabsorbed.

ANION AND OSMOLAR GAPS [46-55]

Anion and to a lesser extent osmolar gaps are considered a valuable clue to the cause of metabolic acidosis. Anion gap is used (to an extent inappropriately) to divide metabolic acidosis into hyperchloraemic and anion gap acidosis.

A higher than normal anion gap is therefore a clue to the presence of organic acidosis.

The concept of anion gap is based on the law of electroneutrality: the sum of cations must equal the sum of anions. Strictly, the term is a misnomer because if all anions and cations are counted no gap exists. The gap exists because all anions and cations are not measured and counted. Unmeasured anions exceed unmeasured cations.

In plasma: $Na^+ + Ca^{2+} + K^+ + Mg^{2+} = Cl^- +$ total $CO_2^- +$ protein$^- + SO_4^{2-} +$ Phosphate$^- +$ organic-acids$^- +$ other anions$^-$.

Negative charges on protein are:

- Albumin ~ 12. Globulin has minimal or no net charge. [46]

- Phosphate is normally approximately 1.8 mEq/L. At the normal pH [H^+] of plasma, phosphate has a ratio of HPO_4^{2-}: $H_2PO_4^-$ of 4:1. Organic acids are normally 2-3 Eq/L. Thus in the above equation with normal values and $SO_4^{2-} \sim 0.5$ mEq/L:

$Na + K^+ + Ca^{2+} + Mg^2 = Cl^- + CO_2 + $ albumin$+ P + (OA, SO_4^{2-} SO_4^{2-} +$citrate$^-)]$
$(4.5 + 4 + 1.5 = 10)$ 12 $1.8 + (8:2$ $)= 22$
OA=organic anions)

Therefore $Na^+ = Cl^- + $ total $CO_2 + (22 - 10) = Cl^- + $ total $CO_2 + 12$.

Therefore Normal <u>Anion gap = $Na^+ - (Cl^- + $ total $CO_2)$. (= 12)</u>.

Values are approximate. There is controversy over normal value for anion gap. Note that electrolytes and <u>Total CO_2</u> are measured on plasma from venous blood—a closed system. Total CO_2 should be used in calculation of anion gap and not bicarbonate measured on arterial blood gas.

There are 2 unsettled issues: the quantity of anionic equivalents on albumin; and whether only the equivalent charges on calcium and magnesium rather than their total concentration should be used: only 50% of calcium and 70% of magnesium are ionised. [44]

However albumin, to which the divalent cations are bound (and to a small extent other anions to which they are complexed), decrease negative charges on albumin. The anion equivalents attributed to each gram/dL (10 g/L) of albumin above and below normal vary between 2.3-2.5mEq [50] although different studies show marked variation.

In most circumstances Na^+, Cl^-, K^+ and total CO_2 are available from standard electrolyte measurements and K+ usually varies by only 1.0 mEq/L. The following is an approximation of the anion gap:

$Na + $ other cations $(10) = Cl^- + $ total $CO_2 + $ other anions.

$Na = Cl^- + $ total $CO_2 + ($other anions—other cations$)$

$Na = Cl^- + $ total $CO_2 + (22 - 10)$

$$\boxed{Na^+ \qquad = Cl^- + TOTAL\ CO_2 + 12}$$

Therefore the anion gap—the difference between unmeasured anions and cations other than Na^+ equals 12 with a range of 8-16. The average anion gap given in the literature varies between 11 and 13. An anion gap outside these limits suggests that an abnormality is present: Increase in unmeasured cations lowers the anion gap whereas an increase in unmeasured anions increases the gap. (Table 3)

LOW ANION GAP [47-49]	HIGH ANION GAP
Hypoalbuminaemia.	Increased albumin.
Increased cations	**Decreased cations**
Hypercalcaemia, Hypermagnesaemia.	↓ serum K^+, Ca^{2+}, Mg^{2+}
Lithium.	
Cationic paraproteins (IgG).	Increased anionic paraproteins
	Increased unmeasured anions
Bromide: overestimation of Cl.	Lactic acid.
	Keto-acids.
Sodium containing drugs eg Carbenicillin	Sulphate, phosphate and organic acids in renal failure
SIADH.	
	Poisons
	Methyl alcohol—formic acid.
	Ethylene glycol Glycolic acid and lactic acid.
Laboratory error or artefact.	D.Lactic acid.
Hyperviscosity.	Salicylate: lactic acid and salicylic acid.
Hyperlipidaemia (↓ Cations).	Pyroglutamic acidaemia.
Overestimation of Cl$^-$.	Hyperglycaemic coma.? Cause.
Leukocyte production of CO_2.	Rhabdomyolysis—organic acids from muscle.

Table 3: Causes of low and high anion gap.

Hypoalbuminaemia is a common cause of low anion gap. [48-53]

Laboratory error is a common cause of low anion gap.[50] It may arise from venous sampling up stream of the vein used for saline infusion (Saline anion gap= 0). In the past bromide ingestion distorted the measurement of sodium because bromide interferes with measurement of chloride and causes a spurious elevation. Using standard bicarbonate, measured on arterial blood but Na^+ and Cl^- on venous blood (total CO_2 is higher) is another source of error.

Hyperlipidaemia may interfere with the colorimetric assay of Cl^-. In severe hypernatraemia sodium may be underestimated.

Increased levels of Ca^{2+}, Mg^{2+} and K^+ are usually apparent and rarely cause analytical problems. Whether ionised rather than total calcium or magnesium should be used is controversial.

Multiple myeloma may sometimes, but rarely, result in marked increase in cations which have positive charges (cationic paraproteins) which lower the anion gap: in one study a reduction in anion gap of 50% resulted from polyclonal IgG gammopathy. [50]

The most important use of a raised anion gap is the clue it gives to the presence unmeasured organic acids: lactic, keto acids organic acids from cell breakdown, especially muscle necrosis, or an unsuspected poison (discussed later).However predictiveness of raised anion gaps for the presence of organic acid is poor unless the anion gap exceeds 30. [41-43] In one study 29% of patients with anion gap between 20-29 did not have lactic or ketoacidosis. [55] In some an abnormal anion gap $\geq$ 5.7 (mean 8.7 mEq/L) was not explained by charges on proteins, phosphate, K^+ and Ca^{2+}. However anion gap $\geq$16+ 0.5 x plasma HCO_3^- strongly suggested an organic acid was present.

A clinical diagnosis of lactic acidosis, keto-acidosis or drug intoxication, based on raised anion gap and exclusion of renal failure is inaccurate. Theoretically if ketoacids or lactic acid is increased the decrease in HCO_3^- should be matched by an increase in anion gap. There are several reasons, well reviewed by Salem and Hujais [55], why the anion gap predicts an organic acidosis inadequately.

* Variations in unmeasured or unconsidered anions such as albumin, phosphate and cations such as K^+, Mg^{2+} and Ca^{2+}.

*   Whether ionised or total calcium and magnesium are used in calculation. [44]
*   Changes in charges on albumin due to alkalaemia (increases negative charges) and acidosis (decreases negative charges).
*   The presence of organic anions other than lactate and keto anions: D lactate, 2OH butyrate, and other unidentified anions which may be particularly important in rhabdomyolysis. In sepsis proteolysis may give rise to a wide variety of different unmeasured organic anions.
*   The volumes of distribution of H^+, HCO_3^- and organic anions vary. [53, 54]
*   In chronic respiratory acidosis using standard HCO_3^-.derived from blood gas measurement, rather than the total CO_2, gives a falsely low anion gap.
*   The variable extent of intracellular buffering.

Thus change in anion gap compared to change in HCO_3^- (Δ AG Δ HCO_3^-) varies between 1-2 in uncomplicated anion gap acidosis. A value of <1:1 suggests a combined hyperchloremic and AG acidosis are present eg hyperchloraemic acidosis due to diarrhoea. A value greater than 2:1, in which the fall in HCO_3^- is less than expected, suggests that metabolic alkalosis was previously present.

The anion gap can be made more predictive by estimating the effects of change in plasma albumin, phosphate and easily measured cations.

Inclusion of plasma, K^+ increases the normal average anion gap to 16 (12 + 4); range 12-20mEq/L.

Deviance of average values of plasma K^+, Ca^{2+} and Mg^{2+} from normal can be used to adjust the expected anion gap.

The expected anion gap can be decreased for hypoalbuminemia or increased if hyperalbuminemia is present from volume depletion: [51-54] albumin contributes 2.5mEq for each lg/dL below or above the normal of 4.2g/dL although the precise value is controversial.

Phosphate deviance from normal can be included—usually only important in renal failure. The charge can be estimated if the pH is normal, by assuming a ratio of HPO_4^{2+}:H_2Po4 of 4:1. This can be estimated by 1.5 x serum phosphate (mmol/L).

Normal fasting SO_4^{2-} is 0.6mEq/L Normal organic acid is 1-6mmol/L.

Formulas based on the Stewart Fencl approach which gives a more accurate estimation of cations and anions, including deviation resulting from a change of pH and variations of water balance, are available but are of questionable clinical usefulness.

The Stewart Fencl approach to acid-base problems is advocated by some Intensivists. Raised anion gap, unexplained by including variables described above, and including lactic and keto-acids occur in critically ill patients and have been reported to predict death better than raised lactic acid and standard AG [56-59]. Base excess and anion gap estimations were changed in 26% of cases by calculation of unmeasured anions by the Stewart-Fencl approach [56]. In a series of critically ill patients accountability for anion gaps were as follows:

- 62% were due to lactate and keto anions.
- 15% were due to changes on proteins, phosphate, K^+, Ca^{2+}
- 23% were unaccounted for.

Several studies have shown a poor relationship between lactic acidosis and anion gap in critically ill patients, [56-59] but others have not. [60, 61] Unmeasured anions or SIG is considered to predict mortality better than either lactate or the anion gap. [56-59]

A positive SIG indicates unmeasured cations are present.

A negative SIG indicates unmeasured anions are present.

However accurate estimation of SIG requires a calculator to solve complex equations. Several intensivists and others advocate using SIG (strong ion gap) believing that it predicts outcome better than either anion gap or plasma lactate level. [44, 56, 57] Others disagree [45, 60, 61] or consider that an anion gap, corrected for deviations of serum ions and albumin, are as predictive.

The most important correction is for albumin. The anion gap should be decreased by 2.5mEq for each gram of albumin below a normal value of 45g/L (4.5g/dL) or increased for each 1.0g/dL above normal. [44,51,53]

Δ Anion Gap Δ HCO_3^-. [62-64]

Another refinement, which is controversial, is the Δ anion gap Δ HCO_3^- ratio: the increment of anion gap above normal compared to the decrement of HCO_3^- below normal.

Theoretically each 1mEq increase in anion gap should be matched by 1mEq decrease in plasma HCO_3^-. The ratio is theoretically 1:1.

For example in anion gap acidosis, a serum total CO_2 of 10mmol/L (15 below a total CO_2 of 25mmol/L) should be accompanied by an anion gap of 12 + 15 = 27. If the ratio is less than this a coexisting hyperchloraemic acidosis or a previous metabolic alkalosis (higher than normal HCO_3^-) is suspected.

Empirically the ΔΔ in lactic acidosis is usually 1.6:1 and in diabetic ketoacidosis 1:1.

There are several reasons why this may not be true apart from the problems with anion gap itself.

Volumes of distribution of protons, associated anions and HCO_3^- may vary. Some anions remain in the ECF while their associated H^+ take several hours to move into cells, a process which is time dependent and may also vary with the particular anion. (Figure 10)

In <u>lactic acidosis</u> [H^+] has a larger volume of distribution than lactate⁻ because of buffering within cells. Lactic acid is efficiently reabsorbed and low renal perfusion also limits urinary excretion. The ΔAG ΔHCO$_3^-$ ratio averages 1.6. [62, 63]

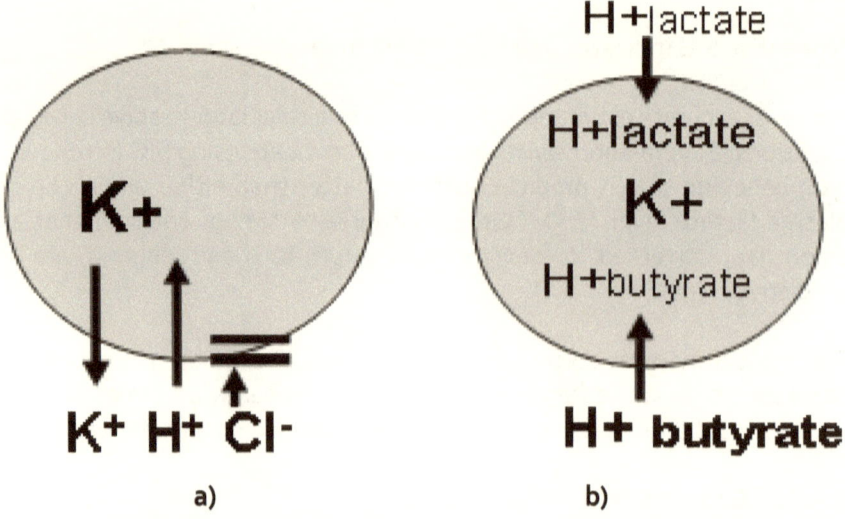

Figure 10: *In a) H^+ exchanges with K^+ because Cl⁻ cannot pass the cell membrane. K efflux and hyperkalaemia accompany acidosis due to HCl. In b) lactate⁻ and butyrate⁻ accompany H^+ into the cell.*

In Diabetic Ketoacidosis loss of ketoanions with cations in urine lowers the anion gap compared to ketoacidosis alone. Indeed diabetic acidosis, often considered as an anion gap acidosis, may present with hyperchloraemic acidosis. [64] Thus the ΔAG $\Delta HCO3-$ ratio varies considerably depending on the extent of ketoacidosis compared to hyperchloraemic acidosis. (See Metabolic acidosis which follows).

Chronic renal failure may present with either a hyperchloraemic or anion gap acidosis depending on the severity and type of renal disease. In early renal failure decreased ability to secrete NH_4^+ may lead to hyperchloraemic acidosis. In the later stages of renal failure retention of phosphate, SO_4^{2-}, uric acid and organic acids cause an anion gap acidosis.

In severe diarrhoea from cholera an increase in albumin and phosphate from haemoconcentration may increase the anion gap and suggest a coexisting organic acidosis is present.

In conclusion the anion gap can be analysed at several levels of sophistication:

- $Na^+ = Cl^- + HCO_3^- + 12$ (normal anion gap).
- $Na^+ + K^+ = Cl^- + HCO_3^- + 16$ (normal anion gap).
- Include all cations and anion deviances from normal. Include Ca^{2+}, Mg^{2+}, K^+ and Phosphate⁻.
- Include albumin in estimation by adding or subtracting 2.5mEq for each 1g/dL below or above normal.
- Include serum lactate—if available.
- Calculate the SIG(strong ion gap).
- Estimate the $\Delta AG:\Delta HCO_3$ ratio although this is probably not useful. [55]

While it may give a useful clue in diagnosis avoid over interpreting the anion gap. Correcting the anion gap for deviations in albumin concentration is the most important.

OSMOLAR GAPS. [65, 66]

Osmotic pressure is due to the total number of particles in solution. NaCl is confined to the water component of plasma, which comprises 93% of water, the remainder being lipids and protein.(discussed in the chapter on Water disorders). Fortuitously the water factor (93% of plasma) roughly compensates for the fact that the dissociation of NaCl is not complete: it gives rise to 1.86 rather than 2.0 particles.

To estimate the plasma osmolality the plasma sodium is doubled to take accompanying anions into account. Thus the plasma osmolality is estimated by:

(2 x Na) + Glucose (mmol/L) + urea (mmol/L). = 2 x Na^+ + 10

Glucose and urea, which are non-ionised, are not doubled because they give rise to 1 particle and do not have accompanying anions.

Osmolality is usually measured by freezing point depression: 1 mole in 1kg H_2O depresses the freezing point of water by 1.86ºC. The osmolal gap is the difference between measured and estimated osmolality.

Osmolal Gap=measured minus estimated osmolality (+ - 15).

A large osmolal gap suggests an unmeasured solute which decreases freezing point of water is present. These include:

Ethyl alcohol; Propyl Alcohol (rubbing alcohol); methyl alcohol (Methanol); Ethylene glycol (antifreeze).

If present: measure plasma ethyl alcohol and test for ketones which suggests propyl alcohol poisoning). Examine for oxalic and hippuric acid crystals which suggests ethylene glycol poisoning.

References at the end of part 2.

METABOLIC ACIDOSIS AND ALKALOSIS; RESPIRATORY ACIDOSIS AND ALKALOSIS. PART 2.

METABOLIC ACIDOSIS: HCO3⁻↓, pH↓, PCO$_2$↓

ORGANIC ANION ACIDOSIS		
Lactic acidosis	L-Lactic Acid (>5mmol/L)	L-LACTIC ACIDOSIS (>5mmol/L) Shock, Hypoxia Sepsis Severe hypoxemia, UNCOMMON
Ketoacidosis	βOH Butyric acid, aceto-acetic acid	Thiamine deficiency Drugs—Metformin Poisons Mitochondrial disorders
Renal failure	Sulphate, phosphate, organic acids, other anions plus mineralacidosis	Hereditary enzyme defects Hepatic failure Leukaemia, lymphoma, malignancy
POISONS		Reyes Syndrome
Alcohol	Ketoacids, lactic acid	Intravenous fructose, sorbitol
Methyl alcohol	Formic, lactic acid, ketones	Malignant hyperthermia LOCAL
Paracetamol	Pyroglutamic acid, Lactic acid	Ischemic Compartmental syndrome Mesenteric infarction
Ethylene glycol	Glycolic acid, oxaloacetic, lactate.	
Cyanide Carbon monoxide Citric Acid poisoning I.V. fructose, sorbitol, alcohol lactic acid, other acids Strong ion gap acidosis in critically ill patients—anions other than lactate Sulphuric acid—ingested sulfur Fatty Acids -Mitochondrial and other abnormalities involved in fatty acid metabolism Hyperalbuminaemia Hyperphosphataemia		

Table 4: Causes of non-Hyperchloraemic (Anion Gap) Acidosis.

Metabolic acidosis may be **hyperchloraemic**- an abnormal increase in Cl⁻ compared to cations; or, **anions other than Cl⁻**. This is referred to as anion gap acidosis (AG).

ANION GAP ACIDOSIS.

Acidosis due to anions other than Cl⁻ (Table 4). A more appropriate term is either non-hyperchloraemic acidosis or organic anion acidosis. However anion gap acidosis can rarely be due to inorganic anions such as phosphate and sulfate. Correlation between the AG and the cause of acidosis is poor. The most common causes are:—lactic acidosis, ketoacidosis and renal failure.

LACTIC ACIDOSIS.[9, 67] (chapter 5). (Figure 11)

Glycolysis occurs in three stages:

1. Anaerobic : production of 2 moles of pyruvate from 1 mole of glucose in the cytosol.
2. Mitochondrial conversion of pyruvate to acetyl coenzyme A (AcCoA), and conversion of AcCoA to CO_2, H_2O and H (hydrogen) in the Tricarboxylic Acid Cycle (TCA)—provided o_2 is available.
3. Transfer of hydrogen (H), H^+ and electrons, liberated from breakdown of AcCoA, to the electron chain for synthesis of ATP.

Only Stage 1, conversion to pyruvate, can proceed without oxygen.

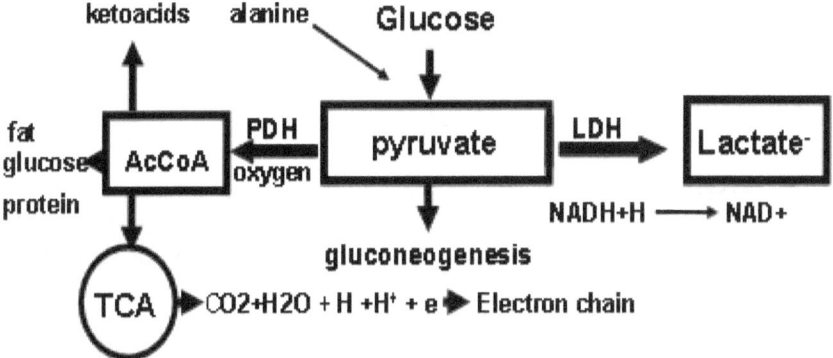

Figure 11: *Simplified model of glucose metabolism.(see text)*

If oxygen is available pyruvate is transported to mitochondria and converted to acetyl coenzyme A (AcCoA), the pivotal substance in aerobic glycolysis.

AcCoA has three fates: metabolism in the Krebs (tricarboxylic acid cycle); conversion to ketoacids; and synthesis of fat, glucose and protein.

Acetyl COA is broken down to CO_2 and Hydrogen atoms (H) in the TCA (Krebs cycle). Hydrogen is the main source of energy which is used to transform ADP to ATP: H, H^+ and electrons (e^-) are transferred to the electron chain by NAD^+ and FAD.

$$2H + NAD^+ \blacktriangleright NADH + H^+.$$

H and e- are added to NAD^+ to give NADH.The e- removed from the other H atom results in H^+.

Electrons pass sequentially down the electron chain, interact with several electron acceptors to the final electron acceptor, molecular oxygen. This is reduced to O^{--} by accepting electrons. Energy released by electrons passing down the chain is used to transport H^+ across the inner mitochondrial membrane into the outer chamber between the inner and outer mitochondrial membranes. A strongly positive proton force develops which intermittently moves H^+ back into the inner mitochondrial space through special channels containing ATPase. In the process ADP is converted to ATP. H^+ then combines with reduced oxygen O^{--} to form water.

$$O^{--} + 2H^+ \longrightarrow H_2O$$

$$C_6H_{12}O_6 + 6O_2 + 36ADP + 36P \rightarrow 6CO_2 + 42H_2O + 36ATP$$

ATP is hydrolysed in carrying out cellular metabolic work.

$$ATP + H2O \longrightarrow ADP + P + H^+ + \text{biological work.}$$

ATP can only be produced from ADP and ADP is only produced by utilisation of ATP, predominantly for operation of $Na^+:K^+$ pumps.

In the absence of oxygen only Stage 1, anaerobic glycolysis, can proceed. Decrease in availability of (oxidised) NAD^+ and FAD decreases transfer of H, H^+ and e^- to the electron chain; aerobic glycolysis ceases ; and pyruvate accumulates. The lactate: pyruvate ratio is proportional to the NADH/NAD^+ ratio in the cytosol. An increase in NADH, compared to NAD^+, increases the <u>redox</u> state (<u>re</u>duction-<u>ox</u>idation) which increases pyruvate conversion to lactate$^-$ by mass action. [8]

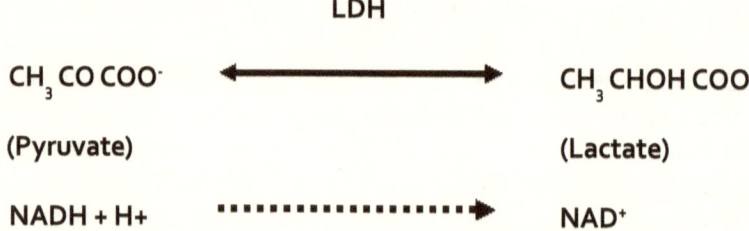

LDH

$CH_3 CO COO^-$ ⟷ $CH_3 CHOH COO^-$

(Pyruvate)   **(Lactate)**

NADH + H+   ⋯⋯⋯▶   **NAD^+**

In the process NADH plus H^+ is converted to NAD^+ and enables anaerobic glycolysis to continue.Normallly the ratio is 10-1 in favour of lactate. Note that it is <u>lactate$^-$ not lactic acid</u> which is formed.

Only 2 moles of ATP are produced from anaerobic glycolysis per mole of glucose compared to 36 moles from aerobic glycolysis. However the small amount of ATP generated is used for vital cellular metabolic work and the NAD^+ generated enables anaerobic glycolysis to continue.

Glucose + 2 ADP + 2P ⟶ 2 lactate$^-$ + 2 ATP + 2 H_2O.
(P = inorganic phosphate)

Each time a molecule of ATP is hydrolysed a proton (H^+) is released, as shown in the following equation. This would lead to increasing cellular acidosis.

$$ATP^{-4} + H_2O \longrightarrow 2ADP^{-3} + P^{-2} + 2H^+ + \text{Biological work}$$

H^+ ions released react with lactate to form lactic acid.

$$H^+ + CH_3 CHOH\ COO^- \text{ (lactate)} \longrightarrow CH_3\ CHOH\ COOH \text{ (lactic acid)}$$

Lactic acid diffuses out of cells to interstitial fluid and circulation. Lactic acid is a strong acid. Buffering by $NaHCO_3$ limits the acidosis that would otherwise occur but at the expense of decreasing extracellular bicarbonate (buffer base).

$$CH_3 CHOHCOO^-H^+ + NaHCO_3 \longrightarrow CH_3 CHOH\ COO^-Na^+ + H_2CO_3 \longrightarrow CO_2 + H_2O$$
$$\text{(Lactic Acid)} \qquad\qquad \text{(Na}^+ \text{ lactate)}$$

If availability of oxygen improves lactate is converted to pyruvate. This is oxidised to CO_2 and H_2O by reverse of the process described and $NaHCO_3$ (buffer base) is restored.

Normally 1000-1500 moles of lactate are produced daily (15-20 mmol/kg/day) by muscle, skin, renal medulla, intestine and brain. Lactate is used as a fuel by myocardium, brain, kidney, and if sufficiently raised, skeletal muscle, and can be converted to glucose in liver and kidney (Cori cycle). Filtered lactate is efficiently reabsorbed by transporters in proximal tubules and only appears in urine when the blood level reaches 6-7mmol/L. Normal blood or plasma lactate is 0.7-2.5 mmol/L but depends on the specific laboratory reference range.

Lactate provides the following advantages. [9]

* Provision of fuel during shock or extreme physical exertion. This can be used by brain, myocardium and kidney to which blood is preferentially delivered (autoregulation).
* Provision of a small amount of ATP. This is crucial for short bursts of extreme physical activity—as in running or fighting, when inadequate oxygen delivery limits glucose oxidation to provide sufficient energy.
* Accepts H^+ from utilisation of ATP in biological work. This decreases cellular H^+ and increases NAD^+ production from NADH which allows anaerobic glycolysis to continue.
* Decreases pyruvate accumulation.

Lactate itself is not harmful: it is infused as Ringers lactate; and during extreme exercise plasma lactate may increase above 20mmol/L. Hyperlactataemia in shock is a beneficial adaption to hypoxia: production by muscle provides fuel utilised by brain and heart. However lactic acidosis is a marker of severity in shock: serum levels >10mmol/L carry a poor prognosis. [10]

Catecholamines, acting on β2 receptors, cause lactic acidosis by stimulating Na^+: K^+ pumps, especially in skeletal muscle [68, 69]. This increases glycolysis and production of pyruvate which contributes to lactic acidosis in shock, sepsis, physical exertion and seizures. Skeletal muscle provides fuel for heart and brain under adverse conditions and lactate⁻ for gluconeogenesis by liver (Lactate Shuttle). [68]

When oxygen supply and ATP production decrease further key metabolic processes, such as operation of membrane pumps, are affected. [1,8] Activity of muscle Na^+: K^+ pumps correlate with lactic acid levels in sepsis.[11, 12] This leads to cellular depolarisation (increased intracellular Na^+ and decreased K^+), calcium influx and apoptosis—the end result in all forms of shock. If oxygen availability improves lactate⁻ is converted to pyruvate⁻ which is oxidised to CO_2 and H_2O by reverse of the process described above; and HCO_3^- is restored. Plasma lactate represents a balance between production and removal. Causes of lactic acidosis are either due to:

- Increased production.
- Decreased removal—liver failure.

Production is increased by:

Catecholamine stimulation of Na^+: K^+ pumps.

Pyruvate accumulation from decreased or abnormal oxidative phosphorylation and accumulation of NADH and excessive pyruvate production.

ATP production is dependent on availability of ADP, which is present in limited amounts in cells [9]. Thus an increase in lactate⁻ production depends on biological work, which converts ATP to ADP, during operation of Na^+: K^+ pumps and other cell functions.

SPECIFIC CAUSES OF LACTIC ACIDOSIS.

Causes of lactic acidosis are often divided into type A and type B: type A is due to hypoxia; type B due to causes other than hypoxia. This approach is not useful however because both are often present in the same condition.

Hypoxia:

The most common cause is inadequate tissue perfusion from hypovolaemia or heart failure but can occur from severe hypoxaemia in respiratory failure, carbon monoxide poisoning and extreme anaemia. During shock catecholamines stimulate muscle lactate production and liver utilisation of lactate decreases from inadequate perfusion. [68]

Sepsis:

Sepsis decreases vascular filling and cardiac function. Hypoxia, due to redistribution of blood flow and microcirculatory failure, was previously considered to be the cause of lactic acidosis in sepsis. However maximising oxygen delivery is ineffective in treatment of septic shock. Although hypoxia, from inadequate tissue perfusion, is the most common underlying cause, metabolic factors associated with the inflammatory response, [70] catecholamines and increased glycolysis are now considered important in pathogenesis: muscle $Na^+: K^+$ pump activity correlates with lactic acidosis in sepsis. [68, 69] Increase in aerobic glycolysis, catecholamine secretion, decreased pyruvate dehydrogenase activity, liver dysfunction, from under perfusion, and hyperventilation may be involved in the pathogenesis of lactic acidosis.

Extreme Physical Exertion and Seizures:

Muscle activity, which exceeds the local supply of oxygen, and the action of catecholamines increase lactate levels during exercise. This can transiently exceed 20mmol/L. [71] Seizures, especially if repetitive, can result in severe lactic acidosis due to muscle spasm and clonic movements in combination with hypoxaemia.

Pheochromocytoma and drugs causing vasoconstriction. Lactic acidosis is probably due to the combination of marked increase in muscle generation of lactate from increased activity of $Na^+:K^+$ pumps, secondary to surges of catecholamine secretion, which decrease tissue perfusion

secondary to severe vasoconstriction. The mechanism of lactic acidosis from amphetamine is probably similar.

Malignant Hyperthermia and Salicylate poisoning

Uncoupling of oxidative phosphorylation from biological work by salicylate or malignant hyperthermia increase oxygen consumption and production and release of muscle lactate.

Liver Disease:

Lactate is used by several tissues. Failure of lactate clearance by liver rarely causes lactic acidosis. Circulatory failure should always be considered before this is diagnosed.

Cancer, Leukaemia, Lymphoma

This rarely causes lactic acidosis in the absence of circulatory failure. The cause has not been established but metabolic abnormalities in cancer tissue, local ischaemia and cellular proliferation have been suggested.

Thiamine Deficiency. [72, 73]

Thiamine, a co-factor for pyruvate dehydrogenase and transketolase, decreases utilisation of pyruvate but rarely causes lactic acidosis. However several cases were caused by a shortage of thiamine in patients on parenteral nutrition. [73, 73]

$$\text{AcCoA} \xleftrightarrow{\text{PDH}} \text{pyruvate} \xleftrightarrow{\text{LDH}} \text{Lactic Acid}$$

Red cell transketolase decreases and is used for diagnosis.

Mitochondrial Disorders. [74]

Various abnormalities in mitochondrial function, which cause dysfunction of oxidative phosphorylation, increase pyruvate and NADH production. [74] Lactic acidosis is characteristically intermittent, in association with a variety of other disorders, such as myopathy, cognitive impairment, stroke, deafness and diabetes.

Cyanide Poisoning. [75] Cyanide causes lactic acidosis by combining with cytochrome oxidase, part of the electron shuttle, and inhibiting oxidation of H^+. Serial blood lactate levels correlate with blood cyanide levels. Measurement may be useful in assessing severity. [75]

Drugs

Metformin	Salicylates
NaHCO$_3$ Infusion	Iron poisoning
Catecholamine infusion	Nucleoside reverse transcriptase inhibitor treatment of AIDS
Fructose infusion	Paraldehyde

Table.5. Drugs causing lactic acidosis.

Metformin

In a systematic review of 176 studies the incidence of lactic acidosis was the same in those taking Metformin compared to sulphonylurea drugs or placebo. [76] However, these studies excluded patients with renal failure or severe co-morbidity. The most important risk factors for metformin induced lactic acidosis are renal failure and shock.

Nucleoside Reverse Transcriptase Inhibitors

Treatment of HIV with Nucleoside Reverse Transcriptase inhibitors has caused lactic acidosis, especially in those with impaired renal function. [77] Those affected usually show mitochondrial myopathy with ragged red fibres. Treatment with Riboflavin, a precursor of Flavin mononucleotide and FAD was reported to be effective in one case. [78]

Fructose Infusions

Fructose, at high concentration, bypasses glucose metabolic control points and increases pyruvate synthesis. This is converted to lactate because its metabolism exceeds the capacity for ATP synthesis.

Respiratory Alkalosis results in small elevations of lactic acid, although levels may be higher if severe volume depletion is present.

Poisons

Lactic acid partly contributes to the acidosis resulting from poisons and is discussed later. Deranged oxidative metabolism is probably responsible.

KETOACIDOSIS. (Ketoacidosis)

Ketoacidosis is due to decrease in insulin secretion from starvation, [79] diabetes, alcohol or poisons. Normal metabolism is shown in figure 12 but is discussed in detail in chapter 13. Production of ketones in Diabetic ketoacidosis (DKA) and fasting are similar and are shown in figure 12.

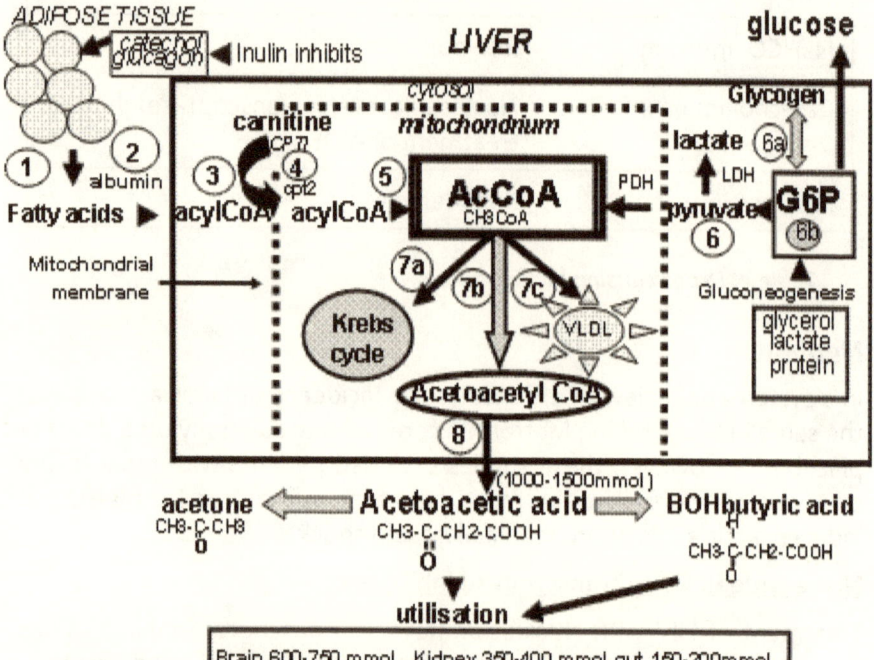

Figure 12: Simplified model showing interrelationships of glucose, fatty acids, acetyl-CoA and production of ketones in liver. The actions occurring in mitochondria are shown in the centre between stipled lines. (Numbers correspond text)

1. Fat breaks down to fatty acids catalysed by hormone sensitive lipase; normally inhibited by insulin and stimulated by catecholamines.

$$\text{Triglyceride} \xrightarrow{\text{lipase}} \text{Glycerol and fatty acids}$$

2. Fatty acids are carried to liver bound to albumin.
3. Fatty acids are converted to <u>acyl-CoA</u> in liver cytosol by acyl-CoA synthetase. (not shown)

Long chain acyl-Coa (or free fatty acids) cannot penetrate the inner mitochondria membrane.

4. Acyl-CoA combines with carnitine forming acyl carnitine, catalysed by carnitine palmitoyl transferase-1 (CPT1). Acyl-CoA is reformed after passing the inner mitochondrial membrane catalysed by CPT-II.

The above process is, in essence, the shuttling of acyl-Coa through the inner mitochondrial membrane using carnitine. (carnitine shuttle)

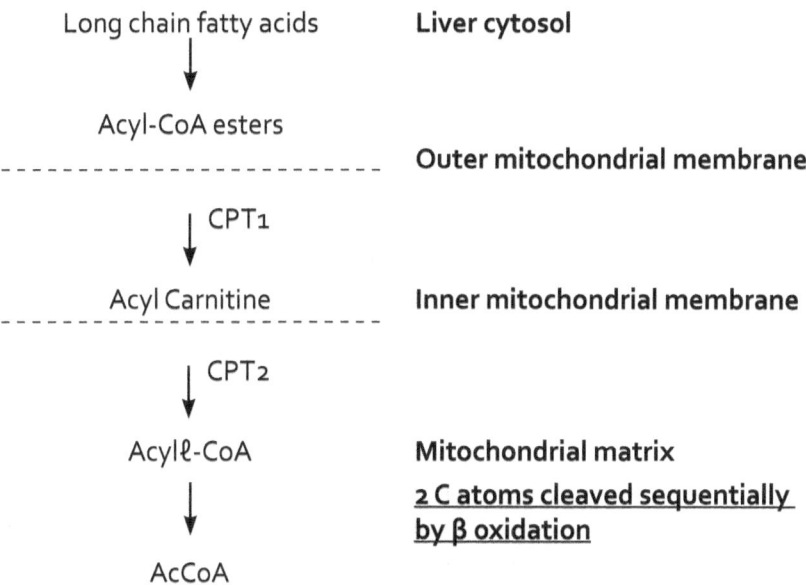

5. In mitochondria oxidation successively removes 2 carbon atoms from the carboxyl end of fatty acylCoA to form Acetyl CoA (AcCoA).
   AcCoA occupies the pivotal position in fuel metabolism.

6. AcCoA is also formed from glucose 6 phosphate (G6P) via pyruvic acid. G6P is derived from either glycogenolysis (breakdown of glycogen), gluconeogenesis from amino-acids, glycerol and lactic acid.

7. AcCoA normally has 3 outcomes:
   a. Oxidation in the citric acid cycle to form ATP.
   b Condensation of 2 molecules to form acetoacetyl COA.
   c Conversion into fatty acids for incorporation into triglycerides as VLDL particles.

8. Acetoacetic acid is reduced to βOH butyric acid and in the process changes NADH to NAD⁺ ; acetoacetic acid converts to acetone.

Diabetic ketoacidosis. [80]

This is an exaggeration of the above. Lack of insulin, which normally inhibits glycogenolysis, gluconeogenesis and lipolysis leads to hyperglycaemia and increased fatty acid production. Fatty acids are transported to liver bound to albumin. Transfer into mitochondria by the carnitine shuttle is increased by glucagon. As in starvation 2 molecules of AcCOA combine to form aceto acetic acid. Acetoacetic acid is reduced to β OH butyric acid, (in the process changing NADH into NAD⁺) and also into acetone.

ACETONE	ACETOACETIC ACID	β OH BUTYRIC ACID
CH_3-C-CH_3 + CO_2 ⟷	CH_3-C-CH_2-COO^-+H^+ ⟷	CH_3-C-COO^-+H^+
	NADH ⟷ NAD	

βOH butyric acid is the main ketone body (ratio 3:1) but may increase to a ratio of 10:1 if lactic acidosis coexists, as occurs if severe hypovolaemic shock or sepsis (reduced redox state favours NADH accumulation) [81]. Keto acids, which are strong acids, are buffered by $NaHCO_3$ in blood.

β (OH) butyric acid + $NaHCO_3$ → Na butyrate⁻ + H_2CO_3 → CO_2 + H_2O

CO_2 is eliminated by ventilation. H⁺ ions are decreased by combining with bicarbonate but at the cost of lowering extracellular HCO_3^- and reducing total body buffering capacity.

Keto anions have 3 possible outcomes:

*   Excretion by kidney with cations, predominately Na⁺ and K⁺. This causes hyperchloremic acidosis. Conceptually, this can be considered to be due to loss of keto anions which would otherwise be used to regenerate (previously consumed) HCO_3^- or due to a decrease in SID (strong ion difference) from cation exceeding chloride losses in urine.
*   Excretion of anions with NH_4^+ produced from glutamine. This has a neutral effect on pH but NH_4^+ synthesis takes time to develop.
*   When GFR decreases further ketoanions are retained in the body and result in anion gap acidosis.

Thus, diabetic ketoacidosis can give rise to anion gap acidosis or hyperchloremic (non anion gap) acidosis or both. On average anion gap acidosis occurs, in which the decrement of HCO_3^- is matched by increase in anion gap (Δ = change). : Δ HCO_3^- Δ anion gap = 1.0 However, there is considerable inter-individual variation [64] which is discussed further in the chapter on Diabetic ketoacidosis. When GFR is relatively normal keto anions are initially excreted with Na^+ or K^+ which lead to hyperchloremic acidosis; when GFR falls significantly, keto anions are retained and cause anion gap acidosis.

Starvation. [79]

During fasting energy needs are provided by glycogenolysis (1-2 days), gluconeogenesis (up to 1 week) and ketosis which starts after 2-3 days, is prolonged, and the main source of energy. [79,80]When glycogen stores are depleted, glycogenolysis in liver is followed by gluconeogenesis using glycerol, lactate and amino-acids. This maintains normal plasma glucose levels. Fat is the main fuel used in starvation. Lipolysis, due to low serum insulin levels, gives rise to fatty acids which are oxidised in the mitochondrial TCA cycle. When oxidation exceeds the capacity of liver to utilise ATP (ADP, an essential precursor, is present in limited amounts) 2 molecules of AcCoA combine to form aceto-acetic acid. This is reduced to βOH butyric acid.

Alcoholic ketoacidosis and lactic acidosis. [82-86]

Ethyl alcohol ▶ Acetaldehyde ▶ acetic acid ▶ Acetyl-CoA ▶ β OHB

NAD^+ ⤸ $NADH + H^+$

Acidosis, in association with excess alcohol, may be due to ketoacids, lactic acid or acetic acid. Metabolism of ethyl alcohol generates $NADH + H^+$ and promotes pyruvate conversion to lactate and aceto-acetate to β OH butyrate. Ketoacidosis may complicate alcohol binges. Various factors, including inhibition of insulin secretion, lack of food intake, hypovolaemia and excessive adrenergic activity may be responsible. Plasma βOH butyrate levels are usually only moderately raised but can exceed 10mmol/L.Lactic acidosis may also occur but serum lactate rarely exceeds 5 mmol/L unless seizures, hypovolaemia or hypoxia occur. Metabolic alkalosis, due to vomiting, may decrease the AG resulting from organic acids. Hyperchloraemic acidosis may result from urinary excretion of keto anions with cations which decrease the anion gap.

POISONS & INTOXICATIONS

Acidosis is due to various organic acids in combination with lactic acid, except for Toluene, which causes hyperchloraemic acidosis.

Methyl Alcohol. [87, 88]:

Methyl alcohol poisoning occurs following ingestion of windshield washer fluid, embalming fluids, methanol for heating and cooking, cleaning fluids and 'Moonshine liquor'. Following ingestion methyl alcohol is metabolised to formaldehyde and formic acid which causes severe anion gap acidosis. Manifestations include inebriation, abdominal pain, increase in serum amylase, anion and osmolar gaps. Pancreatitis may be misdiagnosed because of the combination of abdominal pain and increase in serum amylase. After a latent period brain damage and visual disturbances occur and may lead to optic atrophy and blindness.

Isopropyl alcohol. [9, 10]

This is contained in rubbing alcohol and may mimic diabetic keto acidosis because acetone gives a weak positive reaction to the nitroprusside test.

Ethylene glycol. [88, 89]

This is contained in anti-freeze, thinners, windscreen wash, cleaners, detergents, paints and solar collectors. Ethylene glycol is metabolised to several metabolites including glycolic, oxalic and lactic acids. Glycolic acid may be elevated to 7 mEq/L [89]. A severe anion gap acidosis and osmolar gap results. Oxalic acid combines with calcium to form calcium oxalate and may precipitate in renal tubules. Decrease in mental state, confusion, urinary oxalic acid crystals, renal failure and pulmonary oedema result.

Salicylates. [9, 10]

Salicylates uncouple oxidative phosphorylation. This decreases ATP synthesis, increases oxygen consumption and heat generation. Salicylates cause a mixed disturbance: metabolic acidosis from salicylic and lactic acids and respiratory alkalosis from stimulation of the respiratory centre. Tinnitus, dizziness, hyperventilation and mild anion gap acidosis usually occurs. The combination of fever, hypotension, and AG acidosis mimics septic shock. Pulmonary oedema, seizures and coma occur in severe poisoning.

Pyroglutamic Acidosis (5-oxoproline acidosis). [90]

This rare condition occurs in paracetamol overdose or in those on paracetamol who develop sepsis. Acetaminophen (paracetamol) depletes glutathione stores Decrease in glutathione increases gamma glutamyl cysteine. This is metabolised to pyroglutamic acid (5 oxyproline). Anion gap acidosis, which is common, may be due to 5-oxoproline (pyroglutamic acid) rather than lactic acid as is sometimes alleged. Hereditary deficiency of glutathione synthetase, Vigabactrin and antibiotics are rare causes. However acetaminophen toxicity alone rarely causes pyroglutamic acidosis: other conditions, such as malnutrition, alcohol, underlying liver disease, sepsis, renal failure and drug use may be required to cause this condition. The diagnosis is established by measurement of urine 5 oxyproline.

SUBSTANCE (MW)	ACID. (AG) =anion gap	Osmolal Gap	Plasma ketones	Mental state	Breath odour	Other
Methyl alcohol (32)	Formic, lactic (AG+)	↑	±	↓ Appear drunk	+	Papillitis, abdominal pain, amylase ↑
Ethyl alcohol (46)	βOH butyric, ± Lactic (AG+)	↑	±	↓ Appear drunk		
Isopropyl alcohol (60)	Normal AG	↑	±	↓	Fruity	
Ethylene Glycol (62)	Oxalic, Glycolic (AG+)	↑	-	↓		Urine oxalic acid crystals Renal failure
Salicylate	Salicylic, lactic, keto-acids (AG+)	N	+	↓±		Hyperventilation. Tinnitus. Combined respiratory alkalosis and metabolic acidosis.
Paracetamol	Pyroglutamic (AG+)	N		↓		Hepatitis
Paraldehyde	Acetic, other organic acids (AG+)	N	±	↓	+	
Toluene	Hippuric Hyperchloraemic Normal AG	N	-		+	Hypokalaemia

Table 6:Characteristics of several poisons.AG=anion gap;N=normal

Citric Acid Poisoning. [91]

This rarely causes acidosis. Symptoms are mainly due to ionised hypocalcaemia from complexing of calcium with citric acid. Calcium is infused in treatment.

Toluene Poisoning. [92]

Toluene (methyl benzene), which results from glue sniffing, is metabolised to hippuric acid in liver. Hippurate, an anion, is rapidly excreted with Na^+ or K^+ and therefore causes <u>hyperchloraemic</u>, rather than anion gap acidosis, hypokalaemia and severe sodium depletion. Renal ammonium excretion is normal but the combination of hyperchloremic acidosis and hypokalaemia may cause misdiagnosis as renal tubular acidosis. Whether renal tubular acidosis is really present is controversial [92]. If the GFR decreases from hypovolaemia an anion gap acidosis may also develop as hippurate accumulates.

Treatment of poisoning. [9, 10, 88, 93]

<u>Methyl alcohol and Ethylene glycol</u> are not toxic, but are converted to toxic products by alcohol dehydrogenase (figure13). Therefore ethyl alcohol can be given as an antidote for methyl alcohol and ethylene glycol poisoning to slow their conversion to toxic products. Alcoholic dehydrogenase has a 10-fold greater affinity for ethyl alcohol than for methyl alcohol or ethylene glycol. Alcohol increases the half life of Ethylene glycol by 10 times. [93]

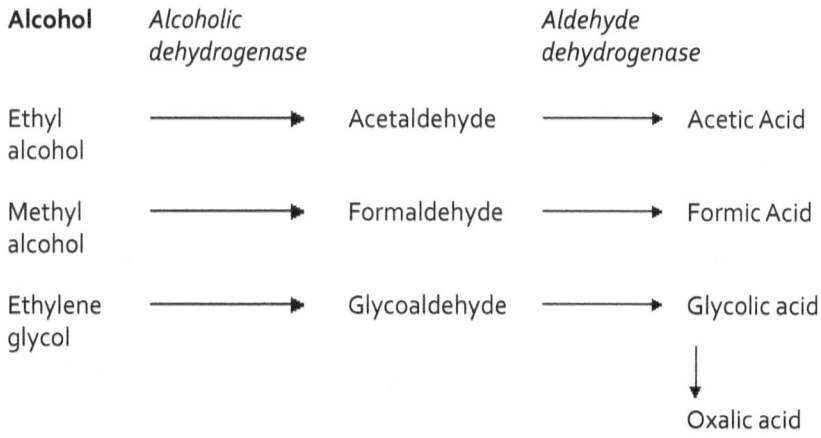

Figure 13. Metabolism of alcohols by alcohol dehydrogenases.

The goal is to achieve an ethyl alcohol level of 22mmol/L (100m/dL). A bolus of ethyl alcohol 0.6g/kg is followed by an infusion of 0.07-0.15g/kg/hour. [10]

4-methyl pyrazole (Fomepizole) potently inhibits alcohol dehydrogenase and reduces formation of toxic metabolites. It is highly effective and safe for treatment of ethylene glycol and methyl alcohol poisoning. [88, 93] It has replaced ethyl alcohol for treatment and decreases need for haemodialysis. The loading dose is 15 mg/kg followed by 10 mg/kg every 12 hours, given intravenously over 30 minutes. Sodium bicarbonate is recommended for treatment of ethylene glycol poisoning to increase elimination of glycolate and inhibit calcium oxalate precipitation. [93]

Both ethylene glycol and methyl alcohol are efficiently cleared by dialysis. Indications for haemodialysis of ethylene glycol poisoning are severe metabolic acidosis, acute renal failure, deterioration or a serum concentration of above 8.0mmol/L. However patients treated with 4-methyl pyrazole early may not require dialysis even if the serum ethylene glycol level is >8.0mmol/L. [93]

Methyl alcohol poisoning

In addition to 4-methyl pyrazole folinic acid, up to 50 mg, the activated form of folic acid, is recommended [88]. Indications for dialysis are severe acidosis, visual impairment or plasma methyl alcohol concentration of >15.6mmol/L (>0.5g/L). [87, 88]

Salicylate poisoning. [9, 10, 93]

Acidosis increases formation of non-ionised salicylic acid. This diffuses into brain faster than ionised salicylic acid.

$$H^+ + salicylate^- \longleftrightarrow H\ salicylate$$

Alkalosis decreases entry of salicylate into brain by increasing ionised salicylate and also increases renal excretion. Levels above 40mg/dL cause toxicity and levels >100mg/dL cause severe toxicity. Serum levels however do not correlate with toxicity if poisoning is chronic. $NaHCO_3$ is given intravenously to raise the arterial blood pH to >7.5. Dialysis is considered for serum salicylate levels >100mg/dL (4mmol/L). A protocol for alkaline diuresis has been suggested. [94]

Ethyl alcohol:

Correct hypovolaemia; give glucose (5-10% dextrose water) and thiamine.

Toluene toxicity. [92]

Correct hypovolaemia and hypokalaemia. Hypovolaemia can be partly corrected with $NaHCO_3$ provided hypokalaemia is also corrected. Saline and KCl further increase hyperchloraemic acidosis because of the high concentration of Cl^- compared to cation.

CRITICALLY ILL PATIENTS AND RHABDOMYOLYSIS.

Critically ill patients and those with rhabdomyolysis may have an anion gap unexplained by serum lactate. This is probably due to several organic acids or other anions released from tissues and muscle. The strong anion gap (SIG) is considered to be a better indicator of prognosis than serum lactate in critically ill patients.

HYPERPHOSPHATAEMIA AND HYPERALBUMINAEMIA

Increase in plasma phosphate and albumin contribute to acidosis and anion gap in Cholera. Anion gap acidosis during Cholera is due to hyperphosphataemia, hyperalbuminaemia, lactic acid due to shock and retained anions from renal failure. [95] Hyperchloraemic acidosis results from loss of bicarbonate in stool. Thus severe acidosis of Cholera is due to combined hyperchloraemic and anion gap acidosis.

NORMAL ANION GAP ACIDOSIS.(HYPERCHLOREMIC ACIDOSIS)

Hyperchloraemic acidosis is due to increased loss of bicarbonate by the intestine; failure of ammonium excretion and renal acidification; endogenous production of acid, which is excreted with cations; or exogenous intravenous or oral intake of acid or potential acid.(table7)

The Stewart-Fencl approach is a conceptually clearer model of hyperchloraemic acidosis: this is considered to be due to either excretion of cations greater than anions or decrease in chloride excretion. It is important to understand that:

- For each H^+ secreted into the tubular lumen new HCO_3^- is formed and reabsorbed into the circulation.
- HCO_3^- reabsorbed without cations must be accompanied by Cl^- excretion or vice versa.
- Loss of organic anions represents loss of potential bicarbonate because bicarbonate has been consumed in their buffering. Their further metabolism, rather than renal loss, regenerates HCO_3^-. The Stewart Fencl model of Acid Base balance, considers loss of cations which accompany organic or inorganic anions as the cause because this decreases the SID (Cations minus Cl^-).

INTESTINAL

Losses of HCO$_3$ (or strong cation losses greater than Cl').
DIARRHOEA.
Ileostomy.
Small bowel disorders, biliary, pancreatic fistulae.
Urinary diversion to bowel.
Laxative abuse.
Cholestyramine resin.

RENAL FAILURE OF ACIDIFICATION   Renal HCO$_3$ loss, failure to excrete H^+ or NH_4^+.
(Loss of strong cations greater than Cl')
Renal tubular acidosis.
Renal failure.

ENDOGENOUS ACID PRODUCTION   loss of potential HCo$_3$
Increased renal loss of cations accompanying anions or loss of organic anions)
Ketoacids—Diabetic, Starvation, Alcoholic intoxication.
D. Lactic acidosis.
Toluene poisoning.

EXOGENOUS INTAKE OF H^+ IONS OR POTENTIAL H^+ IONS
(Intake of anions greater than cations).
NH_4 Cl ingestion.
Intravenous saline infusion.
HCl administration.
Sulphur ingestion.
Cationic amino-acid infusion producing HCl.
Toluene toxicity.

Table 7: Causes of Hyperchloraemic Acidosis: *according to the traditional and Stewart-Fencl model—(in brackets)*

Diarrhoea. (chapter13)

Diarrhoeal stool usually contains sodium and higher concentration of bicarbonate, organic anions, potassium and magnesium than does plasma. Urine shows both a low Na^+ and K^+ from depletion of these cations and low pH. High urinary NH_4^+ levels result in a highly negative urine anion gap.

Biliary secretion contains 60 mmol/L and pancreatic secretion 120 mmol/L of HCO_3^-. Thus fistulas may also cause metabolic acidosis. Volume depletion, acidosis, potassium depletion and less commonly Mg^{2+} depletion occur. In Cholera, hyperphosphataemia, hyperalbuminaemia and lactic acidosis cause an anion gap acidosis as well as hyperchloraemic acidosis [95] from loss of HCO_3^- and organic anions.

Losses from ileostomy or small bowel fistulas are especially likely to cause magnesium deficiency.

Urinary diversion to bowel leads to exchange of Cl^- in urine with HCO_3^- in bowel contents. Urinary diversion may involve an ileal conduit or ureteric implantation into colon (ureterosigmoidostomy).

Cholestyramine resin. [10]

Calcium and magnesium chloride are only partly absorbed during treatment with cholestyramine but Cl^- exchanges with HCO_3^- in bowel. This leads to excretion of Mg and Ca, as bicarbonate and reabsorption of Cl^- and may cause hyperchloraemic acidosis [9].

Renal losses of organic anions (potential HCO_3^- losses or loss of strong cations greater than chloride).

Keto-acids cause acidosis if ketone production exceeds metabolism. Excretion of keto anions with NH_4^+ has a neutral effect on acid base balance. If keto acids are excreted with cations, such as sodium, hyperchloraemic acidosis results; if keto anions are retained, due to decrease in GFR, anion gap acidosis occurs.

Thus diabetic ketoacidosis may cause either hyperchloraemic or anion gap acidosis or both depending on the extent of reduction of GFR from hypovolaemia. If a normal GFR is maintained ketoanions are excreted with cations resulting in hyperchloraemic acidosis.

Anion gap acidosis usually resolves on treatment because ketoanions are metabolised to bicarbonate Infusion of normal saline, which contains more Cl⁻ than Na⁺, compared to plasma, increases hyperchloraemic acidosis.

Poisons.

D-lactic acidosis and toluene poisoning cause hyperchloraemic rather than anion gap acidosis.

D.Lactic Acidosis. [96, 97]

Lactic acid occurs in D or L form. In man only laevo lactic acid normally forms. D lactic acid is produced by gastro-intestinal bacteria: colonic bacteria ferment carbohydrate which favours the overgrowth of acid resistant flora such as lactobacillus. This results in both D lactate and laevo lactate. Filtered laevo lactate but not D Lactate is reabsorbed in proximal tubules by Na⁺ lactate cotransporters. D Lactate is therefore rapidly excreted with cations causing hyperchloraemic acidosis. This decreases SID (strong ion difference). D lactic acidosis presents with encephalopathy, ataxia, confusion, memory loss, fatigue, headache, behavioural abnormalities and nystagmus. D.Lactic acidosis is suspected when acidosis is present but L. lactate is normal in conditions such as short bowel or blind loop syndromes.

Toluene. [92] (discussed previously).

Intake of actual or potential H+ ions or chloride.

Ingestion of NH_4Cl, therapeutic administration of HCl and parenteral administration of cationic aminoacids (arginine and lysine), which give rise to HCl on metabolism, are rare causes of hyperchloraemic acidosis. Sulfur ingestion, a folk remedy, gives rise to H_2SO_4, sulphate⁻ is excreted with Na⁺ and increases loss of cations greater than Chloride.

Saline infusion. [98-100]

Therapeutic administration of normal saline commonly causes hyperchloraemic acidosis. This is not due to an expansion acidosis. There are 2 ways of understand this:

- Saline with a SID of 0 mEq/L is infused into blood with a normal SID of + 40mEq/L: this lowers the (positive) SID and causes acidosis.

- Saline, without HCO_3^-, is infused into blood containing normal plasma HCO_3^- of 24mEq/L and dilutes plasma HCO_3^-.

A randomised study compared infusion of n.Saline with Ringers lactate in women undergoing gynaecologic surgery: those given saline decreased their pH from 7.41 to 7.28 after two hours compared to normal pH in those given Ringers lactate.[98] Hyperchloraemic acidosis is a predictable outcome of saline administration. [99]

1L of normal saline given to normal volunteers increased serum osmolality and decreased arterial blood pH; whereas administration of 1L of Ringers Lactate decreased osmolality and increased arterial blood pH. [100]

Hypoalbuminaemia also results from large volume infusion: this decreases anion charges on albumin, lowers anion gap and causes mild metabolic alkalosis. [99]

The debate about the ideal crystalloid to administer continues because of the different effects of development of hyperchloraemic acidosis following saline but hypoosmolality when other fluids, including Ringers Lactate and Hartman's, are administered. Infusion of fluid with SID of 24mEq/L in rats maintained normal acid-base balance. Higher SID values cause metabolic alkalosis which may be harmful. [101]

Dilutional acidosis.

(Free) water excess (dilutional hyponatraemia) causes slight hyperchloremic acidosis because excess of water with zero SID (or zero HCO_3^-) dilutes plasma with a normal SID of +40mEq/L (or plasma HCO_3^- of 24mEq/L).It is important to emphasise that an increase in plasma volume, in which the concentration of ions and therefore the SID or HCO_3^- does not change, does not cause acidosis.

RENAL TUBULAR ACIDOSIS (RTA). [9, 10, 11, 13, 14, 36, 37,102-105]

A group of disorders characterised by impaired H^+ and or NH_4^+ excretion or impaired HCO_3^- reabsorption out of proportion to reduction in glomerular filtration rate. The kidney performs the following in excreting net acid:

- Reclamation of filtered (HCO_3^-) by proximal tubules.
- Synthesis of NH_4^+ by proximal tubules.
- NH_4^+ transport into the lumen of proximal tubules and transport from the lumen of TALH into the medulla.
- Medullary recycling and concentration of NH_4^+; and its dissociation into NH_3.
- Diffusion of NH_3 from medulla into distal tubular lumens.
- Transport of NH_4^+ from medulla into α intercalated cells by ammonium transporters and secretion of H^+ and NH_4^+ ions by α intercalated cells into distal tubular lumens.
- H^+ combination with HPO_4^- to form $H_2PO_4^{2-}$; and with NH_3 to form NH_4^+; and NH_4^+ combination with Cl^- to form NH_4Cl.
- Excretion of NH_4Cl and H_2PO_4.

There are 2 sources of distal tubular NH_4^+: direct secretion by α cells or diffusion of NH_3 into the tubular lumen from the medulla where it combines with H^+. Causes of renal tubular acidosis are shown in table 8.

PROXIMAL (Type II)	DISTAL (Type 1) Hypokalaemic	DISTAL (Type IV) Hyperkalaemic or normal serum K
Primary—no other dysfunction. Fanconi syndrome. Hypercalcemia. Hyperparathyroidism. Acetazolamide. Vit D deficiency. Vit D resistance. Metal Toxicity. Multiple Myeloma.	Primary Autoimmune. Sjogren's; SLE. Medullary sponge. Kidney. Medullary cystic disease. Transplant rejection. Interstitial kidney disease. Cryoglobulinaemia. Chronic active hepatitis. Primary biliary cirrhosis. Post obstructive uropathy. Sickle cell disease Wilson's disease. Drugs. Amphotericin, Lithium. Analgesic nephropathy.	↓ Aldosterone action. Hyporeninaemic Hypoaldostereonism. Addison's disease. Aldosterone resistance. 21 Hydroxylase deficiency. Interstitial kidney disease. Sickle cell disease. Obstructive uropathy. Drugs. Spironolactone, Amiloride, NSAIDS, Trimethoprim, Heparin. Analgesic abuse Acetazolamide Triamterene, Cyclosporine, Lithium.
Serum K^+ low- normal Min Urine pH < 5.5 Urine Anion Gap normal Urine Osmolal Gap normal Stones, nephrocalcinosis rare	Low, sometimes normal. > 5.5 Positive or low. negative <20 Common	High—normal. < 5.5 Positive or low negative. Variable —

Table 8: Causes of Renal Tubular Acidosis.
(NSAID = non-steroidal anti-inflammatory drugs. SLE = systemic lupus erythematosus. Vit=vitamin)

Proximal RTA—(Type II).

This is due to decreased capacity to reclaim filtered HCO_3^-. Maximum HCO_3^- reabsorption (T max) in proximal tubules decreases, but acidosis is limited because HCO_3^- loss ceases once the threshold of ~15mmol/L, is reached. The defect is isolated or occurs in combination with glucosuria, aminoaciduria and phosphaturia (Fanconi syndrome).Mutations in the $Na^+:HCO_3^-$ cotransporters are one cause and may be associated with blindness. [22]Urine pH, NH_4^+ excretion and urine anion gap are normal.

Hypokalemia results from an increase in distal Na^+ delivery which promotes exchange for K^+ which is then lost in urine. Large doses of HCO_3^- and K^+ are required for treatment. Carbonic anhydrase inhibitors, such as Acetazolamide, produce mild hyperchloraemic acidosis by acting on proximal tubules.

Hyperparathyroidism, Vitamin D deficiency or resistance, metal toxicity and multiple myeloma may cause mild proximal renal tubular acidosis.

Distal renal tubular acidosis. [36, 37,102]

A disorder of distal tubular acidification out of proportion to reduction in glomerular filtration rate [37]. Defective excretion of NH_4^+, the main component of net acid excretion (NAE), with or without inability to maximally acidify urine, is the most important abnormality. Excretion of titratable acid by conversion of HPO_4^{2-} to $H_2PO_4^-$ can only eliminate a maximum of 60-80 mmol H^+ daily compared to NH_4^+ which can eliminate 200-300 mmol H^+ daily.

The Stewart-Fencl model is conceptually sounder than the traditional model: NH_4^+ is produced and excreted to take the place of strong cations such as Na^+ for excretion of Cl^-. This increases SID (strong cations minus Cl^-).Excretion of NH_4Cl is equivalent to excretion of HCl. Defects in NH_4^+ excretion can occur from the following : [36, 37,102]

- Decreased synthesis of NH_4^+ + HCO_3^- in proximal tubules. Hyperkalaemia and a low nephron mass decreases $NH4^+$ synthesis. Hypokalaemia increases NH_4^+ synthesis.
- Disordered function of H^+ ATPase and H^+: K^+ ATPase pumps in α intercalated cells of distal tubules leads to decreased secretion of H^+ into the lumen.

- Decrease in negative lumen potential in distal tubules due to decrease in electrogenic Na^+ reabsorption. Electrogenic Na^+ is provided by:
  - Adequate Na^+ delivery to distal tubules.
  - Normal Na^+ reabsorption without Cl^- by principal cells of distal tubules.
    This is necessary for Na^+ exchange for H^+ or K^+.
- Decrease in Aldosterone and angiotensin 2 secretion or function. Aldosterone stimulates $Na^+:K^+$ pumps which increases the concentration and electrical gradient promoting Na^+ reabsorption; stimulates Na^+ reabsorption by sodium channels (EnaC); and stimulates H^+ and K^+ secretion by channels.
- A luminal membrane which leaks secreted H^+ back into tubular cells or medulla. This decreases availability of H^+ to combine with NH_3
- Decreased cytosolic carbonic anhydrase required for production of HCO_3^- to exchange with Cl^- which is excreted
- Inadequate medullary NH_4^+ concentration and acidity to promote disosciation of NH_4^+ to NH_3. NH_3 diffuses into the collecting duct lumen and combines with secreted H^+. The combination prevents its back leak, lowers luminal NH_3 and H^+ thus promoting further NH_3 diffusion and H^+ secretion. Thus a high concentration of NH_4^+ in the medullary interstitium by NH_4^+ recycling is required.
- Cl^- must be available to accompany NH_4^+ in the lumen via $Cl^- : HCO_3^-$ exchangers on basolateral membranes.

Causes of distal renal tubular acidosis (RTA).

These can be rationalised by considering mechanisms necessary for acid excretion described above, (shown in table 9). Distal RTA is differentiated by serum K^+, low serum K^+ suggests Type 1 and those with a normal or high serum K^+ suggest Type IV is present, however serum potassium may be normal in type 1.

The most common cause of Type 1 RTA in adults, associated with hypokalaemia, is disordered function of $H^+:ATPase$ or $H^+:K^+ATPase$ exchangers [37] in alpha intercalated cells. Autoimmune disease, especially Sjogren's syndrome, is a common caus. [103] The failure of H^+ secretion leads to inability to form NH_4^+ from NH_3 in the tubule lumen. Thus there is a failure both to acidity urine and excrete ammonium. Potassium rather than H^+ or NH_4^+ is therefore secreted in exchange for Na^+ in α intercalated cells.

Type I distal tubular acidosis. [37,103]

Symptoms are due to hypokalaemia—muscle weakness, constipation, fatigue, volume depletion and acidosis. However hypokalaemia is variable depending on whether H^+ ATPase or $H^+:K^+$ pumps are affected. Urine pH is inappropriately high and NH_4^+ low during acidosis. Hypercalciuria, low urine citrate and relatively alkaline urine lead to nephrocalcinosis (60%) and stone formation. Patients with incomplete distal RTA, for example Medullary Sponge and Medullary cystic disease, may be able to acidify urine and maintain normal plasma HCO_3^-, and present with renal stones. Mutations involve H^+: ATPase pumps or Cl^- :HCO_3^- exchangers. (AE1). The latter are also expressed in red blood cells. This causes spherocytosis and South East Asian ovalocytosis but can rarely result in renal tubular acidosis.

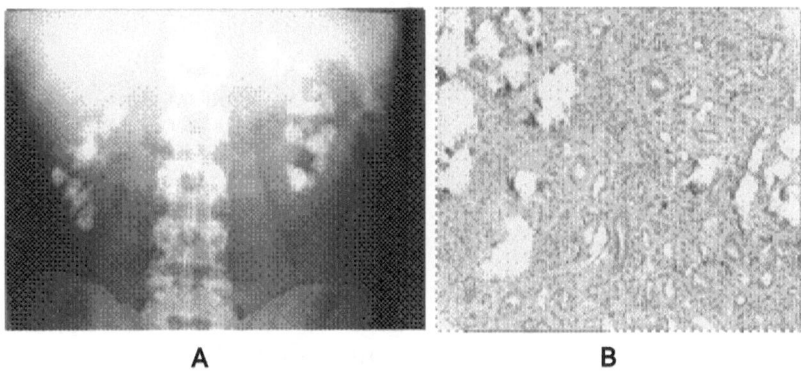

A   B

Figure 14: **Nephrocalcinosis and interstitial fibrosis in a 34-year-old female with Renal Tubular Acidosis due to Sjogrens disease. A shows nephrocalcinosis. B tubular atrophy, fibrosis and mononuclear infiltration in the medulla.** *Presented with inability to stand, symmetric areflexia and paraesthesia. Serum (mmol/L) K1.9, Na129, HCO3⁻ 12,. arterial blood pH 7.28.,* ***ESR 115mm/hour.***

H⁺ ATPase or H :K⁺ ATPase pump dysfunction.	Systemic lupus. Sjogren's syndrome. Mutations: H+ ATPase pumps. Interstitial disease. Medullary sponge or cystic disease. Kidney Transplant resection. Obstructive uropathy.
Back Leak of H⁺.	Amphotericin.
Voltage Defects. Failure of Na⁺ reabsorption to generate negative lumen voltage for K+ secretion.	Na⁺ channel defects. Low cardiac output: decreases Na⁺ delivery to collecting duct. Amiloride, trimethoprim—decreased action of EnaC. Enhanced Cl⁻ transport with sodium rather than Na⁺ :H⁺ exchange.
Aldosterone deficiency or resistance.	Hyporeninaemic hypoaldosteronism. Addison's disease. Pseudohypoaldostereonism.
Decreased NH₄⁺ synthesis.	Hyperkalaemia.
Cytosolic carbonic anhydrase deficiency.	Decreased rate of HCO_3^- synthesis.
Reduced H⁺ conductance.	Toluene.
Normal function of basolateral Cl:HCO3 exchangers.	Hereditary spherocytosis ;ovalocytosis.

Table 9: Diseases causing distal Renal Tubular Acidosis based on mechanisms of acid excretion.
Type IV distal RTA (normal or raised serum K⁺)

COMBINED ALDOSTERONE AND CORTISOL DEFICIENCY.

- Addison's disease
- 21 hydroxylase deficiency.

SELECTIVE ALDOSTERONE DEFICIENCY

Decreased Renin secretion	Hyporeninaemic hypoaldosteronism
Normal or High Renin	Aldosterone receptor defects
	Aldosterone antagonists—spironolactone, heparin therapy
	Converting enzyme inhibitors—ACE inhibitors

Renal medullary interstitial disease, obstructive uropathy [104]

Table 10: Causes of defective secretion or action of Aldosterone.

The most common cause is decrease in mineralocorticoid action on principal cells or drugs interfering with function of sodium channels (ENaC). Aldosterone stimulates H^+:ATPase pumps to secrete H^+ ions; the ENaC sodium channel to reabsorb Na^+; increases the numbers and action of K^+ channels to secrete K^+; and stimulates H^+:K^+ ATPase pumps to secrete K^+ in exchange for H^+. Decrease in aldosterone or its action on receptors therefore leads to decreased H^+ secretion; a less negative luminal voltage because of a decrease in reabsorption of Na^+ in collecting ducts; increased reabsorption of K^+ in exchange for H^+ by H^+:K^+ ATPase pumps; and hyperkalaemia. Hyperkalaemia also decreases NH_4^+ synthesis by proximal tubules and NH_4^+ transport. Distal RTA is differentiated by serum K^+: low serum K^+ Type 1 and those with a normal or high serum K^+ Type IV. However serum potassium may be normal in type 1. Causes of defective action of aldosterone are shown in Table 10.

Hyporeninaemic hypoaldostereonism, which is usually associated with diabetes from dysfunction of renin secreting cells of the juxta glomerular apparatus, is the most important cause. Decreased aldosterone in combination with lack of insulin and acidosis may cause severe hyperkalaemia.

Distal Type IV RTA leads to hyperchloraemic acidosis, volume depletion from decrease in Na^+ absorption, and hyperkalaemia. Urine pH may be appropriately low but NH_4^+ excretion is decreased as shown by low negative or positive urine anion gap. Stone formation is rare [105]. Drugs acting on sodium channels, such as amiloride, may cause distal RTA by decreasing generation of a negative lumen voltage.

RENAL FAILURE. [9, 10, 11, 12, 106, 107]

This may either cause anion "gap" acidosis, hyperchloremic acidosis or both. The following factors are involved in different degrees:

- Low nephron mass decreases NH_4^+ synthesis in proximal tubules. This occurs when GFR falls below 40-50mL/min and decreases Cl^- excretion.
- Interference with medullary recycling of NH_4^+.
- Interference with distal tubular acidification.
- Retention of anions: SO_4^{2-}, phosphate⁻, urate⁻, hippurate⁻ and organic acids⁻ causes a moderate anion gap acidosis.
- H_2SO_4, mainly derived from meat, is buffered by $NaHCO_3$.
  $$H_2SO_4 + NaHCO_3^- \longleftrightarrow Na_2SO_4 + 2H_2CO_3 \longrightarrow 2CO_2 + 2H_2O.$$
  SO_4^{2-} is lost as Na_2SO_4 thus decreasing SID.(strong ion difference).

Early renal failure usually results in hyperchloraemic acidosis. "Anion gap" acidosis increases as renal failure progresses. However the severity of each is also determined by the cause of renal failure: medullary disease causes earlier and more severe renal tubular acidosis because it affects acid excretion—NH_4^+ and H^+. Metabolic acidosis occurs in the majority of patients when GFR decreases to 20% of normal [106]. The plasma HCO_3^- stabilises at a low level because of buffering by bone. However hypercalciuria causes stones and bone disease. Thus even in advanced renal disease serum HCO_3^- rarely falls below 12 mmol/L. [106] Early treatment with $NaCO_3$ is important.

Medullary cystic disease, interstitial nephritis and Lithium toxicity cause RTA by more than one mechanism [36]: defective NH_4^+ synthesis or recycling, distal tubule dysfunction or failure to generate a negative voltage.

APPROACH TO RENAL TUBULAR ACIDOSIS:

- Is the defect isolated or are amino-aciduria, glucosuria or phosphaturia associated. This suggests the diagnosis of proximal RTA.
- What drugs is the patient taking? Can they cause RTA?
- Is the serum K^+ low or high?: Low in proximal and distal Type I; high in distal Type IV.
- Measure urine pH. It is not necessary to pass urine under oil If measured rapidly (ensure NH_3 producing bacterial infection such as from Proteus species are absent)—urine pH is greater than 5.5 despite acidaemia in distal Type I.
- Measure urine anion gap—an estimate of urine NH_4^+ concentration -the key manoeuvre [108,109]. This is rationalised as follows:
  In urine sum of anions must equal sum of cations.
  Major urine cations are Na^+, K^+, Ca^{2+}, Mg^{2+} and NH_4^+.
  Major anions in HCO_3^- free urine are Cl^-, $H_2PO_4^-$, SO_4^{2-} and organic acids. There are usually no major changes in phosphate, SO_4^{2-} and organic acids. Urine Mg^{2+} and Ca^{2+} are present in small amounts and excretion of H_2PO4^-, $SO4^{2-}$ and organic acids are reasonably constant [109]. The average difference between the unmeasured anions and cations is + 80 mmol/L.

$$Na^+ + K^+ + NH_4^+ = Cl^- + 80$$

$$NH_4^+ = Cl^- - (Na^+ + K^+) + 80 \text{ mEq/L}$$

When anion gap is zero ammonium excretion is approximately 80 mEq//L. This is an approximate guide to NH_4^+ excretion.

High urine negative AG suggests adequate NH_4^+ excretion.

High positive or low negative gap during acidosis indicates inadequate NH_4^+ generation. (Chapter 15)

This is misleading if urine anions other than chloride are present in appreciable amounts, for example keto anions and bicarbonate, because these are not measured but obligate cation excretion.

If in doubt, (partial RTA or severe hypokalaemia which can stimulate NH_4^+ synthesis), give <u>furosemide 40-80mg orally.</u> [36, 37]

This increases Na^+ delivery to distal collecting ducts and results in maximum transepithelial voltage because Na^+ is reabsorbed in distal tubules in exchange for H^+. This increases H^+ and NH_4^+ secretion and decreases urine pH to less than 5.5 units 120 -180 minutes following frusemide in normal subjects. [37] In distal RTA (Type I and IV) urine pH does not decrease below 5.5 during acidosis in the majority of cases.

In Type I RTA urine anion gap is low negative or positive indicating low NH_4^+ excretion and urine pH is greater than 5.5 during acidosis. Clinical data and the above response are usually sufficient to establish the diagnosis.

HCO_3^- reabsorption is decreased in proximal RTA but maximum urinary pH is normal or slightly decreased whereas distal RTA has a high urinary pH (>5.5) and low NH_4^+ during acidosis.

Distal RTA (Type I) is associated with hypokalaemia. Positive autoimmune markers should suggest the commonest cause: SLE or Sjogren's syndrome.

Type IV RTA is usually associated with hyperkalaemia: urine pH may be low or high, the urine anion gap is low negative or positive indicating inadequate NH_4^+ excretion and diabetes is commonly present. The most common cause of Type IV distal RTA is Hyporeninaemic hypoaldosteronism, usually associated with diabetes.

Tests in the diagnosis of renal tubular acidosis.

<u>Give Furosemide 40-80 mg</u> orally. Measure pH and urine anion gap for 3 hours. In a recent paper all Type I and IV failed to decrease urine pH below 5.5. [108]

<u>NH_4Cl Loading</u> Give 0.1/kg crushed granules in juice over 1 hour. Collect urine and measure pH (should fall to less than 5.5)

Other tests which are rarely necessary are:

<u>Urine NH_4^+ estimation based on the osmolal gap.</u> [109]

The rationale is based on the number of particles in urine rather than net charge. Urine osmolality is both measured and estimated. Estimated urine osmolality is:

$$2 (Na^+ + K^+) + glucose (mmol/L) + urea (mmol/L)$$

(Na^+ and K^+ are doubled to take account of accompanying anions)

The difference between the measured and estimated osmolality gives an indication of the NH_4^+ present. This is half the difference because NH_4^+ is half of NH_4^+Cl.

$$NH_4 = 0.5 (U. osmol - glucose - urea - 2 (Na + K) [mmol/L]$$

This is not influenced by unmeasured anions which are accounted for by Na^+, K^+ and NH_4^+. Thus if urine anion gap (Net Charge) is positive, which suggests low NH_4^+ excretion, but urine osmolal gap is high (>100mOsmol/kgH$_2$O), which suggests adequate NH_4^+ excretion, unmeasured anions, such as ketoanions, have probably taken the place of Cl^- in accompanying NH_4^+ excretion. This test is useful in ketoacidosis when the calculation of urinary anion gap gives a misleading estimation of ammonium excretion.

Urine: blood pCO2 gradient.

Following infusion of $NaHCO_3$ blood and urine pCO_2 are measured to establish the gradient. H^+ ion combines with unabsorbed HCO_3^- to form carbonic acid and then CO_2 in collecting ducts. This depends on H^+ ion secretion.

$$HCO_3^- + H^+ \longrightarrow H_2CO_3 \longrightarrow CO_2 + H_2O$$

Conversion to H_2CO_3 is slow in distal tubules because carbonic anhydrase is absent. CO_2 is trapped in the tubular lumen. Urinary pCO_2 is normally higher than plasma pCO_2. Reduced urine – blood pCO_2 gradient suggests impairment of H^+ secretion rather than back leak. The gradient is decreased in both Type I and IV RTA (due to defective H^+ ion secretion). The U – P: urine minus plasma pCO_2 in distal RTA (Type I) is <20 and in Type II, proximal renal tubular acidosis, > 20).

TREATMENT OF RENAL TUBULAR ACIDOSIS.

<u>Distal :</u> treat cause and give $NaHCo_3$.

<u>Proximal:</u> much larger amounts of bicarbonate and potassium are required for treatment than for distal RTA

<u>Renal failure:</u> give $NaHCo_3$ early to decrease acidosis.

MANIFESTATIONS OF ACIDOSIS

The most characteristic sign is Kussmaul breathing: highly regular large tidal volume breathing involving both chest and diaphragms. The oxygen cost of breathing is increased, especially in those with underling lung disease. Confusion or decreased consciousness occurs but coma is rare. This is important because the presence of coma should suggest another cause. Myocardial contractility is impaired and arrhythmias occur. [110]

Acidaemia increases sympathetic discharge but attenuates the action of catecholamines on heart and circulation. [110] Increase in serum K^+ occurs in hyperchloraemic but not organic anion acidosis.

Many other symptoms have been described but it is uncertain whether these are due to acidaemia per se or to the underlying cause. Other symptoms are usually due to the condition which causes metabolic acidosis: volume depletion, shock and electrolyte abnormalities.

TREATMENT OF METABOLIC ACIDOSIS. [10.11, 110-116]

Treatment involves correction of the cause, discussed in the chapter on Shock, treatment of specific poisons previously discussed; and chronic treatment of renal tubular acidosis.

Treatment of Acute Metabolic Acidosis with Intravenous $NaHCO_3$, [111-116]

Intravenous sodium bicarbonate for correction of metabolic organic acidosis is not usually used in lactic acidosis or diabetic ketoacidosis because it does not improve outcome. There are several harmful effects of intravenous sodium bicarbonate.

* CO_2 is given off following rapid infusion. CO_2 (but not HCO_3^-) rapidly passes into cells and worsens intracellular acidosis. [10, 11, 12, 111, 112]

  $$Na\,HCO_3^- + H^+ + lactate^- \longleftrightarrow Na\,lactate + H_2CO_3 \longleftrightarrow CO_2 + H_2O$$
  This may not be clinically important if $NaHCO_3$ is infused slowly. [112]

* Bicarbonate administration initially decreases myocardial contractility although this improves with time. [113-115]
* The sodium load may cause or worsen heart failure especially in cardiogenic shock.
* Cardiac arrhythmias are promoted, especially if hypokalaemia is present.
* $NaHCO_3^-$ decreases respiratory drive by modulating the effect of acidosis on peripheral chemoreceptors.
* An increase in pH increases haemoglobin: O2 affinity thus decreasing off loading of oxygen to cells.
* Intravenous hypertonic solutions of $NaHCo_3$ may cause hyperosmolality.
* Ionised hypocalcaemia may result by increasing the binding of H^+ to albumin [9, 10, 11, 12,115] secondary to decrease in $[H^+]$ ($\uparrow$pH). This is important because ionised hypocalcaemia is commonly present before bicarbonate infusion in critically ill patients (see chapter on Calcium disorders).
* Hypokalaemia may worsen in patients with hyperchloraemic acidosis.
* Alkalosis or an increase in pH decreases metabolism of keto acids and lactic acid.

Some advocate bicarbonate therapy to restore HCO_3^- when levels are very low, to prevent further reduction in buffer base to critically low levels. [9,112] Renal replacement therapy, using $NaHCO_3^-$ in exchange, has been reported to be beneficial and may be effective in treatment of metformin associated lactic acidosis.

Intravenous sodium bicarbonate may also be indicated in severe hyperchloraemic acidosis especially if severe hyperkalaemia or renal tubular acidosis is present. [9]

Intravenous sodium bicarbonate is also indicated in some cases of poisoning, such as from salicylate: an increase in pH increases protein binding of salicylate, decreases cerebral transfer of unionised salicylic acid and increases salicylate elimination in alkaline urine.

The amount of sodium bicarbonate given can be estimated by assuming a bicarbonate distribution of 50% of ideal body weight, although this may be higher in severe acidosis. [110,113,117]

HCO_3^- required= <u>increase in HCO_3^- required x weight in kg x 0.5</u>[110].

However follow up measurement of plasma HCO_3^- is important. [110]

METABOLIC ALKALOSIS. [10,118-129] <u>Raised serum HCO_3</u>

<u>Primary metabolic alkalosis</u> = raised serum HCO_3, raised arterial blood pH.

<u>Compensatory to respiratory acidosis.</u>= raised serum HCO_3^-; low arterial blood pH; raised pCO_2.

Metabolic alkalosis is common in hospitalised patients and has adverse effects on patient outcome [10, 11,120,121]. The effects of metabolic alkalosis are similar to respiratory alkalosis but usually less severe because they develop more slowly.

Metabolic Alkalosis causes:

*   <u>Low ionised Ca++.</u>
*   <u>Increase in haemoglobin: O_2 affinity which decreases O_2 release to tissues.</u>
*   <u>Vasoconstriction which decreases oxygen delivery to tissues.</u>
*   Decrease in respiratory response to raised pCO_2.[122].

Manifestations of low ionised Ca^{2+} are tetany–(chapter 10), paraesthesia, dizziness, syncope, seizures, arrhythmias, muscle cramps, weakness and hypoventilation. Vasoconstriction from alkalaemia and increase in haemoglobin: oxygen affinity contributes to these manifestations. Respiratory response to a raised pCO_2 decreases [122] and may be detrimental in those with chronic lung disease.

There may be difficulty in weaning those with chronic obstructive lung disease from ventilators. Alkaline urine predisposes to renal calcium precipitation, stones and nephrocalcinosis. Myocardial contractility decreases. [119,121] Associated manifestations are due to the cause of metabolic alkalosis and associated hypovolaemia, hypertension, hypokalaemia and alkalaemia.

The body therefore defends itself against metabolic alkalosis:

* **Liver converts aminoacids,** which give rise to net carboxyl groups greater than amino groups, to urea. This results in generation of H^+, which combines with HCO_3^- converting it to carbonic acid, which is eliminated as CO_2. [9, 19, 20]

* **Kidney has an enormous capacity to excrete HCO_3^- :** Under normal circumstances once the renal threshold for bicarbonate reabsorption in proximal tubules are exceeded, (Tmax HCO_3^-) reabsorption of HCO_3^- decreases; excess HCO_3^- is rapidly excreted. Normal subjects given 1000 mmol $NaHCO_3$ daily for two weeks only increase serum HCO_3^- to a minor extent [38]. Urinary citrate increases in alkaline urine, decreases calcium precipitation and is also a source of excretion of base. [123]

* The harmful effects of alkalosis on renal calcium precipitation are counteracted by an increase in both citrate and fluid excretion. If hypercalcaemia is present $Ca^{2+}:Mg^{2+}$ sensors (CaSR) inhibit K^+channels, which decrease action of ($Na^+:K^+:Cl^-$) transporters in the TAL. This inhibits Na^+ reabsorption and dilutes tubular fluid.

Respiratory compensation for Metabolic Alkalosis.

pCO2 increases 0.20-1.0mmHg (average 0.7mmHg) for each 1.0 mmol increase in serum HCO_3^-. The response varies and is limited by adverse effects of underventilation, especially in those with disorders of ventilation: pCO2 rarely rises above 55 mm Hg.

Reclamation of HCO_3^-

Excretion of elevated HCO_3^- must decrease to sustain alkalosis. Reabsorption of filtered HCO_3^- is increased in proximal tubules in exchange for H^+, called reclamation. There is considerable controversy about the factors involved and their individual importance. [119,124] These are shown in table 11.

- Decrease in effective blood volume.
- Decrease in GFR.
- Cl- depletion. Chloride is an important modulator of HCO_3 transport (HCO_3- must be absorbed with Na^+ thus increasing $NaHCO_3$ or the SID.
- Potassium depletion.
- Raised pCO_2 and $[H^+]$.

Table 11: Factors in maintenance of metabolic alkalosis

Hypovolaemia increases HCO_3- reabsorption: it lowers GFR, which decreases filtered bicarbonate, and stimulates angiotensin2 and aldosterone secretion which increase Na^+ reabsorption with HCO_3- in proximal tubules.

Metabolic alkalosis can often be corrected by NaCl alone even when moderate hypokalaemia is present [118]. Sodium chloride alone expands extracellular volume, decreases the intense stimulus to proximal $NaHCO_3$ reabsorption, and suppresses aldosterone and angiotensin 2 secretion and potassium excretion. [118,119] However if K^+ depletion is severe KCl is required for correction. However others consider deficiency of Cl- is the important factor in maintenance of metabolic alkalosis. [125] In the Stewart Fencl approach the strong ion Cl- governs metabolic acid-base status. A decrease in Cl- inhibits Cl- : HCO_3- exchange in both proximal and distal tubules.

In distal tubules HCO_3- reabsorption is linked to Cl- excretion: Reabsorption of HCO_3- without cation must lead to Cl- excretion to satisfy electroneutrality. Activity of Na^+:K^+:2Cl cotransporters depend on Cl- availability. A decrease in Cl- sensing by Macula densa cells promotes release of renin, which causes secondary hyperaldostereonism. Chloride administration without volume replacement, corrects metabolic alkalosis [125] provided severe hypokalaemia is absent. [118] When hypokalaemia is severe increased stimulation of H^+:K^+ ATPase pumps increases H^+ secretion which results in acid urine. Other factors involved are hypokalemia which increases proximal tubule HCO_3- reabsorption and stimulates ammoniagenesis; and raised pCO_2 which increases cellular HCO_3- synthesis and reabsorption. [10,119]

The concept of reclamation, compared to generation of metabolic alkalosis is important because alkalosis may remain long after factors generating it have resolved. In HCl acid drainage experiments both volume replacement and Cl⁻ repletion were required before metabolic alkalosis improved despite cessation of HCl drainage.

Renal Regeneration of HCO$_3$ Renal factors which influence distal secretion of H⁺ are:

- Increased activity of Na⁺:K⁺ pumps on basolateral membranes of principal cells.
- Increased delivery of Na⁺ to collecting ducts because absorption of Na⁺ creates a negative gradient facilitating H⁺ and K⁺ secretion.
- Aldosterone [119] or other mineralocorticoids which stimulate H⁺:ATPase pumps in α intercalated cells to secrete H⁺; increase activity and number of sodium channels (ENaC) in Principal cells; increases K⁺ secretion; and activity of Na⁺:K⁺ pumps on basolateral membranes. Local and systemic angiotensin 2 increases H⁺ secretion and HCO$_3$⁻ in both proximal and distal tubule. [24]
- Hypokalaemia stimulates secretion of H⁺ ions by H⁺:K⁺ ATPase pumps thus promoting K⁺ reabsorption in exchange for H⁺;and stimulates ammoniagenesis in proximal tubules. [119]
- Normal function of H⁺ ATPase and H⁺: K⁺ ATPase pumps. Although NH$_4$⁺ is the most important ion in acid excretion H⁺ secretion is required to form an acid lumen to attract
- NH$_3$ diffusion into the lumen from the medulla to bind H⁺. [124]

Pathogenesis of metabolic alkalosis. [118-131]

The usefulness of separating proximal from distal tubular factors in the genesis and maintenance of metabolic alkalosis is questionable given that several of the same factors act on both proximal and distal tubules. The key factors are:

Volume depletion: stimulates HCO$_3$⁻ reabsorption in both proximal [118] and distal tubules [127] (Cl⁻ is deficient) and stimulates synthesis of aldosterone which mainly acts on distal tubules.

Cl- depletion: is probably the most important factor because net HCO$_3$⁻ reabsorption is linked to Cl⁻ excretion; the activity of Na⁺:K⁺:2Cl⁻ transporters depends on Cl⁻ availability and a decrease in Cl⁻ promotes renin release and secondary hyperaldostereonism. Cl^- depletion stimulates proximal HCO_3^- reabsorption. Metabolic alkalosis is much more severe in hypokalaemic subjects on a low, rather than liberal, NaCl diet. [126]

Aldosterone, angiotensin 2: stimulates H^+ secretion by H^+:ATPase pumps in distal tubules [128,129]. Angiotensin 2 stimulates both proximal and distal tubules to reabsorb HCO_3^- and secrete H^+. [24]

Potassium depletion: acts on both proximal and distal tubules to decrease GFR; increases proximal tubule reabsorption of HCO_3^-; stimulates ammoniagenesis in proximal tubules; stimulates H^+:K^+ ATPase pumps to reabsorb K^+ and secrete H^+ ion in α intercalated cells of distal tubules; and inhibits aldosterone secretion.

The cause of metabolic alkalosis is sometimes divided into Cl^- responsive and Cl^- unresponsive. This is unhelpful in practice. Increased mineralocorticoid activity and diuretic therapy are chloride unresponsive. In conclusion: The kidney preserves normal acid-base balance by:

HCO_3^- reclamation in proximal tubules.

HCO_3^- regeneration in distal tubules—the fine tuning of acid-base balance.

Hypovolaemia, Cl^- depletion, aldosterone and hypokalaemia are key factors involved.

SPECIFIC CAUSES OF METABOLIC ALKALOSIS

These are due to increased distal tubule generation of HCO_3^-; loss of HCl or Cl^- in gastrointestinal disorders; administration of alkali; excessive loss of Cl^- in sweat; and in compensation for a raised pCO_2. Specific causes are shown in table 12.

HCl LOSS- vomiting, nasogastric tube aspiration

RENAL CAUSES:

Diuretics. **Mineralocorticoid excess or action** ► Bartter's and, Gitelmans syndrome. Severe K^+ depletion. <u>Poorly absorbed anions</u>. For example Penicillin antibiotics. Following correction of diabetic ketoacidosis.	I.º Hyperaldostereonism. Cortisol excess. ↓11 βOH steroid dehydrogenase 2. ↓11 βOH lase and 17 ∝ hydroxylase. Liddles Syndrome. Liquorice. Apparent mineralocorticoid excess.

IATROGENIC {Citrate infusion in blood (1 unit = 17 mmol citrate), 1 unit packed cells (5.ommol/L citrate), Intravenous $NaHCO_3$, calcium carbonate intake, milk alkali syndrome.
EXCESSIVE SWEAT LOSS: loss of Cl in cystic fibrosis or under extreme environmental conditions.
CHLORIDE LOSING DIARRHOEA.
TREATMENT OF HYPERCAPNIA.
RECOVERY FROM MALNUTRITION.
HYPOALBUMINEMIA.

Table 12: Specific causes of Metabolic Alkalosis.

Loss of HCl.

Gastric juice contains ~ 6omEq/L Na^+, 1omEq/L K^+ and 100-150mEq/L chloride [130,131]. Loss of gastric juice causes:

Cl deficiency.

Volume depletion from Na^+ loss in vomitus and initially with HCO_3^- in urine.

Renin angiotensin aldosterone system activation from volume depletion.

<u>Severe K^+ depletion from urinary loss.</u>

* Each mmol of H^+ and Cl^- secreted into stomach results in the reabsorption of 1mmol $Na^+HCo_3^-$ into the interstitial space and circulation. This generates metabolic alkalosis.
* The kidney initially excretes Na^+ with HCO_3^- because HCO_3^- is a poorly reabsorbable anion. Urine is initially alkaline and contains an increase in sodium bicarbonate.
* Following continued vomiting <u>hypovolaemia</u> increases from loss of sodium chloride in gastric juice and initially from sodium bicarbonate loss in urine.
* Hypovolaemia stimulates the sympathetic nervous system; the renin angiotensin aldosterone system and secretion of AVP.GFR falls and proximal reabsorption of sodium increases
* pCO_2 rises as compensation for metabolic alkalosis and further increases proximal tubule reabsorption of HCO_3^-.

Principal cells in distal collecting ducts increase Na^+ reabsorption in exchange for K^+ which is secreted into the tubular lumen (electrogenic Na^+ reabsorption). This is stimulated by aldosterone and angiotensin 2. Aldosterone causes:

* Increase in activity of basolateral $Na^+ :K^+$ pumps.
* Increase in activity or number of Na^+ channels (ENAC).
* Increase in activity and number of K^+ channels.

The α intercalated cells in collecting ducts increase H^+ secretion which exchanges for sodium, stimulated by aldosterone.

<u>Hypokalaemia is due to urinary not gastric losses of potassium.</u>

When hypokalaemia becomes severe urinary K^+ decreases because $H^+:K^+$ exchangers, rather than $H^+:ATPase$ pumps, increase their activity in α intercalated cells. This increases reabsorption of K^+ in exchange for secreted H^+. Urine therefore becomes acid despite alkalosis. In addition low serum K^+ decreases $Na^+:K^+$ exchange in Principal cells.

Maintenance of metabolic alkalosis is due to an increase in bicarbonate reabsorption in both proximal and distal tubules due to hypovolaemia and a decrease in Cl^- needed for reabsorption with Na^+.

Electrolyte composition of urine varies depending on severity and duration of HCl loss: initially, before full activation of the renin-aldosterone system, HCO_3^- lost in the urine is accompanied by Na^+. Urine is initially alkaline.

Thus urine Na^+ may not be low initially compared to urinary Cl^- which is extremely low.

When volume depletion increases in severity, urine Na^+ and Cl^- both decrease, but urine potassium increases despite hypokalaemia. When hypokalaemia becomes very severe urine K^+ decreases and urine becomes acidic.

DIURETICS. (chapter 14)

Loop diuretics act on $Na^+K^+2Cl^-$ transporters in loops of Henle. Thiazide Diuretics act on Na^+: Cl^+ transporters of distal convoluted tubules and collecting ducts. Diuretics generate alkalosis in the following way:

- Na^+ delivery to more distal tubule sites Increases.
- Loss of sodium causes hypovolaemia and stimulates aldosterone secretion and Na^+ reabsorption in principal cells.
- Increase in lumen negativity increases H^+ and K^+ secretion.
- Aldosterone increases Na^+ exchange for H^+ and K^+.
- Volume depletion, a decrease in GFR, Cl^- depletion, K^+ depletion and Angiotensin2 increase proximal tubule HCO_3^- reabsorption.
- Hypokalaemia decreases GFR, increases HCO_3^- reabsorption and stimulates proximal tubule ammoniagenesis which promote Cl^- excretion.

Bartter's syndrome and Gitelmans syndrome. (chapter 14)

Both syndromes cause chloride resistant metabolic alkalosis.

Bartter's syndrome: is due dysfunction of $Na^+:K^+:2Cl^-$ transporters in ascending loops of Henle and therefore resembles the action of loop diuretic administration.

Gitelmans syndrome: is due to defective $Na^+:Cl^-$ transporters(NCC) in distal convoluted tubules and therefore resembles thiazide diuretic administration.

Excess mineralocorticoid action. (chapter 5)

Increase in action of mineralocorticoids produces volume expansion, hypertension, hypokalaemia and alkalosis. The extent to which hypokalaemia develops depends on the amount of dietary and K^+ intake.

Causes are primary hyperaldosteronism, Cushing's syndrome; deficient action of 11^β and 17α hydroxylase; pharmacological doses of steroids; βOH steroid dehydrogenase 2 deficiency; and liquorice ingestion (Glycyrrhizic acid).

Primary aldostereonism.

Aldosterone acts on aldosterone receptors in principal cells by increasing activity of proton pumps, Na^+ channels, Na^+:K^+ pumps and K^+ channels in luminal membranes. This increases Na^+ reabsorption in exchange for H^+ and K^+which are excreted.

11 β hydroxysteroid dehydrogenase Type II. [132] converts cortisol to inactive cortisone. Cortisol normally acts to an equal extent as aldosterone on aldosterone receptors in collecting ducts. The concentration of cortisol is much higher than aldosterone—micromol compared to nanomol amounts. High doses of steroids exceed the capacity to inactivate corticosteroids. Hereditary defects or inactivation of 11 β hydroxysteroid dehydrogenase type 2 by liquorice results in excessive mineralocorticoid action. [132]

Cortisol excess. occurs in Cushing's syndrome especially when due to paraneoplastic syndrome or high dose corticosteroid therapy. Very high cortisol secretion in paraneoplastic Cushing's syndrome exceeds the capacity of 11 βhydroxysteroid dehydrogenase type 2 to inactivate it. This causes severe hypokalaemia.

Hypertension with secondary hyperaldostereonism. the most common cause is renal artery stenosis.

Renin Secreting Tumours: rare.

Severe Potassium depletion. Potassium depletion increases HCO_3^- absorption in proximal tubules ($\uparrow$ Tm HCO_3^-) and stimulates ammoniagenesis. H^+ secretion increases by H^+:K^+ ATPase pumps In distal tubules and exchanges with K^+ which is reabsorbed. Urine becomes acid and alkalosis develops.

Chloride diarrhoea. [133]

Diarrhoea usually causes metabolic acidosis due to loss of more bicarbonate and organic anions than chloride in diarrhoeal fluid. Chloride diarrhoea

Is a rare hereditary condition which results from a defect of chloride reabsorption in the small and large bowel. Stool Cl^- is raised. Treatment with proton pump inhibitors decreases volume of stool. [133]

Colonic villous adenoma – stool losses are variable but may include large losses of Cl^- rather than HCO_3^-.

Cystic Fibrosis. [134]

The high concentration of sodium and chloride in sweat, (>60mmol/L), compared to normal, leads to volume depletion; metabolic alkalosis from chloride loss greater than the $Na^+:Cl^-$ ratio in extracellular fluid (SID = + 40-42mEq/L).Therefore more chloride than sodium is lost in sweat, in relation to the plasma ratio, and contributes to metabolic alkalosis. Increased aldosterone secretion, secondary to hypovolemia, increases reabsorption of Na^+ in exchange for K^+ and H^+ which are lost in urine. Patients develop metabolic alkalosis, hypokalaemia and hypovolaemia.

Alkali administration. This only occurs if renal failure is present because the capacity to excrete HCO_3^- is so high.

- **Milk alkali syndrome.** [135] This rare condition only occurs in association with renal failure. Ingestion of calcium carbonate and or $NaHCO_3$ causes hypercalcaemia and alkalosis.
- **Ingestion of organic anions such as citrate or acetate** which are metabolised to HCO_3^-.
- **Administration of $NaHCO_3$** by mouth or intravenously.
- **Massive Blood Transfusion:** A high load of citrate is metabolised to bicarbonate. [136]

Delivery of non-reabsorbable anions to distal tubule e.g. carbenicillin and penicillin G in treatment of endocarditis. [137]

Poorly reabsorbed anions, such as penicillinate, obligates Na^+ and/or K^+ excretion to maintain electroneutrality. Thus loss of cations without Cl- increases the SID and may cause metabolic alkalosis.

Following correction of organic anion acidosis. [9, 10]

Bicarbonate infusion may cause metabolic alkalosis following metabolism of lactic or ketoacids to HCO_3^-.

Refeeding Metabolic Alkalosis.

Refeeding following starvation may lead to metabolic alkalosis for unknown reasons. [10]

Compensation for respiratory acidosis. This leads to generation of bicarbonate by distal tubules and increases reclamation by proximal tubules. In both cases this is probably due to the effect of a higher intracellular CO_2 level in increasing synthesis of HCO_3^-. If the condition of the patient improves or if the patient is ventilated pCO_2 may rapidly decrease while extracellular HCO_3^-, which takes time to be excreted, remains raised and causes alkalaemia.

Hypoalbuminemia.

Albumin is a weak acid, an anion with approximately 12 negative charges. A decrease in albumin therefore, results in a slight metabolic alkalosis and a lower anion gap.

The key to understanding metabolic alkalosis is to ask two questions:

> *What generated the alkalosis?*

> *What is maintaining it?*

Factors maintaining alkalosis are hypovolaemia, Cl^- depletion, raised pCO_2, continued excess mineralocorticoid action and severe K^+ depletion. Excess mineralocorticoid activity and continuing diuretic intake cause Cl^- resistant alkalosis. This cannot be corrected by administration of chloride alone.

Stewart Approach to Metabolic Alkalosis.

The Stewart model of metabolic alkalosis is simpler, conceptually clearer and provides easier recall of the causes of metabolic alkalosis than the traditional model.

According to the model there are only two underlying causes of metabolic alkalosis:

> An increase in SID (strong ion difference) : cations >Cl^-

Decrease in ATOT – essentially albumin.

The SID increases from:

- Increased loss of chloride greater than cation. Gastric loss of HCl; increased loss of Cl⁻ from loop or thiazide diuretics; Barrters and Gitelmans syndrome; severe hypokalaemia; compensation for hypercapnia; an increase in mineralocorticoid action; and rarely Cl⁻ losing diarrhoea and cystic fibrosis.
- A gain in cations greater than chloride. Increase in oral or intravenous NaHCO$_3$ intake.

The following is a clinical approach to diagnosis of metabolic alkalosis:

- Look at the arterial blood pH, pCO$_2$ and serum HCO3⁻.
- Is it compensatory to respiratory acidosis: pH low, pCO$_2$ raised and serum HCO$_3$⁻ elevated.
- Is it Primary: pH and serum HCO$_3$⁻ are raised and pCO$_2$ increased: 0.5-0.7mm Hg, on average, for each 1.0 mmol/L rise in HCO$_3$⁻ above normal.
- Are diuretics being taken?
- Is vomiting present?
- Is volume depletion absent or blood pressure raised suggesting mineralocorticoid excess is present?
- What are the urine electrolytes?
  Low or absent urine Cl⁻ suggests HCl loss as in vomiting or naso-gastric suction.
  High Urine Cl⁻ occurs in Diuretics, Bartter's and Gitelmans Syndrome. Barrter's Syndrome, involving defective action of Na⁺K⁺2Cl⁻ transporters in the ascending loop of Henle, resembles the action of frusemide – Urine Ca^{2+} is increased and osmolality low.
  Thiazide diuretics and Gitelmans syndrome involve the diluting segment of distal convoluted tubules and cause high urine osmolality and low urine calcium. Gitelmans syndrome also commonly causes hypomagnesaemia; thiazide diuretics uncommonly do.
  Urine K⁺ is high in vomiting, diuretics, Barrter's, Gitelmans Syndrome and mineralocorticoid excess.

Treatment of metabolic alkalosis.

The treatment is that of the cause.

- Correct volume depletion with normal saline or treat mineralocorticoid excess.
- Correct potassium depletion with KCl.

Cl^- should be given with potassium (KCl). $KHCO_3$ or K citrate will not correct alkalosis or severe potassium deficiency.

Losses of HCl from nasogastric aspiration, vomiting or diuretics, are the most common causes of severe metabolic alkalosis. Proton pump inhibitors decrease the severity of alkalosis by decreasing secretion of HCl and should be considered in those on prolonged nasogastric drainage.

Diuretic induced metabolic alkalosis, associated with hypokalaemia, is treated with either KCl supplements (Slow K 8.0 mmol per tablet or K^+ effervescent 13 mmol per sachet) or potassium sparing diuretics such as amiloride.

Metabolic alkalosis has been safely corrected by HCl (150 mmol/L; maximum infusion 0.2 mmol kg/hour) infused through a central vein [138-140] over 8-24 hours. This is rarely indicated, given availability of proton pump inhibitors.

The amount infused is based on an estimate of the HCO_3^- space as 50% of ideal body weight e.g. to decrease HCO_3^- by 10 mmol/L in a 70 kg male give 10x70x0.5 = 350 mmol.

Specific treatment.

Primary mineralocorticoid excess—aldosterone antagonists [10]

Chronic obstructive pulmonary disease—short course of acetazolamide as a trial when the cause of deterioration has improved and correction is resistant to treatment—but is not evidence based.

RESPIRATORY ALKALOSIS. [141-146]

Primary:

Acute: low pCO_2, raised pH (low [H+]); slightly low serum HCO_3^-

Chronic low pCO_2, raised pH (low [H+], more marked decrease in serum HCO_3^-

Compensatory to metabolic acidosis: high [H+] (low pH), low serum HCO_3^-, low pCO_2

Acute: decrease in pCO_2 initially causes a sight decrease in serum HCO_3^-. Blood and tissue buffers give up H+ and Cl- ions which decrease HCO_3^- further to reach a steady state within minutes. Changes are more pronounced than for metabolic alkalosis because CO_2 rapidly passes through cell membranes. [141,142] The serum HCO_3^- initially falls by 1-3.5mmol/L acutely for every 10mmHg decrease in pCO_2 but rarely decreases below 18mmol/L. [142]

Chronic.

If respiratory alkalosis continues the kidneys respond in1-3 days to excrete HCO_3^- and reabsorb Cl^- [119]. In chronic respiratory alkalosis serum HCO_3^- decreases between 2-5mmol/L for each 10mm fall in pCO_2. Serum HCO_3^- rarely decreases below 12mmol/L. In another study the average [H+] decreased 0.4nmol/L and serum HCO_3^- - 0.41mmol/L for each 1mmHg decrease in pCO_2. [144]

Thus in acute respiratory alkalosis serum HCO_3^- decreases slightly. In chronic respiratory alkalosis serum HCO_3^- decreases more.

Serum phosphate may decrease by up to 0.7mmol/L; the serum K+ decreases by a variable amount. [145] Causes of respiratory alkalosis (hypocapnia) are shown in table 13.

Pulmonary disease is the most common cause of hypocapnia: hypoxaemia stimulates peripheral chemoreceptors which in turn stimulate ventilation. However stimulation of pulmonary receptors from decrease in pulmonary compliance from pulmonary embolism can cause hyperventilation in the absence of hypoxemia; and peripheral chemoreceptors also respond to hypotension in shock.

PRIMARY

<u>Hypoxaemia</u>—pulmonary disease causing true shunts or ventilation: perfusion mismatch, diffusion defects and the effect of altitude

<u>Stimulation of pulmonary receptors</u>—pulmonary disease, pulmonary embolism.

<u>Shock</u>—blood loss, cardiogenic shock or severe sepsis.

<u>Hypoxia</u>: **Carbon monoxide poisoning.**

<u>Psychogenic</u>—panic attacks.

<u>Central nervous system stimulation</u>—brain stem stroke, mass lesions, anxiety, pain, hyperpyrexia.

<u>Drugs</u>—salicylates and theophylline stimulate the respiratory centre.

<u>**Induced or iatrogenic hyperventilation.**</u>

<u>Uncertain cause</u>—liver cirrhosis, pregnancy.

<u>**Recovery from metabolic acidosis.**</u>

<u>**Pseudo alkalosis.**</u>

Compensation to Metabolic acidosis.

Table 13: Causes of Respiratory Alkalosis.

<u>Central stimulation</u> of respiration occurs from stimulation of the respiratory centre from brain stem stroke, cerebral mass lesions, salicylate toxicity and hyperpyrexia.

<u>Psychogenic Hyperventilation</u> occurs in panic attacks, severe anxiety or agitation. An important diagnostic clue is absence of hypoxemia. The combination of decreased 2:3 DPG and vasoconstriction cause a marked decrease in O_2 offloading to tissues.

<u>Iatrogenic.</u>

Iatrogenic hypocapnic alkalosis occurs in those with chronic respiratory acidosis with metabolic compensation (usually due to chronic obstructive lung disease) who are ventilated [121] or improve on treatment: CO_2 may rapidly decrease whereas HCO_3^- excretion (Cl⁻ retention) takes time to occur. Correction of hypovolaemia and administration of Cl⁻ are effective treatment.

Pseudoalkalosis. [146] occurs during cardiopulmonary resuscitation as a result of a marked decrease in pulmonary perfusion but relatively normal ventilation. Central venous blood shows low pH (↑[H+]) and increased pCO_2 while systemic arterial blood shows hypocapnia and a raised pH.

Induced hypocapnia was previously a common treatment of head injury, other forms of coma, anaesthesia, raised intracranial pressure, stroke and in those on ventilators [146]. Lack of evidence of benefit and recognition of harm [146] has led to a decrease in use. Indeed permissive hypercapnia is accepted and may be beneficial in those requiring ventilation for respiratory failure. [147,148]

Compensatory to Metabolic acidosis. (Discussed later).

Effects of acute hyperventilation.

Alkalosis due to acute hypocapnia differs from metabolic alkalosis in its very rapid onset and effect on cellular pH: CO_2 rapidly diffuses into cells and decreases intra cellular [H⁺] while HCO_3^- and H⁺ ions pass cell membranes slowly. Respiratory alkalaemia therefore causes more severe manifestations than does metabolic alkalosis. These are especially apparent in psychogenic hyperventilation from panic attacks. Manifestations of Acute Hyperventilation are shown in table 14.

Hypocapnia has been reported to cause several other adverse manifestations: pulmonary broncho-constriction, which may be important in asthma; decrease in lung compliance; increased intrapulmonic shunting; increase in oxygen demand; increase in anaerobic metabolism causing hyperlactataemia; contribution to lung injury in adult respiratory distress syndrome (ARDS); predisposition to thrombosis; and neurological abnormalities in neonates. The adverse manifestations of altitude sickness are probably due to hypocapnia rather than hypoxaemia. [146]

- Mild hypokalaemia and hypophosphataemia – the extent is controversial. [121]

- Slight increase in ketoacids and lactic acids. the anion gap may decrease due to increase in negative charges on albumin which gives up H+.

- Increased O_2 consumption of muscles involved in hyperventilation.

- Vasoconstriction and decreased peripheral oxygen release cause tissue hypoxia ± intracellular acidosis. Vasoconstriction is worse in respiratory compared to metabolic alkalosis. [121]

- Increase in Haemoglobin: oxygen affinity decreases oxygen offloading to tissues.

- The combination of vasoconstriction and a decrease in offloading oxygen to tissues causes tissue hypoxia. This may cause chest pain, syncope or clouding of consciousness, paraesthesia, tachycardia and cardiac arrhythmia.

- Low ionised calcium. This may cause muscle spasm, tetany, paraesthesia and convulsions. The ECG may show steep T wave inversion and QT prolongation.

- Nausea and vomiting.

Table 14. Effects of acute hyperventilation.

Management is to treat the cause. In functional hyperventilation due to panic attacks reassurance, sedation and rebreathing from a bag to decrease hypocapnia are effective. Antidepressants and cognitive-behavioural therapy often decrease attacks.

RESPIRATORY ACIDOSIS.

Primary: Increase in [H+] (decrease in pH) due to raised pCO_2.

Compensatory: to metabolic alkalosis. Increase in serum HCO_3^-; increase in pH (decrease [H+]; Increase in pCO_2 (see metabolic alkalosis).

PRIMARY RESPIRATORY ACIDOSIS may be acute, chronic or acute superimposed on chronic.

Acute.

High pCO_2; low pH; <u>slight increase HCO_3^-</u>

Increase in pCO_2 decreases pH and raises plasma HCO_3^- slightly. Intracellular acidosis increases rapidly because membranes are rapidly permeable to CO_2. The plasma HCO_3^- rises acutely by 0.25-1.75mmol/L, average 1.0mmol/L, for each 10mm increase in pCO_2.

<u>Blood and tissue buffers</u>: haemoglobin⁻, phosphate⁻ and protein⁻ rapidly take up H^+ ions from H_2CO_3 and increase serum HCO_3^-. Bicarbonate itself cannot participate in buffering because it would lead to H_2CO_3 formation and production of more CO_2.

Increase in pCO_2 and /or decrease in pO_2 stimulate ventilation. CO_2 rapidly passes into the medulla and increases $[H^+]$. This stimulates the respiratory centre to increase ventilation. [10]. In contrast hypoxaemia does not stimulate ventilation by the peripheral chemoreceptors until the pO_2 falls below 60mmHg. [149] The resulting hyperventilation, decreases CO_2 and $[H^+]$ in the medulla.

Chronic respiratory acidosis

High pCO_2; low pH; <u>high HCO_3^-</u>.HCO_3^- increases 3.5-4.0mmol/L for each 10mm rise in pCO_2.

The kidney takes several days to produce new HCO_3^- by excreting Cl^- as NH_4Cl and H^+ as titratable acid($H_2PO_4^-$). Increase in pCO_2 stimulates generation of new HCO_3^- in distal tubules by increasing $[H^+]$ secretion and increases reclamation of HCO_3^- in the proximal tubules. In long standing respiratory acidosis the medullary respiratory centre becomes less sensitive to CO_2 and hypoxaemia becomes the main stimulus to ventilation. Uncontrolled oxygen administration raises pO_2 but may decrease ventilation. Metabolic alkalosis, from an increase in HCO_3^- from renal compensation or from coexistent diuretic use, also decreases respiratory drive. Causes of Acute and Chronic Respiratory Acidosis are shown in Tables 15 and 16.

Chronic obstructive lung disease.

Advanced interstitial lung disease.

Neuromuscular: Motor neurone disease, polymyositis, snake bite.

Central: Brain stem infarction, tumour, bulbar poliomyelitis, sedatives, narcotics, morbid obesity.

Peripheral: Multiple sclerosis, Motor neurone disease, Polymyositis, Cervical cord lesions, Diaphragm paralysis.

Obstructive Sleep Apnoea.

Deliberate hypercapnia in ventilated patients.

Table 15: Causes of Chronic Respiratory Acidosis

Decreased lung compliance.
Massive pulmonary embolism, severe pulmonary oedema, severe pneumonia or aspiration.
Adult respiratory distress syndrome.

Mechanical or airway disorders.
Airway obstruction.
Severe asthma.
Flail chest, tension pneumothorax, and hemothorax.

Neuromuscular
Narcotic overdose. Anaesthesia with muscle relaxants
Guillain Barre Syndrome.
Neurotoxins—botulism, tetanus, organophosphorus poisoning.
Severe hypokalaemia.
Myasthenia gravis.
Cervical cord transection.

Oxygen Treatment of Chronic Hypercapnia.

Table 16: Causes of Acute Respiratory Acidosis.

Treatment of patients with chronic obstructive lung disease with uncontrolled oxygen is a common cause of respiratory acidosis. Patients are dependent on the hypoxemic drive mediated by peripheral chemoreceptors. There is rarely an indication for exceeding an SO_2 >94%: a SO_2 between 85-92% is usually appropriate in acute on chronic deterioration of chronic obstructive respiratory disease.

Hypoventilation decreases clearance of mucus; increases atelectasis; decreases haemoglobin:O_2 affinity; increases ventilation:perfusion mismatch, by decreasing hypoxaemic mediated pulmonary vasoconstriction; and increases blood flow to poorly ventilated areas. Decrease in conscious level from CO_2 narcosis leads to atelectasis from decrease in clearance of secretions.

The initial disturbance in patients with CHRONIC obstructive lung decease is low arterial pO_2. CO_2 diffuses so rapidly that ventilation of relatively normal lung can excrete more CO_2 to compensate for underventilated alveoli. However normal lung cannot increase oxygen uptake because haemoglobin is nearly 100% saturated in these areas.

Raised pCO_2 indicates that asthma, pulmonary oedema and chronic obstructive lung disease are severe.

Clinical Manifestations.

Clinical manifestations are characterised by respiratory acidosis and hypoxaemia. Acute or acute on chronic respiratory acidosis causes early onset mental changes—confusion and somnolence, leading to coma, because CO_2 rapidly passes into brain. The mental state is normal if chronic respiratory acidosis is well compensated by metabolic alkalosis. Headache, high blood pressure, bounding pulse, tremor, asterixis, myoclonus, seizures, tachycardia, arrhythmias and vasodilatation are common.

Severe chronic "stable" respiratory acidosis causes pulmonary hypertension, pulmonary and peripheral oedema if hypoxaemia is severe (oxygen saturation less than 85-90%). Secondary polycythemia, sometimes sufficiently severe to comprise blood flow, is common.

Management

Treat the cause and administer controlled oxygen in chronic obstructive lung disease. Clinical manifestations are usually dominated by hypoxaemia. pCO_2 above 70 mmHg on room air is usually incompatible with life (see following pages on alveolar air equation). Controlled rather than unlimited oxygen, to maintain an SO_2 between 88-94%, is usually adequate.

If metabolic alkalosis is severe acetazolamide 250mg twice daily for 1-2 days may be used cautiously once ventilation improves but evidence of its benefit is lacking.

PRACTICAL APPROACH TO ACID BASE DISORDERS

In the majority of cases clinical data is the most important part of assessment. Never interpret blood gas, pH or serum HCO_3 in isolation. Normograms are rarely available or useful.

Consider reliability

*   Venous rather than arterial sampling results in an inappropriately low pO_2 ~ 40mmHg together with slightly raised pCO_2.
*   Contamination with air (air bubble) increases pO_2 and decreases pCO_2 (air pO_2 = 150mmHg, pCO_2 = ~ 0.)
*   Hyperventilation during arterial puncture may decrease pCO_2 by as much as 10mmHg.
*   Compensate for temperature—severe hypothermia, hyperthermia.
*   Delay in measurement.

ANALYSIS (pH and pCO_2 refers to arterial blood).

*   First look at the pH: This gives one primary disturbance.
*   Look at serum HCO_3 and pCO_2. Which one explains the abnormal pH.
*   Is there compensation for the primary disorder? Look at:
    HCO_3 in primary respiratory disorders.
    pCO_2 in primary metabolic disorders.
    Compensation implies that the disturbance is chronic with the exception of respiratory compensation for metabolic acidosis.

* Search for a cause Even if a primary disturbance +/- compensation seems to explain the disorder always look at the pO_2, anion gap and clinical details to assess if another primary disorder is likely.
  Apply the Alveolar Air equation: What would the pO_2 have been in the absence of hyperventilation; and calculate the Anion gap for a clue to metabolic acidosis.
  pCO_2, if low, may be an appropriate response to hypoxaemia, regardless of compensation, and is thus primary.
  Look at anion gap—if the anion gap is raised a primary metabolic organic acidosis may be inferred even if serum HCO_3^- is normal. If serum HCO_3^- is normal but anion gap abnormally high a previous chronic metabolic alkalosis was probably present.
* Consider rules for compensation.
  Compensation is uncommonly complete- if compensation is complete, consider whether another primary disorder exists? Compensation should be appropriate. However compensation may be complete in chronic respiratory acidosis.
  Acute respiratory acidosis: Acute changes in pCO_2 do not change HCO_3^- appreciably. Serum HCO_3^- increases 0.1mmol per 1 mm Hg increase in pCO2 or 1mmol for each 10mmHg increase in pCO_2.
  Acute respiratory alkalosis—serum HCO_3^- decreases 0.2mmol per 1mmHg decrease in pCO_2 or 2 mmol per 10mmHg decrease in pCO_2.
  Chronic respiratory acidosis: serum HCO_3^- increases 0.4mmol per 1 mm Hg increase in pCO_2 (4mmol per 10mmHg increase in pCO_2).
  Chronic respiratory alkalosis: serum HCO_3^- decreases 0.2–0.4 mmol for an increase in pCO_2 of 1 mm Hg or 2-4 mmol/L per 10 mm decrease.
  Metabolic acidosis—pCO_2 decreases 1mm Hg for 0.2-0.4mmol decrease in HCO_3^- (2-4mmol per 10mmHg decrease in pCO_2). PCO2 should approximately equal the last 2 digits of arterial blood pH. For example pH 7.20 should be associated with pCO_2 of 20 mmHg during metabolic acidosis.
  Metabolic alkalosis—pCO_2 increases 0.7 mmHg (range 0.2-1.0) for each 1.0mmol increase in serum HCO_3^- but pCO_2 rarely exceeds 55mmHg.

Compensation for primary respiratory acidosis takes time for HCO_3 reclamation or excretion. Therefore metabolic compensation for primary respiratory disturbances infers chronicity. In metabolic acidosis respiratory compensation occurs in minutes but complete compensation take several hours.

It is sometimes useful to look at the (abnormal) anion gap reduction and compare this to the decrease in serum HCO_3^-. The Ratio $\Delta HCO_3 \Delta AG$ (Δ= change) is usually between 1 and 2. Theoretically an abnormal anion gap of 1 mEq should be associated with a serum HCO_3^- reduction of 1 mEq. There are several reasons this does not apply-discussed in part 1. The average ratio in lactic acidosis is 1.6. If the ratio is <1 suspect the presence of an additional non anion gap acidosis. If >2.0 suspect a superimposed metabolic alkalosis. However the ΔHCO_3^- : ΔAG is rarely useful.

PRIMARY RESPIRATORY DISTURBANCES.

Look at the pCO_2 and serum HCO_3^-. In interpreting pO_2 it is essential to understand the alveolar air equation which implies that the sum of pCO_2 + O_2 in the alveolus is constant and reciprocally related.

Alveolar air equation.

- $pO_2 = 21\% \times 760$ (barometric pressure at sea level).
  In normal persons atmospheric air becomes 100% saturated with water in the trachea which exerts a pressure of 47mmHg.
- Tracheal $pO_2 = 21\%$ (760-47).
- Alveolar $pO_2 = 21\%$ (760-47) – pCO2 assuming a respiratory quotient of 1.0.
  CO_2 diffuses so rapidly that there is no significant arterial-Alveolar (aA gradient) gradient and therefore alveolar pCO_2 approximates arterial pCO_2.
  The respiratory quotient of 1.0 indicates that 1mole of CO_2 is given off for each 1 mole of O_2 consumed in metabolism. This is true for glucose but metabolism of fat (respiratory quotient 0.7) gives off 0.7 moles of CO_2 per mole of O_2 consumed. This is because some oxygen metabolised from fat is required to combine with excess H^+ atoms to form water so that less CO_2 is formed. Thus under most circumstances:
- Alveolar $pO_2 = 21\%$ (760-47) – 1.25 pCO2.
- Arterial $pO_2 = 21\%$ (760-47) – 1.25 pCO_2 – alveolar arterial oxygen gradient.

The sum of CO_2 + O_2 in alveoli is constant. Therefore the arterial pO_2 must increase or decrease as the pCO_2, which is the same as alveolar pCO_2, decreases or increases. (CO_2 usually diffuses rapidly from alveoli into blood). The changes are slightly greater if the RQ (respiratory quotient) is

<1. Thus a pO_2 of 70mm and pCO_2 20mm implies that the pO_2 would have been less than 50 (70-20) if hyperventilation had not occurred.

RESPIRATORY ALKALOSIS—$pCO_2\downarrow$, pH $\uparrow$

Acute ($\downarrow pCO_2\uparrow pH$, $\downarrow HCO_3^-$): A normal pO_2 corrected for the normal pCO_2 below normal with only a trivial reduction of HCO_3 (1-4 mmol HCO_3) suggests primary functional hyperventilation from either panic attacks or central neurogenic causes is present.

Chronic ($\downarrow pCO_2\downarrow pH$, $\downarrow HCO_3^-$): the commonest cause is from heart failure, pneumonia and other respiratory disorders causing hypoxaemia. Therefore look at the pO_2 and subtract pCO_2 below 40 from it. (Strictly 1.25 x pCO_2) to estimate what the pO_2 would have been if hyperventilation had not occurred. <u>In chronic obstructive lung disease low O_2 precedes a rise in pCO_2.Therefore pO_2 should always be lower than normal.</u>

Compensatory to metabolic acidosis: ($\downarrow pH \downarrow pCO_2\downarrow HCO_3^-$) this is rarely complete. If it is complete (pH normal or inappropriate) consider another condition.

RESPIRATORY ACIDOSIS:$\uparrow pCO_2 \downarrow pH \uparrow HCO_3^-$.

Acute: arterial blood pCO_2 is increased, arterial blood pH decreased, and serum HCO_3^- slightly raised.

Chronic: $\uparrow pCO_2 \downarrow pH \uparrow HCO_3 \downarrow pO_2$). The commonest cause is respiratory failure from chronic obstructive pulmonary disease. The pO_2 will always be low on room air. This is usually compensated by an increase in serum HCO_3^- (sometimes full compensation occurs).

Compensatory to metabolic alkalosis: $HCO_3^-\uparrow pH\uparrow pCO_2\uparrow$ The pCO_2 rarely exceeds 50-55mmHg unless there is coexistent respiratory disease. The pO_2 is normal (minus the raised pCO_2 above 40).

METABOLIC ACIDOSIS: $\downarrow pH \downarrow HCO_3^- \downarrow pCO_2$

* <u>Is compensation appropriate</u>: pCO_2 decreases 1-1.5mm Hg for each 1.0mmol decrease in serum HCO_3; or <u>PCO_2 = last 2 digits of pH).</u>

If it is inappropriate consider if a ventilation problem coexists: arterial blood pO_2 is usually decreased from pulmonary oedema, chronic lung disease etc.

* Is there an abnormal anion gap (>16).
  Anion Gap Acidosis (see causes in previous section).
  Note Urea and creatinine. Is this raised sufficiently to explain the gap (moderately increased in severe renal failure).
  Is there Ketoacidosis. Are urine ketones positive? This tests for acetoacetate and may be negative if the predominant ketone is ßhydroxybutyrate: This may occur in Diabetic keto-acidosis, starvation and alcoholic keto-acidosis. The history is usually diagnostic.
  Is Lactic Acidosis present? This is the commonest cause and is usually inferred if other conditions are excluded on the basis of clinical and laboratory data. Measure serum lactate if available (>5mmol/L for lactic acidosis).
  Poisons (see previous section for more details)
  Methyl alcohol, Ethyl alcohol, isopropyl alcohol.
  Ethylene glycol (antifreeze).
  Toluene Toxicity—Hippuric acid—the anion gap is usually normal. May mimic renal tubular acidosis.
   Paracetamol—Pyroglutamic acid.
* Non anion gap acidosis (Hyperchloraemic Acidosis).
• Can medication or Diarrhoea be the cause?
• Is serum K^+ low or high?
• What is the urine pH :should be < 5.5 during acidosis?
• Is generation of NH_4^+ adequate? Calculate urine anion gap and urine K^+.

Urine anion gap (estimate of NH_4^+) = 0.8 [Cl$^-$ - (Na+ + K+)] + 80

The extent to which Cl$^-$ is higher than Na^+ and K^+ is an estimate of urinary NH_4^+. A positive or low negative anion gap during acidosis indicates inadequate renal excretion of NH_4^+. Urine K^+ will be low in Diarrhoea; high in Type I Distal RTA.

Consider the osmolar gap by calculating and also measuring osmolality by freezing point depression.

Osmolar gap = measured osmolality − 2 x (Na + K) + urea (mmol/L) + glucose (mmol/L) (normal < 15)

If abnormally high are alcohols or ethylene glycol intoxication present?

METABOLIC ALKALOSIS. ($\uparrow$HCO$_{3;}$ $\uparrow$ pH; $\downarrow$ pCO$_2$)

Are diuretics being taken?
Is vomiting present?
Is blood pressure raised? Mineralocorticoid excess?.
Is volume depletion present?
What are the urine electrolytes?

Urine Cl⁻ low or absent—vomiting.
Urine Cl⁻ high—diuretics, Barrters or Gitelmans syndrome.
Urine K⁺ high—vomiting, diuretics and mineralocorticoid.

Remember Barrters syndrome resembles loop diuretics; Gitelmans Syndrome resembles thiazide diuretics. Urine calcium is high in Barrters syndrome and loop diuretic use; low in thiazide diuretic use and Gitelmans Syndrome. The urine osmolality is high in thiazide use; low in loop diuretic use. For a more complete discussion see Urine electrolytes.

REFERENCES

1.   Robinson, James R: Fundamentals of Acid-Base Regulation. Third edition.1967. Blackwell Scientific Publications
2.   Giebisch G, Windhager E Transport of Acids and Bases. p 845 in. Medical Physiology. Ed Boron, WF; Boulpaep, EL, et al.2005.Elsevier Saunders
3.   Marieb, Elaine: Acid Base Balance. p1055-1069. Human Anatomy & Physiology. fifth edition 1995.Benjamin Cummings
4.   Rodwell VW. Water and pH p 15-24 in Harper's Biochemistry. Ed Murray, R; Granner, DK, Mayes, PA, Rodwell VW. 21 edition.2000 McGraw-Hill.
5.   Sherwood, Lauralee: p49-87 Ch3: Fluid and Acid-base balance p 528 in Human Physiology (From Cells to Systems) Ed Sherwood, Lauralee 2005. Brooks/Cole
6.   Ganong, WF: p 271-306. Energy balance, Metabolism & Nutrition. Review of Medical Physiology. 20th Edition 2001.McGraw-Hill:
7.   Porth, Carol M: Alterations in Acid base balance. Ch27: p 625-645. Pathophysiology—Concepts of Altered Health States.5 th edition.1998 Lippincott.
8.   Lehniger, AL; Nelson, D L; Cox MM: Water: It's Effect on Dissolved Biomolecules. Ch 4:p 81-104. Principles of Biochemistry with an

Extended Discussion of Oxygen-Binding Proteins. Second edition.1993 Worth Publishers

9. Halperin, Mitchell L; Goldstein, Marc B: Fluid, Electrolyte, and Acid-Base Physiology. A problem-based approach.3 rd edition1994 WB Saunders

10. Rose, Burton D; Post, Theodore W: Clinical Physiology of Acid-Base and Electrolyte Disorders. 5th Edition.2001 McGraw-Hill.

11. Kaehny WD. Pathogenesis and Management of Metabolic acidosis and Alkalosis p 115-153; Peterson L, Levi M. Pathogenesis and management of Respiratory and Mixed disturbances in Schrier, Robert W: Renal and Electrolyte Disorders. 6th Edition.2003 Lippincott Williams & Wilkins.

12. Androgue, HT: Fluid-Electrolyte and Acid Base Disorders Complicating Diabetes Mellitus; p 2661-2688 in Disease of the Kidney and Urinary Tract. Eds RW Schrier 2001. Lippincott, Williams and Wilkins.

13. Biff P, Alpern RJ. Renal Handling of Hydrogen and Bicarbonate Ions.: p 391-396; Androgue HJ. Normal Chemistry and Physiology of Acid-base Homeostasis in Massry & Glassock's Textbook of Nephrology 4 edition 2001.Eds. Massry SG, Shaul G, GlassockRJ. Williams & Wilkins.

14. Alpern, RJ; Rector, FC. Renal Acidification Mechanisms; in The Kidney p408-471. Vol.1 Ch10:5 th edition.1996 Ed. Brenner, B M.

15. Somero, G: Protons, osmolytes and fitness of internal milieu for protein function. Amer. J. Physiol. 20:R197-213, 1986.

16. Kassirer JP, Bleich HL: Rapid estimation of Plasma Carbon Dioxide Tension from pH and Total Carbon Dioxide Content. NEJM.272 1067-1069.1965.

17. Alpern, RJ: Trade-offs in the adaptation to acidosis. Kidney International 47:1205-1215, 1995.

18. Moe OW, Preisig PA. Dual role of citrate in mammalian urine. Current Opinion Nephrol & Hypert:15:419-424.2006

19. Planelles G.Ammonium Homeostasis and Human Rhesus Glycoproteins. Nephron Physiol.105:11-17.2007

20. Vinay, P, Lemieux G, Gougoux A, Halperin M. Regulation glutamine metabolism in Dog kidney in vivo. Kidney International. 29:68-79, 1986.

21. Wagner CA,Kovicikova J,Stehberger PA et al.Renal Acid-Base Transport: Old and New Players.Nephron Physiology.103:1-6 2006

22. Ibrahim H, Lee YJ, Curthoys NP: Renal response to metabolic acidosis: Role of MRNA stabilization. Kidney Internat. 73:11-18, 2008.

23. Wagner CA: Metabolic acidosis: New insights from mouse models. Current Opinion in Nephrology and Hypertension. 16:471-476, 2007.

24. Ngami GT, Kraut JA.Acid-Base regulation of angiotensin receptors in the kidney. Current Opinion Nephrol Hypertension 19:91-97.2009

25. Kellum, John A: Determinants of Plasma Acid-Base Balance. Critic Care Clinics 21: 329-346 2005.

26. Androgue HJ; Genarri FJ; Galla JH; Madias NE. Assessing acid-base disorders. Kidney International.76:1239-1247 2009

27. Schlichtig, Robert; Grogono, Alan W; Severinghaus, John W: Human PaCO2 and standard base excess compensation for acid-base imbalance. Crit. Care Med. 26:1173-1179, 1998.

28. Simmons, Daniel H: Evaluation of Acid-Base status. Basics of RD. 2(3):1-6.American Thoracic Society. Ed AK Pierce.

29. Dubose, TD: Reclamation of Filtered bicarbonate. Kidney International. 38:584-589, 1990.

30. Soleimani M, Burnham CE: Physiologic and molecular aspects of the Na+ : HCo3- cotransporter in health and disease processes. Kidney Internat. 57:371-384, 2000.

31. Good, DW; Carlton RC ;Dubose T. Transepithelial ammonia concentration gradients in inner medulla of the rat. Amer. J. Physiol. 252:F491-F500, 1987.

32. Wall SM: Mechanisms of NH4 and NH3 transport during hypokalaemia. Acta Physiol. Scand. 179:325-330, 2003.

33. Schuster VL: Organisation of collecting duct intercalated cells. Kidney Internat. 38:668-672, 1990.

34. Wall SM: Recent advances in our understanding of intercalated cells. Current Opinion Nephrology and Hypertension. 14:480-484, 2005.

35. Schwartz JH: Renal acid- base transport: The regulatory role of the inner medullary collecting duct. Kidney Internat. 47:331-341, 1995.

36. Kurtzman, N: Disorders of distal acidification. Kidney International 38:720-727, 1990.

37. Batlle, D, Flores, G: Underlying defects in Renal Tubular Acidosis. Amer. J. Kid. Dis. 27:896-915, 1996.

38. Van Goidsenhoven, G; Gray OV; Price, AV; Sanderson, PH: The effect of prolonged administration of large doses of sodium bicarbonate in man. Clin. Science. 13:383-401, 1952.

39. Hood VL, Tannen RL: Protection of Acid-base Balance by pH Regulation of Acid Production. NEJM. 339:819-826.1998

40. Fencl, Vladimir; Leith, David E: Stewart's quantitative acid-base chemistry: Applications in biology and medicine. Resp. Physiol. 91:1-16, 1993.

41. Sirker, AA; Rhodes A; Grounds RM; Bennett ED. Acid-base physiology: the 'traditional' and the 'modern' approaches. Anaesthesia. 57:348-356, 2002.

42. Gunnerson, Kyle J; Kellum, John A: Acid-base and electrolyte analysis in critically ill patients: are we ready for the new millennium? Crit. Care 9:468-473, 2003.

43. Story, DA; Morimatsu H; Bellomo, R: Strong ions, weak acids and base excess: a simplified Fencl-Stewart approach to clinical acid-base disorders. Brit. J. Anaes. 92(1):54-60, 2004.

44. Kaplan L, Kellum, JA: Strong Ion Gap. Crit. Care Med. 33:266-267, 2005.

45. Dubin, A; Menises, MM; Masevicius FD. Comparison of three different methods of evaluation of metabolic acid-base disorders. Critic. Care Med. 35:1-6, 2007.

46. Poulson WD, Effect of Acute pH Change on Serum Anion Gap. J Am Soc Nephrol.7:357-363.1996.

47. Gabow, Patricia A: Disorders associated with an altered anion gap. Kidney International 27:472-483, 1985.

48. Emmet, M; Narins, RG: Clinical use of the Anion Gap. Medicine 56(1):38-54, 1977.

49. Oh, Man S; Carroll, Hugh J: Current Concepts—The Anion Gap. New Eng. J of Med. 297(15):814-817, 1977.

50. Kraut JA, Madias NE. Serum Anion Gap: Its Uses and Limitations in Clinical Medicine.Clin J Am Soc Nephrol.2:162-174 2007.

51. Figge, J Jabor, A Kazda A; Fencl V: Anion gap and hypoalbuminaemia. Crit. Care Med. 26:1807-1810, 1998.

52. Madias, Nicolaos; Auys, J: Carlos ; Adrogue, Horacio J. Increased Anion Gap in metabolic Alkalosis. The New Eng. J. Med. 300(25):1421-1423, 1979.

53. McAuliffe, John J; Lind, Leonard J; Leith DE; Fencl V. Hypoproteinemic Alkalosis. Amer. J. Med. 81:86-90, 1986.

54. Gabow, Patricia A; Kaehny, William D. Fennessey PV et al.: Diagnostic importance of an increased serum anion gap. New Eng. J. Med. 303(15):854 -858, 1980.

55. Salem, M M; Mujais, S K: Gaps in the Anion Gap. Arch Intern Med. 152:1625-1629, 1992.

56. Balasubramanyan, Napa; Havens, Peter L; Hoffman, George M: Unmeasured anions identified by the Fencl-Stewart method predict mortality better than base excess, anion gap, and lactate in patients in the Paediatric intensive care unit. Crit. Care Med. 27:1577-1581, 1999.

57. Rhodes, Andrew; Cusack, Rebecca J: Arterial blood gas analysis and lactate. Crit Care Med. 6:227-231, 2000.

58. Zaritsky, Arno: Unmeasured anions: Déjà vu all over again? Crit. Care Med. 27:1672-1673, 1999.

59. Kaplan, Lewis J; Kellum, John A: Initial pH, base deficit, lactate, anion gap, strong ion difference, and strong ion gap predict outcome from major vascular injury. Crit. Care Med. 32:1120-1124, 2004.

60. Rocktaeschel, Jens; Morimatsu H, Uchino S; Bellomo R. Unmeasured Anions in Critically ill patients: Can they predict Mortality? Crit. Care Med. 31:2131-2136, 2003.

61. Rinaldi, S; De Gaudio, AR: Strong ion difference and strong anion gap: The Stewart approach to acid base disturbances. Curr. Anaes. & Crit. Care 16(16):395-402, 2005.

62. DiNubile, Mark J: The increment in the anion Gap: Overextension of a concept? The Lancet. 951-953, 1988.

63. Reilly, Robert F; Anderson, Robert J: Interpreting the anion gap. Crit. Care Med. 26:1771-1772, 1998.

64. Adrogue, Horacio J; Wilson, Howard MD et al: Plasma Acid-base Patterns in Diabetic Ketoacidosis. New Eng. J. Med. 307(26):1603-1610, 1982.

65. Gennari, F.John: Serum osmolality—Uses and limitations. NEJM. 310:102-105.1984.

66. Smithline N, Gardner KD: Gaps—Anionic and Osmolal. JAMA. 236:1594-97, 1976.

67. Kellum, John A: Lactate and pHi: Our continued search for markers of tissue distress. Crit. Care Med. 26:1783-1784, 1998.

68. Levy, Bruno: Lactate and shock state: the metabolic view. Crit. Care Med. 12:315-321, 2006.

69. Levy, Bruno; Gibot, Sebastien et al: Relation between muscle Na+K+ ATPase activity and raised lactate concentrations in septic shock: a prospective study. The Lancet. 365:871-875, 2005.

70. Gutierrez, Guillermo; Wulf, Marian E: Lactic acidosis in sepsis: Another commentary. Crit Care Med. 33:2420-2422, 2005.

71. Lindinger, Michael I; Heigenhauser, George JF et al: Blood ion regulation during repeated maximal exercise and recovery in humans. Amer. Physiol. Society.262:R126-R136. 1992.

72. Romanski BA, McMahon MM: Metabolic acidosis and thiamine deficiency. Mayo Clin Proc. 74:259-263, 1999.

73. Centres for Disease Control & Prevention (CDC): Lactic acidosis traced to thiamine deficiency related to nationwide shortage of multivitamins for total parenteral nutrition—United States, 1997. Morbidity & Mortality Weekly Report. 46(23):523-528, 1997.

74. Zeviani, Massimo; Di Donato, Stefano: Mitochondrial Disorders. Brain. 127:2153-2172, 2004.

75. Baud, FJ; Borron, SW Megarbane B; et al: Value of Lactic Acidosis in the assessment of the severity of acute cyanide poisoning. Crit. Care Med. 30(9):2044-2050, 2002.

76. Salpeter, S; Greyber, E ;Pasernak G; Saltpeter E. Review: Metformin does not increase fatal or nonfatal lactic acidosis or blood lactate levels in type 2 diabetes mellitus. ACP Journal Club. 137(3):88, 2002.

77. Bonnet, F; Bonarek, M Morlat P Risk factors for lactic acidosis in HIV-infected patients treated with nucleoside reverse-transcriptase inhibitors: a case-control study. Clin. Inf. Diseases. 36(10):1324-1328, 2003.

78. Fouty, Brian; Freeman Frank; Reves, Randall: Riboflavin to treat nucleoside analogue-induced lactic acidosis. The Lancet. 352(9124):291-292, 1998.

79. Cahill GF: Starvation in Man. Clin. Endocrin and Metab. 5:397-415, 1976.

80. McGarry JD, Foster DW: Ketogenesis and its Regulation. Amer J. Med. 61:9-13, 1975.

81. Marliss EB, Ohman JL, Aoki TT, Kozard GP: Altered redox state obscuring ketoacidosis in diabetic patients with lactic acidosis. NEJM. 283:978-980, 1970.

82. Wrenn KD, Sovbis CM, Minion GE, Rutkowski R: The syndrome of Alcoholic Ketoacidosis. Amer J. Med. 91:119-128, 1991.

83. Fulop, Milford; Bock, Jay; Ben-Ezra, Jonathan et al: Plasma Lactate and 3-Hydroxybutyrate Levels in Patients with Acute Ethanol Intoxication. Amer. J. Med. 80:191-194, 1986.

84. Halperin, ML; Hammeke, M; Josse, RG; et al: Metabolic acidosis in the alcoholic: a pathophysiologic approach. Metabolism: Clinical & Experimental. 32(3):308-315, 1983.

85. MacDonald, L; Kruse, JA; Levy, DB; et al. Lactic acidosis and acute ethanol intoxication. Amer. J. Emer. Med. 12(1):32-35, 1994.

86. Fulop, M; Ben-Ezra, J; Bock, J: Alcoholic ketosis. Alcoholism: Clinical & Experimental Research. 10(6):610-615, 1986.

87. Kruse, JA: Methanol Poisoning. Int. Care Med. 18:391-397, 1992.

88. Brent J. Fomepizole for Ethylene Glycol and Methanol Poisoning. N Engl J Med. 360:2216-2223. 2009

89. Gabow, Patricia A; Clay, Keith; Sullivan JB; Lepoff R. Organic Acids in Ethylene Glycol Intoxication. Annals of Intern. Med. 105:16-20, 1986.

90. Fenves AZ, Kirkpatrick HM, Patel VV et al. Increased Anion Gap Metabolic Acidosis as a Result of 5-Oxoproline (Pyroglutamic Acid): A role for Acetaminophen. Clin J Am Soc Nephrol.1:441-447 2006

91. DeMars CS ; Hollister K ;Tomassoni A et al. Citric acid ingestion: A life threatening cause of metabolic acidosis. Annals Emergency Medicine. 38:588-591.2001

92. Carlisle EJF, Donnelly SM, Vasuvattakul KS et al. Glue –Sniffing and Distal Renal Tubular Acidosis: Sticking to the Facts. J. Am.Soc. Nephrol.1:1019-1027.1991.

93. Megarbane, Bruno; Borron, Stephen W; Baud, Frederic J: Current recommendations for treatment of severe toxic alcohol poisonings. Int. Care Med. 31:189-195, 2005.

94. Gordon, IJ; Bowler, CS; Coakley, J; Smith, P: Algorithm for modified alkaline diuresis in salicylate poisoning. Brit. Med. Journal. 289:1039-1040, 1984.

95. Wang F, Butler T, Rabbanig H, Jones PK: The Acidosis of Cholera. Contributions of Hyperproteinuria, Lactic acidema and Hyperphosphataemia to an Increased Serum Anion Gap. NEJM. 315:1591-5, 1986.

96. Uribarri, Jaime; Oh, Man S; Carroll, Hugh J: D-Lactic Acidosis: A Review of Clinical Presentation, Biochemical Features, and Pathophysiologic Mechanisms. Medicine. 77(2):73-82, 1998.

97. Halperin, Mitchell;, Kamel KS: D-lactic acidosis: turning sugar into acids in the gastrointestinal tract. Kidney International. 49:1-8, 1996.

98. Sceingraber, Stefan; Rehm, Markus; Sehmisch, Christiane; Finsterer Udilo; et al: Rapid Saline Infusion Produces Hyperchloraemic Acidosis in patients Undergoing Gynaecological Surgery. Anaesthesiology. 90(5):1265-1270, 1999.

99. Prough, Donald S; Bidana, Akhil: Hyperchloraemic Metabolic Acidosis Is a Predictable Consequence of Intraoperative Infusion of 0.9% Saline. Anesthiology. 90(5):1247-1249, 1999.

100. Williams EL, Hildebrand KL, McCormick SA et al: The effect of Intravenous lactated Ringers Solution Versus 0.9% sodium chloride solution on serum osmolality in human volunteers. Anaesthesia and Analgesia. 88:999-1103, 1999.

101. Morgan TJ, Venkatesh B, Beindorf A, Hall AJ Acid-base and bio-energetics during balanced versus unbalanced normovolaemic haemodilution. Anaesth Intensive Care. 35:173-179, 2007.

102. Smulders, Y M; Frissen J; Slaats, E H; Silberbusch J. Renal Tubular Acidosis—Pathophysiology and Diagnosis. Arch Intern Med. 156:1629-1636, 1996.

103. Niewold, Timothy B; Short, Daniel K; Albright, Robert C: 27-year-old Woman With Numbness and Weakness of the Extremities. Mayo Clin. Proc. 78:95-98, 2003.

104. Batlle, DC; Arruda, JAL; Kurzman, NA: Hyperkalaemic Distal Renal tubular Acidosis associated with obstructive uropathy. NEJM. 304:373-380, 1981.

105. Uribarri, J; Oh, MS; Pak, YC: Renal stone risk factors in patients with Type IV Renal Tubular Acidosis. Amer. J. Kid. Dis. 23:784-787, 1994.

106. Kraut, JA; Kurtz, I: Metabolic acidosis of CKD: diagnosis, clinical characteristics, and treatment. Amer. J. Kidney Diseases. 45:978-993, 2005.

107. Warnock DG: Uremic Acidosis. Kidney Internat. 34:278-287, 1988.

108. Goldstein, MB; Bear, R; Richardson, RMA et al: The Urine Anion Gap: A clinically useful index of Ammonium excretion. Amer. J. Medical Sciences. 292:198-201, 1986.

109. Kamel, KS, Ethier, JH; Richardson, RM, et al: Urine electrolytes and osmolality when and how to use them. Amer. J. Nephrol. 10:89-102, 1990.

110. Adrogue, Horacio J; Madias, Nicolaos E: Management of Life-Threatening Acid-Base Disorders. New Eng. J. Med. 338(1):26-32, 1998.

111. Ritter, JM; Doktor, HS; Benjamin, N: Paradoxical effect of bicarbonate on cytoplastic pH. The Lancet. 335:1243-1246, 1990.

112. Cuhaci, Bulent; Lee, Jean; Ahmed, Ziauddin: Sodium bicarbonate and intracellular acidosis: Myth or reality? Crit Care Med. 29(5):1088-1090, 2001.

113. Bersin, Robert M; Chatterjee, Kanu; Arieff, Allen I: Metabolic and Haemodynamic consequences of Sodium Bicarbonate Administration in Patients with Heart Disease. Amer. J. Med. 87:7-13, 1989.

114. Ayus, J. Carlos; Krothapalli, Radha K: Effect of Bicarbonate Administration on Cardiac Function. Amer. J. Med. 87:5-6, 1989.

115. Cooper, D. James; Walley, Keith R; Wiggs, Barry R; et al: Bicarbonate Does Not Improve Haemodynamics in Critically Ill Patients Who Have Lactic Acidosis. Annals of Internal Med. 112(7):492-498, 1990.

116. Stacpoole PW. Lactic Acidosis: The Case against Bicarbonate Therapy. Annals of Internal Med. 105(2):276-279, 1986.

117. Fernandez PC, Cohen RM, Feldman GM: The concept of bicarbonate distribution space: The crucial role of body buffers. Kidney Internat. 36:747-752, 1989.

118. Seldin, Donald W; Floyd C Rector: The generation and maintenance of metabolic alkalosis. Kidney International. 1:306-321, 1972.

119. Sabatini, Sandra: The cellular basis of metabolic alkalosis. Kidney International. 49:906-917, 1996.

120. Hodgkin, John E; Soeprono, Fred F; Chan, David M: Incidence of metabolic alkalaemia in hospitalized patients. Crit. Care Med. 8(12):725-8. 1980.

121. Adrogue, Horacio J; Madias, Nicolaos E: Management of Life-Threatening Acid-Base Disorders. New Eng. J. Med. 338(2):107-110, 1998.

122. Heinemann, Henry O; Goldring, Roberta M: Bicarbonate and the Regulation of Ventilation. Amer. J. Med. 57:361-363, 1974.

123. Coe, Fred; Parks, Joan H: Defenses of an unstable compromise: Crystallization inhibitors and the kidney's role in mineral regulation. Kidney International. 38:625-631, 1990.

124. Levine, David Z: Single-nephron studies: Implications of acid-base regulation. Kidney International. 38:744-761, 1990.

125. Rosen, Randy A; Julian, Bruce A; Dubovsky, Eva V; et al: On the Mechanisms by Which Chloride Corrects Metabolic Alkalosis in Man. Amer. J. Med. 84:449, 1988.

126. Hernandez RE, Schambelan M, Cogan MG et al: Dietary NaCl determines severity of potassium depletion—induced metabolic alkalosis. Kidney Internat. 31:1356-1367, 1987.

127. Wesson, D: Augmented bicarbonate reabsorption by both the proximal and distal nephron maintains chloride—deplete metabolic alkalosis in Rats. J. Clin. Invest. 84:1460, 1989.

128. Stone, DK; Xie, XS: Proton translocating ATPases: Issues in structure and function. Kidney Int. 33:767, 1988.

129. Garg, LC; Narang, N: Effects of aldosterone on NEM sensitive ATPase in rabbit nephron segments. Kidney Int. 34:13, 1988.

130. Condon, R; Nius, L: Manual of Surgical Therapeutics. 9th Ed, 1996. Ed. Boston Little Brown.

131. Humphreys, MH: Fluid and Electrolyte Management. P147 in Current Surgical Diagnosis and Treatment. Ed. Way, LW, Doherty, GM, 11th Edition. 2003. Lange Medical Books/McGraw Hill.

132. Hierholzer, Klaus; Siebe, Harald; Fromm, Michael: Inhibition of 11β-hydroxysteroid dehydrogenase and its effect on epithelial sodium transport. Kidney Int. 38:673-678, 1990.

133. Aichbichler, Berendt W; Zerr, Charles H; Santa Ana, Carol A; et al: Proton-Pump Inhibition of Gastric Chloride Secretion in congenital Chloridorrhoea. New Eng. J. Med. 336:106, 1997.

134. Kennedy, JD; Dinwiddie, R; Daman-Willems, C; et al: Psuedo-Bartter's syndrome in cystic fibrosis. Arch. Dis. Child. 65:786-787, 1990.

135. Orwoll ES: the Milk-Alkali Syndrome: Current Concepts. Ann Int Med. 97:242-248, 1982.

136. Barcenas CG, Fuller TJ, Knochel JP: Metabolic Alkalosis after massive blood transfusion—Correction by Haemodialysis. JAMA. 236: 953-954, 1976.

137. Brunner, FP; Frick, PG: Hypokalaemia, Metabolic Alkalosis, and Hypernatraemia due to 'massive" Sodium Penicillin Therapy. Brit. Med. J. 4:550-552, 1968.

138. Abouna, G.M., Veazey, P.R., and Terry, D.B., Jr., Intravenous infusion of hydrochloric acid for treatment of severe metabolic alkalosis. Surgery, 1974. 75(2): p. 194-202.

139. Knutsen, Olav H: New Method for Administration of Hydrochloric Acid in metabolic Alkalosis. The Lancet 1. 953-956, 1983.

140. Brimioulle, Serge; Vincent, Jean-Louis, Defaye, Phillipe; et al: Hydrochloric acid infusion for treatment of metabolic alkalosis: Effects on acid-base balance and oxygenation. Crit Care Med. 13(9):738, 1985.

141. Editorial: The Concept of bicarbonate distribution space : The crucial role of body buffers. Fernandez, PC; Cohen, RM; Feldman, GM. Kidney International. 36:747-752, 1986.

142. Madias, Nicolaos E; Adrogue, Horacio J; Horowitz, Gary L; et al: A redefinition of normal acid-base equilibrium in man: Carbon dioxide tension as a key determinant of normal plasma bicarbonate concentration. Kidney Int. 16:612-618, 1979.

143. Gledhill, N; Beirne, GJ; Dempsey, JA: Renal response to short term hypocapnia in man. Kidney Int. 8:376, 1975.

144. Gennari, FJ, Kaehny WD, Levesque, PR; et al. Acid-base response to chronic hypocapnia in man. Clin. Res. 28:533, 1980.

145. Krapf, Reto; Beeler, Iris; Hertner, Daniel; Hulter, Henry N: Chronic Respiratory Alkalosis. New Eng. J. Med. 324:1394, 1991.

146. Laffey, John G; Kavanagh, Brian P: Hypocapnia. New Eng. J. Med. 347(1):43-52, 2002.

147. Laffey, John G; Kavanagh, Brian P: Carbon dioxide and the critically ill—too little of a good thing? The Lancet. 354:1283-1286, 1999.

148. Amato, Marcelo Britto Passos; Barbas, Carmen Silvia Valente; Medeiros, Denise Machado; et al: Effect of a Protective-Ventilation Strategy on Mortality in the Acute Respiratory Distress Syndrome. New Eng. J. Med. 338(6):347-354, 1998.

149. Weir, E. Kenneth; Lopez-Barneo, Jose; Buckler, Keith J; Archer, Stephen L: Acute Oxygen-Sensing Mechanisms. New Eng. J. Med2042-2055, 2005.

POTASSIUM

(25% in Earth's crust (General References 1-6).

'Far better an approximate answer to the right question, than an exact answer to the wrong question'. John Wilder Turkey.

Exchangeable total body potassium (TBK) 30-50mmol/kg ~ 1500-5000 mmol.

Fat Free potassium 68mmol/kg (98% intracellular).

Total extracellular potassium 40 - 60mmol (4.0 x Extracellular Volume (10-15L).

Cellular potassium ≈ 150mmol/L.

Plasma potassium ~ 4.0mmol/L (3.5-5.0 mmol/L).

Ratio intracellular/extracellular K^+ = ~ 30-37:1.

Food intake 0-400 mmol/ day Average 70- 100 mmol/day.

Overall absorption > 90% absorption in small bowel; secreted in colon. Normal faecal loss 5-8% of food intake or 5 - 10mmol/day.

TOTAL BODY POTASSIUM (TBK).

The majority of potassium is contained in muscle (~70%), brain and viscera. A lesser amount is contained in red cells, collagen and bone and very little is present in adipose tissue. Estimation of TBK should be based on ideal body weight because adipose tissue has a low potassium concentration. Normal potassium fat free mass is approximately 68 mmol/kg.

Average males, with higher muscle but lower adipose tissue mass, have higher TBK, ~ 50mmol/kg, than females, ~ 40mmol/kg, and children ~ 40mmol/kg.

TBK declines with age and malnutrition as muscle mass decreases. (Table 1).Total body potassium is much less in those with malnutrition [12-16] and chronic diseases [17] and increased in those with large muscle mass. [18]

Potassium is not only important as the main cation in cells and in growth but the intracellular—extracellular K^+ ratio is vital in propagation of nerve impulses and muscle contraction.

LARRSON[7] n = 736 healthy subjects (Male n = 325, female n = 411) K^{40} Gamma Ray counting

Age intervals (years)	37 - 41	42 - 46	47 - 51	52 - 56	57 - 61
M mmol/kg	54	53	52	51	50
F mmol/kg	47	45	43	42	42

M (Mean Age 49) ;mean TBK = 52mmol/kg. F (Mean Age 42), mean TBK = 44mmol/kg

Novak[8] n = 520 healthy subjects (n = 215 M, 350 F)

Age intervals (years)	18-25	23-25	35-45	45-55	55-65	65-85
M mmol/kg	56	53	53	49	48	43
F mmol/kg	46	46	44	39	38	38

Gallagher[9] healthy volunteers (n = 473) (M 204, F 269) K^{40} Gamma Ray counting.

M	Mean Age 47.7years	K 49.0mmol/kg	Weight 77.7kg	BMI 25.2
F	Mean Age 50.0years	K 34.0 mmol/kg	Weight 70kg	BMI 23.4

Kehayias[10] n = 188 healthy volunteers (K40 Gamma Ray counting).

Age intervals (years)	20– 29	30–39	40–49	50–59	60–69	70–79	80-89
M mmol/kg	53	49	44	43	44	40	37
F mmol/kg	43	41	36	35	35	32	32

Skrabal[11] n=287 normal healthy volunteers. (K^{43})

M mmol/kg	46
F mmol/kg	35

Table 1: Total body potassium abstracted from several sources. M = Male; F = Female. BMI = Body Mass Index.

Potassium is contained in cells at a concentration of approximately 150mmol/L, [1] the same as sodium in interstitial fluid. Note that plasma water, without lipid and protein, has a higher concentration of sodium ~ 150mmol/L than does plasma. In comparison the intracellular sodium concentration is ~ 10mmol/L and extracellular potassium 4.0mmol/L. A model of the electrolyte distribution in the cell is shown below.

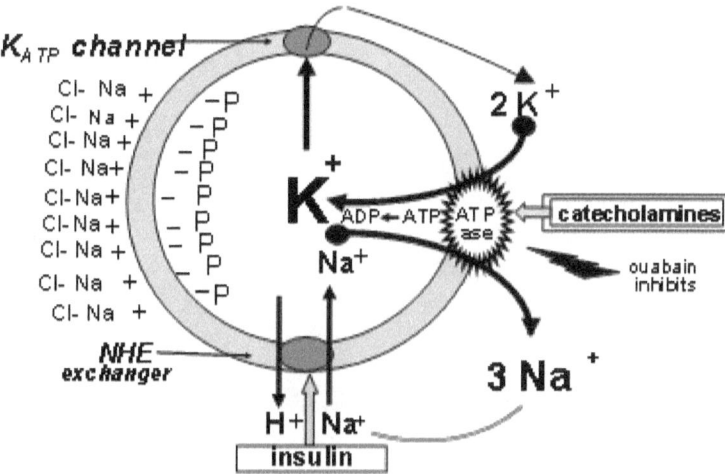

Figure 1: *Simplified Model of electrolyte distribution and mechanisms of electrolyte movement into and out of cells.*

P = both organic phosphate⁻ and protein⁻ which counterbalance positive charges on K^+, Mg^{2+} and other cellular cations. Intracellular anions are repelled by K^+ and align along the inner cell membrane while Na^+ aligns along the outer membrane. Na^+: K^+ pumps transfer $3Na^+$ out of cells in exchange for $2K^+$. This, requires ATP as a source of energy and Mg^{2+} as cofactor. Pumps are stimulated by catecholamines and insulin. [19, 20] A potassium channel (K_{ATP}) and Na: $^+H^+$ exchangers (NHE) are shown at opposite ends of the cell. The Na^+:H^+ exchanger, which transports Na^+ into the cell in exchange for H^+, is stimulated by insulin. Potassium channels leak K^+ which generates negative electrical potential because cellular anions do not diffuse out of the cell. [19]

Changes in extracellular potassium concentration are vital because the difference in K^+ concentration between inside and outside cells makes the most important contribution to the electromotive potential force (EMF) across cell membranes. This is vital for excitability, function of nerve and muscle. The electromotive force (EMF) is generated as follows [19] (figure 1):K^+ moves out of cells through potassium channels (K^+_{ATP}) in membranes due to its high concentration gradient across cell membranes. Na^+ is much less permeable and lesser amounts diffuse into cells. Potassium channels which leak also provide K^+ in the vicinity of cell membranes for continued activity *of* $Na^+:K^+$ pumps. Movement of positive charges out of cells increases net negative charges on protein and phosphate within cells. (By convention when a cation leaves the cell the intracellular potential is called negative).

The cell interior becomes increasingly negative as a result and the electrical force attracting K^+ back into the cell increases. Potassium efflux ceases when the force due to the concentration gradient moving K^+ out of cells is balanced by increase in negative potential in the cell. At the balance point EMF is given by the NERNST equation:

$$
\begin{aligned}
\text{EMF} \quad &= \quad -61 \log (K (i) / K (o)) \ (i = \text{inside}; o = \text{outside cell}) \\
&= \quad \sim -61 \log 150/4.0 \\
&= \quad -61 \times \log 37.5 = -61 \times 1.574 \\
&= \quad \sim 96 \text{ mV}
\end{aligned}
$$

However, ions other than K^+, which move into or out of cells, also exert an EMF. The transmembrane potential depends on their:

- <u>Concentration difference across membranes.</u>
- <u>Permeability across membranes.</u> Although transcellular concentration gradient of Na^+ is approximately $10(i)/150_{(o)}$ its contribution to EMF is lower than K^+ because its permeability is much lower.
- <u>Polarity.</u> For example Na^+, which enters rather than leaves cells, exerts a positive EMF. The components of EMF of most cells is: [19]

K^+	-96mV
Na^+	+ 10mV
<u>Na^+K^+ ATPase pump</u>	<u>- 4mV</u>
Net EMF	-90mV

Note that $Na^+:K^+$ pumps exert a negative potential because 3 Na^+ ions are transported out of cells in exchange for 2K^+ into cells.

The leak of K^+ and Na^+ would eventually lead to equilibrium, with equal concentrations of Na^+ and K^+ inside and outside cells, and would dissipate the cellular negative potential. An energy requiring pump, utilising ATP, pumps 3 Na^+ out of cells in exchange for 2 K^+ into cells and thus maintains normal ionic concentrations.

The combination of leak and rectifying Na$^+$:K$^+$ pumps maintain the transmembrane voltage to which the leak contributes 95% and pumps 5%.

Depolarisation is the process of rapid dissipation of negative potential in cells. Na$^+$ channels are activated by voltage gates in nerve and muscle which open in response to decrease in voltage. When a specific lower voltage is reached, spontaneously or due to a stimulus, Na$^+$ moves much more rapidly into cells and decreases intracellular negative potential—called depolarisation. The sudden conformational change in Na$^+$ channels, which leads to marked increase in sodium permeability, occurs when voltage decreases to approximately -50 to -70mV—called the threshold electrical potential. Excitability of muscle and nerve is mainly due to the difference between resting and threshold potential.

Increase in cell Na$^+$ activates potassium channels which increase K$^+$ efflux out of cells, thus restoring the original negative potential.—called **Repolarisation**. However the negative potential is now due to an increase in Na$^+$ and decrease of K$^+$ ions inside cells.

Finally Na$^+$:K$^+$ pumps are intensely stimulated by an increase in intracellular Na$^+$ concentration and restore normal K$^+$ and Na$^+$ concentrations inside cells.- called **Recharging**

The most important contribution to the resting cellular EMF is the transcellular concentration ratio of potassium.

Extracellular fluid contains a total of only 40-70mmol of potassium (70kg male=15L x 4.0mmol/L).Thus large losses or gains of potassium must be buffered by cells. For example, gain of 60mmol K$^+$ in a single meal or loss of 60mmol in 1L of diarrhoeal stool, without transcellular K$^+$ exchange, would change extracellular K$^+$ to ~8.0 and ~0mmol respectively in a 70kg man. This would have a catastrophic effect on transcellular EMF. Thus potassium transfer into and out of cells is crucial.

Potassium Transfer into and out of Cells.

Net K$^+$ losses are buffered by transfer of cellular K$^+$ into ECF.

Potassium transfer into or out of cells either has to be accompanied by an anion or exchange with a cation to satisfy electroneutrality. Intracellular protein and organic phosphate anions cannot diffuse through cell membranes. Potassium transfer is mainly achieved by exchange with Na^+ due to action of $Na^+ K^+$ pumps. [21-24].

When potassium depletion is corrected cellular Na^+ transfers back into extracellular fluid, in exchange for extra cellular K^+, which moves into cells. This initially increases extracellular sodium, plasma volume and tonicity.

The extent to which H^+ rather than Na^+ exchanges with K^+ is controversial and may depend on acid-base balance. [4, 21 25, 26] Basic amino acids also exchange with K^+ but probably only cause hyperkalaemia when infused. [4, 27, 28]

Potassium may also move into cells in the formation of glycogen, which takes up potassium and phosphate in its formation. Fenn [29] reported that 0.36 mmol K^+ was associated with 1 gram of glycogen. This is released on glycogenolysis, although this is controversial.

Thus most cellular K^+ loss is achieved by exchange with Na^+, although this may be less if sodium depletion is associated. [30]

Given that the intracellular potential is proportional to the gradient across membranes, variations of extracellular K^+ (4.0mmol) alters this ratio much more than equivalent changes in intracellular K^+ at 150mmol/L.

Therefore extracellular K^+ is strenuously defended.

Until recently salt was often unavailable and highly valued. Food eaten in the past consisted of vegetables, leaves and fruit, containing high potassium concentrations with accompanying organic anions rather than Cl^-. [31, 32] Meat (K^+ approximately 100mmol/Kg) was eaten intermittently. The Paleolithic diet contained, on average, 12.6 times more potassium than sodium [32] and often only ~30mmol sodium for mixed diets and 6-7mmol for vegetarian diets. Breast milk contains only 5-6mmol/L of sodium.

Animals, including man, who alternate between starvation and gorging, had to deal with large loads of potassium. [33] Even during starvation breakdown of body tissues release large amounts of potassium, approximately 100mmol per kilogram of muscle. During a gorge more than 300mmol potassium could be ingested and was rapidly absorbed. This entered an extracellular space containing only 50-60mmol of potassium! Despite this, ingestion of 300mmol potassium over 6 hours, leads to an elevation of plasma K^+ to only 5.3mmol/L. [34] Administration of single doses of 205-232 mmol of potassium in 7 volunteers did not increase serum K^+ appreciably. A daily intake of 644 mmol in one subject did not cause symptoms. [35] A daily potassium load of 800 mmol/L is tolerated by potassium adapted individuals. [34]

Moreover the kidney filters approximately 25,000 mmol sodium compared to only 700mmol of potassium daily.

Thus man has evolved to give <u>priority to sodium reabsorption while redistributing and efficiently excreting potassium.</u>

This is achieved by <u>rapid redistribution of K^+ into cells</u> followed by <u>efficient renal excretion</u>.

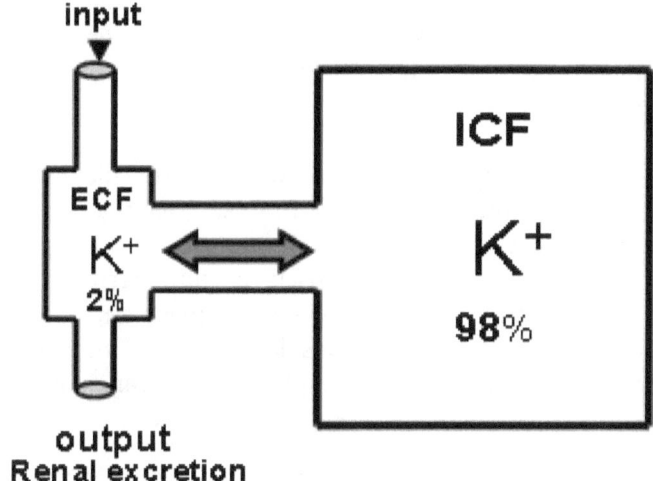

Figure 2. Model of distribution of potassium between cells and extracellular fluid.

Cells contain approximately 98% of TBK (68mmol/kg lean body mass) and ECF 2%. Input is usually oral or intravenous but can include potassium released from cellular necrosis, such as from rhabdomyolysis, sepsis and chemotherapy. A small amount of dietary intake is also lost in faeces.

Redistribution into cells occurs by increased activity of individual $Na^+:K^+$ pumps, numbers of pumps or both. [6, 36] $Na^+: K^+$ pumps are stimulated by hyperkalaemia, catecholamines, acting on $\beta 2$ receptors, and by an increase in intracellular Na^+ concentration [6, 36-38]. A sufficiently high extracellular K^+

also stimulates pumps [36-38] and increases the number of K$^+$ channels in cell membranes. [36-38] Low extracellular K$^+$ decreases pump activity.

Insulin [6, 20, 36, 38-44]

Genetic economy suggests that insulin, secreted in response to meals to dispose of nutrients, should also promote movement of K$^+$ from meals into cells. Insulin does this by activating Na$^+$: K$^+$ pumps. Insulin secretion is stimulated by hyperkalaemia itself, if serum K$^+$ is sufficiently high, [34, 39, 40, 42] but a smaller rise of serum K$^+$ of 0.3-0.7 mmol/L has no effect. However a small increase in serum K$^+$ could increase insulin in portal rather than systemic blood to stimulate insulin release. [39] Portal insulin is normally considerably higher than systemic levels because insulin is degraded on passing through liver.

Potassium is initially transferred to liver and then moves into muscle. The extent that insulin lowers extracellular K$^+$ depends on the amount of insulin administered or secreted. This has implications for treatment of hyperkalaemia.

During an insulin clamp technique, in which serum glucose was kept constant and insulin infused at different rates, 70% of potassium moved into liver during the first hour; and then into muscle during the second hour of insulin infusion, so that muscle became responsible for the continued fall in plasma potassium. The fall in plasma K$^+$ was related to the amount of insulin infused: serum insulin of 37μU/mL reduced serum K$^+$ by 0.5mmol/L, 100μU/mL (in the upper physiological range) by 1.0mmol/L and 1200μU/mL (pharmacological range) by 1.5mmol/L. [44]

MEAN PLASMA INSULIN (μU/mL)	INSULIN UNITS PER HOUR	SERUM K DECREASE mmol/L
27	1.2	0.58
51	2.4	0.62
100	4.8	1.09
428	24	1.44
1,191	70	1.54

Table 2: Insulin infusion rate in 29 male volunteers. Modified from De Fronzo (assuming theoretical average weight of 70kg.) [44]

Glucose metabolised also correlated with reduction in plasma K^+. Decrease in basal insulin increases plasma K^+ [44]. Insulin acts by stimulating Na^+:K^+ pumps, mainly in skeletal muscle and liver. Two mechanisms may be involved:

- Insulin stimulates Na^+:H^+ exchange via Na^+:H^+ exchangers (Fig 1). Increase in intracellular Na^+ concentration intensely stimulates activity of Na^+: K^+ pumps.
- Insulin translocates Na^+:K^+ pumps from the cell interior, where they are inactive, to cell membranes where they are active [43].

During potassium deprivation muscle uptake of glucose and K^+ may be regulated independently by insulin and not necessarily by Na^+:K^+ pumps. [45] Insulin is responsible for retaining an amount of potassium in cells: removal of the pancreas results in transfer of potassium into the extracellular space and decreases the homeostatic response to a potassium load. [42]

During phosphorylation 1mole of glucose binds 4 moles of potassium phosphate. [46] A fixed quantity of K^+ is incorporated in tissue glycogen. Therefore external potassium is utilised when glycogen is formed as a result of the action of insulin; and potassium is released on glycogenolysis.

Catecholamines [6, 36-38, 45, 47-50]

Marked increase in interstitial K^+ occurs on exercise.

Catecholamines promote movement of K^+ into cells (Figure 1). Recall is facilitated by considering that catecholamines are secreted during exercise and counteract the effects of exercise on potassium transfer into interstitial fluid and circulation. β agonists stimulate K^+ uptake by muscle by acting on β receptors and decrease extracellular K^+ [36, 37]. This is achieved by increasing activity of Na^+: K^+ pumps and is abolished by β blockers, but less by $β_1$ selective blockers. [50] β blockers, such as propanolol, increase serum K^+ by approximately 0.3mmol/L. [36, 47]

On the other hand α adrenergic agonists increase serum K^+ concentration by acting on alpha receptors. Adrenaline acts on both alpha and beta receptors: [48] infusion immediately raises and then, decreases serum K^+ proportional to the duration of infusion. [37] Serum K^+ decreases by 0.8mmol/L, on average, and remains low following discontinuation.

Catecholamine secretion from stress, such as from delirium tremens, [6, 36, 38] trauma, labour[49] and acute myocardial infarction cause hypokalaemia. [6, 36] $\beta 2$ agonists given for asthma also lower serum K^+. [36] β_2 agonists also stimulate glycogenolysis and gluconeogenesis. Increase in extracellular glucose concentration stimulates insulin secretion which reduces serum K^+. In a study, using ritodrine and terbutaline, serum K^+ decreased by 0.9mmol/L before serum glucose rose and decreased further to a serum K^+ of 2.5mmol/L as a result of insulin secretion. [49] The combination of β_2 receptor agonists and insulin, which act by different mechanisms, [36] lower serum K^+ more than either alone.

Exercise

Following depolarisation, in the process of muscle contraction, the resting membrane potential (RMP) collapses as K^+ moves out of cells. Normallly K^+ enters T tubules prior to transfer back into cells and little enters interstitial fluid. [36,38] However during intense exercise the capacity of Na^+:K^+ pumps to re-accumulate K^+ in muscle is exceeded and potassium concentration of interstitial fluid surrounding muscle may reach over 8.0mmol/L. [51] This decreases depolarisation, excitability and contractile force, limits exercise capacity and correlates with the rate of increase of muscle interstitial potassium. [51]

Exercise increases K^+ loss from skeletal muscle depending on its extent and duration. Serum K^+ increases by 0.3-0.4 mmol/L after 1 hour of free walking. [2] Exhaustive exercise, however, increases serum K^+ by as much as 3.0mmol/L to a level of 7.0mmol/L [38, 51, 52]. The electrocardiogram shows peaked T waves. [52]

β Blockade increases peak plasma K^+ during severe exercise [50, 51] but selective β blockers cause less hyperkalaemia [50]. This is important in patients with renal failure.

Serum K^+ falls precipitously below the resting level within minutes of stopping exercise and may fall below normal after exercise is completed: [38, 51] in one study to 3.2mmol/L. [38] Thus in games, such as squash, [53] characterised by intermittent bouts of intense activity followed by relative rest, serum K^+ fluctuates from high to low and may predispose to sudden death. [53]

Aldosterone

Rise in plasma K^+ of 0.1 mmol/L increases aldosterone secretion within thirty minutes. The role of aldosterone in moving K^+ into cells is controversial [36, 38, 39] because skeletal muscle, the main K^+ containing tissue, lacks aldosterone receptors. Thus the main role of aldosterone in potassium balance is to <u>increase renal potassium excretion.</u>

Acid base balance [54-64]

H^+ ion concentration (pH) influences transcompartmental distribution of K^+. Hyperchloraemic acidosis causes efflux of cellular K^+ while alkalosis causes influx. The original theory that K^+ simply exchanges with H^+ remains unproven. Studies relating K^+ movement to changes in pH have been carried out in animals using different methods to produce pH changes. The highly variable results may have been confounded by the effects of anaesthesia, co-administration of fluids, especially dextrose containing solutions, variations in tonicity from hypertonic fluid infusion, (sodium bicarbonate for example); changes in pCO_2; catecholamine secretion in response to hypercarbia; renal excretion of K^+; and duration of alkalosis and acidosis.

The few studies in humans have been done on few subjects (only 5 in the original study by Burnell et al). [54)] Most studies, mainly in animals, have been reviewed by Androgue and Madias. [55)]

The balance of evidence suggests that <u>hyperchloraemic acidosis</u> increases plasma K^+ appreciably, probably by decreasing activity of Na^+: K^+ pumps. [57)] However, <u>organic acidosis</u> does not. [55-59)] This is probably due to impermeability of cell membranes to Cl^- anions, compared to lactate$^-$ and ketoanions$^-$, which are free to enter cells with H^+.

A unifying explanation for changes in extracellular K^+, secondary to changes in arterial blood pH, is that H^+ transfer across cell membranes must be accompanied by cations: a ratio. $[H^+]i:[H^+]o$ (i=inside, o=outside) exists as there is for K^+.[55,56)] Thus hyperchloraemic acidosis results in efflux of K^+ as H^+ is buffered in cells but this does not occur when H^+ enters cells accompanied by lactate or ketoanions, shown in figure 3.

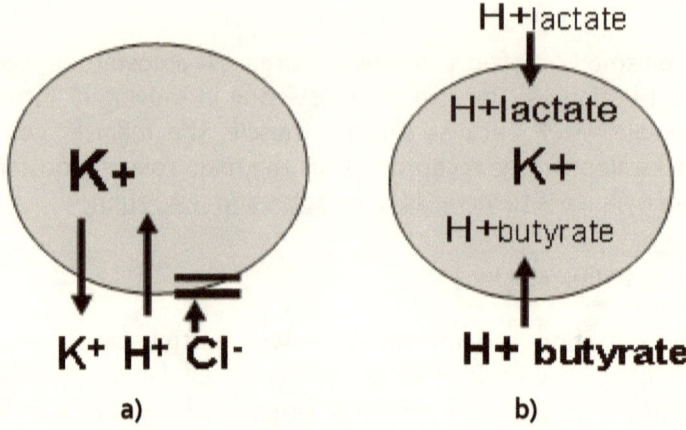

Figure 3: *In a) H+ exchanges with K⁺ because Cl⁻ cannot pass cell membranes. K⁺ efflux and hyperkalaemia accompany acidosis due to HCl. In b) lactate and butyrate can enter cells with H⁺. K⁺ efflux does not occur. Acidosis from β hydroxybutyric and lactic acid do not cause K⁺ efflux from cells and hyperkalaemia does not occur.*

Thus, in buffering, H⁺ must exchange with K⁺ in hyperchloremic acidosis to maintain electro neutrality but keto⁻ and lactate⁻ anions freely pass cell membranes with H⁺ ions. [57] Several studies have shown that plasma K⁺ does not increase during lactic acidosis from seizures or ketoacidosis. [58, 59]

CO_2 passes rapidly into cells during respiratory acidosis or alkalosis: cells share in buffering and do not require H⁺: K⁺ exchange.

The quantitative aspects—the extent plasma K⁺ changes due to change of pH from hyperchloraemic acidosis, is variable in studies in both animal models and man, and a reliable relationship has not been established. The effect of hyperchloraemic acidosis depends on its duration, extent of respiratory compensation and renal bicarbonate retention. Acidosis produced by NH_4Cl in six healthy human male volunteers did not increase serum potassium. [61] However, acidosis produced was mild; hyperkalaemia may have not had time to develop; and glucose given during the experiment may have decreased serum potassium by increasing insulin secretion. Decrease of 0.1 pH unit increased serum K⁺ by 1.6mmol/L In dogs [60]. In most studies serum K⁺ rose appreciably.

Acute respiratory acidosis

This increases plasma K^+ but to a much smaller extent than occurs in hyperchloremic acidosis and is highly variable in different studies. [55] Respiratory acidosis increased plasma potassium by 0.7mmol/L per 0.1 unit decrease in arterial blood pH in anephric dogs, but no increase occurred in rat or rabbit. [62] Respiratory acidosis, to a pH 7.15-7.20, increased serum K^+ from 4.0 to only 4.3mmol/L in human volunteer's. [63]

Metabolic alkalosis and respiratory alkalosis

The majority of studies during alkalosis, mainly in animals [55], show a small decrement in plasma K^+ due to transcellular shifts during alkalosis. Studies in passively hyperventilated patients showed a decrease in plasma potassium but were highly variable. [55] Moreover use of muscle relaxants may have contributed. Treatment of severe metabolic alkalosis with HCl in patients did not increase serum potassium. [64]

The smaller change in serum K^+ during alkalosis, compared to acidosis, may be due to distortion created by the pH scale: For example, an <u>increase</u> in pH 0.3 unit produces a rise in $[H^+]$ of 20 nmol/L compared to decrease in pH 0.3 unit which results in an increase of $[H^+]$ of 40 nmol/L-double the change of the former.

In conclusion evidence suggests that transcellular shifts cause a substantial:

- <u>Increase in serum K^+ in hyperchloraemic but not organic acidosis.</u>
- <u>Slight or no increase in respiratory acidosis.</u>
- <u>Small or moderate decrease of plasma K^+ in respiratory or metabolic alkalosis from transcellular shifts.</u> Changes in serum K^+ from metabolic alkalosis are mainly due to renal losses of potassium.

Hypoxia

<u>Severe</u> hypoxia causes hyperkalaemia by inhibiting $Na^+:K^+$ pumps and potassium channel opening. [38]

Tonicity

Hypertonicity, which causes water loss and potassium efflux from cells to ECF, increases serum K$^+$. [36] This probably causes potassium loss from K$^+$ channels by 2 mechanisms: secondary to a rise in cellular K$^+$ as water transfers to ECF, which increases the concentration gradient and results in cellular efflux of potassium; or by water efflux (solvent drag) –dragging K$^+$ through water channels. In man a modest increase in tonicity (10 - 20mOsmol/kg H$_2$0) increases serum K$^+$ by 0.5-0.7mmol/L. [36] Infusion of hypertonic sodium bicarbonate, glucose, in the absence of insulin secretion, hypertonic saline or mannitol increase serum K$^+$. [36]

Infusion of glucose raised serum K$^+$ between 0.2 and 1.0 mmol/L In insulinopenic diabetic patients and correlated with serum glucose and osmolality following infusion. [65]This is clinically important because infusion of hypertonic glucose increases plasma K$^+$ in diabetics who are insulinopenic. Oral glucose or meals in insulin dependent diabetics may also increase serum K$^+$ by the same mechanism. Intravenous hypertonic glucose, given without insulin to insulinopenic diabetics to decrease serum potassium, may actually increase hyperkalaemia. Infusion of 5% saline, 6mmol/kg body weight, [66] over 120 minutes in patients with chronic renal failure, increased serum K$^+$ between 0.3-1.3mmol/L. [66]

Hypothermia [67-69]

Hypothermia may cause serum K$^+$ levels to fall below 2.5mmol/L from shift of K$^+$ into cells [67] and may cause cardiac arrhythmias. [67, 68] Body temperature correlates with serum K$^+$ levels in postoperative hypothermia. [68]Treatment with potassium may result in hyperkalaemia and arrhythmias on rewarming. [67]

On the other hand hyperkalaemia may develop from rhabdomyolysis, other tissue destruction, hypoxia and severe acidosis, if hypothermia is severe, and is a marker of a poor outcome or death. [69]

K$_{ATP}$ channels [70-72]

ATP-sensitive potassium, channels (K$^+_{ATP}$) are important in secretion of insulin by β cells: inhibition of K$^+$ efflux by sulfonylurea drugs leads to insulin secretion. [70]ATP-sensitive K$^+$channels have diverse functions in other cells, including extracellular K$^+$ balance, K$^+$ excretion, maintenance of vascular tone and preconditioning. [71] Channels are activated (opened) by hypoxia, H^+, lactate⁻, adenosine and low ATP, for example in septic shock, leading to vasodilation. Some drugs, such as non-steroidal antiinflammatories, nicorandil, nitrates and volatile anaesthetic agents also activate K^+_{ATP} channels. [72] These rarely cause hyperkalaemia or decrease vascular reactivity. [71, 72] Sulphonylurea drugs, caffeine, theophyline and barium [73] block ATP sensitive K^+ channels. In practice only Barium and theophylline (in poisoning) and large amounts of caffeine cause hypokalaemia. [73, 74] However glybenclamide has been used to attempt reversal of K^+_{ATP} channel activation from drugs and sepsis. [71, 72]

Theophyline and caffeine. [75, 76]

Theophyline [75] and caffeine are methylxanthine derivatives with similar structure to adenosine. [76,] Adenosine normally inhibits catecholamine secretion. Occupation of adenosine receptors by caffeine, including its metabolite paraxanthine, and theophylline increases catecholamine secretion. This stimulates activity of Na^+: K^+ pumps. Inhibition of phosphodiesterase, which increases cAMP, also decreases metabolism of catecholamines but is less important. In addition activity of K^+ channels, which transfer potassium out of cells, is normally increased by adenosine. [76] Caffeine and theophylline cause hypokalaemia by both decreasing activity of potassium channels and by increasing catecholamine driven Na^+:K^+ pump activity.

Magnesium [77-86]

Magnesium is a cofactor required for activity of Na^+:K^+ pumps. Complete correction of cellular potassium decreases in animal models with magnesium depletion and is postulated to occur in man by decreasing density and activity of Na^+:K^+ pumps in skeletal muscle. [77-79] The speed of K^+ movement in cardiac muscle is influenced by Mg^{2+} acting on K^+ channels.

Magnesium deficiency is postulated to cause kaliuresis [80] and hypokalaemia. [77, 81, 82] However severe hypomagnesaemia did not prevent normalisation of plasma potassium when combined deficiencies were present in children with malnutrition [83] and infants with gastroenteritis. [84] Recently magnesium deficiency was shown to increase urinary potassium excretion, by decreasing inhibition of K^+ channels (ROMK) in membranes of distal tubules, but did not cause hypokalaemia. [85] There is inadequate evidence that magnesium causes hypokalaemia [85, 86] although deficiency may lower cellular K^+.

Na$^+$:K$^+$ ATPase pumps [36, 38, 51 52]

Skeletal muscle plays a dominant role in short term adjustment of plasma potassium [36, 38, 50, 51] because it contains 70% of total body Na$^+$:K$^+$ pumps and these are more active compared to other tissues. Muscle tissue contains billions of Na$^+$: K$^+$ pump molecules per gram wet weight. [51] The effect of potassium in exercising skeletal muscle, which in extreme cases increases plasma K^+ to 7.0-8.0 mmol/L, [38,51,52] is counteracted by catecholamine stimulation by β_2 adrenoreceptors. This increases adenyl cyclase mediated stimulation of Na$^+$:K$^+$ pumps. Fatigue occurs from an accumulation of interstitial potassium, which can reach 10mol/L in extreme cases, if pumps are overwhelmed. [36, 38, 51]

Three factors govern the extent of potassium lowering by muscle:

- The quantity of muscle
- The concentration of Na$^+$ K$^+$ pumps per muscle. [36,38]
- The activity level of each pump. [36,38]

Changes in the number of Na$^+$:K$^+$ pumps synthesised varies in different conditions (table 3).

Potassium deficiency is an important cause. There is marked loss of Na$^+$:K$^+$ pumps from skeletal muscle, smooth muscle and to a lesser extent heart muscle within 3 days of potassium depletion. Skeletal muscle acts as a buffer to defend the K_i:K_o ratio. Full recovery takes 6 days. During potassium deficiency activity of pumps also decrease [79] and is half maximal when serum K^+ falls below 3.5mmol/L.[36] This has implications for treatment of K$^+$ depletion because transfer of potassium into cells decreases until Na$^+$: K$^+$ pumps are resynthesised. During potassium repletion the high intracellular Na$^+$, (from Na$^+$ previously transferred into the cell in exchange for K$^+$) increases Na$^+$: K$^+$ exchange and large deficits are rapidly replaced. However once intracellular K^+ normalises and intracellular Na$^+$ decreases further uptake of K^+ is slowed until pumps are resynthesised. This may take several days and may predispose to hyperkalaemia in the interim. [36]

Increase in Na+ K+ pumps .	Decrease in Na+ K+ pumps.
Hyperkalaemia.	Hypokalaemia, potassium
deficiency.	
Thyrotoxicosis.	Hypothyroidism.
Physical training.	Immobility and inactivity.
	Starvation.
	Diabetes.
	Chronic renal failure.
	Magnesium depletion.

Table 3: Causes of change in number of Na$^+$:K$^+$ ATPase pumps. [36,38]

Hyperkalaemia increases the number and activity of pumps. Increased activity is probably at least partly due to stimulation of Na$^+$:H$^+$ exchange, because it can be blocked by amiloride.

In conclusion extracellular K$^+$ concentration depends on:

Total body K$^+$ and extent to which it fills or exceeds K$^+$ capacity.

Distribution of K$^+$ between the extra and intracellular compartment.

Which depends on both the number and activity of Na$^+$:K$^+$ pumps.

Redistribution of potassium is a temporary solution to k+ loads. ultimately excess k+ must be excreted.

The kidney has a remarkable capacity to excrete excess potassium.

RENAL CONTROL OF POTASSIUM. [1-3, 5, 45, 87-96]

Potassium is competed filtered. On a daily intake of 100mmol, approximately 700 -800mmol of K$^+$ are filtered each day. In general > 90% of filtered K$^+$ is reabsorbed and urinary potassium is due to potassium secretion by distal tubules. (Figure 4)

65 -70% is reabsorbed in proximal tubules, 20-25% in thick ascending limbs loops of Henle and 5-10% in cortical and medullary collecting ducts.

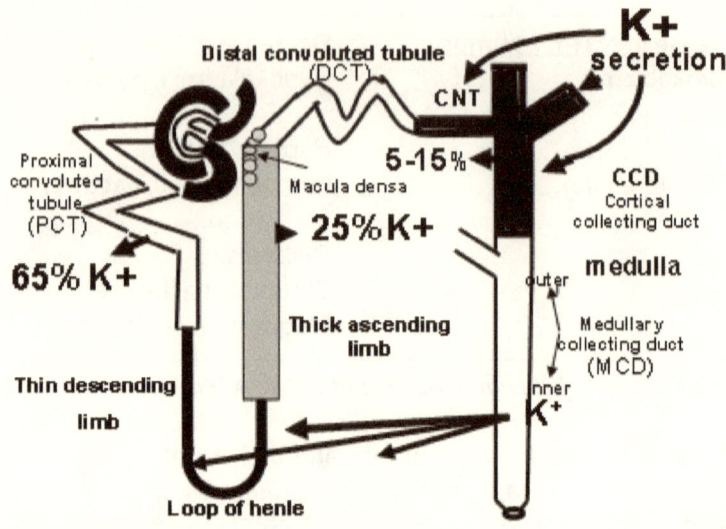

Figure 4: K⁺ reabsorption and secretion.

K⁺ is recycled from medullary CD to interstitium and descending limbs loop of Henle. 65-70 % reabsorption occurs in proximal tubules, 25 % in ascending limbs loop Henle and 5-15% in cortical and medullary CD. Urine K⁺ is mainly due to secretion in connecting tubules and cortical CD -shown as the blacked out area.

Potassium Recycling. [87]

Some K⁺ is reabsorbed in medullary collecting ducts, probably by H⁺: K⁺ pumps, [33] trapped in medullary interstitium by counter current exchange, and secreted into the end of proximal tubules and descending limbs loops of Henle. [87] Recycling conserves potassium during low dietary K⁺ intake or water diuresis.

Cellular mechanisms of potassium reabsorption.

Most potassium is reabsorbed proximal to distal tubules. Alpha intercalated cells in connecting tubules, cortical and medullary collecting ducts only reabsorb 5-15%, but this is where fine tuning of potassium homeostasis takes place. Reabsorption increases during potassium deficiency.

Alpha Intercalated cells in collecting ducts reabsorb K⁺ from the tubular lumen in exchange for H⁺ by H⁺:K⁺ pumps, figure 5. These become more active than H⁺ pumps during K⁺ deficiency. H⁺ secretion into the lumen acidifies urine. K$^+$ with HCO$_3^-$ exits from basolateral membranes. Low activity of Na$^+$:K$^+$ pumps and NH$_4^+$ substitution for K$^+$ on Na$^+$:K$^+$ pumps [88] decreases K$^+$ transfer into cells and enhances K$^+$ conservation. Potassium deficiency also stimulates synthesis of NH$_4^+$ and decreases K$^+$ secretion by collecting duct principal cells.

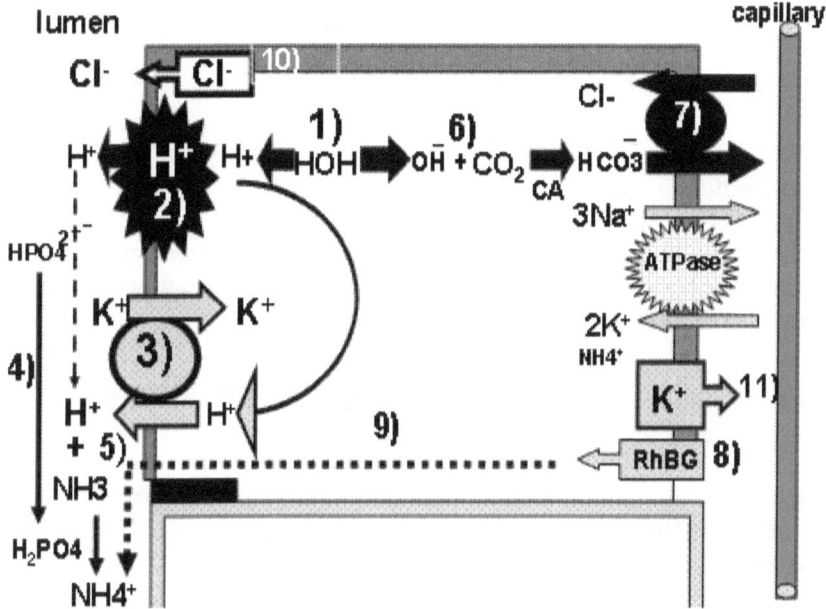

Figure 5: α Intercalated cell. (Numbers correspond to text below).

1. H$^+$ and OH$^-$ ions are generated from dissociation of H$_2$O.
2. H$^+$ is secreted by proton (H$^+$ ATPase) pumps or
3. in exchange for K$^+$ on H$^+$:K$^+$ ATPase pumps.
4. H$^+$ either combines with HPo$_4^-$ to form H$_2$Po$_4$
5. or with NH$_3$ to form NH$_4$. NH$_3$ diffuses into the tubule lumen from the medulla and combines with H$^+$ to form NH$_4^+$. Non lipid NH$_4^+$ prevents its back leak into the cell.
6. CO$_2$ in cell combines with OH$^-$, remaining from dissociation of H$_2$O, to form HCO$_3^-$, catalysed by carbonic anhydrase: CO$_2$ + OH$^-$ = HCO$_3^-$.
7. HCO$_3^-$ exits the cell on Cl$^-$:HCO$_3^-$ exchangers.
8. NH$_4^+$ enters the cell via NH$_4^+$ transporters, (RhBG) by substituting for K$^+$ on Na$^+$:K$^+$ pumps or basolateral Na$^+$:K$^+$:2Cl$^-$ transporters. (not shown)
9. NH$_4^+$ enters the tubular lumen by NH$_4^+$ transporters.(RhBC)
10. Cl$^-$ enters tubular lumen$^+$ via Cl$^-$ channels to accompany NH$_4^-$.
11. Potassium exits cell in basolateral K$^+$ channel.

The ability to decrease urine K^+ when dietary intake decreases may take several days and is associated with decreased aldosterone secretion. [89] When sodium depletion coexists K^+ is conserved, despite an increase in aldosterone secretion, [90] because Na^+ reabsorption proximally limits Na^+ available for exchange with K^+ in distal tubules.[89, 90] Metabolic alkalosis is more severe when NaCl and K^+ are both restricted compared to potassium restriction alone. [89, 91]

Potassium secretion.

Given that most filtered potassium is reabsorbed urinary potassium concentration is due to K^+ secretion.

Principal cells in collecting ducts and connecting tubules secrete K^+ in exchange for Na^+ (Figure 6). [1-5,32,45,92,] Na^+ is absorbed by 2 mechanisms in connecting tubules and collecting ducts.

Electro neutral, Na^+ is accompanied by Cl^- reabsorption via the paracellular route.

Electrogenic: Na^+ is reabsorbed without accompanying anions [1, 3, 33, 45, 93]. This increases the negative potential in the tubular lumen and promotes K^+ secretion—in exchange for reabsorbed Na^+.

It is important to emphasise that K^+ secretion only occurs from electrogenic Na^+ reabsorption - Na^+ reabsorbed without anions. Even during salt poor diets, as occurred in the past, there was a need to deliver 1mmol Na^+ to the cortical collecting duct for each 1mmol of K^+ secreted[32]. There are 2 important clinical implications:

Anions which are poorly reabsorbed, such as HCo_3^-, sulphate$^-$ and organic anions promote K^+ secretion in exchange for Na^+ reabsorption. [92] Decrease in Na^+ delivery to distal nephrons, when cardiac output decreases from hypovolaemia or cardiac failure, limits Na^+:K^+ exchange and potassium excretion. K^+ secretion is carried out by principal cells of collecting ducts shown in Figure 7.

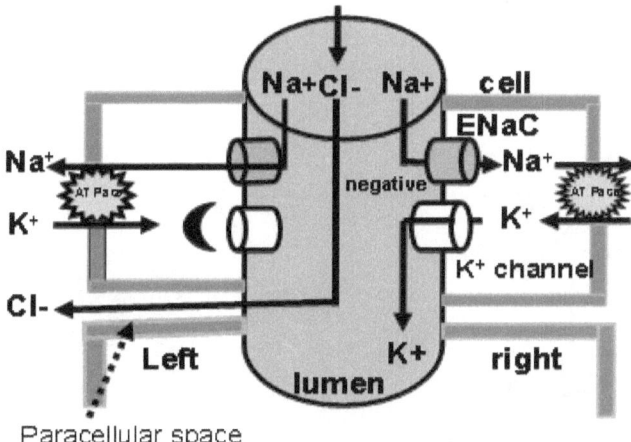

Paracellular space

Figure 6: *Showing Na$^+$ reabsorption in collecting duct: left side electro neutral; right side electrogenic. In electrogenic reabsorption Na$^+$ is reabsorbed through the Na$^+$ channel (ENaC) and K$^+$ is secreted (exchanged) in response to the negative luminal potential created. In electro neutral reabsorption (left side) Na$^+$ is reabsorbed with Cl$^-$, which is reabsorbed through the paracellular space.*

K$^+$ excretion is increased by both high serum K$^+$ and aldosterone. Aldosterone can act as a Na$^+$ conserving or K$^+$ losing hormone. [45] K$^+$ conservation is more easily achieved when hypovolaemia coexists but K$^+$ excretion is not dependent on Na$^+$ balance, intravascular volume or renin secretion. [39, 96] Aldosterone secretion is stimulated by both angiotensin II and directly by raised serum K$^+$. Both are synergistic in stimulating secretion [99]. Aldosterone has the following actions:

* Increases Na$^+$ reabsorption by stimulating sodium channels (EnaC) and H$^+$ ATPase pumps which exchange H$^+$ for Na$^+$:
* Increases Na$^+$ extrusion from basolateral membranes by stimulating Na$^+$: K$^+$ pumps;
* Increases K$^+$ efflux from K$^+$ channels.

Aldosterone acts by inducing a kinase, SgK1, which phosphorylates Nedd 4[97]. Phosphorylation inactivates Nedd 4, a cytoskeletal protein, which normally retrieves Na$^+$ channels (EnaC) and NaCl cotransporters (NCC) from luminal membranes. Their continued occupancy of membranes, due to action of aldosterone, increases sodium reabsorption and K$^+$ excretion via K$^+$ channels. The aldosterone receptor responds to both cortisol and aldosterone. Cortisol, which is present at approximately 1000 times the concentration of aldosterone (μmol compared to nmol amounts), would, if allowed to act, result in severe sodium retention. However cortisol is inactivated to cortisone [97, 98] by 11 ß hydroxysteroid dehydrogenase II (BOHD) before it can occupy the receptor.

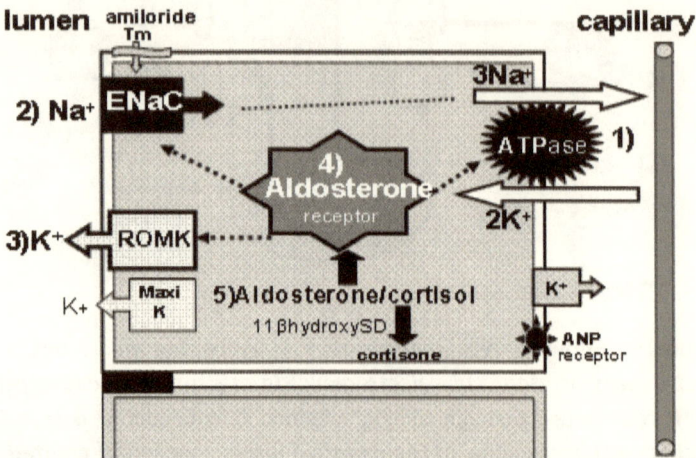

Figure 7. Model of Principal Cell in Collecting Duct. (Excluding water reabsorption). Numbers corresponds to text. ENaC = sodium channel. ROMK= K⁺ channel with high open probability. Maxi K = K⁺ channel with high flow. Tm = trimethoprim-inhibits ENaC. ANP = Atrial natriuretic peptide receptor. IIßhydroxySD= 11 ß hydroxysteroid dehydrogenase type 2.

1. *Activity of basolateral Na⁺:K⁺ pumps generate negative intracellular potential and low Na concentration gradient.*
2. *This increases tubular Na⁺ reabsorption through sodium channels—EnaC. Transfer of Na⁺ from lumen to cell increases negative potential in the lumen.*
3. *K⁺ is transported into tubular lumen by K⁺ channels (in exchange for Na⁺) in response to the negative lumen potential. Na⁺ exits and K⁺ enters cells by Na⁺: K⁺ pumps.*
4. *The aldosterone receptor stimulates activity of ENaC channels, K⁺ channels and Na⁺ K⁺ pumps.*
5. *Cortisol, which acts with equal affinity to aldosterone on the aldosterone receptor, is converted to inactive cortisone by 11 ß hydroxysteroid dehydrogenase type II.*

WNK₄ (with no lysine kinase) and other WNKs modulate the action of aldosterone by:

* Inhibiting action of NCC (Na^+ Cl^- transporters) in the DCT (distal convoluted tubule) thus increasing NaCl delivery to collecting ducts (CD).
* Inhibiting K^+ secretion by collecting duct principal cells by phosphorylating K^+ channels.
* Stimulating paracellular Cl^- conductance, thus increasing Na^+ reabsorption with Cl^- rather than electrogenic Na^+ reabsorption in exchange for K^+.

Mutations of WNK_4 increase NCC activation in the DCT and decrease K^+ secretion in principal cells. This leads to hypertension, hyperchloraemic acidosis and hyperkalaemia—Gordon's syndrome. [45, 94, 97] Gordon's syndrome is due to overactivity of NaCl transporters (NCC) but due to mutations of WNK_4 rather than NCC transporters. [45, 94, 97] Gitelman syndrome is due to mutations which decreases activity of NCC transporters.

Modulation of K+ Secretion by Poorly Reabsorbable Anions

Excretion of K^+ is increased by K^+ exchange with Na^+ and is promoted if poorly reabsorbable anions such as HCO_3^-, phosphate$^-$, sulphate and organic anions are present in the CCD. Na^+ cannot be reabsorbed with these anions so that it must exchange with K^+ or Na^+. [1-3, 33, 92]. Hyperkalaemia inhibits HCO_3^- reabsorption in proximal tubules: delivery of poorly reabsorbable HCO_3^- increases K^+ secretion in exchange for Na^+. Decrease in Cl^- delivery to the CCD in metabolic alkalosis also increases electrogenic Na^+ reabsorption—in exchange for K^+.

Potassium Excretion and Acid-Base Balance [45, 88]

Hyperkalaemia promotes hyperchloraemic acidosis and hypokalaemia promotes metabolic alkalosis. Hyperkalaemia decreases and hypokalaemia increase synthesis of $NH_4^+HCO_3^-$ in proximal tubules. During hyperkalaemia NH_4^+ can take the place of K^+ on $Na^+:K^+:2Cl^-$ cotransporters in the TAL, thus decreasing K^+ reabsorption. (Chapter 6)

Hyperkalaemia due to disorders of cortical collecting ducts.

Failure to secrete K^+ into the tubular lumen of the CCD causes hyperkalaemia. This may be due to:

* Inadequate Na^+ delivery to principal cells to exchange with K^+.

- <u>Abnormal function of epithelial sodium channels</u> (ENaC)from mutations or drugs such as amiloride or triamterene
- <u>Defective action of aldosterone from</u>:
  * Decreased secretion.
  * Receptor defects.
  * Receptor blocking—spironolactone, Eprelenone.
- <u>Low flow rate</u>. This limits K^+ secretion because of build up of high luminal K^+ concentration. Low flow due to ADH is compensated by the action of ADH in increasing K^+ secretion in distal tubules. [1] Urea recycling increases the concentration of urea in collecting ducts which traps water, increases tubular flow and facilitates K^+ excretion. Thus K^+ excretion is facilitated by intake of a high protein -potassium diet.

Role of K+ sensors: response to potassium in food and to extracellular K+. [96,100,101]

Marked increase of dietary potassium increases K^+ excretion independently of aldosterone.[100] Extracellular potassium elicits responses to conserve or excrete K^+ by acting on distal nephrons. In order for excretion to occur extracellular K^+ has to increase above normal-a classical system of negative feedback control. Rabinowicz first proposed the existence of a kaliuretic reflex: potassium in food is sensed by the splanchnic bed or stomach [100] and causes increased potassium excretion by distal tubules <u>before</u> an increase of extracellular K^+ occurs, described as <u>feed forward</u> control. [96,101] During low K^+ containing meals progesterone secretion increases and stimulates K^+ reabsorption from collecting ducts in the absence of hypokalaemia. Progesterone may therefore be an important potassium conserving hormone. [101]

Defence of Hypokalaemia. [96]

Hypokalaemia or intake of low potassium containing food decreases synthesis of aldosterone, Na^+:K^+ pumps in muscle and inactivates maxi K^+ channels by phosphorylating and internalising them. Na^+: K^+ pumps in muscle become resistant to insulin mediated transfer of K^+ into cells but not to glucose transfer. [96] Secretion of K^+ by principal cells decreases. Activity of H^+:K^+ pumps increase in α intercalated cells which increase reabsorption of K^+ in exchange for H^+. Synthesis of NH_4HCO_3 increases in proximal tubule cells which allows substitution of NH_4^+ for K^+ on basolateral Na^+: K^+ pumps or Na^+:K^+:$2Cl^-$ transporters distally. This limits K^+ entry into α intercalated cells. Aldosterone secretion, in response to Na^+ depletion does not cause an increase in K^+ secretion because Na^+ reabsorption is increased proximally, delivery to principal cells decreases and limits exchange with K^+. Progesterone secretion increases in male subjects on a low potassium diet or during hypokalaemia. This may act by increasing activity of $H^+:K^+$ exchangers in the CCD:[101]

Defence of Hyperkalaemia. [96,101]

The response of gastrointestinal K^+ sensors promotes excretion of K^+ from potassium containing meals even before plasma K^+ increases as described.[96] Insulin secretion increases transfer of K^+ into cells. Synthesis of aldosterone, $Na^+:K^+$ pumps and K^+ channels increase in response to either hyperkalaemia or high potassium containing meal.[96] Secretion of K^+ by principal cells increases from action of both aldosterone and raised extracellular potassium. Reabsorption of K^+ by α intercalated decreases due to decreased activity of $H^+:K^+$ pumps; and NH_4 substitutes for K^+ on luminal NCC transporters in ascending limbs loops of Henle, so that K^+ reabsorption decreases there.

Potassium homeostasis in renal failure. [102-106]

Impaired capacity to excrete potassium in renal failure is due to decrease in the number of relatively normal functioning nephrons. However, the failing kidney has a remarkable capacity to deal with potassium loads despite a marked reduction in nephrons. [34,104,106] This is achieved by an increase of $Na^+:K^+$ pumps in basolateral membranes and K^+ channels in luminal membranes [104,106]. Collecting ducts in cortex and medulla increase K^+ secretion and K^+ concentrates in the medulla by recycling.[87] Both raised extracellular K^+ concentration and aldosterone play a role. Aldosterone is important for adaption to potassium loads, but not essential: K^+ secretion [100,102-104] increases from high serum K^+ alone.

High excretion of urea per nephron increases flow rate in the CCD and facilitates K^+ secretion by decreasing K^+ concentration in tubular fluid. [104-106] This is important because many foods containing high K^+ also contain high potential urea content which increases flow down tubules. [105]

Uptake of K^+ by non-renal cells increases and K^+ excretion increases 3-4 times above normal in colon. This is an appreciable percent of K^+ excretion between dialyses. [104]

The extent to which internal redistribution contributes to potassium disposal is less than in normal subjects: $Na^+:K^+$ pump activity decreases in renal failure and translocation of administered K$^+$ to cells is less. [104,106] Insulin secretion increases in response to hyperkalaemia [39 104,106] but probably only when this is severe [103] and an increase within the physiological range may not be clinically important. [39] However hyperkalaemia may be more effective in stimulating insulin secretion than serum levels suggest because levels in portal blood are 3-10 times higher than in systemic blood. [106]

Feeding, which stimulates insulin secretion, the sympathetic nervous system and catecholamine secretion in response to exercise, are important in limiting hyperkalaemia. [106]

Feeding is more effective than intravenous glucose in decreasing hyperkalaemia because insulin secretion is greater from the incretin effect of food; and potassium in food stimulates distal tubule secretion of K$^+$ by feed forward control as described. Oral glucose blunts the rise in serum K$^+$ [107] but serum K$^+$ increases in insulinopenic patients. Intravenous glucose in insulinopenic patients is especially dangerous. Beta blockers should be avoided and insulin compliance promoted in diabetic patients.

The capacity to take up further K$^+$ is limited once serum K$^+$ rises above normal: [102] a small additional load of potassium of only 0.25mmol/kg may cause severe hyperkalaemia in diabetics. [102]

To summarise K$^+$ excretion is driven by both aldosterone and high extracellular K$^+$ concentration.

Conclusion

The following diagram, figure 8, summarises homeostasis of potassium. Most ingested K$^+$ is absorbed. Considerable losses of K$^+$ occur from diarrhoea. Breakdown from starvation, rhabdomyolysis or other causes, especially during hypermetabolic states, such as infection, causes appreciable release of potassium.

Cells "buffer" both excess and deficiency of potassium by altering the extracellular-intracellular ratio of potassium to prevent the resting membrane potential (RMP) changing catastrophically. Serum K$^+$, insulin and catecholamines are the most important factors in internal redistribution. Cells have an enormous capacity to store excess K$^+$ temporarily following a high K$^+$ intake or cell lysis—as much as five times the total extracellular potassium.

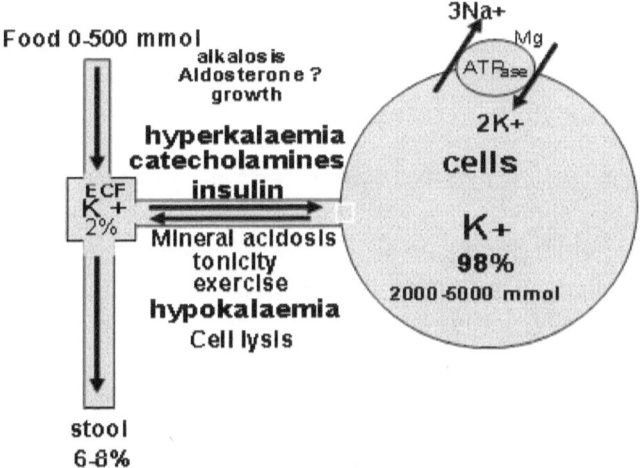

Figure 8: Mechanisms responsible for distributing potassium between cells and extracellular fluid.

Cells contain 98% of total body potassium (TBK), approximately 68 mmol kg lean body mass. ECF contains only 2% of TBK, approximately 45-60 mmol. Input of K^+ occurs from food but may follow severe cellular necrosis from rhabdomyolysis, sepsis, ischaemia and cancer chemotherapy. Factors influencing internal distribution between intracellular and extracellular fluid are shown. Internal redistribution is a temporary solution for potassium homeostasis: potassium must be excreted or conserved by the kidney.

Oral intake of 400 mmol potassium daily in normal subjects increased serum K^+ from 3.8 to only 4.8mmol/L. Plasma aldosterone increased 2½ times in the first two days. The serum K^+ decreased to 4.2mmol/L by 20 days of continued high intake [108]. A daily potassium load of 800mmol is tolerated by potassium adapted subjects.[35] However renal excretion is the only route by which K^+ is permanently eliminated.

Two main factors govern K^+ excretion: serum K^+ and aldosterone. Both high serum K^+ and aldosterone are required for maximum excretion. Low serum K^+ and low aldosterone are required for maximum conservation of potassium.

The final urinary concentration of potassium is mediated by two types of cells in distal nephrons, located mainly in connecting tubules (CNT) and cortical collecting ducts (CCD).

Principal cells—Secretion by principal cells in CD and connecting tubules are responsible for almost all urinary potassium.

Alpha Intercalated cells—reabsorb potassium from tubular fluid.

CAUSES OF HYPOKALAEMIA AND HYPERKALAEMIA

Changes in serum potassium are due to alterations in the potassium load, the transcellular distribution of potassium (internal redistribution) or external potassium losses or gain.

Scribner and Burnell introduced the concept of potassium capacity—the sum of anions that normally associate with K^+. [109] This is equivalent to the total body potassium (TBK) when neither deficiency nor excess is present.

Potassium deficiency is present if TBK is less than K capacity (K.C) and potassium excess when TBK exceeds K capacity (K.C).

Following muscle loss from malnutrition or muscle wasting TBK decreases due to decrease of potassium capacity (tissue loss) and does not indicate that potassium depletion is present[109]. Considerable misinformation resulted in the past because low TBK was used as a measure of potassium depletion. Indeed it is a measure of lean body mass.

On the other hand hyperkalaemia may develop in renal failure because TBK exceeds K^+ capacity following destruction of body tissue. [109] Causes of both hypokalaemia and hyperkalaemia are facilitated by considering factors which are common to both:

* Redistribution of potassium between cells and extracellular fluid—physiological or pathological.
* External losses or gains of potassium:
  Failure of excretion or increased loss by the kidney.
  Non-renal losses: diarrhoea and intestinal disorders.
* Intake of potassium:
  Excess K^+ intake in diet, intravenous K^+ or tissue destruction.
  Decreased K^+ intake: or relative deficiency during rapid tissue formation.

Causes of hypokalaemia and hyperkalaemia are shown in table (4):

EXTERNAL – INTERNAL REDISTRIBUTION	HYPOKALAEMIA	HYPERKALAEMIA
PHYSIOLOGICAL		
Insulin	Increased Insulin	Decreased insulin
Catecholamines	β agonists,	β Blockers
Tonicity		Hypertonicity
Hypoxia, hypothermia	Early Hypothermia	Late hypothermia Hypoxia
Acid-Base	Metabolic and Respiratory alkalosis	Mineral acidosis— respiratory acidosis
Exercise	Post exercise	During exercise
PATHOLOGICAL		
Periodic paralysis	Familial and thyrotoxic	Familial hyperkalaemic
Poisons	Barium, Chloroquine, verapamil	Depolarising Drugs: Succinylcholine
Drugs	Several (see text)	β Blockers, Digoxin, others
Diabetic ketosis	Following treatment	Before treatment

RENAL CAUSES	HYPOKALAEMIA	HYPERKALAEMIA
Renal excretion	Increased—osmotic diuresis, diabetes	Decreased—renal failure
Mineralocorticoid	Hypoaldostereonism	Addison's Disease
Aldosterone Receptor	Gain in function	Loss of function— Pseudohypoaldostereonism.
Corticosteroids	High dose Tumours—ACTH secretion	Adrenal steroid Suppression
Hereditary enzyme	11β + 17α OH lase	21 hydroxylase, others
Renin	Secreting tumours	Hyporeninaemic hypoaldosteronism
11β OH S D2	Deficiency, liquorice	-
DIURETICS	loop, thiazide	Amiloride Spironolactone

OTHER DRUGS	Fludrocortisone Poorly absorbed anions e.g. Penicillin	Inhibition of Aldosterone Synthesis Heparin, Cyclosporine, Ketoconazole NSAIDS, ACE, ARB
TUBULAR DISORDERS		
Hereditary	Barrters, Gitelmans	Gordon's Syndrome (WNK)
Renal tubular acidosis	Type I and II	Type IV. Tubulointerstitial
Acquired tubulointerstitial	Several causes following treatment	Hyporeninaemic Hypoaldosteronism
OTHER	Vomiting Metabolic Alkalosis Non-Reabsorbable Anions	

NON-RENAL CAUSES	**HYPOKALAEMIA**	**HYPERKALAEMIA**
DIET	Low potassium	High K^+ foods, salt substitutes, herbs, intravenous K^+
Tissue Formation/ Destruction	Refeeding syndrome, B12 treatment Post exercise recovery	Rapid Destruction Severe hyper catabolism Tumour lysis syndrome During exercise Rhabdomyolysis
DIARRHOEA Magnesium depletion	several causes ↓cellular repletion	

Table 4: *Causes of hypokalaemia and hyperkalaemia. (Some may have multiple causes)* Pseudohypo = Pseudohypoaldostereonism. ACE = angiotensin converting enzyme blockers. ARB = ACE receptor blockers. NSAIDS = non-steroidal antiinflammatory drugs.

Mild hypokalaemia results from physiological redistribution—extracellular shifts of potassium into cells, from an inadequate dietary intake or rapid reformation of tissue.

Severe Hypokalaemia, however, is usually due to losses from either kidney or intestine.

POTASSIUM SHIFTS

Physiological shifts due to insulin, alkalosis, caffeine and catecholamines were discussed previously. Insulin is especially important in hypokalaemic patients who receive glucose infusions or even following meals.

Although hypokalaemia due to catecholamines is mild, this may be important in specific clinical settings, such as acute coronary syndromes [110-112] or in patients with mild pre-existing hypokalaemia from diuretic treatment. [111] Adrenaline infusion may decrease Serum K^+ by 0.8 mmol and may add to pre-existing hypokalaemia in those on diuretics. [111] Serum K^+ decreased to 3.4mmol/L in volunteers following thiazide diuretics for one week; and then decreased to 2.7mmol/L following adrenaline infusion. [111]

Mild hypokalaemia is common following admission to hospital. [112,113] This may be due to stimulation of catecholamines by trauma, infection, delirium tremens [113] or other stress.

Fluctuations in serum K^+ due to catecholamines have been suggested as a cause of sudden death during strenuous exercise, especially in squash players, who alternate extreme bursts of activity with rest. [53,110] Marked decrease in serum $K^+ > 1.0$mmol/L, in some subjects, occurred following the end of a rally compared to an increase during the rally. [110]

In conclusion β adrenergic agents or sympathetic activity may cause hypokalaemia and promote arrhythmias by two mechanisms: direct stimulation of $Na^+:K^+$ pumps and by indirect $Na^+:K^+$ pump stimulation secondary to insulin release: this either increases Na^+ entry into cells by $Na^+:H^+$ exchangers- a potent stimulus for $Na^+:K^+$ pump activity, or transfers $Na^+:K^+$ pumps from cytoplasm to cell membranes.

Pathological Shifts

β agonists Mild hypokalaemia due to β agonist treatment of asthma may, in combination with hypoxaemia or diuretics, predispose to arrhythmia. [114] Terbutaline and Ritodrine, given for prevention of pre-term labour [49] decreased serum K^+ by 0.9mEq/L in the first 30 minutes of administration and then to serum K^+ of 2.5mEq/L at four hours, due to increase in insulin secretion secondary to glycogenolysis. Three of 14 women developed cardiac arrhythmias. Serum lactate also increased from 1.0 to 4.5mmol/L. [49] The hypokalaemic effect of β agonists varies: fenoterol decreases serum K^+ more than salbutamol or terbutaline for similar bronchodilator action. [115]

Dobutamine may decrease serum K^+ by 0.4mmol/L and increases the frequency of ventricular arrhythmias. [116]

Theophylline and caffeine are methylxanthine derivatives with a similar structure to adenosine. [76,117,118] Adenosine normally inhibits catecholamine secretion. Occupation of adenosine receptors by caffeine or theophylline, including its metabolite paraxanthine, increases catecholamine secretion. This stimulates activity of Na^+: K^+ pumps (figure 9). Inhibition of phosphodiesterase, which increases cAMP, may also decrease metabolism and increase catecholamine levels, but is probably less important. [117] In addition activity of K^+ channels, which transfer potassium out of cells, is normally increased by adenosine. [76] Caffeine and theophylline therefore decrease activity of potassium channels which normally leak K^+ to extracellular fluid. This promotes hypokalaemia. Caffeine also increases insulin secretion secondary to hyperglycaemia and stimulates respiration. [117] Insulin and respiratory alkalosis increase cellular influx of potassium.

Caffeine decreases plasma K^+ by 0.2-0.4 mmol/L depending on the amount. Volunteers given 180mg of caffeine decreased serum K^+ by 0.26 mmol/L but after 360 mg by 0.8 mmol/L. [119] An average cup of coffee contains 120 mg of caffeine [119]. Thus several cups can cause an appreciable decrease in serum potassium. Over the counter medications may contain up to 200 mg of caffeine. [117]

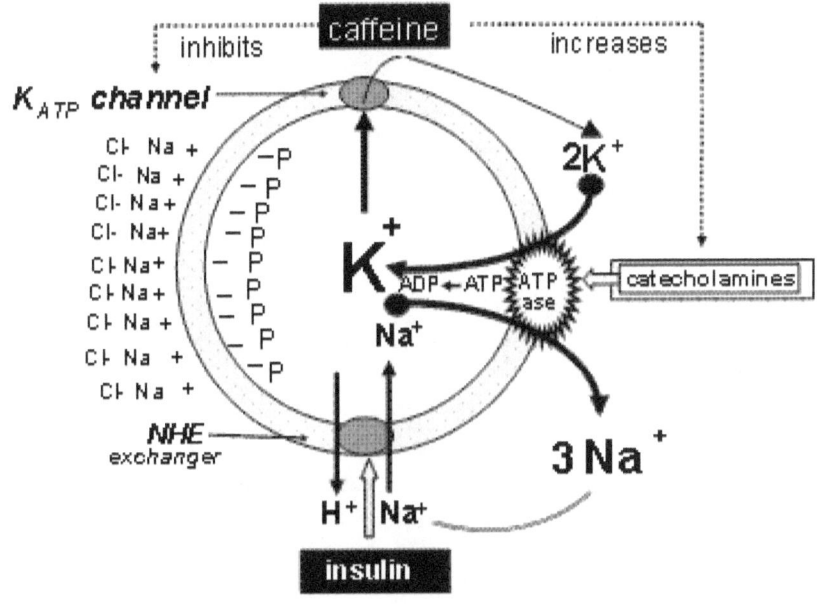

Figure 9 A: *Mechanisms causing hypokalaemia from caffeine.*

P = both organic phosphate⁻ and protein which counterbalance positive charges on K⁺ and other cell cations. The intracellular anions are repelled by K⁺ and align along the inner cell membrane while Na⁺ aligns along the outer membrane. Na⁺:K⁺ pumps transfer 3Na⁺ out of cells in exchange for 2K⁺. Potassium channels leak K⁺ which generates negative electrical potential [19] *A potassium channel and Na:⁺H⁺ antiporter, which transports Na⁺ into the cell in exchange for H⁺, are shown at opposite ends of the cell. Pumps are stimulated by catecholamines and sodium entry into the cell is stimulated by insulin.* [19, 20] *Caffeine inhibits K_{ATP} channels and increases stimulation of Na⁺: K⁺ pumps by catecholamines.*

Consumption of soft drinks, which contain glucose and caffeine, may cause severe hypokalaemia. [76] Ingestion of several litres of coca- cola, which contains caffeine (180-360 mg/L), has caused life threatening hypokalaemia with paralysis due to both caffeine and sugar. Sugar adds to hypokalaemia induced by caffeine by causing K⁺ loss from osmotic diuresis and by stimulating insulin secretion. [76] This has been called coca-cola paralysis.

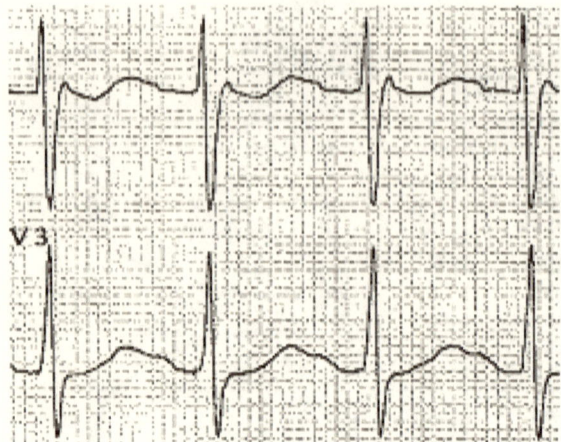

Figure 9B. *ST-T changes and U waves in a 27 year old man who was unable to get out of bed from paralysis caused by intake of 5 L coca-cola the afternoon before. Serum K+ = 1.9 mmol/L Examination showed symmetrical weakness and decreased limb reflexes but sparing of cranial nerves and respiration. Two similar episodes had occurred in the past. A relatively small amount of K⁺, ~ 120 mmol corrected the deficiency. This suggested that external-internal redistribution was the most important cause.*

Barium, (contained in pesticides and depilatories), blocks K⁺ channels and prevents both renal excretion and potassium efflux from cells. [36, 73, 74,]

Sulphonylurea drugs and verapamil. [120] also block K⁺ channels but do not cause hypokalaemia in pharmacological doses. However hypokalaemia has been reported in severe verapamil [120] and chloroquine[121] poisoning. Chloroquine poisoning caused hypokalaemia—below 2.0mmol/L in 11% of 191 consecutive cases, probably by blocking K⁺ channels. [121] Non-polarising muscles relaxants such as tubocurarine and gallamine cause a decrease of serum K⁺ by 1.0mmol/L in dogs. [122]

Hypothermia, discussed previously, probably causes hypokalaemia by moving extracellular K⁺ into cells.

Hypokalaemic periodic paralysis (FPP)

Familial hypokalaemic periodic paralysis is an autosomal dominant disorder usually involving the receptor for the Ca²⁺ channel of skeletal muscle. [123] Serum K⁺ usually decreases to 1.5-2.5mmol/L during attacks and may be accompanied by hypomagnesaemia and hypophosphatemia

[124]. Symptoms are more severe, for a particular serum K^+ level, than for external K^+ losses because extracellular K^+ decreases in association with an increase in cellular K^+ ;whereas both cellular and extracellular K^+ decrease together in other causes of hypokalaemia. Therefore, in Familial periodic paralysis, the K_i/K_o ratio (i=inside; o=outside) increases more for a particular serum K^+ than occurs from external losses; and hyperpolarises cell membranes to a greater extent.

Attacks of paralysis last minutes or days but cranial nerves and respiration are usually spared. Attacks are precipitated by meals, emotion and exercise. [124] A high transtubular K^+ gradient (TTKG), which is inappropriate for hypokalaemia, is a clue to diagnosis. [124] Treatment is relatively ineffective but dichlorphenamide; acetazolamide and Pinacidil may have some effect. [125]

Periodic paralysis, associated with thyrotoxicosis, is much more common, especially in males (10-1) of Asian [126] and Polynesian [127] descent. This has been reported to occur in as many as 15-20% of Chinese males with thyrotoxicosis but is much less common in females. [126] Cranial nerves and respiratory muscles are usually spared as in Familial Periodic Paralysis. [126-128] Thyrotoxicosis may be misdiagnosed because manifestations are few and family history absent. Activity of $Na^+:K^+$ pumps increase. [129]. Thyrotoxic Periodic Paralysis usually occurs at night and is precipitated by meals and exercise. [126-128]

Two consecutive cases, referred to the author, were initially diagnosed as Transverse myelitis and Guillain Barre syndrome respectively. Clues to the diagnosis were the abrupt onset, despite previous apparent normal health, sparing of respiration and cranial nerves, despite total limb paralysis, Japanese ethnicity and tachycardia due to Thyrotoxicosis. Complete resolution of hypokalaemia and paralysis followed 40 mmol K^+ orally and propranalol.

Beta blockers and potassium shorten attacks but may lead to rebound hyperkalaemia following treatment. [126,127] This occurred in 22% of those receiving a median dose of 124mmol K^+ compared to none who received 68 mmol. [127] Combination of β blockers and potassium are especially dangerous. [127] β blockers are effective in both prevention and treatment of acute attacks without risk of rebound hypokalaemia. [126,130]

Dietary intake and tissue reformation

Mild potassium deficiency occurs when potassium intake decreases because full adaption to low potassium intake takes several days. Urinary K^+ conservation becomes more efficient and can decrease to 5-15mmol/day when more marked losses occur. [89,131,132]

Renal conservation of potassium is more efficient when Na^+ and K^+ deficiencies occur together [83, 84] because less Na^+ is delivered to collecting ducts to exchange with K^+. Mean urine K^+ on presentation was 2.5mmol/L in infants with both deficiencies due to diarrhoea (mean serum K^+ 2.4mmol/L) [84] and 2.9mmol/L in malnourished children with both Na^+ and K^+ depletion. [83] Inadequate calorie intake or starvation limits development of hypokalaemia because K^+ is released from tissue catabolism.

Dietary potassium is especially important in two conditions: when potassium losses occur from diarrhoeal disorders and when tissue growth is rapid. The incidence of hypokalaemia in malnourished children in developing countries is not due to malnutrition per se but related to the amount of potassium in diet. [83] Hypokalaemia was common in West Africa, where cassava and rice, each of low potassium content, were main food staples, compared to countries where food staples contain a higher K^+ content. [83] Breast milk only contains 5-6mmol Na^+ and 10mmol K^+ per litre. Thus infants who receive "demand" breast feeding during diarrhoea develop severe losses of Na^+;and K^+ and develop severe hypokalaemia.

Refeeding Hypokalaemia

Refeeding without adequate potassium or phosphate, especially during parenteral nutrition, is an important hazard in malnourished adults or children. Rapid reformation of tissue can precipitate severe hypokalaemia, hypophosphataemia and hypomagnesaemia. [133] Anorexia nervosa and psychiatric disease may result in severe hypokalaemia. [134] Hypokalaemia may follow rapid formation of red cells following vitamin B^{12} treatment of pernicious anaemia [135] or white cells following treatment by granulocyte macrophage colony stimulating factor. [136]

Recovery of muscle following rhabdomyolysis. [137-139]

Visible urinary myoglobinuria occurs when over 100g muscles are destroyed and serum myoglobin levels exceed 0.5-1.5mg/dL. [138]Rhabdomyolysis is especially common in untrained persons undertaking exhaustive exercise; [137] in hyperpyrexia; crush injury; compartment syndromes; coma; following falls in the elderly; metabolic myopathy; and alcoholism. [137,139]. K+ phosphate and magnesium released from necrosed muscle are initially excreted to maintain normal extracellular levels. Sodium and water losses may be severe. Severe hypokalaemia, hypomagnesaemia and hypophosphataemia occur as muscle reforms. [137-139]

Geophagia is a rare condition in which ingestion of clay binds and thus limits potassium absorption. [140]

Hypokalaemia due to Dialysis.

Patients are often dialysed against a low K+ solution which produces mild potassium depletion Additional potassium losses or inadequate dietary potassium may lead to hypokalaemia. [141]

Losses of Potassium due to Sweating. [142,143]

Sweating under hot, humid environmental conditions, especially in subjects with cystic fibrosis, [142,143] causes sodium, chloride and potassium losses. This may lead to sodium depletion, metabolic alkalosis and hypokalaemia. However sweat contains only 5-15mmol/L K+ compared to 25-50mmol/L sodium and chloride. A more likely mechanism for hypokalaemia is urinary loss of K+ from exchange with Na+ in distal tubules due to sodium depletion, hyperaldosteronism and metabolic alkalosis. Metabolic alkalosis is due to losses of chloride in relative excess of sodium compared to the extracellular concentration.

NON RENAL EXTERNAL LOSSES OF POTASSIUM

Diarrhoeal disorders (chapter 12).

Fluid in small intestine has low K+ concentration. Thus ileostomy losses uncommonly cause potassium depletion. Colonic exchange of Na+ for K+ and Cl- for organic anions and HCO_3^- lead to losses of Na+, K+ and bicarbonate in diarrhoeal disorders. The frequency and severity of hypokalaemia is related to the site of bowel affected, the organism involved, severity of water and electrolyte losses, which determines Na+ exchange for K+ in colon, and composition of the diet.

Thus cholera, a small intestinal disease, characterised by rapid transfer of water and sodium into small bowel, leads to diarrhoeal stools with a much lower concentrations of K+ and higher concentrations of sodium and chloride. [144] Stool K+ losses due to other causes of diarrhoea in children are higher, but variable: K+27-60mmol/L, (mean 44.0mmol/L). Diarrhoeal stool potassium was only 20mmol/L.In demand breast feeding infants. Less severe diarrhoea, colonic disorders such as inflammatory colitis, malabsorption, laxative abuse and villous adenoma allow Na^+/K^+ exchange to occur in colon and may result in severe potassium and sodium depletion.

Laxative use may not be volunteered. The clue to diagnosis is low urinary potassium and presence of hyperchloraemic acidosis.

RENAL LOSSES OF POTASSIUM

Vomiting.

Paradoxically hypokalaemia results from <u>renal</u>, not gastrointestinal losses of potassium. Gastric juice contains only 2-10mmol/L of K^+. Less than 100mmol of K^+. is probably lost in 10 L of vomitus. Approximately 1-2L of gastric juice, containing an average of 122mmol Cl^-, 60 mmol Na^+ but only 10mmol K^+, is secreted daily depending on pH: Gastric juice of low acidity contains more sodium and less H^+.

Loss of gastric juice in vomiting, regurgitation or nasogastric aspiration results in sodium depletion, metabolic alkalosis and hypokalaemia. The pathogenesis of these disturbances are as follows:

- Each mmol of H^+ and Cl^- secreted into stomach results in reabsorption of 1mmol HCO_3^- into the interstitial space. This generates metabolic alkalosis.
- The kidney initially excretes Na^+ with HCO_3^- because HCO_3^- is a poorly absorbable anion. Urine is initially alkaline and contains an increase in sodium and bicarbonate concentration but low Cl^-.
- Following continued vomiting hypovolaemia increases from loss of Na^+ Cl^- in gastric juice and initially from sodium bicarbonate loss in urine.
- Hypovolaemia stimulates the Sympathetic nervous system, Renin Angiotensin Aldosterone system and ADH (AVP) secretion. GFR falls, proximal tubule reabsorption of Na^+ increases and extracellular bicarbonate rises from increased HCO_3^- reabsorption in place of Cl^- in proximal tubules. Principal cells, in distal collecting ducts, increase electrogenic Na^+ reabsorption in exchange for K^+ secretion, stimulated by aldosterone, because HCO_3^- is a poorly reabsorbed anion,. This causes:

* Increase in activity of basolateral Na^+: K^+ pumps.
* Increase in activity and or number of Na^+ channels (ENAC) and H^+ ATPase pumps.
* Increase in activity and number of K^+ channels.

K^+ is reabsorbed in exchange for H^+ which is secreted by the H^+:K^+ ATPase pumps in alpha intercalated cells if severe hypokalaemia develops and urine becomes acid despite alkalosis. Low serum K^+ decreases Na^+:K^+ exchange in Principal cells because of hypovolaemia.

<u>Maintenance of metabolic alkalosis is due to increased bicarbonate reabsorption in both proximal and distal tubules.</u>

The electrolyte composition of urine varies depending on the severity and duration of HCl loss: In the initial stages, before the renin-aldosterone system is fully activated, HCo_3^- lost in urine is accompanied by Na^+. Urine is initially alkaline. Thus urine Na^+ may not be low initially compared to urinary chloride which is extremely low. When volume depletion increases in severity urine Na^+ and Cl^- both decrease but urine potassium increases despite hypokalaemia. Hypokalaemia increases in severity urine potassium decreases and urine becomes acidic. This increases metabolic alkalosis.

<u>The cause of hypokalaemia is urinary ; not gastric loss of K^+.</u>

Increased secretion or action of Mineralocorticoids. (1-5[145-150])

Mineralocorticoids, such as aldosterone and deoxycorticosterone, increase Na^+ reabsorption in distal tubules in exchange for K^+, which is lost in urine. This results in hypertension, hypokalaemia and alkalosis. The causes may be primary or secondary to increased renin secretion. The underlying mechanisms are increased activation of aldosterone receptor either from a gain of function; increased mineralocorticoid secretion; or failure to inactivate corticosteroids which act on the aldosterone receptor.

Primary Hyperaldosteronism. [145,146]

This common cause of hypertension is due to an aldosterone secreting adenoma, carcinoma or bilateral adrenal hyperplasia. Familial and more common sporadic form occurs. Increasing numbers of cases without hypokalaemia are now recognised because of availability of a simple test: aldosterone—renin ratio [147].This shows high serum aldosterone but low renin levels.

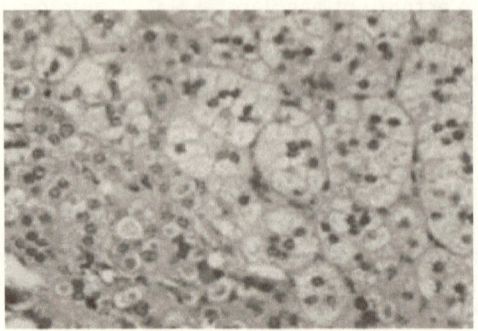

Figure 10. Adenoma of adrenal gland.

Mineralocorticoids other than aldosterone. (145[,146])

DOCA producing tumours are rare.

Congenital Adrenal Hyperplasia. [145,148] Enzyme deficiencies in the cascade leading to cortisol synthesis result in low cortisol secretion. This increases secretion of ACTH which stimulates synthesis of deoxycorticosterone. [97,145] This causes hypertension, hypokalaemia and suppresses renin and aldosterone secretion. The most common causes are:

11 β hydroxylase deficiency: adrenal androgens are also increased by ACTH and result in virilisation.

17 α hydroxylase deficiency: this also decreases sex hormone synthesis, which results in ambiguous genitalia in males and decreases secondary sexual characteristics in females.

Decreased action of II β hydroxysteroid dehydrogenase. (97, 98, 145, 149, 150) (Apparent mineralocorticoid excess).

Cortisol acts with equal affinity to aldosterone on aldosterone receptors, but its concentration is approximately 1000 times higher (aldosterone picomol/L, cortisol micromol/l). Cortisol is converted to inactive cortisone by ß hydroxysteroid dehydrogenase Type II, before it acts on receptors. Rare hereditary defects of II ß hydroxysteroid dehydrogenase and liquorice, [149] which inactivates the enzyme, may cause hypokalaemia and hypertension.

Corticosteroid Excess.

Pharmacological doses of corticosteroids may overwhelm the capacity of the enzyme to inactivate cortisol.

Corticosteroids increase GFR and delivery of sodium to distal tubules which facilitate exchange for potassium. Cushing's disease and treatment with corticosteroids may result in mild hypokalaemia. Severe hypokalaemia is more common in paraneoplastic Cushing's syndrome because ACTH hypersecretion results in extremely high cortisol levels. [151]

Aldosterone-cortisol hybrids—Glucocorticoid Remedial Hypertension. (97,145,152)

Aldosterone is normally produced in the adrenal zona glomerulosa following stimulation by angiotensin II and hyperkalaemia; whereas cortisol is produced in the zona fasciculata stimulated by ACTH.

A genetic defect results in synthesis of a C18 cortisol—aldosterone hybrid in the zona fasciculata, driven by ACTH. Thus ACTH, rather than Angiotensin II, stimulates aldosterone secretion. Increase in aldosterone secretion causes hypertension and hypokalaemia. A small dose, 0.5 mg, of dexamethasone suppresses ACTH stimulated aldosterone secretion and decreases hypokalaemia and blood pressure.

Glucocorticoid resistance.

Decreased function of the glucocorticoid receptor to cortisol increases ACTH secretion. This stimulates secretion of cortisol, mineralocorticoids and androgens. Hypertension, hypokalaemia, fatigue and hyperandrogenism result. [97]

Secondary Hyperaldosteronism.

Autonomous renin secreting tumours of juxta-glomerular apparatus are rare. [153]

Malignant hypertension.

High renin secretion, due to renal ischaemia, increases aldosterone secretion and causes hypokalaemia.

Renovascular hypertension. [154]

Inadequate renal perfusion stimulates renin secretion in the kidney with renal artery stenosis. This increases angiotensin 2 secretion and causes secondary hyperaldosteronism. Both serum renin and aldosterone levels increase. High blood pressure to the normal kidney increases excretion of sodium (pressure natriuresis). Volume depletion, secondary to this, may become sufficiently severe to cause hyponatraemia. Both hyponatremia and hypokalaemia may occur in comparison to primary mineralocorticoid hypertension.

Diabetic ketoacidosis. [155] (chapter 13)

Urinary losses of Na^+ and K^+ result from osmotic diuresis induced by glucose and ketonuria. K^+ losses, from exchange with Na^+ in distal tubules, result from increased delivery of Na^+ to principal cells and raised aldosterone secondary to volume depletion. In addition K^+ is excreted with ketoanions which are poorly absorbed.

Plasma K^+ is usually normal or high on presentation from a combination of volume depletion, hypertonicity, deficiency of insulin and hyperchloraemic acidosis which are present to a variable extent. In a study of 142 presentations of Diabetic ketoacidosis serum pH, anion gap, and extent of hyperglycaemia were the most important variables influencing the initial serum potassium and extent of insulin deficiency. [155] Severe hypokalaemia commonly results following rehydration, ongoing urinary potassium losses, insulin treatment, reformation of glycogen and correction of acidosis

Diuretics and hereditary tubular disorders. (chapter14)

Diuretics are common causes of potassium deficiency.

Loop diuretics.

Furosemide and Bumetanide block Na^+:K^+:$2Cl^-$ cotransporters in thick ascending loops of Henle (TALH). This increases Na^+ and Cl^- excretion in urine because a marked increase in Na^+ delivery to principal cells exceeds their reabsorptive capacity. Hypovolaemia stimulates aldosterone secretion. Increased Na^+ delivery to principal cells and raised serum aldosterone increase tubular K^+ exchange for Na^+. Increased losses of chloride in urine promote bicarbonate reabsorption to accompany Na^+ and causes metabolic alkalosis. Calcium excretion increases because its absorption is linked to Na$^+$ reabsorption. Saline depletion, metabolic alkalosis, hypokalaemia and hypercalciuria result.

Thiazide and Indapamide.

Thiazide diuretics block sodium chloride transporters (NCC) in distal convoluted tubules (DCT) and collecting ducts. This increases Na$^+$ delivery to collecting ducts. Loss of K$^+$, in exchange for Na$^+$, occurs in principal cells of collecting ducts as described above. Thiazide diuretics are less potent than loop diuretics because they act on DCT, where only 5 % of sodium is reabsorbed, compared to 25% in the TALH. There are 2 other major differences: calcium excretion is decreased, not increased; and urinary dilution, which continues in the DCT by absorption of sodium without water is decreased.

Loop diuretics are used in treatment of hypercalcaemia and sometimes severe hyponatraemia due to inappropriate ADH secretion, because urinary sodium concentration is usually half that of serum sodium. Thiazide diuretics, although less potent, are also used to decrease urinary calcium excretion in stone formers. They are much more likely to cause hyponatraemia. There are 3 methods for reducing potassium loss from diuretics apart from giving supplemental potassium: use of low doses reduced Na $^+$ intake, because this limits K$^+$:Na$^+$ exchange in distal tubules, and use of potassium sparing diuretics.

Hereditary tubular disorders. (chapter 14)

Bartter's and Gitelmans Syndrome.

These hereditary syndromes cause dysfunction of Na$^+$:K$^+$:2Cl$^-$ cotransporters and NaCl cotransporters of ascending limbs loop of Henle and distal convoluted tubules (DCT) respectively. For ease of recall Bartter's syndrome resembles the action of loop diuretics, because both interfere with function of Na$^+$:K$^+$:2Cl$^-$ cotransporters; while Gitelman syndrome resembles thiazide diuretics because both block NaCl transporters (NCC) of the DCT.

Gain of function of sodium channels in distal tubules—Liddle's Syndrome. [97,156-157]

Gain in function of ENaC sodium channels in luminal membranes of Principal cells increases Na$^+$ reabsorption and K$^+$ secretion into the distal tubular lumen. This results in hypertension, hypokalemia but low serum renin and aldosterone. Amiloride is effective for treatment.

The gain in function is due to mutations in the beta or gamma subunits of the EnaC, which interact with Nedd4, a cytoskeletal protein. This normally retrieves EnaC from the apical membranes where it acts. Defective mutations of Nedd 4 decreases retrieval of EnaC from cell membranes: increased occupancy promotes reabsorption of sodium. K^+ is lost downstream in electrogenic exchange for Na^+. [97]

Acquired renal tubular disorders.

Renal tubular acidosis (type I distal and type II proximal).

Type I—Distal Renal Tubular Acidosis (chapter 6).
A disorder of H^+: ATPase or H^+: K^+ ATPase pumps in α intercalated cells of distal nephrons results in failure to excrete H^+ and NH_4^+ ions. This leads to both acidosis and increased loss of K^+ rather than H^+ in exchange for Na^+.

Type II—Proximal Tubular Acidosis.(chapter 5).
Decreased HCO_3^- reabsorption in proximal tubules causes increased Na^+ delivery to distal tubules where Na^+ is reabsorbed in exchange for K^+.

Non-Reabsorbable Anions. [158,159]

Anions other than Cl^-, such as HCO_3^-, SO_4^{2-}, penicillinate$^-$, carbenicillin and keto anions, are reabsorbed poorly in distal tubules. Na^+: K^+ potassium exchange results in excretion of poorly absorbable anions with K^+.

Excessive consumption of dietary organic anions, low salt intake and sweating has been suggested as a cause in a young woman with hypokalaemia. [160] Increased excretion of organic anions obligated excretion of Na^+ and K^+ in distal tubules.

Medications

Drugs may cause hypokalaemia from transcellular shifts; by causing diarrhoea; by increasing mineralocorticoid secretion; causing urine loss of K^+; or a combination of these. These are summarised in the table 5.Acetaminophen overdose may cause hypokalaemia [161]. B12 administration [135] or granulocyte colony stimulating factor [136] rarely cause hypokalaemia from rapid reformation of cells.

Transcellular Shifts	β agonists, theophylline, caffeine, muscle relaxants, insulin, dobutamine.
Diarrhoea	Laxatives, bowel preparations.
Increased Renal Loss	Diuretics—loop, thiazide and acetazolamide, Non-reabsorbable anions, Aminoglycosides, cisplatinum, amphotericin.
Mineralocorticoid action	Fludrocortisone, liquorice, gossypol, high dose glucocorticoid.

Table 5: *Hypokalaemia due to Medications*

In conclusion: the most common causes of severe hypokalaemia are external losses from diarrhoea or renal losses of potassium. The most common renal losses result from vomiting, diuretics, Diabetic ketoacidosis and from primary or secondary hyperaldosteronism. Internal redistribution of K^+ causes mild hypokalaemia or contributes to hypokalaemia produced by external losses of potassium.

INTERPRETATION OF HYPOKALAEMIA

Figure 11 shows a theoretical approach to diagnosis of hypokalaemia. This is usually short circuited because the diagnosis is usually apparent from the history. The most important, if the cause is uncertain, are analysis of urine electrolytes, serum bicarbonate and measurement of blood pressure.

The most important clues, if the diagnosis is uncertain following clinical assessment, are the presence of hypertension, alkalosis, urine electrolytes and analysis of medication use.

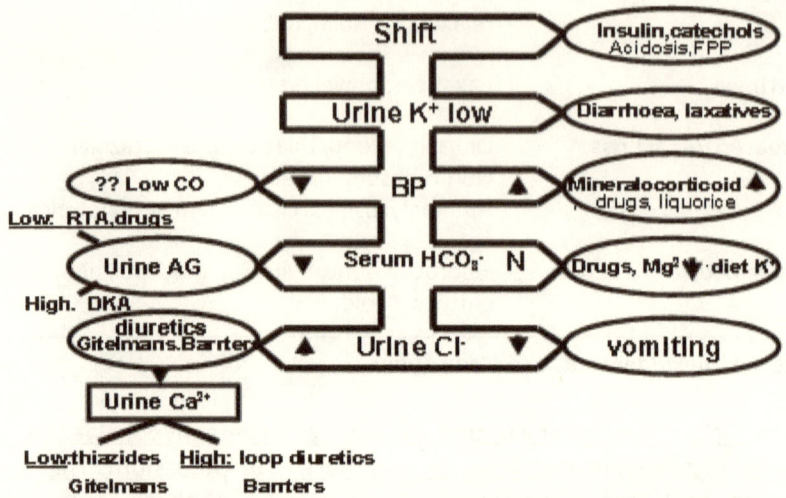

Figure 11. Pathway for analysis of the cause of Hypokalaemia. CO= cardiac output; AG= anion gap; FPP= Familial Periodic Paralysis; catechols =catecholamines.

Pseudohypokalaemia is a rare condition due to increased uptake of potassium by leukemic blood cells when blood is allowed to stand at room temperature. [1]

SERUM BICARBONATE.

Low.

Renal tubular acidosis Type 1 (non-anion gap acidosis).

Diabetic ketoacidosis—serum glucose elevated.

Diarrhoea—non-anion gap acidosis.

High -Vomiting or diuretic use.

Hypertension—suggests mineralocorticoid excess or action or Liddles syndrome. (Table 6).

	ALDOSTERONE	RENIN	CORTISOL
Primary Hyperaldosteronism	↑	↓	N
ENaC Gain of function *(Liddle's Syndrome)	↓	↓	N
ß hydroxysteroid dehydrogenase 2 deficiency	↓	↓	N
Paraneoplastic ACTH	↓	↓	↑
Apparent Mineralocorticoid excess	↓	↑	N
Secondary Hyperaldosteronism	↑	↑	N
Other Mineralocorticoid excess	↓	↓	Variable
Congenital adrenal hyperplasia (11βOHlase,17αOHlase deficiency)	↓	↓	↓
Glucocorticoid remedial hypertension	↑	↓	
Glucocorticoid receptor resistance	↑	↓	↑

Table.6: Differential diagnosis of Hypertension with Hypokalaemia.

Diuretics cause loss of Na^+, K^+ and Cl^- in urine. However if diuretics are discontinued uncorrected hypovolaemia and potassium depletion result in low levels of urinary Na^+, K^+ and Cl^-.

Bartter's and Gitelman's syndrome resemble Loop and Thiazide diuretic action respectively, but are rare. Urine calcium is raised from use of Loop diuretics but low from use of Thiazide diuretics. Thus Bartter's syndrome shows hypercalciuria, Gitelmans syndrome hypocalciuria. Hypomagnesaemia is common in Gitelmans Syndrome.

Vomiting has three phases. An early phase before severe sodium depletion occurs. Urine Cl^- is low but urine Na^+ may not be low because HCO_3^- excretion obligates Na^+ excretion. The second phase occurs when Na^+ depletion is present. Proximal tubule reclamation of HCO_3^- increases and alkalosis progressively increases. Urine K^+ is high because it exchanges with Na^+ in distal

Tubules stimulated by aldosterone. Urinary K^+ loss is the cause of severe potassium depletion—not gastric losses.

In the third phase hypokalaemia becomes sufficiently severe that K^+ is reabsorbed in exchange for H^+ in distal tubules: urine becomes acid and K^+ loss in urine decreases.

Diarrhoea has a high negative urine AG because excretion of NH_4^+ is increased due to acidosis from HCO_3^- loss in stool.

URINE ELECTROLYTES AND URINE ANION GAP (AG). Table 7

		Na^+	K^+	Cl^-	AG (pH)	Serum HCO_3
DIARRHOEA		↓	↓	N or ↑	High Negative (acid)	↓
VOMITING	Early	N	↓	↓	Positive (Alkaline)	↑ or N
	Mid	↓	↑	↓	Positive	↑
	Late	↓	↓	↓	Negative (acid)	↑
DIURETICS		↑	↑	↑		↑
Post Treatment		↓	↓	↓		↑ or N
BARRTERS		↑	↑	↑		↑
GITELMANS		↑	↑	↑		↑
RENAL TUBULAR ACIDOSIS	Distal	↑	↑	↓	Positive (>5.5)	↓
	Proximal	↑	N or ↑	↓	Positive (normal)	↓ or N

Table 7. Urine electrolytes, urine anion gap and serum HCO_3^- in diarrhoea, vomiting, diuretics, and tubular disorders. Urine anion gap = $Na^+ + K^+ - Cl^-$). High negative urine AG suggests a high level of NH_4^+ excretion (the cation NH_4^+ accounting for the gap in positive charges). A positive or low negative AG suggests a low level of NH_4^+ excretion. Urine Ca^{2+} is low in Gitelman syndrome and thiazide diuretics.

Other Drugs and conditions.

β agonists, insulin, barium toxicity, low K^+ intake, marked tissue reformation (refeeding syndrome) administration of high dose antibiotics with unabsorbable anions have been discussed.

Measurement of serum aldosterone, renin and renin-aldosterone ratio are important screening tests if hypertension is present.

A refinement in the assessment of hypokalaemia is calculation of the TTKG (transtubular K^+ gradient) discussed later in the section on hyperkalaemia. When hypokalaemia occurs potassium, secreted into the CCD lumen, should decrease and the TTKG should be low (TTKG <2.0) in non renal causes of hypokalaemia. This is useful in the early diagnosis of Periodic paralysis because high doses of potassium should be avoided in treatment. [162]

HYPERKALAEMIA

Hyperkalaemia is produced by three mechanisms:

- Increase in potassium load from diet or tissue breakdown.
- Shift of potassium from cells to ECF.
- Decrease in renal excretion.

The former two are uncommon if renal function is normal.

Man has a remarkable capacity to deal with potassium loads—more than five times the total extracellular potassium can be accommodated without developing severe hyperkalaemia. The following mechanisms are involved in causing hypokalaemia.

> ### External – Internal Potassium Redistribution

Physiological shifts. These contribute to but are rarely the sole cause of severe hyperkalaemia, although serum potassium can rise above 7.0mmol/L transiently during extreme exercise. [51, 52] Alpha adrenergic agents, such as adrenaline, transiently increase but then decrease serum potassium levels and cause hypokalaemia following exercise. [110,163]

Pathological shifts

β blockers, hypertonicity and acidosis contribute to development of hyperkalaemia when other causes are present.

β blockers, especially non-selective, may elevate serum K^+ by 0.7mEq/L in patients on dialysis. [36] In healthy subjects serum potassium increased ~0.7mmol/L more from β blockers and exercise than exercise alone. [163-165] $β_2$ [163,164] but not $β_1$ blockers [165] increase serum K^+ appreciably on exercise.

Tonicity

Modest increase in tonicity (10 - 20mOsmol/kgH$_2$O) increases serum K^+ by 0.5-0.7mmol/L. [36] Infusion of 5% saline, 6mmol/kg body weight over 120 minutes, increased serum K^+ between 0.3-1.3mmol/L, (average 0.6mmol/L), in patients with chronic renal failure [66] and correlated with serum osmolality. Infusion of glucose, hypertonic sodium bicarbonate, or mannitol also increases serum K^+. [36] Hypertonic saline, used in intensive care and neurosurgery, may increase serum K^+ by 0.5-0.7mEq/L. [36]. Hypertonicity, but not hyperosmolality, increases serum K^+. [66]

Glucose infusions given to insulinopenic diabetic patients raises serum K^+ between 0.2 and 1.3 mmol/L and correlate highly with serum glucose levels and osmolality following infusion. [65]

Intravenous glucose, used for suspected hypoglycaemic coma in insulinopenic diabetics, can be dangerous. [65] Intravenous glucose, given without insulin to diabetics, to decrease serum potassium, increases rather than decreases serum K^+. Oral glucose or meals in insulinopenic diabetics also increases serum K^+ by the same mechanism. [65,107]

Hyperchloraemic acidosis, but not organic acidosis, increases serum K^+ appreciably as discussed previously. [55, 56]

Digoxin Toxicity.

Digoxin inhibits Na^+:K^+ pumps in a dose dependent manner [166] but only causes hyperkalaemia in severe poisoning. [166,167] Excretion of K^+ may lead to hypokalaemia on recovery.

Cationic aminoacids. (28)

Cationic amino acids exchange with K^+ in cells. Infusion of 30- 60 gm arginine increased serum potassium by 1.0 mmol/L.

Succinylcholine

Succinylcholine depolarises cell membranes and causes K^+ efflux into the extracellular fluid. Serum K^+ usually rises less than 0.5mmol/L. The rise is much greater and may be life threatening in those with neuromuscular disorders, burns and severe trauma. [168]

Familial hyperkalaemic periodic paralysis. [169,170]

Most cases are due to an autosomal dominant abnormality of Na^+ channels· Attacks of paralysis are milder and shorter than familial hypokalaemic paralysis and mild myotonia may also occur. Cranial nerve and respiratory paralysis does not occur. Attacks are induced by exercise and ingestion of potassium. Treatment with β_2 agonists is effective in limiting attacks. [170] Low potassium containing meals, limitation of exercise, mild hypokalaemia, induced by thiazide diuretics and fludrocortisone decrease episodes.

Hypothermia. [67-69]

Hypokalaemia initially develops from transfer of potassium into cells. Prolonged and severe hypothermia causes efflux of K^+ from cells, possibly from hyperchloraemic acidosis, hypoxia and tissue damage. Prognosis is related to serum K^+. This may reach 14.5mmol/L in severe cases. [69]

Marine Toxins.

Toxins of some marine animals, which inhibit $Na^+:K^+$ pumps or block Na^+ channels, is a rare cause of hyperkalaemia.

Diabetic ketoacidosis. (Chapter 13)

The most important shift occurs in diabetic ketoacidosis: normokalaemia or even hyperkalaemia occurs on presentation despite potassium depletion. Lack of insulin, hyperchloraemic acidosis, hypercatabolism, hyperosmolality, hypovolaemia, prerenal failure and glycogenolysis contribute to varying degrees. Insulin deficiency is the most important. [39-42,155] These variables rapidly resolve on treatment.

Cellular potassium uptake is impaired chronically unless adequate insulin is taken. Fasting may increase serum potassium levels in diabetics on dialysis because an insulin dependent pool of intracellular K^+ is retained in cells. [42]This is especially important if Hyporeninaemic hypoaldosteronism or renal failure is present. In the absence of insulin a K^+ load may be confined to the extracellular space alone. [102] Administration of glucose without insulin is dangerous in diabetics because hyperosmolality increases serum K^+. [65,107,171-174] 35 grams of intravenous glucose increased serum K+ from 6.5 to 8.4 mmol/L in one diabetic.[174]

TISSUE DESTRUCTION.

Shift of potassium from cells to extracellular fluid occurs in rhabdomyolysis, severe sepsis, ischaemic necrosis and tumour lysis. Hyperkalaemia may occur before K^+ is excreted; and renal failure from myoglobinuria may decrease K^+ excretion.

Tumour Lysis Syndrome. [175-177]

Anticancer therapy against sensitive rapidly proliferating and bulky tumours releases cellular contents into interstitial fluid and circulation. Acute renal failure, hyperuricemia, hyperkalaemia, hyperphosphataemia, hypocalcaemia, elevation of serum LDH (lactic dehydrogenase) and acidosis may occur [176]. Risk factors are pre-treatment renal insufficiency, elevated lactic dehydrogenase, and hyperuricemia [176]. Allopurinol is protective. [175]

Rhabdomyolysis. [137-139,178]

This has many causes including alcohol and illicit drugs ; medication, especially neuroleptics and statins; seizures; compartment syndromes; coma; crush injuries; mitochondrial disorders; myopathies; and extreme exertion- especially in hot conditions.

Recurrent episodes occur from muscle enzyme deficiencies, myopathies and mitochondrial muscle disorders. Potassium and phosphate are released from necrosed muscle. Renal failure from myoglobinuria increases risk of life threatening hyperkalaemia. Visible myoglobinuria occurs when urinary myoglobin exceeds 250μg/ml equivalent to >100g of muscle necrosed. [178]

The main cause of hyperkalaemia is defective function of K+ secretion by principal cells of cortical collecting ducts.

RENAL CAUSES OF HYPERKALAEMIA.

- Secretion of potassium requires:
- Adequate Na^+ and fluid delivery to CCD to exchange with K^+.
- Electrogenic Na^+ exchange with K^+ in principal cells.
- Adequate action of aldosterone.
- Normal K^+ channel function.
- Adequate flow rate.

Inadequate Na+ and fluid delivery to cortical collecting ducts.

This results from low cardiac output from cardiac failure, hypovolaemia or intrinsic renal failure.

Low Cardiac Output.

Hypovolaemia or primary cardiac disorders [179,180] decreases GFR and increases Na^+ and water reabsorption in proximal tubules. This decreases Na^+ delivery to distal tubules [179] and limits K^+ secretion in exchange for Na^+. This is exacerbated by ACE (angiotensin converting enzyme) inhibitors and β blockers used for cardiac disease. [179]

Renal Failure. (discussed earlier)

Smaller numbers of nephrons are available to excrete potassium in chronic renal failure. Adaption to high K^+ loads prevents hyperkalaemia, in the absence of another cause, until GFR falls below 15mL/minute. Adaption is achieved by increased excretion of K^+ by remaining nephrons, due to increase in activity of Na^+:K^+ pumps, [108] stimulated by both hyperkalaemia and aldosterone. The colon also increases K^+ excretion 3-4 times above normal. Internal redistribution does not increase and may decrease as renal failure progresses. [102 106,107]

Once hyperkalaemia develops the capacity to take up further K^+ is limited. A K^+ load in diabetics may be confined to the extracellular space alone. [102] In mild renal failure hyperkalaemia usually only develops in association with another cause such as:

- Massive cell necrosis.
- Hypoaldostereonism.
- Marked increase in potassium intake.
- Drugs which increase serum K$^+$.
- Hypovolaemia or cardiac failure.

DISORDERS OF ALDOSTERONE. [145,156, 181]

These are shown in table 8. Aldosterone secretion requires a normal adrenal zona glomerulosa, functioning enzymes in the pathway to aldosterone synthesis and appropriate secretion of renin. Aldosterone secretion is normal but its action is defective in Pseudohypoaldostereonism.

PRIMARY ADRENAL DISEASE [145]

Acquired

Autoimmune disease, Aids and tuberculosis are the most common causes. Autoimmune disease is probably due to antibodies directed against 21β hydroxylase, an enzyme required for both aldosterone and cortisol synthesis. [145]

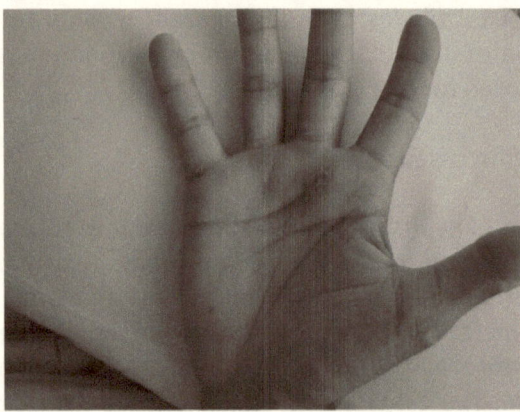

Palm of a 32 year male showing increased pigmentation of creases due to adrenal failure from autoimmune 21 hydroxylase deficiency. He collapsed after operation: BP=85/65; serum$^+$=119 mmol/L ;K$^+$= 7.1 mmolL.

Low cortisol from Hypopituitarism does not cause hyperkalaemia because aldosterone secretion is normal.

Transient hypoaldostereonism and hyperkalaemia may follow surgical removal of an aldosterone secreting adenoma. [182]

Hereditary. Aldosterone Synthetic Enzyme Defects (figure 12)

Disorders involving enzymes in boxes on the left hand side of the table cause hypoaldostereonism. The most common is 21 hydroxylase deficiency (autosomal recessive).

Deficiencies of 3β hydroxylase, 11β hydroxylase and 21β hydroxylase also cause cortisol deficiency because both are required for cortisol synthesis. 3 β hydroxylase and 21β hydroxylase deficiency also lead to increased androgen production driven by ACTH. [181]

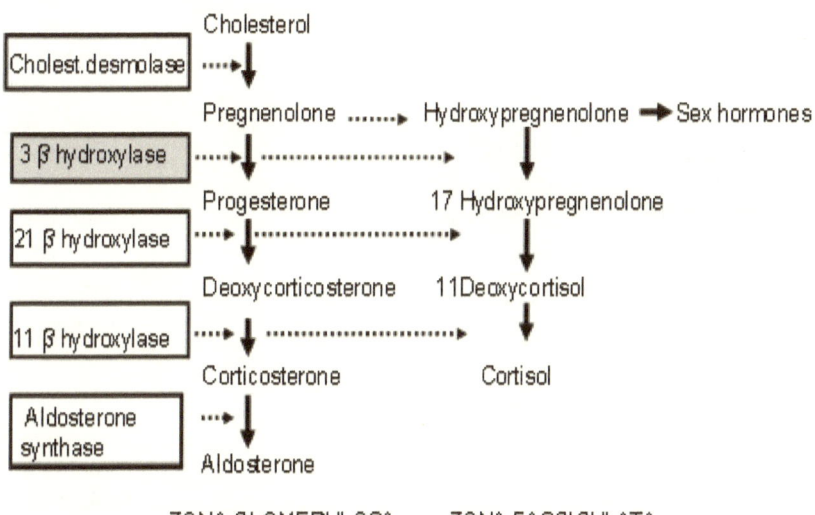

Figure 12: *Synthetic cascade of aldosterone, cortisol and sex hormones. Stippled arrows show that cortisol synthesis is affected in addition to aldosterone. Deficiencies cause both hypocortisolaemia and hypoaldostereonism.*

Pseudohypoaldostereonism. [156]

A term applied to inability of aldosterone to produce its major physiological effects [156] despite normal secretion. Aldosterone secretion is normal, hence pseudo, but its action is defective: either because of defective aldosterone receptors; defective function of ENaC (sodium) channels; of uncertain cause; or because of generalised disease of colleting ducts.

Type I: Loss of Function of Na+ channels and Aldosterone Receptor. [145,156]

These rare disorders cause Pseudohypoaldostereonism and clinically resemble hypoaldostereonism by causing sodium depletion, hyperkalaemia and hyperchloraemic acidosis, but in association with raised aldosterone and renin levels. Decrease in function of the ENaC (sodium channels) or aldosterone receptors decreases reabsorption of Na$^+$ which decreases potassium and H$^+$ secretion. Several recessive mutations, which decrease function of ENaC channels, (pseudoaldostereonism Type I) and four different mutations affecting mineralocorticoid receptors have been described. Carbenoxolone, which inhibits 17β hydroxy steroid dehydrogenase Type II, is partially effective in treatment.

	RENIN	ALDOSTERONE	OTHER
Primary Adrenal disease	↑	↓	↓Cortisol
Hyporeninaemic Hypoaldostereonism	↓	↓	Diabetes
Aldosterone enzyme synthetic defects	↑	↓	± ↓Cortisol ± Sex changes
*Pseudohypoaldostereonism			
ENaC dysfunction	↑	↑	Recessive
Aldosterone receptor defect	↑	↑	Dominant Hypertension
Gordon's Syndrome	↓	↓	Acidosis

Table 8: *Causes of decrease in secretion or action of aldosterone (excluding drugs).* Pseudohypoaldosteronism: a collective name applied to inability of aldosterone to produce its major physiological effects.* [156]

Type II Pseudohypoaldostereonism. Gordon'sSyndrome. [45, 97,183-185]

This autosomal dominant disorder may be asymptomatic and present in adults. [183] It is the physiological counterpart of Gitelman syndrome and due to increased activity of NaCl cotransporters (NCC) in distal convoluted tubules. Increased NaCl reabsorption, proximal to the CCD, decreases sodium delivery to principal cells. Chloride reabsorption also increases by paracellular pathways and decreases electrogenic sodium reabsorption. [45,184,185] This decreases the negative lumen potential necessary for tubular K^+ secretion and results in hyperkalaemia. An increase in Na^+ and Cl^- reabsorption causes hypertension, hyperchloraemic acidosis and decreases renin and aldosterone secretion. Thiazide diuretics, which decrease action of NCC transporters, are effective in treatment. [45,183-185]

Although Gordon's syndrome is due to an increase in activity of NaCl cotransporters, it is not due to a mutation of NCC transporters, but to mutations in WNK4 and WNK1 (with no lysine kinase). WNKs modulate the action of aldosterone by inhibiting NCC in the DCT. This increases NaCl delivery to collecting ducts; [97,185] inhibits K^+ secretion in collecting duct principal cells by phosphorylating and thus inactivating K^+ channels; and stimulates paracellular Cl^- conductance. This increases Na^+ reabsorption with Cl^- rather than in exchange with K^+ and leads to hypertension, hyperkalaemia and metabolic acidosis. [45, 97,185]

Type III Pseudohypoaldostereonism. (chapter 15)

A group of acquired diseases which predominantly affect collecting ducts and interstitium of kidney. Some causes are obstructive uropathy, [186,187] AIDS, [188,189] interstitial nephritis due to drugs, medullary cystic disease and autoimmune disease, [190] sickle cell disease and renal transplantation.

Aids.

There are several causes of hyperkalaemia in addition to tubulointerstitial disease. This includes adrenal infection, drugs such as trimethoprim, which inhibit the EnaC sodium channels, and a decrease in response to aldosterone. [188,189]

Hyporeninaemic hypoaldostereonism. [1-6, 191-194]

Defective renin secretion by juxtaglomerular cells is the commonest cause of hypoaldosteronism. It is usually associated with diabetes, tubulointerstitial disease, autoimmune disorders or heparin therapy. Mild-moderate renal failure or other cause is necessary for hyperkalaemia to develop. Defective secretion of aldosterone, in response to angiotensin II, has been reported in some cases. [192]

Asymptomatic hyperkalaemia, usually with hyperchloraemic acidosis, is the most common presentation. [192] Treatment is:

• Avoidance of drugs which predispose to hyperkalaemia.

- Low potassium diet.
- Administration of loop or thiazide diuretics.
- ± Fludrocortisone. [193]

Both Pseudohypoaldostereonism and Hypoaldosteronism are characterised by defective K^+ secretion; abnormal Na^+ losses and metabolic acidosis: $Na^+:K^+$ exchange, H^+ and NH_4^+ excretion are defective. Hyperchloraemic acidosis is due to inhibition of NH_4^+ synthesis from hyperkalaemia in proximal tubules.[191] However normal acid urine (pH < 5.3) can usually be excreted. [195] Correction of hyperkalaemia alone restores urinary ammonium excretion. [191]

DRUGS. [2, 3, 196] (Table 9)

Drugs rarely cause hyperkalaemia unless other factors, such as mild renal failure or Hyporeninaemic hypoaldostereonism are present, but are important contributory causes.

EXTRACELLULAR POTASSIUM SHIFTS

Digoxin:

causes dysfunction of $Na^+:K^+$ pumps in proportion to the serum level. Poisoning by various herbs, [197,198] including foxglove, milkweed, hawthorn berries and Chinese extracts from animals, which contain cardiac glycosides, may cause hyperkalaemia. [198]

β blockers:

block β2 mediated cellular uptake of K^+ and inhibit renin release.

Succinyl Scoline:

DepolarisescellmembranesandreleasesK^+.Lifethreateninghyperkalaemia may occur in those with neuromuscular disease and burns. [36,168]

Infusion of cationic amino-acids: Arginine and lysine can enter cells in muscle in exchange for K^+. [27 28,]

Inhibition of Aldosterone Synthesis.

Heparin inhibits aldosterone synthesis within days of treatment which is independent of its anticoagulant effect or route of administration.

Prolonged use causes a marked decrease in the mass of the adrenal Zona glomerulosa. Raised serum K^+ occurs in 7% but is usually mild unless other factors affecting K^+ secretion are present. [199] Low molecular weight heparin causes hyperkalaemia [200] but less than standard heparin. [201]

INTERFERENCE WITH RENAL EXCRETION.

- **Inhibition of aldosterone synthesis**–Heparin, Ketoconazole.
- **Inhibition of aldosterone synthesis and decreased GFR** ACE inhibitors, Angiotensin receptor blockers. (ARB's), β blockers. Non-steroidal antiinflammatory drugs.
- **Inhibition of aldosterone synthesis and principal cell dysfunction** Calcineurin inhibitors: Cyclosporin, Tacrolimus.
- **Blocking the aldosterone receptor**—spironolactone or eprelenone.
- **Blocking of principal cell epithelial sodium channel**– amiloride, triamterene, high dose trimethoprim.

INTRACELLULAR-EXTRACELLULAR K^+ SHIFTS.

Digoxin	decreased function $Na^+:K^+$ pumps.
β Blockers	inhibit action of $Na^+:K^+$ pumps.
Succinyl scoline	depolarises cell membranes.
Cationic amino acid infusion	exchange for cell K^+.
Glucose in diabetics	K^+ efflux from cells.

Intravenous potassium containing antibiotics and potassium.

Table 9: *Hyperkalaemia due to drugs.*

Inhibition of Aldosterone Synthesis and decreased GFR. [202-205]

ACE inhibitors decrease Angiotensin II (A2) synthesis. This causes hypoaldostereonism and decreases GFR. When renal perfusion decreases severely, as in severe congestive cardiac failure, intense proximal reabsorption of Na^+ limits its availability for Na^+: K^+ exchange in distal tubules. [202,203] Therefore hyperkalaemia is more common in those with mild renal failure and cardiac failure but can occur in those with normal renal function. [202] ACE receptor blockers (ARB) increase serum K^+ to the same extent as ACE inhibitors. [203, 204] Hyperkalaemia developed in 10 %

within one year of prescription of these drugs. [203] Very low doses of ACE inhibitors decrease the risk of hyperkalaemia. [205] The combination of ACE inhibitors, spironolactone and β blockers, often used in heart failure, is especially likely to cause hyperkalaemia. [204]

Non-Steroidal Anti-Inflammatory Drugs (NSAIDs). [206-208,]

Non steroidal antiinflammatory drugs increased serum K^+ by 1.0mmol/L above normal in 23% of 50 patients admitted to a medical service. [206] 26% of patients in one study developed an increase of serum K^+ greater than 1.0mmol/L [207] although selection bias may have inflated the incidence. NSAIDs depress renal function by inhibiting synthesis of prostaglandins and induce Hyporeninaemic hypoaldosteronism in those with renal disease by interfering with the stimulatory effect of prostaglandins on renin release. [206] In addition decrease in urine K^+ excretion may also occur due to decrease in flow rate in distal tubules [206] and decreased activity of high conductance K^+ channels. [206]

β Blockers cause hyperkalaemia by two mechanisms: [196]

- Inhibition of renin secretion.
- Blocking shift of K^+ into cells.

Inhibition of Aldosterone synthesis plus Principal Cell Dysfunction.
[202,208,209]

Calcineurin inhibitors, cyclosporin and tacrolimus, probably cause hyperkalaemia and hyperchloraemic acidosis [196] by inhibiting Na^+:K^+ pump activity in cortical and outer medullary collecting ducts. [209] Cyclosporine also inhibits apical (luminal) K^+ channel activity in Principal cells. [196] Interstitial fibrosis may inhibit aldosterone synthesis and function of K^+ channels.

Blocking of Aldosterone Receptors—Spironolactone,

The frequency of hyperkalaemia increased following the RALES study which popularised use of spironolactone to modify cardiac remodelling in heart failure. [210] The majority of these patients were also taking ACE inhibitors and β blockers. [211] Eprelenone also causes hyperkalaemia but not gynaecomastia. [212] Mortality from hyperkalaemia may outweigh the benefits of combined treatment with ACE inhibitors and spironolactone in high risk patients.

Blocking Principal Cell Sodium Channels (ENaC)

Amiloride and triamterene [213] block ENAC in the distal nephron and prevent electrogenic Na$^+$ reabsorption and thus K$^+$ secretion.

Trimethoprim. [214-217]

Trimethoprim, an organic cation, acts like amiloride by blocking luminal sodium channels. [216] High doses used in the treatment of Pneumocystis carinii pneumonia in AIDS patients has resulted in life threatening hyperkalaemia. [214] However mild hyperkalaemia may occur in those on standard drug therapy with mild renal failure.[215] Trimethoprim, for urine infections, and spironolactone or ACE inhibitors, for cardiovascular diseases, are commonly used together. Both combinations increase admission to hospital for hyperkalaemia. In one study: the former by 12 times and the latter 6 times compared to normal.(BMJ 343:544.2011)

Increased Intake of Potassium.

- Dietary.
- Infusion of potassium penicillin.
- Blood transfusion.
- Infusion of potassium chloride or phosphate in treatment.
- Oral potassium supplements.

Oral potassium supplements.

Potassium supplements, which are over prescribed, based on highly questionable data,[218] are an important cause of hyperkalaemia. Hyperkalaemia may occur in the absence of renal failure if considerable amounts are taken.[219,220] Adverse reactions, most commonly hyperkalaemia, occurred in 5.8% of 16,000 consecutive patients given potassium chloride in one drug surveillance programme.[220] Hyperkalaemia was more common in those taking potassium orally than intravenously. Hyperkalaemia may also occur from excessive use of salt substitutes containing potassium. [220,221] Diet is an important cause of hyperkalaemia, especially if renal failure is present. It is insufficiently realised that oral potassium is well absorbed and is probably a more common cause of hyperkalaemia than intravenous potassium in patients with renal failure.

Increased dietary intake of potassium

This is important when GFR decreases below 30mL/min. Use of salt substitutes which contain potassium, over the counter NSAIDs and herbal remedies may not be volunteered by patients. Some examples are shown in table10. Noni juice from fruit of the Noni tree (Och plant, Nonu, Nhau, cheese fruit), a popular herbal product contains 56mmol/L of potassium, and has caused hyperkalaemia in those with chronic renal failure. [222]

SOURCE	POTASSIUM
Potassium supplements	Slow K (8mmol tab; effervescent 13mmol/sachet
Salt substitutes	10—13mmol/1000mg [208]
Seaweed	25mmol/100g
Dried figs	25mmol/100g
Dried fruits, nuts avocados, bananas	12.5mmol/100g
Vegetables, other fruits	6.0mmol/100g
Oranges	5.5mmol/100g
Tomatoes	10mmol/100g
Bananas	12mmol/100g
Meats	6.0mmol/100g
Orange juice	51.0mmol/L
Canned Pineapple juice	34mmol/L [221]
Grapefruit juice	43mmol/L [221]
Tomato juice	58mmol/L [221]
Noni juice	56mmol/L [221]
Apple juice	28-32mmol/L

Table 10: *Potassium content in several foods and supplements (from several sources).*

Hyperkalaemia Developing in Hospital.

Hyperkalaemia may follow treatment of hypokalaemia in hospitalised patients due to large doses of potassium given in treatment; continuing potassium supplements; and sometimes in combination with drugs which promote hyperkalaemia. [220, 223]

Hyperkalaemia may occur despite [219,220] absence of renal failure. [220, 224] This has occurred during intravenous therapy, [220,224,225] following intraperitoneal infusion [226] and even oral ingestion. [23,220,227-229] The ECG (Figure 13) showing hyperkalemia, in the section which follows, was from a child who took large amounts of orange juice and bananas during the recovery phase of acute tubular necrosis. Interestingly the potassium concentration of bananas is 2.23 mmol per inch. [230] Oral potassium is especially dangerous in the setting of digitalis toxicity and diseases involving the cardiac conducting system. [229]

The safety of oral compared to intravenous potassium replacement has been overemphasised. Absorption of oral potassium is rapid and largely complete. In the seminal study by Darrow reporting the importance of potassium replacement in dehydrated children without renal failure, ten of 14 infants were hyperkalaemic at the end of their balance studies. Serum K^+ was 9.6mmol/L in one [227,228]. K^+ supplementation by mouth was a more common cause of hyperkalaemia in the surveillance study referred to above. [220].

A single abnormality rarely causes hyperkalaemia in absence of severe renal failure. Multiple causes are usually present.

The following groups of patients are particularly prone to develop hyperkalaemia because of the presence of multiple risk factors and the need to use drugs which promote the development of hyperkalaemia.

Diabetic Patients

Decrease in insulin secretion.

Reduced GFR from diabetic nephropathy.

Volume depletion from osmotic diuresis or ketonuria.

Hyporeninaemic hypoaldostereonism and Tubulointerstitial disease.

Risk factors from other co-morbidity: Congestive cardiac failure, myocardial infarction, stroke.

Risk factors from commonly used drugs: ACE inhibitors, β blockers, aldosterone antagonists, potassium sparing diuretics

Table 11: Risk factors for hyperkalaemia in diabetics

ACE inhibitors are important because they decrease progression of renal disease in diabetes. Low dose ACE inhibitor reduces proteinuria without causing hyperkalaemia. [205] Fasting in diabetic patients with end stage renal disease increases serum K+ due to insulinopenia and decrease in sympathetic activity. [20] In one study the mean serum K+ increased by 0.5 mmol/L during fasting. This is important in those undergoing surgery or procedures. Intravenous and oral glucose increase serum potassium and can be hazardous in insulinopenic patients. [65,171, 172]

Insulin deficiency severely impairs cellular uptake of potassium: when serum K+ is slightly raised an added load may be confined to the extracellular space alone. [102]

Patients with cardiac failure

ACE inhibitors commonly cause hyperkalaemia [203,231)] but their administration improves prognosis and symptoms of heart failure. However the combination of ACE inhibitors and angiotensin receptor blockers may cause harm without benefit. [232] Life threatening hyperkalaemia can develop when ACE inhibitors are combined with spironolactone. [211,233]

- Decrease in GFR due to low cardiac output.
- Increased sodium reabsorption proximal to distal nephrons limits K+ secretion in exchange for Na+ .

Rick factors from drugs used in heart failure [196 202 204 210 230 232]
  * Inhibition of aldosterone secretion from ACE inhibitors or its action by angiotensin receptor blockers.
  * Use of potassium sparing diuretics which decrease K+ secretion in principal cells.
  * β blockers – inhibit renin release and adrenergic mediated cellular K+ uptake.
  * Digoxin: decreases activity of the Na+K+ pumps.
  * Potassium replacement.

Risks from associated diseases:

Diabetes and renal failure.

Table 12. Risk factors for hyperkalaemia in heart failure.

Therapeutic trials, which showed a low incidence of hyperkalaemia from ACE inhibitors or spironolactone, are misleading because of enrolment of patients at low risk; relatively normal renal function, and more frequent monitoring under experimental rather than real life conditions. A Canadian study reported a marked increase in hospitalisation for hyperkalaemia from increased use of spironolactone following the RALES trial [210] although its clinical significance was disputed. Spironolactone improves outcome in advanced heart failure [204] and may decrease progression of renal disease. [231] However the dose should be kept low and serum creatinine monitored. Only a minority need discontinuation [204] but use of spironolactone should be considered carefully if GFR decreases below 30 mL/minute. [233] β blockers block the release of renin and interfere with cellular uptake of K^+ by decreasing activity of $Na^+:K^+$ pumps. β blockers, spironolactone in low dose and ACE inhibitors, all three of which block the RAAS system, are beneficial in most heart failure patients, but in combination, increase risk of hyperkalaemia and require careful monitoring.

> **Patients with mild chronic renal failure or Hyporeninaemic hypoaldosteronism who take medication promoting hyperkalaemia**

Medications which interfere with K^+ secretion in principal cells increase risk of hyperkalaemia in those with mild renal failure or reduced GFR. It is important to calculate GFR in elderly and malnourished patients because serum creatinine levels are misleading as an indication of GFR. Special care should be taken in prescribing drugs which interfere with potassium transfer or excretion in patients with diabetes, heart disease and renal failure when GFR decreases below 30ml/minute. [233] The following medications shown in table 13 are important:

* <u>Potassium sparing diuretics</u> – amiloride, spironolactone, triamterene and heparin.

* <u>Drugs interfering with aldosterone synthesis or action</u>. ACE inhibitors or ARB blockers.

* <u>Non steroidal antiinflammatory drugs</u>: interfere with prostaglandin stimulation of renin secretion.

* <u>β blockers</u>: block the sympathetic nervous system by inhibiting renin release and cellular uptake of potassium.

Table 13. Drugs predisposing to hyperkalaemia in patients with mild renal failure or Hyporeninaemic hypoaldostereonism.

The combination of ACE inhibitors and spironolactone should be considered carefully in renal failure [211,231] and monitored closely. The use of ACE inhibitors and aldosterone blockade [231] are important in preserving renal function so that they should be tried, monitored carefully and continued provided serum creatinine levels do not exceed 30% of base line. A rise of less than this is usually due to dysfunction of autoregulation rather than structural renal disease and does not indicate they should be stopped. [234]

Risk from associated diseases: (diabetes, heart failure, tubulointerstitial disease are commonly present).

Risks for hyperkalaemia in tubulointerstitial disease and Transplant patients are shown in tables 14 and 15.

- Dysfunction of principal cells interferes with K^+ and H^+ secretion in the absence of severe renal failure.

- Reduced GFR.

Risks from medication

- ACE inhibitors, spironolactone or β blockers predispose to hyperkalaemia.
- Use of Trimethoprim in AIDS and Cyclosporin in transplantation cases.

Risks from associated disease
- Diabetic nephropathy with Hyporeninaemic hypoaldosteronism may coexist. Sjogren's syndrome, systemic lupus erythematosus, sickle cell disease, obstructive uropathy, AID's and renal transplantation may cause interstitial disease.

Table 14. Hyperkalaemia from tubulointerstitial disease.

Transplant patients:

- Tubulointerstitial disease – risks as above.

- Risks from drugs – as above.

- Cyclosporin and tacrolimus suppress renin release and interfere with K^+ secretion in collecting ducts [209]. Hyperkalaemia develops in 44-73% of transplant patients on Cyclosporin or Tacrolimus. [196]

Table 15. Risks of hyperkalaemia in transplant patients.

APPROACH TO Hyperkalaemia

PSEUDOHYPERKALAEMIA

This is usually due to loss of K^+ from platelets, red or white blood cells following blood sampling or from exercising muscles. Exercise or use of a tourniquet to improve blood sampling and difficult venipuncture can cause a considerable error in serum K^+ measurement. [235-237] Plasma K^+ levels are lower than serum levels [235] and arterial blood has lower plasma K^+ than venous levels. In one study venous plasma levels were 0.23mEq/L higher than arterial. [241]

Storage and cooling of blood:

Cooling of blood during storage results in loss of K^+ from cells at 0.1-0.3mEq/L/hour for 48 hours and leads to plasma levels several times the original concentration. [238,-239]

Loss of Potassium from red cells, platelets and white cells:

Platelets are the main cause of K^+ losses on storage [235]. In disorders of platelet function, such as thrombocythemia or leukaemia K^+ loss begins immediately and may result in spurious hyperkalaemia even without storage. Collection in plasma, using heparin as anticoagulant, may decrease artefactual elevation, but not completely, in conditions such as thrombocythemia. Just visible haemolysis increases plasma K^+ by 0.2mEq/L. [240]

Familial Pseudohyperkalaemia.

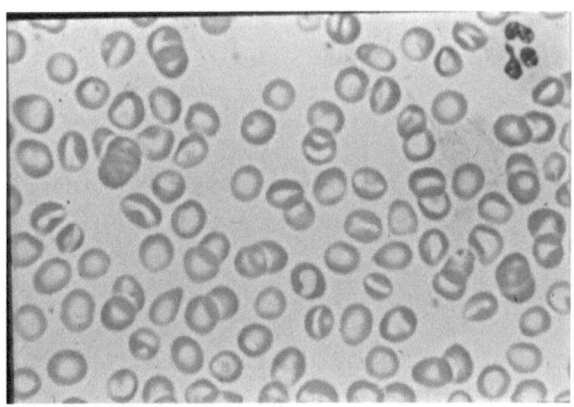

__Blood film of Hereditary Stomatocytosis.__

Inherited Pseudohyperkalaemia, probably autosomal dominant, is due to abnormal leak of K^+ from red blood cells. [242] Hereditary Stomatocytosis is due to mutations of the HCO_3^- :Cl^- exchanger. Red cells leak K^+ in Hereditary Stomatocytosis and other disorders of red cell membranes and may cause pseudohyperkalaemia.[242-243,244] The test should be repeated without exercise, with minimal tourniquet time, preferably using heparin as anticoagulant and measuring plasma rather than a serum sample. An ECG alerts to spurious hyperkalaemia if there is doubt about the validity of raised serum K^+. [235]

TRUE HYPERKALAEMIA

- *Look at serum creatinine* and if slightly or moderately raised estimate glomerular filtration rate by a validated formula. This is especially important in malnourished and elderly. Look for a cause in addition to renal impairment if there is only mild or moderate impairment in GFR > 20—30mls/min.
- *Review all medications*: note their potential to impair potassium excretion or intracellular transfer of K^+.
- *Look at Dietary contributions*. (table10) The patient may not volunteer these.
- *Look at serum bicarbonate and anion gap*.

If hyperchloraemic acidosis is present consider:
- tubulointerstitial renal disease
- Hyporeninaemic hypoaldosteronism or Addison's disease
- Aids, renal transplantation., SLE.
- Gordon's syndrome.
- *Is heart failure or volume depletion present?* This contributes to hyperkalaemia.
- *Is the patient in an at risk group.*

Diabetic.

Establish if Hyporeninaemic hypoaldosteronism, insulin deficiency, volume depletion or drugs are present—ACE inhibitors, NSAIDS, β blockers.

Chronic heart failure.

This causes inadequate distal Na^+ delivery which is needed for exchange with K^+. Consider the effects of drugs—ACE, ARBs, Spironolactone and β blockers.

Tubulointerstitial disease.

Is there evidence of tubulointerstitial disease: Sjogren's syndrome, AIDS, renal transplant etc? Are there manifestations of hyperkalaemia, hyperchloraemic acidosis, decreased urine concentration, polyuria, pyuria, eosinophilia and decreased GFR? Are drugs implicated? Remaining causes are rare.

Even if there is an adequate reason for hyperkalaemia always enquire about contributory factors such as medications and diet

In unusual or unexplained cases calculation of the transtubular potassium gradient (TTKG) and urine anion gap may aid diagnosis.

TTKG. [1]

The majority of cases of severe hyperkalaemia have a defect in K^+ secretion in cortical collecting ducts (CCD). The gradient between cortical collecting duct tubular fluid and plasma K^+, in the presence of hyperkalaemia, should reach 7-10 on a normal diet and >11 if hyperkalaemia is present. Water abstraction from medullary collecting ducts, without potassium reabsorption, increases urine potassium by the difference in osmolality between the CCD osmolality (assumed to be 300mOsmol/kg H_2O) and urine osmolality. The TTKG (transtubular K^+ gradient can be estimated as follows:

The K^+ concentration in the CCD can be estimated by dividing the CCD osmolality—assumed to be 300mOsmol/kg H_2O, by urine osmolality. This is based on two assumptions: provided some ADH is present osmolality in the CCD is ~ 300mOsmol/kg H_2O because more dilute tubular fluid will come into equilibrium with renal cortex with an osmolality of 300mOsmol/Kg H_2O). Only slight K^+ absorption occurs distal to the CCD. (These assumptions may not be correct.)

For example if serum K^+ is 6.0 mmol/L, the urine potassium 80 mmoL/L and urine osmolality 1200mOsmol/kg H_2O:

The CCD K^+ = 300/1200 x 80mmol/L = 20 mmol/L

TTKG = urine osmolality/ 300 x urine K^+ / serum K^+. =20/6.0 = 3.33.

This level is much less than the expected level of >10 in the presence of hyperkalaemia and therefore suggests renal potassium secretion is defective.

Urine anion or osmolar gaps, discussed previously, give an estimation of urine NH_4^+ excretion. This is decreased in disturbances of secretion or action of aldosterone. (Type IV renal tubular acidosis). The use of urine anion gap estimation suggests the diagnosis of renal tubular acidosis: in normal volunteers given NH_4Cl and 8 patients with diarrhoea urine anion gap was negative (-27 and -20) whereas it was positive (+23; +30; +39) in patients with classic renal tubular acidosis (RTA); hyperkalaemic distal RTA; or selective aldosterone deficiency. [195] (Chapter 6)

Diagnosis of hypoaldostereonism and pseudoaldostereonism and their differential diagnosis can be facilitated by measuring aldosterone and renin, their ratio and serum cortisol (Table 8).

CLINICAL MANIFESTATIONS

HYPERKALAEMIA.

Increase in extracellular K^+, which decreases the K^+i /K^+_o ratio, (becomes less negative) lowers the transmembrane resting potential (TRP) [246-250] of atrium, ventricle and Purkinje system and shortens duration of the action potential in all cardiac tissues. [249] This initially allows less intense stimuli to evoke action potentials and predisposes to arrhythmia, skeletal muscle twitching and paraesthesia. Atrioventricular (AV) conduction is initially accelerated and then progressively decreases as serum K^+ rises. [247-250]

When serum K^+ increases further the duration of the action potential shortens, conduction velocity decreases and rate of repolarisation increases. [249] Calcium does not decrease TRP but decreases depolarisation caused by high serum K^+. [248-249] Increasing extracellular K^+ has a biphasic effect on impulse formation and conduction: initially increasing and then causing a profound decrease in impulse formation and conduction in all cardiac tissues. This progresses to heart block and asystole. [249,250]

Changes are not only dependent on serum K^+ but also on the speed of development of hyperkalaemia. [247,249] Indeed if serum K^+ rises sufficiently rapidly bradycardia, heart block and asystole can result from change of serum K^+ from low to normal (Zwaardemaker-Librecht phenomenon). [247,249, 250,] Administration of potassium is particularly prone to cause heart block in digitalised patients. Gradual increase in serum K⁺ may cause ventricular and junctional ectopic beats, ectopic tachycardias and, although uncommon, ventricular fibrillation. [249]

Peaked T waves, due to early repolarisation, are the first ECG change. Atrial muscle is especially vulnerable to hyperkalaemia but fibres of the SA and AV nodes are more resistant. Therefore, although P waves disappear, conduction continues by atrial fibre pathways which are relatively resistant to hyperkalaemia. [249,250] A rapid heart rate, without P waves, but wide QRS complexes are usually due to nodal or sinus tachycardia rather than ventricular tachycardia. [249]Peaked T waves are characterised by similar slopes for the up and down stroke of the T wave (Figure 13).

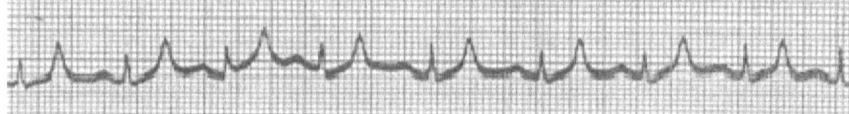

Figure 13: Peaked T waves in an 8 year old child with plasma K 7.1mmol/L recovering from acute tubular necrosis following peritoneal dialysis. Hyperkalaemia was due to ingestion of excessive intake of bananas and fruit juice.

The PR interval lengthens and QRS widens from a decrease in conduction in His Purkinje fibres. The P wave decreases in amplitude, then disappears and AV junctional escape is common. The widened QRS merges with T waves giving rise to a sine wave pattern: <u>all 3 portions of the QRS are equally affected compared to the middle and terminal segments in bundle branch block.</u> [247,249]

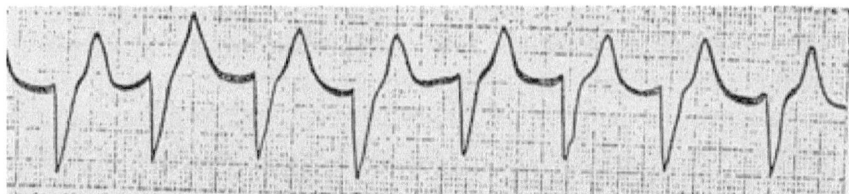

Figure 14: ECG before treatment with glucose insulin. Initial serum K 9.1mmol/L. The P wave is absent in the above tracing and QRS prolonged. Following treatment P waves reappeared.

Uncommonly a pseudoinfarction pattern shows ST segment elevation over precordial leads. [246 250,251] However peaked T waves are usually present in other leads. [249,251]. (Figure 15.)

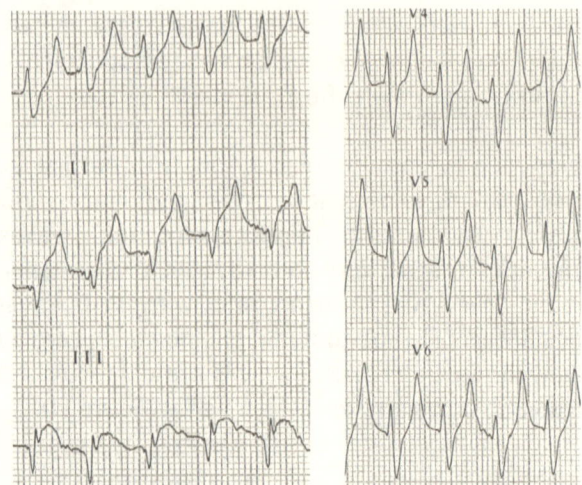

Figure 15: Pseudo infarct pattern due to hyperkalaemia.
Tall T waves in leads, V5, V6 and Q waves in leads, 2,3.

Cardiac arrest from asystole, pulseless electrical activity, or ventricular fibrillation, may occur in the absence of ECG changes, especially in those with underlying heart disease. Indeed there is limited correlation between serum levels and ECG changes. Ventricular fibrillation is more common when hyperkalaemia develops rapidly while asystole is more common when it develops slowly. [249] Cardiac manifestations are also related to underlying cardiac disease, rapidity of development of hyperkalaemia and other electrolyte disturbances. Hypocalcaemia or low ionised Ca^{2+} from or alkalosis [249] increases the toxic effects of hyperkalaemia.

Hyperkalaemia may depress conduction at several levels. [249,252] It is important to emphasise that heart block, without T or QRS changes, may be the first manifestation of hyperkalaemia in those with underlying conduction abnormalities. [252] Indeed treatment of hypokalaemia to normal in such persons may precipitate complete heart block (personal observations). The sudden appearance of heart block in patients at risk should alert to the possibility of hyperkalaemia. [252] Although the pacing threshold increases pacing may be successful. [249]

Potassium should be used cautiously in those with conduction defects or digoxin toxicity because complete heart block may result [229,252]. Oral potassium may be as hazardous as intravenous potassium. [229] The ECG has poor sensitivity for diagnosis. [4,252,253]

Neuromuscular manifestations Paraesthesia, weakness of limbs, muscle fatigue, cramps, fasciculations and areflexia.

Hyperchloraemic acidosis occurs because hyperkalaemia inhibits NH_4^+ synthesis in proximal tubules.

MANIFESTATIONS OF HYPOKALAEMIA

Information on signs of hypokalemia has usually been reported from observations on human volunteers or small numbers of patients with conditions where other electrolyte disturbances may have been responsible for the signs described. The following is based on reported data combined with observations on large numbers of severely hypokalemic infants and children in an area of West Africa where severe hypokalemia was common. [224]The main manifestations of hypokalaemia are <u>cardiac, neuromuscular and gastrointestinal</u>.

CARDIAC

Hypokalaemia increases the resting membrane potential (hyperpolarisation), duration of the action potential and duration of the refractory period. [246,255] A stronger impulse is required to bring TRP to threshold potential. [247] This predisposes to re-entrant tachyarrhythmia and automaticity which increases as serum K decreases. [255] Murmurs, collapsing pulses, [256-259] and arrhythmias [255-268] —ventricular arrhythmias, [247,260-262,268] ventricular fibrillation, [261,266] Torsades de Pointes [263] and atrial tachycardia [224,262] have been reported in hypokalaemic subjects. Atrial tachyarrhythmias are more common in children. [224] Ventricular tachycardia and ventricular fibrillation may be more common in adults, especially in those with underlying heart disease. Hypokalaemia is a risk factor for arrhythmias and predisposes those taking diuretics to increased frequency and complexity of paroxysmal ventricular ectopics. [263-266]

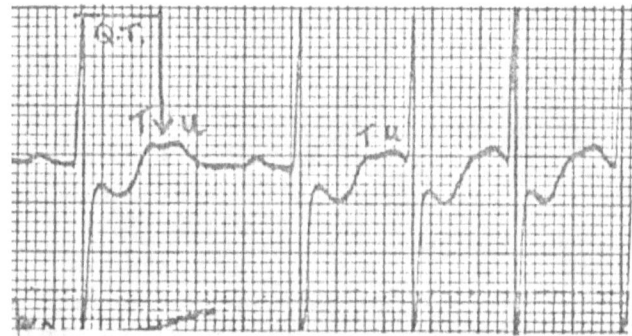

Figure 16. ECG leads showing sinus rhythm with ST depression, T and U waves followed by supraventricular tachycardia. Plasma K^+ 1.0 mmol/L; Na^+ 116 mmol/L; arterial blood pH 7.44.

ECG manifestations of hypokalaemia.

Hypokalemia mainly affects the repolarising phase of the cardiac cycle: ST segment, T and U waves. QRS and P wave changes have been described infrequently. [246,247,255,262]

T and U wave changes. (figure 13).

The T wave decreases and U wave increases as plasma potassium falls. Discrete T and U waves may occur, either of which may be larger; and occasionally a second U wave occurs. T and U waves may interact: complete fusion gives the impression of a single wave which may be mistaken for a normal T wave; partial fusion—termed superimposition—gives rise to a variety of patterns where separation of waves may be easy, as in the hump back configuration, or difficult where only a slight notch between the two is apparent. Fusion is more likely to occur if the QT interval is prolonged—as in hypocalcaemia or alkalemia. The U wave may fuse with the P wave if the cardiac cycle is short. [269-271]

ST segment changes.

The QT interval is not prolonged from hypokalemia per se, but may be prolonged from associated alkalosis which lowers ionised extracellular Ca^{2+}. ST depression increases in severity as hypokalemia increases. A variety of patterns result from the interaction of the ST segment, T and U waves. The most common is a diphasic pattern resembling the letter S on its side.

The three components of the ventricular complex, ST, T and U show maximal changes in different leads: the maximal elevation of U occurs in transition zone V3-V4. Furthermore, the voltage of T and U waves may vary in the same lead.

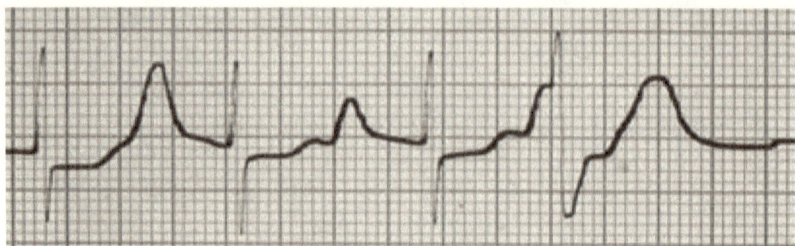

Figure 17. V4 of the ECG of a patient with plasma K⁺ 1.8 mmol/L. Note various patterns of fusion of T with U wave in the same lead. The second complex shows a small T followed by a larger U wave ;the first complex shows a giant U wave.

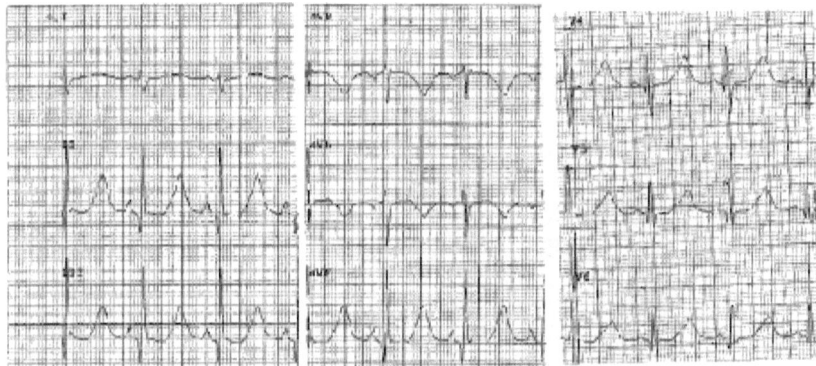

Figure 18. Giant U waves in a young female due to hypokalaemia from vomiting: serum K⁺ 1.6 mmol/L. This gives the appearance of a prolonged QT interval but T waves are absent.

The following are useful in interpretation.

- ECG changes are <u>generalised</u> and not confined to one anatomical area.
- Analysis of all leads, because the patterns produced vary. Lead aV_L, for example, usually has the lowest U wave and V_3-V_4 the highest. There is usually at least one lead where it is possible to separate the T and U components of a fused or superimposed T-U complex.
- U wave > T wave in the same lead, a U wave > 1mm in V_3, and ST depression > 0.5mm.
- The most common causes of misinterpretation is to mistake T-U and P-U fusion waves for T waves; to fail to realise the significance of an early broad T wave; and to mistake the initial positive component of a positive-negative diphasic ST complex for a T wave.
- Recording the ECG at double voltage and half speed.

NEUROMUSCULAR MANIFESTATIONS. [224,272-282]

Fatigue, limb weakness, myalgia, fasciculations, muscle cramps, paraesthesia and areflexia are characteristic. [224 257,259 274] Limb paralysis and inability to walk are uncommon except for attacks of Familial Periodic Paralysis and severe hypokalaemia (serum < 2.0mmol/L). [224]

Paralysis may mimic conditions such as Guillain-Barré syndrome, porphyria and poliomyelitis. Coma does not occur even in severe hypokalaemia. [224] Respiratory failure and rhabdomyolysis occur [224,256,257,273-282,] but are rare.

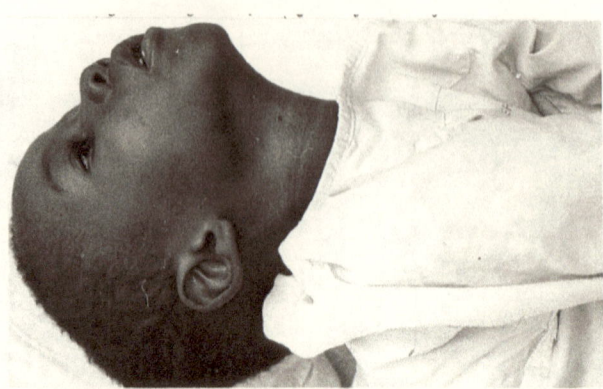

Figure 19: *6-year old child referred with a diagnosis of poliomyelitis. Inability to support head on pulling the child forward. He was unable to walk. Plasma K 1.4mmol/L, Na125 mmol/L; arterial blood pH7.44. Serum CPK = 1,100 U/L*

GATROINTESTINAL MANIFESTATIONS

Constipation, abdominal distension and ileus are common during severe hypokalaemia [4,224,264,283,284] and are probably due to decreased intestinal mobility. Abdominal distension and ileus respond dramatically (within hours) to adequate intravenous K⁺ replacement. [15,224,264,283] Even mild potassium deficiency in post operative ileus should be rigorously treated.

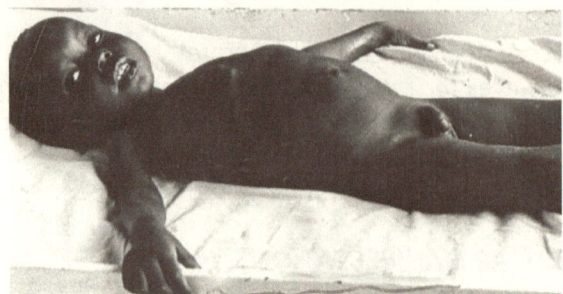

Figure 20: *Showing severe apathy, muscle weakness with areflexia and abdominal distension in a child 5 years of age. Plasma K⁺ 1.0 mmol/L, Na⁺ 116 mmol/L,*

Severity of hypokalaemia

Moderate hypokalaemia commonly causes weakness, apathy and hypo-reflexia. More serious manifestations occur uncommonly if plasma K⁺ is greater than 2.5mmol/L [22, 23,132,224]—apart from periodic paralysis. Severe hypokalaemia (K+ < 2.0 mmol/L) causes more serious manifestations. In my observations all recorded cases of cardiac arrhythmia and paralysis occurred in children whose plasma potassium was < 2.0mmol/L. Cardiac arrhythmias, abdominal distension, ileus and muscle weakness rapidly responded to intravenous K+ with the exception of muscle weakness when rhabdomyolysis was present. [224] There are four factors which govern the frequency of manifestations besides the severity of hypokalaemia:

- Rapidity of development.
- Presence of other electrolyte abnormalities.
- Presence of underlying cardiac disease.
- Infusion of low K+ containing glucose fluids.

My observations in children indicate that the frequency of serious manifestations and death showed a marked increase when severely hypokalemic subjects were treated with glucose, low potassium containing, infusions: respiratory paralysis, coma myotonic twitching, severe abdominal distension, ileus, and cardiac arrhythmias preceded death before intravenous potassium became available for use. [224]Many accounts of respiratory failure due to hypokalemia have been described in diabetic patients during treatment with glucose saline, or sodium bicarbonate without K+. [224,256,273 275,276-, 280, 285] Cardiac arrhythmias, cardiac dilatation, systolic murmurs, collapsing pulse have usually been described during glucose infusion. [256,257-259, 279] For example the sudden onset of respiratory and limb paralysis coincided with infusion of 5% glucose solution to potassium depleted subjects.[224,256, 259,273-280,286]

Severe ventricular tachycardia was reported by Kunin et al [260] in two hypokalemic patients who received glucose infusion containing K+ at a concentration of 20mmol/L. This prompted them to examine the effects of 5% glucose solutions containing concentrations of K+ of 20 and 40mmol/L on the plasma K+ of normokalemic and hypokalemic subjects. Both solutions depressed plasma potassium for periods up to 1 hour. Cardiac arrhythmia developed in two patients who received the weaker potassium solution. When a similar K+ concentration was infused in mannitol the plasma potassium rose in all cases.

Glucose given orally may also decrease serum potassium [23,287], cause heart block[229] and ECG changes [249,287] Post prandial electrocardiographic T wave changes are probably due to a similar mechanism. [287]

RENAL AND PHYSIOLOGICAL MANIFESTATIONS

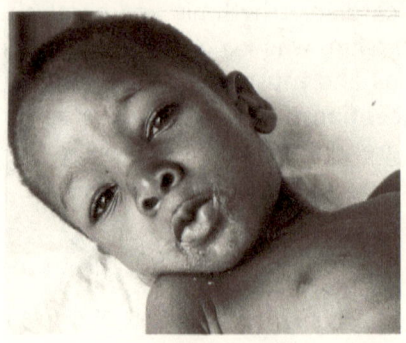

Figure 21. Showing tetany of facial muscles, due to metabolic alkalosis, following treatment of hypokalaemia.

Metabolic alkalosis often accompanies potassium depletion. This is due to associated loss of chloride, as in vomiting, hypovolaemia, diuretic use or increased bicarbonate reabsorption. NH_4HCO_3 synthesis increases during hypokalaemia; NH_4^+ is excreted with Cl^- and $KHCO_3$ is reabsorbed. This is discussed further, with references, in chapter 6. Tetany may accompany severe K depletion, but is due to associated metabolic alkalosis which decreases ionised calcium. [224] Tetany is masked by hypokalaemia and often develops when hypokalaemia resolves. [4] (Figure 21) A long QT interval is also due to low ionised calcium and does not occur from hypokalaemia per se.

Hypokalaemia causes polydisia due to an increase in thirst [4,288], possibly from action of angiotensin 2 on the hypothalamic thirst centre, and polyuria [4,288] resistant to ADH. [288]

Thirst precedes the defect in concentration. [288] A characteristic vacuolar change, which is reversible,[4] occurs in tubules in rare cases. [4, 224, 289] (Figure 22). Vacuolar nephropathy was found in 1 of 9 consecutive children with plasma K^+ of less than 2.1mmol/L who died. [224]

Hypokalaemia increases NH_4^+ synthesis and urinary ammonium chloride excretion.[88] Ammonia may worsen hepatic encephalopathy and hypokalaemia may have other adverse effects in liver cirrhosis. [2] This increases proteolysis to provide amide precursors for glutamine synthesis.

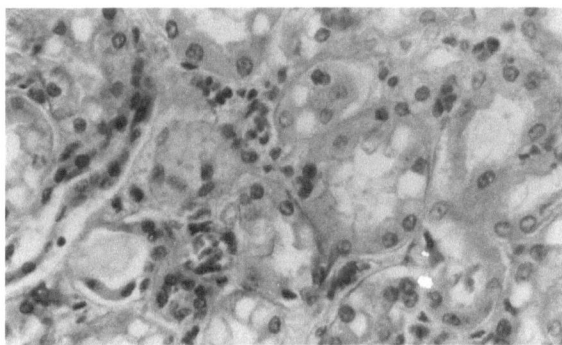

Figure 22: Vacuoles are present in many cells of proximal tubules in a child with severe hypokalaemia and kwashiorkor.

Hypokalaemia causes severe vasoconstriction of preglomerular arterioles and decreases G.F.R. Intercalated cells in distal tubules hypertrophy and numbers of H^+: K^+ pumps in luminal membranes increase. This increases K^+ reabsorption and H^+ secretion. Na^+: K^+ pumps decrease in muscle and other tissue. [36] This may limit the ability to excrete potassium following recovery. Glycogen synthesis, which requires potassium, may decrease.

TREATMENT OF POTASSIUM DISORDERS

HYPERKALAEMIA

PREVENTION IN PATIENTS AT RISK OF HYPERKALAEMIA

- Establish a complete risk profile for each patient: both diseases and drugs which interfere with K^+ excretion—especially renal failure, diabetes, heart failure, Hyporeninaemic hypoaldosteronism and drugs which interfere with K^+ excretion or K^+ transfer from extracellular fluid to cells.
- Estimate GFR using a validated formula. Do not rely on using serum creatinine alone, especially in elderly or malnourished patients.
- If GFR is less than 30mL/minute be cautious in use of drugs which block the Renin-angiotensin aldosterone system: ACE inhibitors, β blockers and spironolactone or Eprelenone.
- Use spironolactone in low dose (25mg daily) or Eprelenone (50mg/day) and start ACE inhibitors or Angiotensin receptor blockers at low dose. Consider using loop diuretics when GFR decreases below 30mL/minute and sodium bicarbonate to treat hyperchloraemic metabolic acidosis. Avoid use of β blockers, especially non-selective, in patients with renal failure who exercise.

- Ask patients about "over the counter" herbal remedies, which may contain potassium or cardiac glycosides, salt substitutes and NSAIDs. For example cardiac glycosides are contained in Chan Su, an aphrodisiac, milkweed, lily of the valley, hawthorn berries, Siberian ginseng and foxglove.
- Educate patients and provide information sheets on K^+ content of foods, avoidance of herbal remedies and salt substitutes. Inform about fluctuations in heart and renal failure and to seek medical attention early if these occur.
- Avoid fasting, for example before operation, or give insulin glucose in diabetics with end stage renal disease because insulin deficiency [20,290,291,292] and sympathetic nervous system activity [292] increases serum K^+. The serum K^+ increased 0.58mmol following 18 hours fasting in diabetics with chronic renal failure. [290].
- Maintain optimum management of chronic renal failure by using sodium bicarbonate to correct acidosis. Sodium bicarbonate is especially effective because of delivery of poorly reabsorbed anions (HCO_3^-) with Na^+ to distal tubules.
  Use loop rather than thiazide diuretics.
  Use low rather than high dose ACE inhibitors.
- Monitor serum K^+ initially and if deterioration occurs.
- Take special care in treatment of hypokalaemia in those with risk factors for hyperkalaemia—especially with renal dysfunction. Aim to correct serum K^+ to 3.0mmo/L and then reconsider. This applies as much to oral potassium supplements.
- Avoid using drugs which interfere with K^+ excretion: K^+ sparing diuretics, trimethoprim, non-steroid anti-inflammatory drugs (NSAIDS) and heparin.

ACUTE TREATMENT OF HYPERKALAEMIA.

The ECG has poor sensitivity for hyperkalaemia and does not correlate well with serum levels. [253, 254 293,] Underlying heart disease is a risk for arrhythmias. The severity and speed of development of hyperkalaemia are important in development of manifestations. [247,294]

<u>Treatment of Factors Contributing to Hyperkalaemia.</u>

- Stop drugs interfering with cellular shift and excretion of K^+.
- Stop high potassium containing foods or fluids.

- Treat hypovolaemia and heart failure if present. Give IV 100-200mg furosemide or other loop diuretic in heart failure.
- Give corticosteroids and fludrocortisone if adrenal dysfunction is present and oral fludrocortisone 0.1mg if Hyporeninaemic hypoaldosteronism is present.

Decrease Serum Potassium or its harmful effects.

- Stabilise the myocardial membrane with calcium.
- Promote K$^+$ entry into cells to improve the transcellular gradient.
- Eliminate K$^+$ from the body by:
  * Resins to exchange Na$^+$ or Ca^{2+} for K$^+$.
  * Increase urinary excretion of K$^+$ - loop diuretics or correction of hypovolaemia.
  * Dialysis.

Calcium.

Use of Ca^{2+} for initial treatment is based on expert opinion, its physiological effects in antagonising K$^+$ and its membrane stabilising effects in decreasing the arrhythmia threshold in animal models and tissues. However the concentration of calcium used in these studies was considerably higher than are used in man from expert recommendations. [295] High doses of calcium, well above the amount from recommended doses, were used in papers cited as evidence for use of calcium. The evidence for benefit is highly questionable. For example, Chamberlain [296], quoted in several reviews, reported 5 "anecdotal" cases in which calcium was used in severe hyperkalaemia:

90mL calcium gluconate given over 5 minutes was used in Case 1.

30mL calcium gluconate in Case 2 who died 1 hour later. Improvement in ECG changes was not convincing.

Intracardiac calcium chloride was injected in case 3 who died following electromechanical dissociation.

60mL calcium gluconate was given to Case 4. Improvement in ECG changes was unconvincing.

5mL intracardiac calcium chloride was injected in Case 5 followed by 90mL intravenously. The serum Ca^{2+} following resuscitation was 4.0mmol/L.

Evidence, frequently cited in his paper, should not be used to support the administration of calcium for treatment of hyperkalaemia.

Merrill et al [297] found no benefit from using intravenous calcium in 9 of 10 cases of hyperkalaemia and doubtful benefit in one case; whereas sodium and glucose insulin infusion were beneficial.

No deaths occurred in 242 consecutive hospitalised patients with hyperkalaemia despite suboptimum treatment which included use of calcium in only 36% of episodes. [291]

Whether calcium should be used routinely and the dose, which is effective and safe, has not been established. Some experts only use calcium if arrhythmias or severe ECG changes are present. Hypercalcaemia is difficult to avoid or control [296,297] and is potentially dangerous. However hypocalcaemia may accompany renal failure and its replacement, if present, may improve ECG changes of hyperkalaemia. [298]

An intravenous bolus of 10mL of calcium gluconate (4.5mmol) is recommended, repeated once if required. This may be followed by an infusion, if hypocalcaemia is present, to prevent recurrence.

Promotion of K+ entry to cells.

There are no randomised controlled trials using outcomes such as arrhythmia or death as an end point. Randomised trials using reduction of serum K^+ as the end point are few, subject numbers low, methods flawed and all have been carried out in subjects with chronic renal failure.

A Cochrane Collaboration systematic review of treatment of hyperkalaemia included 12 randomised or quasi- randomised studies using Salbutamol, Glucose-insulin, bicarbonate, the combination and theophylline (1 study) [299] This concluded that:

- β_2 agonists were effective, by any route: intravenously, by nebuliser or spacer.
- There were few side effects from β2 agonists but documentation of these was unreliable.
- Both β blockers and insulin were equally effective in reducing hyperkalaemia.
- Both together decreased potassium more than either alone.

- β blockers caused transient hyperkalaemia and sometimes took 30 minutes to be effective compared to 15 minutes for glucose-insulin.
- The single study comparing theophylline with glucose insulin showed that both were equally effective.
- Bicarbonate was ineffective in decreasing serum potassium.
- Resins were ineffective at 4 hours.

However exclusion of studies which were not randomised and which included some of the best data was surprising given that the outcome assessed was a change in serum potassium rather than morbidity or mortality: it is very unlikely that measurement of serum K^+, given independent laboratory Quality Control, would be subject to bias. The exclusion of good evidence based data in this way could be labelled 'randomisation bias'. Moreover several conclusions were liable to mislead: Although 'β agonists were effective by any route they were clearly less effective by spacer than nebulisation. Beta blockers were not as effective as insulin in that some patients did not respond.

A major limitation of the study, which was not sufficiently emphasised, was that in most studies $β_2$ agonists were given at 4-8 times the dose usually used in asthma; and that insulin was usually given as a single bolus whereas it may be more effective as a continuous infusion.

INSULIN.

Insulin has a very short half life of 3-4 minutes. [300] It is ineffective in decreasing serum K^+ by intramuscular or subcutaneous routes. [301] Following 7 units given intravenously serum insulin reaches ~ 2000 μu/mL after two minutes but then rapidly decreases. [300]. Hypoglycaemia occurs unless glucose is given within 15-30 minutes. Insulin acts by increasing activity of Na^+:K^+ pumps either by increasing Na^+: H^+ ion exchange in cells or by translocating cytoplasmic Na^+:K^+ pumps to cell membranes.[43]The best evidence for effectiveness of insulin in decreasing serum K^+ in normal subjects derives from De Fronzo et al: [44] reduction of serum potassium depended on the rate of insulin infused. I have reformulated the data from De Fronzo et al in table 16 below using the mean weight (78kg) of his subjects; calculating the insulin infused per hour and the glucose as the volume of 10% glucose administered.

The data in the groups from Table 16 have been combined as suggested by De Fronzo in the following table 17:This shows that insulin given at approximately 2 units/hour decreased serum K^+ by 0.6mmol/L; 5 units/

hour by 1.0-mmol/L; and 47 units/hour by 1.5mmol/L. Approximately 100mL, 200mL and 500mL of 10% dextrose water per hour respectively were required to maintain euglycaemia. Excessive water intake and rapid decrease in osmolality limit the use of the higher insulin dose.

	Insulin/Units infused/Hour	Mean Plasma Insulin µU/mL	Change Plasma K⁺ mmol/L	Glucose (g) Infused/hour	10% DW/mL infused/hour
1)	1.2	27	0.58	7.5	75
2)	2.4	51	0.62	15	150
3)	4.8	100	1.09	20	200
4)	24	428	1.44	44	440
5)	70	1,191	1.54	54	540

Table 16: *Change in plasma potassium for different insulin infusion rates in 29 healthy subjects, modified from data by De Fronzo et al.* [44] *Insulin infusion has been changed to units per hour and glucose infused to grams/hour using the mean weight of 78kg for the different groups. The last column shows the mL of 10% dextrose water (DW) required to deliver glucose infused.*

Insulin Units Infused/hour (mean)		Change in Plasma K⁺ mmol/L	10% DW (mL) Infused/hour
1+2	(1.8)	0.6	117
3	(4.8)	1.09	200
4+5	(47)	1.49	490

Table 17: *Results from Table 10 combining groups 1 and 2 and 4 and 5.*

Insulin is also effective in end stage renal failure and decreases serum K⁺ by 0.6-1.0mmol within one hour. [300-304] A continuous infusion, maintaining serum insulin of 100mu/mL in subjects with end stage renal disease and controls, decreased serum potassium by 0.98 mmol/L and 0.95mmol/L, remarkably similar to that reported by De Fronzo in normal subjects for similar serum insulin levels. [305] Insulin given as a bolus of 10 units with glucose decreases serum potassium within 15-30 minutes; results in a maximum decrease of serum K⁺ in one hour; and has an effect for 2-3 hours, despite its short half life. [302,303] A bolus of 10 units of insulin decreases serum K⁺ by approximately 1.0mmol/L in severe renal failure- similar to non-renal failure controls, but glucose mediated uptake is impaired. [305]

There are three potential problems in using insulin—glucose:

Hypertonicity, secondary to hyperglycaemia, may increase serum K^+. Inadequate glucose infused may result in hypoglycaemia. The water needed to deliver glucose may lead to rapid change in serum osmolality.

Hypoglycaemia developed one hour following an intravenous bolus of 10 unit's of insulin with 25g glucose in the study by Allon and Copney [303] and 20% of subjects given a similar amount in another study; [304] but not following 40g glucose and 10 units insulin in a study by Lens. [302]

Blumberg [304] reported slight hypoglycaemia in 5 of 10 patients given a continuous infusion of 5mU/kg/min of insulin in 20% glucose water (In a 70kg subject equivalent to 21 unit's insulin/hour). Serum insulin levels reached 354μU/L. As a result they recommended a considerable decrease of insulin to 50U in 500mL of 20% glucose·

To avoid these problems:

- At least 35-50g glucose rather than 25g should be given following a bolus of 7-10 units insulin, the amount depending on the initial serum glucose level.
- Insulin should be given first followed by glucose to avoid hyperosmolar induced increase in serum K^+.
- Glucose should be given as a 10% solution for continuous use (or a higher concentration by central line) and the total amount of water administered carefully considered.

Based on data in Table 17 decrease in plasma K^+ of 1mmol can be achieved with 5 unit's insulin with 200mls 10% dextrose water given per hour safely over a short duration to avoid water excess.

The maximum reduction of potassium of 1.5mmol required ~ 50 units/hour and ~ 500 mL 10% dextrose water per hour.

β2 Agonists. [106,302-304,306-312]

These decrease serum K^+ by increasing activity or numbers of $Na^+:K^+$ pumps [36,38] and perhaps by increasing plasma glucose mediated insulin release. [307] Salbutamol, Terbutaline and Fenoterol are equally effective. [115] β_2 agonists transiently increase serum K^+, [106,299] but may take up to 30 minutes following administration to work, have a substantial effect for at least two hours[303] and some effect for 6-8 hours. [304,308] However serum K⁺ may show a minimal decrease in a small minority, perhaps from resistance to β agonists in uraemia. [106, 303]

$β_2$ agonists are effective by intravenous injection, nebulisation and spacer. Nebulisation [309,310] is more effective than spacers, [311] but at considerably higher doses (10-20mg) than are used in asthma and intravenous injection seems to be more effective than nebulisation of 20mg. [308] A metered dose inhaler (1200ug) decreased serum potassium by 0.5mmol/L.[311] Fenoterol, Salbutamol and Terbutaline by puffer (up to 18 puffs) decreased serum potassium by 0.76, 0.46 and 0.52mmol/L respectively. [115]

Intravenous Salbutamol, given as a 0.5mg bolus, decreased serum K⁺ by 1.4mmol/L at 30 minutes and 1.0mmol/L at 180 minutes [302] and a dose of 4ug/kg in children decreased serum K⁺ by 1.48mmol/L at 40 minutes and 1.6mmol/L at 120 minutes. [308]

$β_2$ agonists cause sinus tachycardia, predispose to arrhythmias, [312] although these have not been observed in reported studies in man. They theoretically increase oxygen consumption in the high doses used and increase glucose and insulin secretion.[307] The advantages and disadvantages of $β_2$ agonists and insulin are shown in table 18.

$β_2$ blockers	Glucose insulin
Less reliable. [106,303]	Potential hypoglycaemia.
Initial increase in serum K⁺. [106,299]	Water overload at high dose insulin administration.
Slower to work (~30 mins). [302,306]	Hyperkalaemia if hyperosmolality is induced by glucose.
Tachycardia and increase in oxygen consumption. [307]	
Potentially Arrhthmogenic. [312]	
Extremely high dose required.	

Table 18: *Disadvantages of β blockers compared to insulin for treating hyperkalaemia.*

Studies comparing insulin with β_2 agonists show that the combination lowers serum K^+ more than either alone [299,303,304,306]. β_2 agonists also increase serum glucose levels, perhaps by stimulating gluconeogenesis and glycolysis, [106] and decrease hypoglycaemia resulting from glucose insulin infusions.

Sodium bicarbonate. [304,313,314]

There is controversy over its effectiveness but sodium bicarbonate probably has minimal potassium lowering effect in chronic renal failure. [304] A slight decline of plasma K^+ from 6.04mmol/L to 5.44mmol/L, at 4-6 hours, followed bicarbonate (290mmol) infusion but half the reduction was considered to be due to volume expansion. [313] Bicarbonate was ineffective in lowering serum potassium in the only placebo controlled trial [314] and did not add to the potassium reducing effect of either insulin or Salbutamol. [304,314] However treatment with bicarbonate in uraemic patients with hyperchloraemic acidosis for hyperkalaemia has not been studied and would theoretically be expected to decrease serum potassium.

Bicarbonate has the following potential problems:

- Hypertonicity resulting from infusion of hypertonic sodium bicarbonate may increase serum potassium initially.
- Decrease in intracellular pH occurs initially because of conversion of HCO_3^- to CO_2 which rapidly passes cell membranes causing intracellular acidosis.
- It may compromise cardiac function and decrease oxygen release to tissues by increasing haemoglobin-oxygen affinity.
- It may cause congestive cardiac failure in those with euvolaemia and underlying cardiac disease.
- A rapid change in osmolality from hypertonic sodium bicarbonate may cause cerebral neurones to shrink.
- Ionised Ca^{2+} decreases and is important if hypocalcaemia is present beforehand as a result of renal failure.

It may be effective in hyperchloraemic metabolic acidosis. It is contraindicated in heart failure but, if volume depletion is present, part correction of the sodium depletion can be given as isotonic sodium bicarbonate to prevent an increase in hyperchloraemic acidosis from saline infusion.

Elimination of Potassium from the body.

A trial of volume replacement should be considered if hypovolaemia cannot be excluded (Chapter 11). Furosemide 100-200mg should be given intravenously if congestive cardiac failure is present. Furosemide can also be given once hypovolaemia is corrected.

Cation Exchange Resins (Na+ or Ca2+ Polystyrene Sulphonate.

The effectiveness of resins are based on limited data and have not been subjected to controlled trials. Resins are usually combined with sorbitol to decrease constipation. Colonic ulceration is an important complication. Resins in the sodium cycle (sodium polystyrene sulphonate, (Resonium A) contain 3.2mmol Na^+ per gram. Cation exchange resins exchange approximately 1.2mmol potassium per gram of resin. [315] 20-60 grams of oral sodium cycle polystyrene cation exchange resin decreased serum K^+ by ~ 1.0mmol/L [315] by 24 hours. However glucose infused in the study may have contributed. Berlyne warned of the risk of cardiac failure resulting from use of Na^+ containing resin: 120-180mmol of Na^+ could be absorbed daily. [317] Calcium resins avoid this potential problem. Resin in the Ca^{2+} cycle bound 0.9mmol K^+/gram of resin. Berlyne et al reported K^+ decreased by 1.35mmol/L in patients given 60 gram of calcium resin/day. [316] Resin can be given orally in a dose of 20-30 gram six hourly in the Na^+ or Ca^{2+} phase with sorbitol 20% in 100-200mL water. [295] Resin given by retention enema is also effective and decreased serum K^+ by 0.8mmol/L. [315] Resins are not effective, however, for several hours.

SUMMARY :EMERGENCY TREATMENT OF HYPERKALAEMIA

- Give calcium gluconate 1 ampoule (2.25mmol) if cardiac arrhythmia, asystole, widening of the QRS complex, absent P waves or hypocalcaemia are present. Repeat in 15 minutes if indicated. If hypocalcaemia is present, as a complication of renal failure, correct and consider maintaining normal serum calcium by infusion.
- Give Salbutamol 1200ug, inhaled by spacer, often more readily available, 10mg by nebuliser or IV 0.25mg-0.5mg bolus.(or other β_2 agonist).
- Insulin Glucose—give a bolus of insulin 0.1u/kg (or approximately) 7-10 units immediately followed by 35-50g of 50% glucose depending on initial serum glucose level and extent of coexisting malnutrition (increases insulin sensitivity).This lasts several hours and is often

sufficient in combination with ß agonists. This can be followed by: 1L 10% dextrose water in 4-6 hours, depending on severity of hyperkalaemia and water status, with a side arm delivering insulin to maintain serum glucose at 4-8mmol/L. Start at 5 units/hour (approximately results in serum insulin of 100μu/ml) and infuse 200mL 10% dextrose water per hour to maintain euglycaemia. 50 units of insulin/hour require approximately 500mls/hour of 10% dextrose water to maintain euglycaemia and decrease serum K^+ by ~ 1.5mmol/L.

Give Kayexalate calcium or (sodium polystyrene sulphonate + 20% sorbitol), 15-60g in 100-200mL, every 4-6 hours or retention enema 50g.

- Treat volume depletion with saline ± isotonic sodium bicarbonate rapidly. No more than 1L sodium bicarbonate should be given, but only if heart failure is absent, to prevent worsening of hyperchloraemic acidosis.
- Treat cardiac failure with 100-200mg of intravenous furosemide.
- Stop dietary potassium and drugs promoting hyperkalaemia such as βblockers, ACE inhibitors, potassium sparing diuretics and implement general measures listed previously.

DIALYSIS

This is the main method of eliminating potassium from the body. [304] The Nephrology service should be contacted early.

TREATMENT OF HYPOKALAEMIA

Information on treatment of hypokalaemia is confusing, contradictory and unreliable. There are no randomised studies on the amount and rate of potassium replacement and observational studies are methodologically flawed. Important questions in treating hypokalaemia are:

1.) How much potassium is needed in treatment? This is based on:
   * Serum potassium.
   * The normal total body potassium of the subject. (K^+ capacity).
   * Cause and duration of hypokalaemia and extent of internal redistribution of potassium (cellular—extracellular K^+ redistribution).
   * Ongoing losses of potassium.

2) **What factors are important for both safety and effectiveness of potassium repletion?**
   The morbidity and mortality of hypokalaemia and effects of delay in correction.
   Rate of potassium correction.
   Factors which lead to overcorrection and to hyperkalaemia.

3) **What fluid should be used for potassium administration:** **intravenous normal saline, ½normal saline, 5 % dextrose water, oral tablets or sachets.**

4) **What route should be used for administration:** **central, peripheral line or oral?**

5) **What is the correlation between serum K+ and extent of total potassium depletion?**

CORRELATION BETWEEN PLASMA K$^+$ AND K$^+$ DEPLETION.

The correlation between serum K$^+$ and extent of depletion– the extent to which serum potassium can guide therapy is controversial. The relationship between serum K$^+$ and quantity of depletion has often been distorted by grouping mean serum K$^+$ rather than individualising levels; by considerable differences in the normal total body potassium between subjects; the speed of development of potassium depletion; acid base balance; and cause of hypokalaemia.

Several experts consider that the plasma potassium is a good guide to depletion. (Figure 23) This does not apply to extracellular/intracellular shifts of K$^+$ due for example, to periodic paralysis.

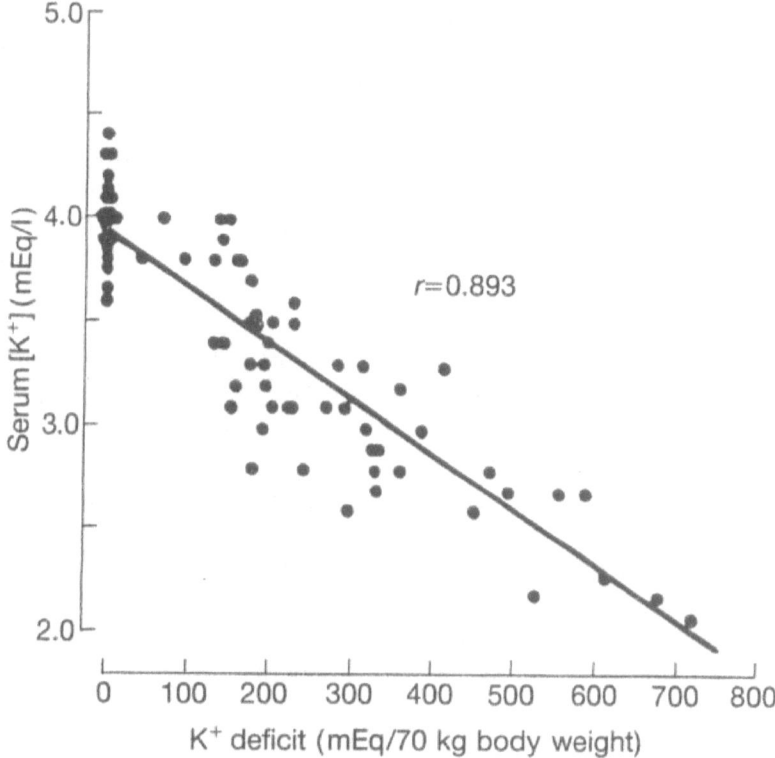

Figure 23: [6] Effect of uncomplicated K+ depletion on plasma K+ based on 7 balance studies for 24 subjects. In 6 studies, K+ depletion was induced in normal volunteers without caloric or nitrogen depletion; 2 data points were available for each of 11 subjects in 3 of these studies and 3 to 5 data points for each of 11 subjects in others. In the remaining study, recovery from potassium depletion in 2 subjects yielded 7 and 10 data points per subject. This article was published in Medicine. Sterns, R.H., Cox M, Feig, PU, Singer I.. Internal potassium balance and the control of the plasma potassium concentration. Medicine. 60(5). 339-54, Copyright Elsevier 1981, by permission.

Scribner and Burnell [109] and Swartz and Relman [23] considered that reduction of serum K+ from 4.0mmol/L to 3.0mmol/L was associated with a deficit of 100-200mmol and a serum K+ of 2.0mmol/L with a total deficit of 400-600mmol/L. These were based on small numbers of subjects.

The fall in serum K+ was 0.27mmol/L per 100mmol potassium deficit There was a good correlation between serum K+ and the extent of deficiency of potassium (r = 0.893).

Kruse [318] observed an increase of potassium of 0.25mmol/L following infusion of 20mmol potassium in one hour to patients with serum K^+ levels of approximately 3.0mmol/L.

It is important to relate the extent of K^+ deficiency to the normal total body potassium because this shows considerable variation between subjects. Scribner and Burnell [109] introduced the term, potassium capacity: the total body K^+ when potassium homeostasis is normal, to enable comparison of potassium deficiency between subjects and studies.

I reviewed 9 studies of chronic potassium depletion of 1-3 weeks duration in 35 subjects reported in the literature [22,23,131,132,320-324] to derive potassium deficiency as a percentage of an estimated potassium capacity (normal total body K^+) to aid in treatment of large numbers of subjects with potassium depletion. A theoretical potassium capacity was assigned. This is tabled in the appendix at the end of this section. These showed increasing deficiency as serum potassium decreased.

In 20 subjects with serum potassium levels between 2.8-3.2mmol/L (mean 3.0mmol/L) the average deficit was 6.4% of potassium capacity (estimated normal total body potassium).

In 4 subjects with serum K^+ levels between 2.6-2.7mmol/L the average deficit was 11% of the theoretical potassium capacity.

In 2 subjects with a mean serum K^+ of 1.8 mmol/L the average deficit was 28% of potassium capacity.

The data derived from these balance studies involved different causes of potassium depletion; of variable duration; variations in pH and tonicity; and depended on theoretical estimation of potassium capacity in all except 2 cases.

However the level of serum K^+ is clearly related to the extent of depletion.

I carried out [224] acute (up to 24 hour) balance studies in children with severe hypokalaemia and sodium depletion due to diarrhoea who were treated with intravenous potassium and sodium containing fluids, but no oral fluids, in West Africa. This was done, in the absence of published data, to provide a future guide for the amount of potassium required in treatment of large numbers of children with severe hypokalaemia.

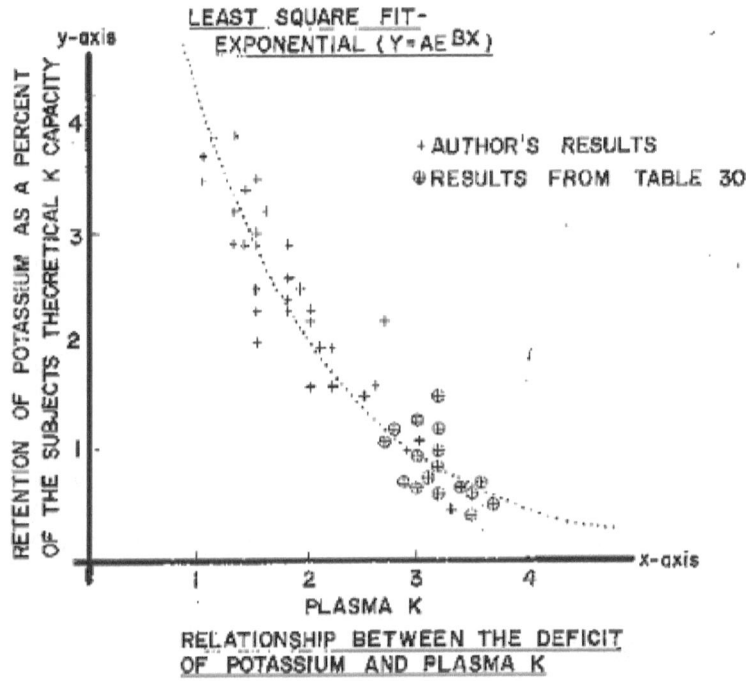

Figure 24: Potassium retention as a percent of K⁺ capacity (estimated normal TBK) plotted against initial serum K levels in 24 children who achieved a normal serum K⁺ at the end of the balance. K⁺ =serum potassium mmol/L. KR   =retention of K⁺ (K⁺ administered IV minus urine K⁺) KC=estimated K capacity (normal total body K⁺ for the subject)

A theoretical K⁺ capacity, based on body weight and nutritional status, was estimated <u>before treatment</u> to aid in estimating the amount of potassium needed to correct the deficiency (details given in the appendix).The results of potassium retention (as a percentage of estimated K⁺ capacity) for initial plasma K^+ levels of 24 children whose plasma K⁺ was normal at the end of the balance period are shown in figure 24 below. The results from the 9 studies of chronic potassium depletion are also plotted because there were few children with initial serum potassium levels of 2.8-3.2 mmol/L who were treated with intravenous K⁺. Short balance periods had the advantage that potassium losses in urine were very low, in comparison to the severity of K⁺ depletion; and stool losses ceased because nothing was given orally while children were seriously ill. Despite considerable imperfections a correlation between serum K⁺ and extent of depletion is apparent. This data was found to be useful in practice, in treating large numbers children with severe hypokalaemia due to diarrhoea in West

Africa and contributed to reduction in mortality from approximately 10% to 1%.It was subsequently found to be a useful guide for treatment in hypokalaemic adults. Scrutiny of individual results, including potassium retention before potassium normalised (appendix), suggests there is a reasonable correlation between the level of plasma K^+ and extent of depletion in children with diarrhoea. Combining broadly similar K^+ levels in this study:

Plasma K^+ mmol/L		K^+ retention as % KC (K^+ capacity)
1.3-1.5	(n= 8)	28%
1.6-1.9	(n= 4)	22%
2.0-2.8	(n= 7)	14%
2.9-3.0	(n= 2)	10.5%

However the measurement on an arterial plasma sample, rather than venous and the gradual development of potassium depletion may have been associated with larger deficiencies than would occur from a more acute onset or other conditions.

Potassium capacity.

Estimation of the potassium capacity (normal TBK of the particular patient) is important in assessing potassium needed in treatment because this varies considerably. Measurements in healthy young volunteers, which are reasonably consistent, show that average young males and females have normal total body K^+ of 50-53 and 43-47mmol/kg respectively although other methods of measurement give lower values. This decreases with age and malnutrition due to loss of muscle. Studies have not been done in hospitalised patients, but potassium capacity is probably much lower because of muscle wasting. The K^+ capacity is approximately 30-35mmol/kg in malnourished subjects. Measurements in 188 older healthy volunteers showed the following:: [10]

	≤ 40-69 years	70-79 years	80-89 years
Male.	44mmol/kg	40mmol/kg	37mmol/kg
Female.	36mmol/kg	32mmol/kg	32mmol/kg

Ideal body weight should be used in estimation of potassium capacity because adipose tissue contains little potassium. The importance of estimating normal total body potassium (KC) is shown in the following example:

Malnourished female 30kg body weight	80kg 40yr old male with no malnutrition
K^+ capacity (normal total/body K^+) 30mmol/kg = 30 x 30 = **900mmol**	= 50mmoll/kg = 80 x 50 = **4000 mmol**

Potassium needed for replacement varies over four times between the patients if serum K^+ is the same in each case.

CAUSES AND RAPIDITY OF ONSET OF HYPOKALAEMIA.

Internal redistribution of potassium

Various factors, discussed previously, may change plasma K^+ from internal redistribution independently of external losses or gain of K^+.

Decrease in serum K	Increase in serum K
Alkalosis (metabolic, respiratory)	Hyperchloraemic metabolic acidosis
Caffeine	Hypertonicity
Insulin	Severe insulin lack
β_2 Agonists	β_2 blockers

The quantitative aspects of internal redistribution of potassium have not been established with reasonable certainty, but are probably small except for Periodic paralysis, hyperchloraemic acidosis, diabetic ketoacidosis and severe insulin deficiency. β agonists and adrenaline, however, can decrease serum K^+ to 2.8-3.2mmol/L in the absence of external losses. Hyperchloraemic, but not organic acidosis, increases plasma potassium levels. Change in pH showed a marked effect on reducing plasma potassium in sodium depleted children. [224]

External causes of potassium losses.

The relation between severity of hypokalaemia and extent of potassium deficiency may vary depending on the cause, for example, vomiting, diarrhoea, hyperaldosteronism; and rapidity of onset, but comparisons have not been reported.

For example serum potassium increases from hyperchloraemic acidosis in diarrhoea, independently of external losses, whereas serum K^+ decreases due to metabolic alkalosis from vomiting. Thus the same low serum potassium level may be associated with greater overall potassium depletion from diarrhoea than from vomiting.

Diabetic ketoacidosis shows the highest potassium depletion for a particular serum K^+ level at presentation: Moderate potassium depletion should be suspected when serum K^+ is normal at presentation and severe potassium depletion suspected when mild hypokalaemia is present. This is probably due to a combination of factors which increase internal redistribution of potassium from cells to extracellular fluid: insulinopenia, increased tonicity, cell lysis or ischaemia, hyperchloraemic acidosis and glycogenolysis.

Several studies on diabetic ketoacidosis have shown severe K^+ deficiency is present when serum K^+ is low on admission, often associated with severe symptoms, despite aggressive potassium replacement. [273,325-328] In six reported cases with hypokalaemia 467 mmol K^+, on average, was given within 14 hours to raise serum K^+ to 3.7mmol/L. [326-328] Following rehydration and insulin-glucose infusion a marked decrease in serum K^+ results: dilution from fluids alone; continuing urinary losses as high as 30-40% of administered potassium; from glycogen reformation, which requires potassium phosphate in it's formation and from shift of K^+ into cells from correction of hyperchloraemic acidosis; the effects of insulin; and decrease in serum osmolality.

Rapidity of development of potassium depletion.

Severity of symptoms during episodes of Periodic paralysis, despite only mild-moderate hypokalaemia, is probably due to both the rapidity of onset and increase in cellular K^+ in association with low extracellular K^+. This hyperpolarises cell membranes to a greater extent than when both the cellular and extracellular K^+ decrease together from external K^+ losses. Apart from this, rapid onset of K^+ losses may decrease time for adaption by down regulating Na^+:K^+ pumps, increasing activity of K^+ channels, decreasing aldosterone secretion and increasing numbers or activity of H^+:K^+ exchangers in α intercalated cells of distal tubules.

Ongoing losses of potassium.

On going urinary losses of K^+ are important for estimating the amount of potassium required for treatment. Severe ongoing K^+

losses are especially common during treatment of Diabetic ketoacidosis, ongoing or recent diuretic use, vomiting, continuing diarrhoea and hereditary tubular disorders. In some cases measurement of urine K^+ may alert to the need for increasing K^+ administration.

FACTORS IMPORTANT IN THE SAFETY AND EFFECTIVENESS OF TREATMENT OF POTASSIUM DEPLETION.

Untreated or inadequately treated hypokalaemia.

Serious manifestations of hypokalaemia are rare when serum K^+ is above 3.0mmol/L and are uncommon above 2.0mmol/L. [224] These become increasingly common as plasma K^+ falls below 2.0 mmol/L: cardiac arrhythmias and neuromuscular, including respiratory paralysis, are the most important. There is concern that mild hypokalaemia in those with underlying cardiac disease or on diuretics may contribute to sudden death or arrhythmias. [265-267,329,330] Mild hypokalaemia may also predispose to hypertension. [331] However others consider routine use of potassium supplements is unwarranted in those on diuretics. [331]

The setting in which hypokalaemia occurs should govern the urgency and speed of K^+ replacement. In postoperative patients hypokalaemia predisposes to ileus. [224 283,333] Rapid resolution of ileus followed aggressive K^+ replacement in children. [224] Hepatic failure may be precipitated by hypokalaemia in patients with cirrhosis. Correction of hypokalaemia is important in those with respiratory failure or severe respiratory disease.

Hypokalaemia increases the incidence of ventricular tachycardia and ventricular fibrillation which correlate with serum K^+ in patients with myocardia infarction. [334]

Preoperative hypokalaemia predisposes to cardiac arrhythmias and death [333], although this has been disputed, provided hypokalaemia is mild. [335,336] Hypokalaemia associated arrhythmias, especially in patients taking digitalis, should be treated rapidly. However caution should be exercised in those with dysfunction of the conducting system because complete heart block may follow treatment in the absence of hyperkalaemia. [229,252 personal observations]

However the margin of safety for potassium excess is small.

In excess, potassium may distribute equally between extracellular and intracellular water compared to the disproportionate contribution from cellular potassium during depletion. In chronic renal failure, during potassium excess, cells may take up less potassium, [101,102,104,108] perhaps equivalent to the extracellular volume alone. [102,108,268]

The potassium deficit associated with a plasma K of 3.0mEq/L maybe quantitatively similar to potassium excess associated with a plasma K^+ of 10.0 mEq/L. Because of this and the rarity of serious manifestations, (with few exceptions), resulting from serum potassium of 3.0mEq/L a considerable margin of safety results if hypokalaemia is initially corrected to a plasma K^+ of 3.0mEq/L.

Metabolic Acidosis

Apart from the effects of mineral acidosis in producing cellular efflux of K^+ there may be resistance to cellular influx in acidosis. [224]

RATE AND MAXIMUM CONCENTRATION OF K^+ INFUSED.

Recommendations on the maximum concentration of potassium infused vary considerably from 40 to over 80mmol/L. [318] Kruse et al [318] administered 1351 bolus infusions of 20mmol K^+, concentration 200mmol/L, in one hour to patients with mild hypokalaemia (mean serum $K^+ \sim 3.0$mmol/L). 23%were administered by peripheral vein. There were ten instances of mild hyperkalaemia. Following criticism 'the study was repeated with more frequent monitoring in 40 cases, 14 via peripheral vein. Severe hyperkalaemia did not develop and there were no cases of venous pain, peripheral vein thrombosis or arrhythmias. [337]

The rate at which potassium can be infused safely is also controversial, but clearly depends on the severity of hypokalaemia.

Kruse et al [318] infused 20 mmol in one hour to patients with potassium levels greater than 3.0mmol/L. The maximum increase of serum potassium was 0.48mmol/L and average increase 0.25mmol/L 10 minutes following discontinuation.

Hamill RJ et al [339] infused 20, 30 and 40mmol potassium in 100mls saline (concentration 200-400 mmol/L) over one hour via a central venous line to subjects with serum potassium levels between 2.8-3.2mmol/L. Hyperkalaemia did not occur. In these studies, reviewed by Kruse et al, the recommended maximum rate of potassium infusion varied between

10-100mmol/hour with the majority recommending in the range of 10-30mmol/hour.

In hypokalaemic children, managed by the author, [224] rates of initial potassium infusion between 0.5-2.0 mmol/kg/hour did not cause hyperkalaemia.

Cardiac arrest and ventricular fibrillation can theoretically result from very fast rates of potassium infusion even though plasma K remains below normal. (Zwaardemaker—Librecht phenomenon):[250] cardiac arrest occurred when potassium was increased rapidly to a cardiac preparation, perfused with a fluid containing low potassium concentration. [249,250] Surawicz and Gettes [250] attributed this to a selective inhibition of pacemaker activity due to the inhibition of diastolic depolarisation of pacemaker fibres—perhaps due to temporary imbalance between intra and extracellular K^+ concentration. Correction of hypokalaemia to normal may precipitate complete heart block in those with disorders of the conduction system and digoxin toxicity. [Personal observations, 229]

There is rarely a need to administer potassium at a rate greater than 20 mmol/hour.

SOLUTIONS USED FOR ADMINISTRATION.

Volume status and tonicity

An important factor in intravenous potassium correction, including the rate at which potassium can be infused, is the effect this will have on volume status and tonicity. Infusion of dextrose water as the vehicle for potassium may cause or worsen existing hypotonicity. On the other hand if severe hypovolaemia accompanies potassium depletion and potassium is added to normal saline or Hartmans solution a hypertonic infusion results and rapid administration may shrink cells, correct hypotonicity or increase serum K^+ too rapidly.

For example addition of 40 mmol KCl to 1L of normal saline increases effective osmolality of fluid infused to 380 mOsmol/kgH$_2$O compared to normal serum osmolality of 289 mOsmol/kgH$_2$o. Rapid infusion of this solution predisposes to osmotic demyelination if severe hypotonicity is present before infusion (chapter4). On the other hand sodium may need restriction if heart failure is present. Administration of potassium without Na^+ increases extracellular sodium from cellular K^+: Na^+ exchange.

Potassium chloride also contributes to hyperchloraemic acidosis in the same way as normal saline.

Infusion of K⁺ free fluids containing glucose is dangerous when hypokalaemia is present: this may result in myotonic twitching, coma and ileus in addition to arrhythmias and paralysis. [224] These and depression of serum K⁺ may occur even when glucose is infused with K⁺ at a concentration of 20mmol/L. [260] Kunin [260] observed ventricular tachycardia in 2 hypokalaemic patients receiving 5% dextrose water containing K⁺ 20mmol/L. Infusion of both 20mmol/L and 40mmol/L K⁺ in 5% dextrose water to volunteers depressed serum K for up to one hour and cardiac arrhythmia developed in two subjects given the weaker solution. In 21 patients with serum K⁺ concentrations between 1.9-4.7mmol/L who were administered 20-40mmol/L K⁺ in 10% dextrose water, serum K⁺ levels decreased in 10 and remained normal in 8. The authors advised infusing a minimum of 40mmol/L K⁺ when glucose was infused.

Observations in West Africa, before potassium was available for intravenous use, showed that respiratory paralysis, myotonic twitching, ileus, coma and cardiac arrhythmias occurred in severely hypokalaemic children given glucose containing solutions without potassium. My review of several papers reporting these manifestations, including death due to hypokalaemia, showed that glucose was being infused. Most accounts of respiratory failure due to hypokalaemia have been described in diabetic patients during treatment with glucose containing fluids without potassium. [256,258,259,272,273,275-278]

Bolus administration of K⁺ is usually unnecessary and potentially dangerous. Rapid correction predisposes to heart block and asystole even when serum K+ is normal: high concentration in the vicinity of the cardiac tissue predisposes to arrhythmias. [249] Very rapid administration of K⁺ should not be given unless indicated. [249]

In conclusion the vehicle for administration and potassium concentration should be governed by the need to restrict sodium or water or to limit rise in tonicity.

Potassium in glucose containing fluids, given to subjects with hypokalaemia, should not be less than 40mmol/L. This has practical implications because glucose solutions may be infused to maintain an intravenous line. Glucose given orally also decreases plasma potassium. [287]

ROUTE OF POTASSIUM ADMINISTRATION: PERIPHERAL OR CENTRAL LINE; OR ORAL POTASSIUM.

There is controversy about whether a central or peripheral line should be used [318] because of the potential for thrombophlebitis and pain along the course of the vein during infusion. Pain is due to the potassium concentration rather than tonicity of the solution: infusion of isotonic KCl in volunteers caused excruciating pain along the vein whereas isotonic saline did not. [35]

There were only 3 instances of venous pain (2.6%) which led to discontinuation in the initial study by Kruse et al in which K+ was infused at a concentration of 200 mmol/L. In a second study pain and thrombophlebitis did not occur in 14 cases in which a peripheral vein was used to infuse KCl at a concentration of 200 mmolL.

Infusion of potassium at a concentration of 60mmol/L in saline or dextrose water rarely caused venous pain or thrombophlebitis and at 80mmol/L uncommonly did in hypokalaemic children. [224]. Heparin and lignocaine added to the infusate decreases pain along the vein. [338, personal observations].

Kruse et al [318] listed 37 studies in a systematic review in which potassium was administered intravenously. In nine studies, using peripheral veins, the K+ concentration was greater or equal to 60mmol/L in seven.

Given the advocacy by some to avoid the peripheral route for potassium infusions above 40mmol/L it is important to emphasise the trade off between the delay, pain of the procedure and complications of central venous catheter insertion compared to the uncommon complications, immediate availability and ease of insertion by using peripheral veins. Many other intravenous drugs cause venous pain. Central line administration has the following disadvantages:

* Complications and pain of the procedure.
* Thrombophlebitis is much more serious in large rather than peripheral veins.
* Delay in administration while the procedure is pending.
* High concentration of K+ adjacent to cardiac tissue can cause cardiac asystole and heart block:
* Greater surveillance needed.
* Increased and wasted resources.

Bolus infusions of isotonic KCl are more dangerous and should not be carried out outside of Intensive care or High dependency Unit.

Oral potassium replacement is appropriate for the majority of patients with mild hypokalaemia and can supplement intravenous therapy of severe hypokalaemia unless there is vomiting, inability to take oral fluids or cardiac arrhythmia. Oral potassium also allows less water intake than occurs when potassium is infused and avoids unplanned increase in potassium infusion. There are two main preparations of oral potassium:

Slow K   8mmol KCl per tablet

Effervescent potassium   14mmol KCl, 8.0mmol Cl, ~6mmol bicarbonate

Slow K may cause intestinal ulceration with prolonged use.[340] Effervescent potassium may not be palatable, and may not be appropriate if severe metabolic alkalosis coexists because of its lower chloride content. Potassium can be given as the citrate or bicarbonate salt if hyperchloraemic acidosis is present, as in renal tubular acidosis.

The tendency to give 1 tablet of oral potassium 2-4 times daily when serum K is < 2.8mmol/L is inadequate because correction is long delayed. One tablet or sachet can be given ½ hourly or hourly and the serum K^+ measured after 10 doses. [341]

However the safety of oral compared to intravenous potassium replacement has been overemphasized: the absorption of oral potassium is rapid and virtually complete. Hyperkalaemia may follow oral potassium replacement given to hypokalaemic subjects (personal observations). Indeed most cases of hyperkalaemia now occur in association with potassium tablets or high potassium containing foods in combination with other factors.

For example a considerable increase in hospitalisations for hyperkalaemia followed the use of spironolactone for the treatment of heart failure. [210]

Oral potassium, which is well absorbed, may be as hazardous as intravenous potassium [220] although gastrointestinal osmoreceptors and K^+ sensors may give some protection.[100,295] Oral potassium also requires surveillance during treatment in patients with renal dysfunction.

Considerable care in potassium replacement is clearly indicated in renal failure. Correction to a slightly low serum K$^+$ gives a considerable margin of safety. Even in its absence, hyperkalaemia may develop when potassium deficiency is treated. Ten of the 14 infants in the seminal study by Darrow were hyperkalaemic at the end of their balance studies—one had plasma K of 9.6mmol/L [227,228] Twenty of 653 subjects treated for hypokalaemia developed hyperkalaemia in another study. [225] Although the amount of K$^+$ given to the subjects was usually higher than required for treatment it was within the normal renal excretory capacity.

Adaptive responses for excretion of excess potassium may take time to develop. There are several potential reasons: the down regulation of Na$^+$:K$^+$ pumps, which occurs during K$^+$ deficiency, may take time to normalise and secretion of aldosterone, synthesis of receptors or channels in principal cells and K$^+$:H$^+$ exchangers in intercalated cells, may take time to develop. Despite this hyperkalaemia rarely develops in the absence of renal failure unless large amounts of K$^+$ are given.

Other factors which decrease cellular uptake should be considered when potassium is administered. There may be resistance to potassium transfer to cells, in hyperchloraemic acidosis, in critically ill patients (personal observations) or in patients on some drugs (for example β blockers). Only a small amount of potassium (50-90mmol) should be given during Hypokalaemic periodic paralysis to avoid rebound hyperkalaemia following redistribution on recovery.

IN CONCLUSION in treating hypokalaemia:

Estimate amount required for correction.

Decide on peripheral, central vein infusion and or oral route.

Choose the appropriate fluid for infusion.

Consider the appropriate speed of correction.

Estimate amount of potassium required for correction.

Estimate Potassium capacity (normal TBK (Based on ideal body weight)

Years of age	Normal male	Female
<60	50mmol/kg	45mmol/kg
Chronic disease	45	40
>60	40	35
>80	35	30
Severe under nutrition	35-40	30-35

Plasma K^+.

Consider the role of external- internal redistribution because, by itself, this may decrease the serum K^+ to ~3.0mmol/L in the absence of deficiency. Consider acid-base status, especially hyperchloraemic acidosis, serum tonicity, associated volume depletion, the effects of insulin and catecholamines, the cause of deficiency and rapidity of development.

Estimate K^+ deficiency as a % of KC (potassium capacity) based on serum K^+.

The following information is based on the authors experience and review of the literature.

Plasma K mmol/L.	K deficiency as a % K.C
3.0	0-5% (+-5). depending on the role
2.5-3.0	5-10% (+-5). of internal redistribution
2.0-2.5	10-15% (+-5).
1.5-2.0	10-20% (+-5).

The potassium deficit, as a percentage of potassium capacity, probably varies considerably depending on acid-base changes, osmolality, insulin status, the cause and duration of hypokalaemia

Consider ongoing losses of potassium.

Consider the importance of the speed of correction.

Estimation of potassium deficiency is clearly approximate. Remeasure plasma potassium regularly especially when half the estimated deficit of potassium has been given.

The need for early potassium administration should be anticipated if a normal serum K^+ is present on presentation in severe diabetic ketoacidosis.

A slightly low serum K$^+$ suggests that severe deficiency is present which may indicate that potassium administration should be given with initial saline infusion. K+ should be given early in postoperative ileus due to hypokalaemia.

Route of potassium correction.

Administer potassium orally if vomiting is absent to supplement intravenous administration.

Give 1 sachet of K effervescent or Slow K tablets, KCl, every half to one hour and remeasure plasma K when half the estimated potassium has been given.

Intravenous potassium: peripheral vein-up to 60-80 mmol/L, or central line.

Intravenous K$^+$ is given if oral potassium is contraindicated, vomiting present, there are serious manifestations or potentially severe manifestations of hypokalaemia, urgency or a plasma K+ < 2.0-2.5mmol/L is present.

The vehicle for intravenous potassium depends on coexisting fluid electrolyte disorders. If severe hypovolaemia coexists with hypokalaemia 20 mmol/L, rarely 40 mmol/L, potassium in normal saline can be administered. If sodium is not required, heart failure is present or rapid change in tonicity is a risk, give KCl, 40-80 mmol/L in 5% dextrose water depending on the severity of potassium depletion.

If there is minimal risk of heart failure or mild –moderate sodium depletion is present potassium, 40-70 mmol can be added to 1L of half strength saline to give a solution of relatively normal tonicity e.g. 60mmol KCl added to 1L of half normal saline gives a (Na$^+$ and K$^+$) concentration of ~130mmol/L.

Do not give a concentration of potassium lower than 40mmol/L in glucose containing solutions to hypokalaemic patients.

If oral potassium is not contraindicated give oral potassium with intravenous potassium. This increases the speed of potassium replacement while avoiding potential problems of fluid infusion.

Administration via a peripheral vein is appropriate for most cases.

Intermittent boluses of KCl (10mmol/10 mL or 100 mmol/L with 50 mmol sodium chloride in 100 mL) are theoretically more likely to cause pain along veins; to be more hazardous in causing hyperkalaemia and heart block and asystole in the presence of a normal serum K^+; and require greater surveillance. They have a place, however, if both sodium and water require restriction.

Heart failure.

There may be a need to restrict fluid. Thus a potassium concentration of 80 mmol/ in 5% dextrose water may be required if hypokalaemia is present. Preferably use oral potassium.

Hyponatraemia.

Administration of electrolyte free fluid may need to be restricted. On the other hand K^+ added to saline may result in over rapid correction of hypotonicity: if K^+ is retained Na^+ released from cells contributes to tonicity and increases extracellular sodium.

Rate of intravenous potassium administration

- The following rates of initial potassium infusion are usually effective, but safe, for initial correction of severe hypokalaemia.
- Severe hypokalaemia. Serum K^+ less than 2.0 mmol/L: Potassium 0.20-0.5mmol/kg hour (based on ideal body weight) but 20mmol potassium per hour should rarely be exceeded.
- If chronic renal failure is present or oliguria persists, plan to under correct potassium depletion—to a plasma K of approximately 3.0mmol/L.
- Avoid giving potassium greater than estimated because adaption to excess potassium may be delayed.

Appendix

	Weight	K.C. (TBK)	Serum K	K Retention	K depletion as? KC
1)	Mean of 5 healthy males HCl depletion				
	64.8	3240	3.2	175	5.4%
2)	Mean 9 males (21-38yrs) HCl depletion				
	70.5	3525	3.1	189	5.4%
3)	2 healthy males. Diuretics and DOCA			9 balances data given for 2	
	73.7	3685	2.8	191	5.2%
	68.4	3442	2.8	237	6.9%
4)	2 healthy males. Low potassium diet by resin				
	70.2	3510	3.0	268	7.6%
	68	3400	3.2	289	8.5%
5)	3 studies on 2 healthy males. Low K diet with resin.				
	82.17	4108	2.9	330	8.0%
	83.9	4195	3.1	266	6.3%
	85	4250	3.2	162	3.8%
6)	6 males 26-36years. Diet and resin and diuretic.				
	54	2700	2.6	350	13%
	70	3500	3.1	203	6%
	80	4000	2.8	277	7%
	65	3250	3.4	134	4%
	73	3650	2.6	311	8.5%
	67	3350	2.7	316	9.4%
7)	2 of 11 volunteers. Diet and resin.				
	76.8	3840	2.8	399	10.4%
	85.8	4290	3.0	244	5.7%
8)	4 balances in 3 healthy males. Diet with resin				
	69.8	3490	3.1	221	6.3%
	68.4	3420	2.7	320	9.4%
	74.0	3700	3.0	407	11%
	63.7	3185	2.7	502	16%
9)	2 females with laxative abuse				
	43.6	1744 *	2.1	25.5%	
	44.5	1659 *	1.6	31%	

Potassium balance studies in nine publications

Data recalculated to derive potassium depletion as a percent of theoretical K.C. (normal total body potassium).

Theoretical assigned KC   50mmol/kg   males

                                 45mmol/kg   females

* Total body K measured by isotope

1)   Kassirer and Schwartz [319]   2)   Kassirer et al [320]

3)   Relman and Schwartz [321]   4)   Black and Milne [322]

5)   Wormersley and Darragh [131]   6)   Kaess et al (323)

7)   Squires and Huth [132]   8)   Schwartz and Relman [23]

9)   Huth, Squires, Elkinton (22)

Mean K Retention as % of KC in Study 1 and 2	serum K 3.1-3.2 = 5.4%
Mean K Retention as % of KC in 5 other subjects	serum K 3.1-3.2 = 6.18%
Mean K Retention as % of KC in 6 subjects	serum K 2.8-3.0 = 7.5%
Mean K Retention as % of KC in 4 subjects	serum K 2.6-2.7 = 11%
Mean K Retention as % of KC in 1 subject	serum K 2.1 = 25.5%
Mean K Retention as % of KC in 1 subject	serum K 1.6 = 31%

Weight kg	K.C mmol/ kg	K.C Total body potassium	Total K.R	K.R KR/KC%	Serum				K. rate mmol/kg	I.V at sampling
					K_1	K_2	P^H_1	P^H_2		
				*independent	* dependent					
6.5	35	230	90	39	1.3	4.0	7.37	7.45	.4	No IV 2h
7.5	35	262	70	27	1.3	3.6	7.42	-	.38	40/5%
6.0	30	180	52	29	1.4	4.1	7.03	7.42	.1	20/5%
15	30	450	111.5	25	1.4	4.0	7.44	7.52	.47	44/5%
6.3	30	189	42	22	1.5	3.9	7.64	7.60	.22	5% 2h
5.3	30	185	42.5	23	1.5	4.1	B 60		.43	20/5%
6.5	35	195	39.5	20	1.5	4.3	7.52	7.35	.31	Nil
4.7	35	164	46	27	1.6	3.5	7.31	7.36	.26	15%
7.7	35	270	55	20	1.7	4.8	7.32	7.49	.29	No IV ½h
5.0	35	175	21	21	1.8	3.5	7.30	7.38	.36	20/5%
3.2	35	112	22	20	1.9	3.5	7.35	7.45	.28	Blood 2.5h
5.3	35	185	22.5	12.0	2.2	4.1	-	-	.40	20/5%
4.7	35	164	25.5	15.5	2.2	5.4	7.40	7.50	.30	Nil 2h
4.8	30	144	22	15	2.5	4.1	7.48	7.48	.37	Nil 1h
5.8	40	230	27.5	12	2.6	3.9	7.18	7.29	.23	Nil 1h
4.6	40	184	19	11	3.0	3.9	7.30	7.41	.23	Nil ½h
5.3	40	212	18.5	18.5	2.1	3.9	7.33	7.38	.3	20mmol in 5%
5.8	35	203	13	13	2.0	5.0	7.43	7.43	.58	40mmol/kg
3.0	35	105	10.5	10	2.5	5.2	7.28	7.47	.90	35mmol/kg
7.1	35	250	26	10	2.9	4.2	7.31	7.37	.35	No IV
5.1	35	178.5	76	42	1.5	3.7	B20	20	.39	Nil

Potassium retention (IV K minus urine K) **in children with severe hypokalaemia given intravenous potassium and achieving normal plasma potassium levels**. Retention is expressed as a percent of an assigned potassium capacity (estimated normal total body potassium) KC = estimated K capacity KR = retention potassium (K infused minus urine K) KR KC% = K retention divided by K capacity as a percent. K_1 = initial plasma K^+;. K_2 = final plasma potassium at end of balance.

pH1 and pH2—initial and pH at end of balance.

K rate = rate of potassium infusion since the start of treatment to end of balance.

IV at sampling: 40/5% = 40mmol in 5% dextrose water h = hour
5% = 5% dextrose water B = plasma bicarbonate
35 = 35mmol KCl in Darrows solution.

The studies shown above were carried out on seriously ill children who were given nil by mouth until they were out of danger (less than 24 hours). All had severe sodium depletion. Only two children passed more than a single stool because they were not initially fed.

Potassium capacity was assigned before treatment as follows.

Children with no malnutrition	40mmol/kg
Mild/moderate kwashiorkor or marasmus	35mmol/kg
Children with severe kwashiorkor	30mmol/kg

The K capacity rarely falls below 30mmol/kg in kwashiorkor and is higher in marasmus than kwashiorkor.

Weight	K.C mmol/kg	K.C total	Total K.R	K.R mmol/kg	KR %KC	K_1	K_2	PH_1	PH_2	K. rate	I.V. at sampling
10.8	30	320	80	7.4	25	1.1	3.1	7.45	7.53	.47	Nil ½h
7.8	30	234	48	6.15	20.5	1.3	3.1	7.45	7.45	.40	40/5%
7.5	35	260	67.5	9.0	26	1.4	3.3	7.50	7.53	.28	Nil ½h
8.5	30	255	47.5	5.59	19	1.8	3.1	7.45	7.51	.30	40/5%
7.5	30	225	28	3.7	13	1.8	2.9	7.41	7.52	.30	No IV ½h
6.3	30	190	20	3.2	11	2.0	2.8	7.41	7.52	.35	40/5%
5.6	35	196	14	2.5	7	3.0	3.3	7.47	7.52	.11	5%
10.0	30	300	54	5.4	18	1.0	2.1	7.37	7.49	.5	5% DW 1.5h
5.9	30	180	32.5		18	1.1	1.9	7.28	7.49	.43	5% 1h
9.8	30	290	52	5.3	18	1.5	2.3	7.33	7.52	.35	5% 1h
6.3	40	252	19.5	3.2	8	1.4	2.5	7.41	7.47	0.7	35
8.0	40	320	42	5.25	13	1.5	2.4	7.18	7.43	.17	Blood 4h
5.3	35	185	25		13.5	1.5	2.2	-	-	.40	20/5%
9.0	30	270	17	1.9	6	1.8	2.3	7.48	7.47	.20	Nil
5.0	35	175	6	Not steady 1.2	4	1.8	2.2	7.30	-	.37	35
5.2	35	177	8	1.54	4.5	1.9	2.2			0.5	35mmol / no DW
6.2	30	186	17	0.9	9.2	2.0	2.6	7.16	7.42	.40	20/5%
7.0	30	210	17	2.4	8	2.0	2.5	7.15	7.40	.39	20/5%
5.7	40	228	18	3.16	8	1.5	2.3	7.33	7.50		No IV ½h
2.9	35	100	7.5	2.6	7.5	2.2	2.8			0.6	35
4.1	35	143	5.5	1.34	4	2.5	3.4	7.31	7.48	0.6	35
3.3	35	15	11	33	9.5	2.6	3.3	7.30	7.44	0.5	35

Balance studies in children who did not reach a normal plasma K at end of balance.

References

General references

1. Kamel, K.S., et al., Disorders of potassium balance in Brenner and Rector's the kidney, B.M. Brenner and F.C. Rector, Editors. 1996., W.B. Saunders: Philadelphia. p. 999-1037.

2. Introduction to Disorders of Potassium p826-835. Potassium Homeostasis p372-402, Hypokalaemia p836-887, Hyperkalaemia p888-930, In Acid, Base and Electrolyte Disorders. Ed. Rose BD, Post TW, 5th Edition. 2001 Saunders WB.

3.   Peterson, L.N. Levi, M, Disorders of potassium metabolism. p. 171-215 in Renal and electrolyte disorders, R.W. Schrier, Editor. 2003, Lippincott Williams & Wilkins: Philadelphia

4.   Welt, L.G ;Hollander W ;Blythe W.B; Chapel Hill N.C. The Consequences of Potassium Depletion. J Chronic Dis.1960. 11:213-254

5.   Sansom, S.C., Shigaki M, and Giebisch, G, Potassium homeostasis -. p. 276-289. in Massry & Glassock's textbook of nephrology, Editors S.G. Massry and R.J. Glassock,fourth edition. 2001. Lippincott Williams & Wilkins. Philadelphia

6.   Sterns, R.H. Cox M, Feig, PU, Singer I. Internal potassium balance and the control of the plasma potassium concentration. Medicine, 1981. 60(5). 339-54,

Specific

7.   Larsson, I., Lindroos,A K, Peltonen, M, Sjostrom, L, Potassium per kilogram fat-free mass and total body potassium: predictions from sex, age, and anthropometry. American Journal of Physiol Endocrinol & Metabolism, 2003. 284 E416-E423.

8.   Novak, L.P., Aging, total body potassium, fat-free mass, and cell mass in males and females between ages 18 and 85 years. Journal of Gerontology, 1972. 27(4): p. 438-43.

9.   Gallagher, D., Visser, M, Wang, Z, et al., Metabolically active component of fat-free body mass: influences of age, adiposity, and gender. Metabolism: Clinical & Experimental, 1996. 45(8): p. 992-7.

10.   Kehayias, J.J., Fiatarone, MA, Zhuang, H, Roubenoff, R, Total body potassium and body fat: relevance to aging. American Journal of Clinical Nutrition, 1997. 66(4): p. 904-10.

11.   Skrabal, F, Arnot R.N., and Joplin, G.F., Equations for the prediction of normal values for exchangeable sodium, exchangeable potassium, extracellular fluid volume, and total body water. British Medical Journal, 1973. 2(5857): p. 37-8.

12.   Electrolyte Metabolism in Severe Infantile Malnutrition. Ed. Garrow, JS, Smith, R, Ward, EE, Permagon Press.1968

13.   Alleyne, GAO, Studies on total body potassium in malnourished infants. Factors affecting potassium repletion. British Journal of Nutrition, 1970. 24(1):p. 205-12.

14.   Smith, R. and Waterlow, J.C., Total exchangeable potassium in infantile malnutrition. Lancet, 1960. 1: p. 147-9.

15.   Garrow, J.S., Total body-potassium in Kwashiorkor and Marasmus. Lancet, 1965. 2: p. 455-8.

16.   Alleyne, G.A., Millward, D.J., and Scullard, G.H., Total body potassium, muscle electrolytes, and glycogen in malnourished children. Journal of Pediatrics, 1970. 76(1): p. 75-81.

17.   Maniyan, C.G., Pillai MG, Sujata, R, et al., Measurement of 40k as an indicator of body potassium: implication for diabetes and other disease conditions. Radiation Protection Dosimetry, 2003. 104(1): p. 71-6.

18.   Cohn, S.H., Varstsky, D, Yasumara, S, et al., Indexes of body cell mass: nitrogen versus potassium. American Journal of Physiology, 1983. 244(3): E305-310

19.   Guyton, A.C. and Hall, J.E., Membrane potentials and action potentials. p. 57-71. in Textbook of medical physiology, A.C. Guyton and J.E. Hall, Editors. 2006., Elsevier Saunders: Philadelphia

20.   Allon, M. Treatment and prevention of hyperkalemia in end-stage renal disease. Kidney International, 1993. 43(6): p. 1197-209.

21.   Darrow, D.C. and Yannett, H., The changes in the distribution of body water accompanying increase and decrease in extracellular electrolyte. Journal of Clinical Investigation, 1935. 14266.

22.   Huth, E.J., Squires, R.D., and Elkinton, J.R., Experimental potassium depletion in normal human subjects. II. Renal and hormonal factors in the development of extracellular alkalosis during depletion. Journal of Clinical Investigation, 1959. 38(7): p. 1149-65.

23.   Schwartz, W.B. and Relman, A.S., Metabolic and renal studies in chronic potassium depletion resulting from overuse of laxatives. Journal of Clinical Investigation, 1953. 32(3): p. 258-71.

24.   Heppel, L.A., The electrolytes of muscle and liver in potassium depleted rats. American Journal of Physiology, 1939. 127 385.

25.   Burnell, J.M. and Dawborn, J.K., Acid-base parameters in potassium depletion in the dog. American Journal of Physiology, 1970. 218(6): p. 1583-9.

26.   Sanslone, W.R., et al., Amino acid content of muscle and plasma with altered pH. Metabolism: Clinical & Experimental, 1970. 19(2): p. 179-86.

27.   Eckel, R.E., Norris, J.E., and Pope, C.E. Basic amino acids as intracellular cations in K deficiency. American Journal of Physiology, 1958. 193(3): p. 644-52.

28.   Dickerman, H.W. Walker, W.G, Effect of cationic amino acid infusion on potassium metabolism in vivo. American Journal of Physiology, 1964. 206: p. 403-8.

29.   Fenn, W.O., Deposition of potassium and phosphorus with glycogen in rat livers. Journal of biological chemistry, 1939. 128(297).

30.   Leibman J; Edelman IS. Interrelations of plasma potassium concentration, plasma sodium concentration, arterial pH and total exchangeable potassium J Clin Invest 38:2176-2188 1959

31. Eaton, S.B. and Konner, M., Paleolithic nutrition. A consideration of its nature and current implications. New England Journal of Medicine, 1985. 312(5): p. 283-9.

32. Halperin, M.L., Cheema-Dhadi, S, Lin, SH, Kamel S, Control of potassium excretion: a Paleolithic perspective. Current Opinion in Nephrology & Hypertension, 2006. 15(4): p. 430-6.

33. Silva, P., Brown, R.S., Epstein, F.H., Adaptation to potassium. Kidney International, 1977. 11(6): p. 466-75.

34. Metabolic Homeostasis. Limits of Body tolerance for Potassium. P40 Ed Talbot, N.B., Richie, R.H., Crawford, J.D. Harvard University Press 1969.

35. Keith, N.M; Osterberg, A.E; Burchell, H.B. Some effects of Potassium Salts in Man. 1942. Ann Int Medicine 16 879-892

36. Sterns, R.H. and Spital, A., Disorders of internal potassium balance. Seminars in Nephrology, 1987. 7(4): p. 399-415.

37. Brown, M.J., Brown, D.C., Murphy, M.B., Hypokalemia from beta2-receptor stimulation by circulating epinephrine. New England Journal of Medicine, 1983. 309(23): p. 1414-9.

38. Clausen, T. and Everts, M.E., Regulation of the Na,K-pump in skeletal muscle. Kidney International, 1989. 35(1): p. 1-13.

39. Cox, M., Sterns, R.H., and Singer, I., The defence against hyperkalemia: the roles of insulin and aldosterone. New England Journal of Medicine, 1978. 299(10): p. 525-32.

40. Knochel, J.P., Role of glucoregulatory hormones in potassium homeostasis. Kidney International, 1977. 11(6): p. 443-52.

41. Hiatt, N, Yamakawa T, Davidson M.B, Necessity for insulin in transfer of excess infused K to intracellular fluid. Metabolism: Clinical & Experimental, 1974. 23(1): p. 43-9.

42. Pettit, G.W; Vick, R.L, Contribution of pancreatic insulin to extrarenal potassium homeostasis: a tow-compartment model. American Journal of Physiology, 1974. 226(2): p. 319-24.

43. Hundal, H.S;Marette A;Mutsumoto Y et al., Insulin induces translocation of the alpha 2 and beta 1 subunits of the Na+/K(+)-ATPase from intracellular compartments to the plasma membrane in mammalian skeletal muscle. J. Biol. Chem, 1992: p. 5040-3.

44. DeFronzo, R.A., Felig, P, Ferrannini E, Wahren J., Effect of graded doses of insulin on splanchnic and peripheral potassium metabolism in man. American Journal of Physiology, 1980. 238 E421-E427.

45. Giebisch, G, Krap, R, Wagner, C, Renal and Extrarenal regulation of potassium. Kidney Internat, 2007. 72:397-410.

46. Bessman, SP, Pel, N., Phosphate Metabolic Control of Potassium Movement—its effect on osmotic pressure of the cell in Phosphates and Minerals in Health and Disease. p175-186. Eds. Massry, SG, Ritze, Jahn, H. Plenum Press. New York and London.

47.   Rosa, R.M., Silva, P, Young, JB, et al., Adrenergic modulation of extrarenal potassium disposal. New England Journal of Medicine, 1980. 302(8): p. 431-4.

48.   Williams, M.E., Rosa R.M., Silva, P et al., Impairment of Extrarenal Potassium Disposal by α-Adrenergic Stimulation. New England Journal of Medicine, 1984. 311: p. 145-9.

49.   Braden, G.L., Von Oeyen, PT, Germaine, M.J., et al., Ritodrine- and terbutaline-induced hypokalemia in preterm labor: mechanisms and consequences. Kidney International, 1997. 51(6): p. 1867-75.

50.   Castellino, P., Bia, M.J., and DeFronzo, R.A., Adrenergic modulation of potassium metabolism in uremia. Kidney International, 1990. 37(2): p. 793-8.

51.   Clausen, T, Role of Na^+K^+ pumps and transmembrane Na^+K^+—distribution in muscle function. Acta Physiologica, 2007. 192:339-349.

52.   Coester, N., Elliott, J.C., and Luft, U.C., Plasma electrolytes, pH, and ECG during and after exhaustive exercise. Journal of Applied Physiology, 1973. 34(5): p. 677-82.

53.   Struthers, A.D., Quigley, C., and Brown, M.J., Rapid changes in plasma potassium during a game of squash. Clinical Science, 1988. 74(4): p. 397-401.

54.   Burnell, J.M; Villamil MF; Uyeno BT et al., The effect in humans of extracellular pH change on the relationship between serum potassium concentration and intracellular potassium. Journal of Clinical Investigation, 1956. 35(9): p. 935-9.

55.   Adrogue, H.J. and Madias, N.E., Changes in plasma potassium concentration during acute acid-base disturbances. American Journal of Medicine, 1981. 71(3): p. 456-67.

56.   Brown, E.B., Goot, B, Intracellular hydrogen ion changes and potassium movement. Amer. J. Physiol, 1963. 204:765-770.

57.   Graber, M., A model of the hyperkalemia produced by metabolic acidosis. American Journal of Kidney Diseases, 1993. 22(3): p. 436-44.

58.   Orringer, C.E., Eustace, J.C., Wunsch, C.D., Gardner, L.B., Natural history of lactic acidosis after grand-mal seizures. A model for the study of an anion-gap acidosis not associated with hyperkalemia. New England Journal of Medicine, 1977. 297(15): p. 796-9.

59.   Fulop, M., Serum potassium in lactic acidosis and ketoacidosis. New England Journal of Medicine, 1979. 300(19): p. 1087-9.

60.   Oster, J.R., Perez, G.O., and Vaamonde, C.A., Relationship between blood pH and potassium and phosphorus during acute metabolic acidosis. American Journal of Physiology, 1978. 235(4): p. F345-51.

61.   Wiederseiner, J.M., Muser J, Lutz, T, et al., Acute metabolic acidosis: characterization and diagnosis of the disorder and the plasma potassium

response. Journal of the American Society of Nephrology, 2004. 15(6): p. 1589-96.

62. Poole-Wilson, P.A. and Cameron, I.R., Intracellular pH and K+ of cardiac and skeletal muscle in acidosis and alkalosis. American Journal of Physiology, 1975. 229(5): p. 1305-10.

63. Brackett, N.C., Jr., Cohen, J.J., and Schwartz, W.B., Carbon dioxide titration curve of normal man. Effect of increasing degrees of acute hypercapnia on acid-base equilibrium. New England Journal of Medicine, 1965. 272: p. 6-12.

64. Abouna, G.M., Veazey, P.R., and Terry, D.B., Jr., Intravenous infusion of hydrochloric acid for treatment of severe metabolic alkalosis. Surgery, 1974. 75(2): p. 194-202.

65. Viberti, G.C., Glucose-induced hyperkalaemia: A hazard for diabetics? Lancet, 1978. 1(8066): p. 690-1.

66. Conte, G., Canton, A.D., Imperatore, P, et al., Acute increase in plasma osmolality as a cause of hyperkalemia in patients with renal failure. Kidney International, 1990. 38(2): p. 301-7.

67. Koht, A, Cane, R, Cerullo, L.J., Serum potassium levels during prolonged hypothermia. Intensive Care Medicine, 1983. 9:275-277.

68. Bruining, H.A., Goelhouwer, R.U., Acute Transient Hypokalaemia and Body Temperature. Lancet, 1982. 2:1283-1284.

69. Schaller, M.D., Fischer, A.P., Perret, C.H., Hyperkalaemia. A prognostic factor during acute severe hypothermia. JAMA, 1990. 264;1842-45.

70. Boyd, A.E., Aguilar-Bryan, L., Nelson, D.A., Molecular mechanisms of action of glyburide on the beta cell. American Journal of Medicine, 1990. 89(2A): (suppl) 3S-7S.

71. Singer, M; Coluzzi F; O'Brien A; Clapp LH; et al., Reversal of life-threatening, drug-related potassium-channel syndrome by glibenclamide. Lancet, 2005. 365(9474): p. 1873-5.

72. O'Brien A.J; Thakur G; Buckley JF et al., The pore-forming subunit of the K(ATP) channel is an important molecular target for LPS-induced vascular hyporeactivity in vitro. British Journal of Pharmacology, 2005. 144(3): p. 367-75.

73. Bahlmann, H., Lindwall, R., and Persson, H., Acute barium nitrate intoxication treated by hemodialysis. Acta Anaesthesiologica Scandinavica, 2005. 49(1): p. 110-2.

74. Berning, J. Hypokalaemia of barium poisoning. Lancet, 1975. 1(7898): p. 110.

75. Kearney, T.E., Monoguerra, A.S., Curtis, G.P., Ziegler, M.G., Theophylline Toxicity and the Beta-Adrenergic System. Ann. Int. Med., 1985. 102:766-769.

76. Alazami M, Lin S-H, Cheng C-J et al. Master classes in Medicine. Unusual causes of hypokalaemia and paralysis J Med 2005.99:181-192

77. Whang, R., Whang, D.D., and Ryan, M.P., Refractory potassium repletion. A consequence of magnesium deficiency Archives of Internal Medicine, 1992. 152(1): p. 40-5.

78. Shils, M.E., Experimental human magnesium depletion. Medicine, 1969. 48(1): p. 61-85.

79. Dorup, I., Skajaa, K, Clausen, T, Kjeldsen, K., Reduced concentrations of potassium, magnesium, and sodium-potassium pumps in human skeletal muscle during treatment with diuretics. British Medical Journal(Clinical Research Ed), 1988. 296(6620): p. 455-8.

80. Kelepouris, E. Cystolic Mg2+ modulates whole cell K+ and Cl current in cortical thick ascending limb (TAL) cells of rabbit kidney. Kidney International. 1990. 37:564.

81. Rodriguez, M., Solanki, D.L., and Whang, R., Refractory potassium repletion due to cisplatin-induced magnesium depletion. Archives of Internal Medicine, 1989. 149(11): p. 2592-4.

82. Webb, S. and Schade, D.S., Letter: Hypomagnessemia as a cause of persistent hypokalemia. JAMA, 1975. 233(1): p. 23-4.

83. Kingston, M., Electrolyte disturbances in Liberian children with kwashiorkor. Journal of Pediatrics, 1973. 83(5): p. 859-66.

84. Kingston, M.E., Biochemical disturbances in breast-fed infants with gastroenteritis and dehydration. Journal of Pediatrics, 1973. 82(6): p. 1073-81.

85. Huang, C.L., Cuo, E., Mechanisms of hypokalaemia in magnesium deficiency. J. Amer. Society Nephrol., 2007. 18:2649-2652.

86. Dyckner, T., Wester, P.O., Ventricular extrasystoles and Intracellular electrolytes before and after potassium and magnesium infusions in patients on diuretic treatment. Amer Heart J.1979. 97:12.

87. Jamison, R.L., Potassium recycling. Kidney International, 1987. 31(3): p. 695-703.

88. Zubida, K., Szutkonsa, M., Vernimmen, C, Bichara, M., Renal handling of NH_3/NH_4^+: Recent Concepts. Nephron. Physiol., 2005. 101:77-81.

89. Johnson, B.B., Lieberman, A.H., and Mulrow, P.J., Aldosterone excretion in normal subjects depleted of sodium and potassium. Journal of Clinical Investigation, 1957. 36(6 Part 1): p. 757-66.

90. Field, M.J. and Giebisch G.J., Hormonal control of renal potassium excretion. Kidney International, 1985. 27(2): p. 379-87.

91. Hernandez, R.E; Shambelan M; Cogan MG, et al., Dietary NaCl determines severity of potassium depletion-induced metabolic alkalosis. Kidney International, 1987. 31(6): p. 1356-67.

92. Carlisle, E.J.F., Donnelly, S.M., Ethier, J.H. et al. Modulation of the secretion of potassium by accompanying anions in humans. Kidney Int., 1991. 39:1206-1212.

93. Giebisch, G., Renal potassium channels: function, regulation, and structure. Kidney International, 2001. 60(2): p. 436-45.

94. Rodan AR, Huang C-L. Distal potassium handling based on flow modulation of maxi-K channel activity. Current Opinion in Nephrol Hypertens. 2009 18:1-6.

95. Cheema-Dhadli S;Linsh; Keong-Chong C et al., Requirements for a high rate of potassium excretion in rats consuming a low electrolyte diet. Journal of Physiology, 2006. 572(Pt 2): p. 493-501.

96. Greenlee M, Wingo CS, McDonough AA et al.Narrative Review: Evolving Concepts in Potassium Homeostasis and Hypokalemia. Ann Int Medicine. 2009 150:619-625.

97. Achard J-M, Hadchouel J, Faure S, JeunemaitreX.Inherited Sodium Avid States. Advances in Chronic Kidney Disease 2006 13:118-123.

98. Edwards, C.R.W., Stewart, P.M., Burt, D. et al, Localisation of 11 β Hydroxysteroid dehydrogenase—Tissue Specific Protector of the Mineralocorticoid Receptor. Lancet,2 1988. 986-9.

99. Pratt,J.H.,Rothrock,J.K.,Dominguez,J.H.,Evidence that angiotensin-11 and potassium collaborate to increase cytosolic calcium and stimulate the secretion of aldosterone. Endocrinol, 1989. 125:2463-9.

100. Rabinowitz, L, Aldosterone and potassium homeostasis. Kidney International, 1996. 49(6): p. 1738-42.

101. Wingo CS, Greenlee M.Progesterone:not just a sex hormone anymore? Kidney International. 2011.80:231-233

102. Sterns, R.H; Feig PU; Pring M et al., Disposition of intravenous potassium in anuric man: a kinetic analysis. Kidney International, 1979. 15(6): p. 651-60.

103. Sugarman, A. Brown, R.S., The role of aldosterone in potassium tolerance: studies in anephric humans. Kidney International, 1988. 34(3): p. 397-403.

104. van Ypersele de Strihou, C., Potassium homeostasis in renal failure. Kidney International, 1977. 11(6): p. 491-504.

105. Halperin, M.L., Gowrishankar, M, Mallie, J.P. et al., Urea recycling: an aid to the excretion of potassium during antidiuresis. Nephron, 1996. 72(4): p. 507-11.

106. Salem, M.M., Rosa, M.R., Battle, D.C., Extrarenal Potassium Tolerance in Chronic Renal Failure: Implications for the Treatment of Acute Hyperkalaemia. Amer. J. Kidney Dis., 1991. 18:421-440.

107. Allon, M.E., Dansby, L., Shanklin, N., Glucose Modulation of the Disposal of an acute potassium load in patients with end-stage renal disease. Amer. J. Med., 1993. 94:475-89.

108. Rabelink, T.J., Koonans, H.A., Hene, R.E. et al, Early and late adjustment to potassium loading in humans. Kidney International, 1990. 38(5): p. 942-7.

109. Scribner, B.H. and Burnell, J.M., Interpretation of the serum potassium concentration. Metabolism: Clinical & Experimental, 1956. 5(4): p. 468-79.

110. Brown, M.J., Hypokalemia from beta 2-receptor stimulation by circulating epinephrine. American Journal of Cardiology, 1985. 56(6): p. 3D-9D.

111. Struthers, A.D., Whitesmith, R., and Reid, J.L., Prior thiazide diuretic treatment increases adrenaline-induced hypokalaemia. Lancet, 1983. 1(8338): p.1358-61.

112. Morgan, D.B. and R.M. Young, Acute transient hypokalaemia: new interpretation of a common event. Lancet, 1982. 2:751-2.

113. Manhem, P., et al., Hypokalaemia in alcohol withdrawal caused by high circulating adrenaline levels. Lancet, 1984. 1:679.

114. Lipworth, B.J., D.G. McDevitt, and A.D. Struthers, Prior treatment with diuretic augments the hypokalemic and electrocardiographic effects of inhaled albuterol. American Journal of Medicine, 1989. 86 : p. 653-7.

115. Wong, C.S; Pavord ID; Williams J, et al., Bronchodilator, cardiovascular, and hypokalaemic effects of Fenoterol, salbutamol, and terbutaline in asthma. Lancet, 1990. 336(8728): p. 1396-9.

116. Goldenberg, I.F; Olivari HT; Levine TB; Cohen JN., Effect of dobutamine on plasma potassium in congestive heart failure secondary to idiopathic or ischemic cardiomyopathy. American Journal of Cardiology, 1989:63 p. 843-6.

117. Benowitz N Al. Clinical Pharmacology of Caffeine. Annu Rev.Med.1990. 41:277-88

118. Hall, K.W; Dobson KE; Dalton JG, et al., Metabolic abnormalities associated with intentional theophylline overdose. Ann Internal Medicine, 1984. 101(4): p. 457-62.

119. Passmore, A.P., Kondowe, G.B., and Johnston, G.D., Caffeine and hypokalemia. Annals of Internal Medicine, 1986. 105(3): p. 468.

120. Minella, R.A., Shulman, D.S., Fatal Verapamil toxicity and hypokalaemia. Amer. Heart J., 1991. 121:1810-12.

121. Clemessy, J.L; Favier C; Borron SW et al., Hypokalaemia related to acute chloroquine ingestion. Lancet, 1995. 346(8979):. 877-80.

122. Wong, K.C et al., Hypokalemia during anaesthesia: the effects of d-tubocurarine, gallamine, succinylcholine, thiopental, and halothane

with or without respiratory alkalosis. Anaesthesia & Analgesia, 1973. 52(4): p. 522-8.

123.   Tricarico, D; Servdei S;Tonali P et al., Impairment of skeletal muscle adenosine triphosphate-sensitive K+ channels in patients with hypokalemic periodic paralysis. Journal of Clinical Investigation, 1999. 103(5): p. 675-82.

124.   Lin, S.H., Lin, Y.F. Halperin, M.L., Hypokalaemia and paralysis. QJM, 2001. 94(3): p. 133-9.

125.   Sansone, V., Meolag, Links, T.P. et al, The Cochrane Database of Systemic Reviews. Treatment of Periodic Paralysis. The Cochrane Library, 2008. Reviews 2.

126.   Ko, G.T; Chow CC; Yeung VTF; et al., Thyrotoxic periodic paralysis in a Chinese population. QJM, 1996. 89(6): p. 463-8.

127.   Elston, M.S; Orr-Walker BJ; Dissana Y AM; Conaglen JV, Thyrotoxic, hypokalaemic periodic paralysis: Polynesians, an ethnic group at risk. Internal Medicine Journal, 2007. 37(5): p. 303-7.

128.   Tran, H.A; Kay SE; Kende M et al., Thyrotoxic, hypokalaemic periodic paralysis in Australasian men. Internal Medicine Journal, 2003. 33(3): p. 91-4.

129.   Chan, A; Shinde R; Chew CC et al., In vivo and in vitro sodium pump activity in subjects with thyrotoxic periodic paralysis BMJ, 1991. 303: 1096-9.

130.   Lin, S.H. Lin, Y.F. Propranolol rapidly reverses paralysis, hypokalemia, and hypophosphatemia in thyrotoxic periodic paralysis. American Journal of Kidney Diseases, 2001. 37(3): p. 620-3.

131.   Womersley, R.A. and Darragh, J.H., Potassium and sodium restriction in the normal human. Journal of Clinical Investigation, 1955. 34(3): p. 456-61.

132.   Squires, R.D. and Huth, E.J., Experimental potassium depletion in normal human subjects. I. Relation of ionic intakes to the renal conservation of potassium. Journal of Clinical Investigation, 1959. 38(7): p. 1134-48.

133.   Weinsier, R.L. and C.L. Krumdieck, Death resulting from overzealous total parenteral nutrition: the refeeding syndrome revisited. American Journal of Clinical Nutrition, 1981. 34(3): p. 393-9.

134.   Wolff, H.P; Vecsei P; Kruck F et al., Psychiatric disturbance leading to potassium depletion, sodium depletion, raised plasma-renin concentration, and secondary hyperaldosteronism. Lancet, 1968. 1: p. 257-61.

135.   Lawson, D.H., Murray, R.M., and Parker, J.L., Early mortality in the megaloblastic anaemias. Quarterly Journal of Medicine, 1972. 41(161): p. 1-14.

136. Viens, P; Thyss A; Garner G et al., GM-CSF treatment and hypokalemia. Annals of Internal Medicine, 1989. 111(3): p. 1.

137. Knochel, J.P., Catastrophic medical events with exhaustive exercise: "white collar rhabdomyolysis". Kidney International, 1990. 38(4): p. 709-19.

138. Bosch X; Poch E; Grau JM. Rhabdomyolysis and acute kidney injury. New Engl J Med.2009.361:62-72

139. Vanholder R, Sever MS, Erek E; Lamere N Rhabdomyolysis. Am Soc Nephrol.11:1553-1561 2000

140. Gonzales JJ; Owens W; Ungaro PC et al, et al., Clay ingestion: a rare cause of hypokalemia. Annals of Internal Medicine, 1982. 97(1): p. 65-6.

141. Morgan, A.G; Burkinshaw L; Robinson PJA; Rose NSM Potassium balance and acid-base changes in patients undergoing regular haemodialysis therapy. British Medical Journal, 1970. 1: p. 779-83.

142. Johnson, D.W;Parnham A; Herzig K; Wittman J. Sunshine, sweating, and main d'accoucheur. Lancet, 1999. 353: p. 1.

143. Dave, S., Honney, S, Flukme, R.J. et al., An unusual presentation of cystic fibrosis in an adult. American Journal of Kidney Diseases, 2005. 45(3).e 41-4

144. Wang, F., Butler, T., Rabrani, G.H, The Acidosis of Cholera. NEJM, 1986. 315:1591-1595.

145. White, P.C., Disorders of aldosterone biosynthesis and action. New England Journal of Medicine, 1994. 331(4): p. 250-8.

146. Blumenfeld, J.D., Sealey, J.E., Schlussel, Y., et al., Diagnosis and treatment of primary hyperaldosteronism. Annals of Internal Medicine, 1994. 121(11): p. 877-85.

147. Weinberger, M.H. and Fineberg, N.S., The diagnosis of primary aldosteronism and separation of two major subtypes. Arch Intern Med, 1993. 153(18): p. 2125-9.

148. White, P.C. New M.I, Dupont, B., Congenital adrenal hyperplasia. (1). New England Journal of Medicine, 1987. 316(24): p. 1519-24.

149. Farese, R.V., J; Biglieri EG; Shakelton CHL. et al., Liquorice-induced hypermineralocorticoidism. NEJM, 325: 1223-7. 1991

150. Clore, J; Schoolwerth A; Watlington, C.O., When is cortisol a mineralocorticoid. Kidney Internat. 1992. 42:1297-1308.

151. Gomez-Uria, A. and A.G. Pazianos, Syndromes resulting from ectopic hormone-producing tumors. Medical Clinics of North America, 1975. 59(2): p. 431-40.

152. Rich,G.M,UlickS,CookS,et al.,Glucocorticoid-remediable aldosteronism in a large kindred: clinical spectrum and diagnosis using a characteristic biochemical phenotype. Annals of Internal Medicine, 1992. 116(10): p. 813-20.

153. Corvol, Pinet F, Galen FX,Plouin PF et al, Seven lessons from seven renin secreting tumors. Kidney International. Supplement. 25: S38-44. 1988

154. Bonnin, J.M; Edwards RG; Scroop GC et al., Hyponatraemia and renovascular hypertension. Case report with plasma renin and vascular sensitivity studies. Australasian Annals of Medicine, 1968. 17(4): p. 315-9.

155. Adrogue, H.J; Lederer ED; Suki WN; Eknoyan G Determinants of plasma potassium levels in diabetic ketoacidosis. Medicine, 1986. 65(3): p. 163-72.

156. Stokes, J.B., Disorders of the epithelial sodium channel: insights into the regulation of extracellular volume and blood pressure. Kidney International, 1999. 56(6):p. 2318-33.

157. Mulatero P,Verhovez A, MorelloF, Veglio F. Diagnosis and treatment of low-renin hypertension. Clinical Endocrinology. 2007 67:324-334

158. Brunner, F.P. and Frick, P.G., Hypokalaemia, metabolic alkalosis, and hypernatraemia due to „massive" sodium penicillin therapy. British Medical Journal, 1968. 4: p. 550-2.

159. Cabizuca, S.V., Dresser, K.B., Carbenicillin Associated Hypokalaemic Alkalosis. JAMA, 1976. 236:956-7.

160. Kamel, K.S; Ether J; Levin A ;Halperin ML et al., Hypokalemia in the „beautiful people". American Journal of Medicine, 1990. 88(5): p. 534-6.

161. Waring, W.S., Stephen, A.F.L., Malkowska, A.M., Robinson, O.D., Acute acetaminophen overdose is associated with dose-dependent hypokalaemia: a prospective study of 331 patients. Basic and Clinical Pharmacology and Toxicity, 2008. 102:325.

162. Lin, S.H., Lin Y F., Chen, D.T. et al., Laboratory tests to determine the cause of hypokalemia and paralysis. Archives of Internal Medicine, 2004. 164(14): p. 1561-6.

163. Williams, M.E.,Gervino, E.V.,Rosa, R.M.et al.,Catecholamine modulation of rapid Potassium shifts during exercise. NEJM, 1984. 311(3): p. 145-9.

164. Lim, M ; Linton RAF; Wolff CB et al., Propranolol, exercise, and arterial plasma potassium. Lancet, 1981. 2: p. 12.

165. Carlsson, E., Fellenius, E., Lunborg, P., Svengson, L. et al., beta-Adrenoceptor blockers, plasma-potassium, and exercise. Lancet, 1978. 2(8086): p. 424-5.

166. Smith, T.W., Digitalis. Mechanisms of action and clinical use. New England Journal of Medicine, 1988. 318(6): p. 358-65.

167. Smith, T.W; Butler VP; Haber E et al., Treatment of life-threatening digitalis intoxication with digoxin-specific Fab antibody fragments: experience in 26 cases. New England Journal of Medicine, 1982. 307(22): p. 1357-62.

168. Cooperman, L.H., Succinylcholine-induced hyperkalemia in neuromuscular disease. Jama, 1970. 213(11): p. 1867-71.

169. Fontaine, B., et al., Periodic paralysis and voltage-gated ion channels. Kidney International, 1996. 49(1): p. 9-18.

170. Wang, P. and Clausen, T., Treatment of attacks in hyperkalaemic familial periodic paralysis by inhalation of salbutamol. Lancet, 1976. 1: p. 221-3.

171. Goldfarb, S; Cox M; Singer I et al., Acute hyperkalemia induced by hyperglycemia: hormonal mechanisms. Annals of Internal Medicine, 1976. 84(4): p. 426-32.

172. Nicolis, G.; Sanchez A; Gabrilove JL., et al., Glucose-induced hyperkalemia in diabetic subjects. Archives of Internal Medicine, 1981. 141(1): p. 49-53.

173. Perez, G.O; Lespier L; Knowles R, et al., Potassium homeostasis in chronic diabetes mellitus. Archives of Internal Medicine, 1977. 137(8): p. 1018-22.

174. Ammon RA, Stratford-May W, Nightingale D Glucose induced Hyperkalemia with Normal Aldosterone levels. Annals Intern Medicine.1978.89:349-351.

175. Hande, K.R; Garrow G.C, Acute tumor lysis syndrome in patients with high-grade non-Hodgkin's lymphoma. American J Medicine, 1993. 94(2): p. 133-9.

176. Nicholaou, T., Wong, R., and Davis, I.D., Tumour lysis syndrome in a patient with renal-cell carcinoma treated with sunitinib malate. Lancet, 2007. 369: p. 1923-4.

177. Kalemkerian, G.P., Darwish, B., and Varterasian, M.L., Tumor lysis syndrome in small cell carcinoma and other solid tumors. American Journal of Medicine, 1997. 103(5): p. 363-7.

178. Melli G Chaudhry V, Cornblath DR. Rhabdomyolysis. An evaluation of 475 Hospitalised patients Medicine2005. 84:377-385.

179. Oster, J.R. and Materson, B.J., Renal and electrolyte complications of congestive heart failure and effects of therapy with angiotensin-converting enzyme inhibitors. Archives of Internal Medicine, 1992. 152(4): p. 704-10.

180. Danovitch G.M, Bourgoignie J, Bricker, NS. Reversibility of the „salt-losing" tendency of chronic renal failure. New England Journal of Medicine, 1977. 296(1): p. 14-9.

181. White, P.C., New, M.I., and Dupont, B., Congenital adrenal hyperplasia. (2). New England Journal of Medicine, 1987. 316(24): p. 1580-86.

182. Taniguchi, R; Koshiyama H; Yamauchi M et al., A case of aldosterone-producing adenoma with severe postoperative hyperkalemia. Tohoku Journal of Experimental Medicine, 1998. 186(3): p. 215-23.

183. Flatman PW.Cotransporters, WNKs and hypertension: an update. Current Opinion Nephrol Hypert: 17: 186-192 2008

184. Take, C; Kurasawa T; Kurokawa K et al., Increased chloride reabsorption as an inherited renal tubular defect in familial type II pseudohypoaldosteronism. New England Journal of Medicine, 1991. 324(7): p. 472-6.

185. Huang, C.L., Kuo, E., Toto, R., WNK kinases and essential hypertension. Current Opinion in Nephrology, 2008. 17:133-137.

186. Batlle, D.C., Arruda J.A.,. Kurtzman N.A, Hyperkalemic distal renal tubular acidosis associated with obstructive uropathy. New England Journal of Medicine, 1981. 304(7): p. 373-80.

187. Sabatini, S. and N.A. Kurtzman, Enzyme activity in obstructive uropathy: basis for salt wastage and the acidification defect. Kidney Intern, 1990. 37(1): p. 79-84.

188. Glassock, RJ. Human immunodeficiency virus (HIV) infection and the kidney; Annals of Internal Medicine, 1990. 112(1): p. 35-49.

189. Caramelo, C; Bello E; Ruiz E et al., Hyperkalemia in patients infected with the human immunodeficiency virus: involvement of a systemic mechanism. Kidney International, 1999. 56(1): p. 198-205.

190. Lee, F.O; Quismorio FP; Troum OM, et al., Mechanisms of hyperkalemia in systemic lupus erythematosus. Archives of Internal Medicine, 1988. 148(2): p. 397-401.

191. Szylman, P; Better OS; Chaimowitz C; Roster A, Role of hyperkalemia in the metabolic acidosis of isolated hypoaldosteronism. New England Journal of Medicine, 1976. 294(7): p. 361-5.

192. Kokko, J.P., Primary acquired hypoaldosteronism. Kidney International, 1985. 27(4): p. 690-702.

193. Sebastian, A; Schambelan M; Lindenfeld S et al., Amelioration of metabolic acidosis with fludrocortisone therapy in hyporeninemic hypoaldosteronism. New England Journal of Medicine, 1977. 297(11): p. 576-83.

194. DeFronzo, R.A., Sherwin, R.A., Felig, P. et al., Nonuremic diabetic hyperkalemia. Possible role of insulin deficiency. Archives of Internal Medicine, 1977. 137(7): p. 842-3.

195. Batlle, D.C; Hizon M ;Cohen E et al., The use of the urinary anion gap in the diagnosis of hyperchloremic metabolic acidosis. New England Journal of Medicine, 1988. 318(10): p. 594-9.

196. Perazella, M.A., Drug-induced hyperkalemia: old culprits and new offenders. American Journal of Medicine, 2000. 109(4): p. 307-14.

197. Miller, L.G., Herbal medicinals: selected clinical considerations focusing on known or potential drug-herb interactions. Archives of Internal Medicine, 1998. 158(20): p. 2200-11.

198. Cheng, T.O. Herbal interaction with cardiac drugs. Arch. Int. Med., 2000. 160:870.

199. Oster, J.R., Singer, I., and Fishman, L.M., Heparin-induced aldosterone suppression and hyperkalemia. Amer J Medicine, 1995. 98(6): p. 575-86.

200. Koren-Michowitz, M., Avni, B., Michowitz, Y., et al., Early onset of hyperkalemia in patients treated with low molecular weight heparin: a prospective study. Pharmacoepidemiology & Drug Safety, 2004. 13(5): p. 299-302.

201. Canova, C.R., Fischler, M.P., and Reinhart, W.H., Effect of low-molecular-weight heparin on serum potassium Lancet, 1997. 349(9063): p. 1447-8.

202. Reardon, L.C. and Macpherson, D.S., Hyperkalemia in outpatients using angiotensin-converting enzyme inhibitors. How much should we worry? Archives of Internal Medicine, 1998. 158(1): p. 26-32.

203. Palmer, B.F., Managing hyperkalemia caused by inhibitors of the renin-angiotensin-aldosterone system. New Engl J Medicine, 2004. 351(6): p. 585-92.

204. Shlipak, M.G., Pharmacotherapy for heart failure in patients with renal insufficiency. Annals of Internal Medicine, 2003. 138(11): p. 917-24.

205. Keilani, T; Danesh FR; Schlueter WA et al., A subdepressor low dose of ramipril lowers urinary protein excretion without increasing plasma potassium. American Journal of Kidney Diseases, 1999. 33(3): p. 450-7.

206. Schlondorff, D., Renal complications of non-steroidal anti-inflammatory drugs. Kidney Internat., 1993. 44:643-53.

207. Zimran A,Kramer M; Plaskin M, Hershko C. Incidence of hyperkalaemia induced by indomethacin in a hospital population. BMJ, 1985. 291:107-8.

208. Garella S; Matarese Al.Renal effects of prostaglandins and clinical adverse effects of non steroidal antiinflammatory drugs. Medicine. 1984 63: 165

209. Tumlin, J.A. and Sands, J.M., Nephron segment-specific inhibition of Na+/K(+)-ATPase activity by cyclosporin A. Kidney International, 1993. 43(1): p. 246-51.

210. Juurlink, D.N ;Mamdani MM; Lee DS., et al., Rates of hyperkalemia after publication of the Randomized Aldactone Evaluation Study. New England Journal of Medicine, 2004. 351(6): p. 543-51.

211. Schepkens, H; Vanholder R; Billiouw JM ;Lameire N. Life-threatening hyperkalemia during combined therapy with angiotensin-converting enzyme inhibitors and spironolactone: an analysis of 25 cases. American Journal of Medicine, 2001. 110(6): p. 438-41.

212. Karagannis, A., Tziomatos, K., Papageogu, A. Papageogiou A et al., Spironolactone versus eprelenone for the treatment of idiopathic

hyperaldostereonism. Expert Opinion in Pharmacotherapy, 2008. 9:509-15.

213. Frelin, C., Vigne, P., Barbry, P., Lazdunski, M., Molecular properties of Amiloride action and of its Na$^+$ transporting targets. Kidney Int., 1987. 32:p. 785-93.

214. Greenberg, S; Reiser IW; Chou S-Y; Porush JG. Trimethoprim-sulfamethoxazole induces reversible hyperkalemia. Annals of Internal Medicine, 1993. 119(4): p. 291-5.

215. Mori, H., Kuroda, Y., Imamura, S. et al., Hyponatremia and/or hyperkalemia in patients treated with the standard dose of trimethoprim-sulfamethoxazole. Internal Medicine, 2003. 42(8): p. 665-9.

216. Velazquez, H; Parazella MA; Wright FS; Ellison DH et al., Renal mechanism of trimethoprim-induced hyperkalemia. Annals of Internal Medicine, 1993. 119(4): p. 296-301.

217. Alappan, R., Perazella, M.A., and Buller, G.K., Hyperkalemia in hospitalized patients treated with trimethoprim-sulfamethoxazole. Annals of Internal Medicine, 1996. 124(3): p. 316-20.

218. Harrington, J.T., Isner, J.M. Kassirer, J.P., Our national obsession with potassium. American Journal of Medicine, 1982. 73(2): p. 155-9.

219. Illingworth, R.N. Proud foot, A.T., Rapid poisoning with slow-release potassium. British Medical Journal, 1980. 281(6238): p. 485-6.

220. Lawson.DH. Adverse Reactions to Potassium Chloride. The Boston Collaborative Drug Surveillance Programme, Boston University Medical Centre. Quarterly J Medicine.1974.43:433-440

221. Hoyt, R.E. Hyperkalemia due to salt substitutes. Jama, 1986. 256(13): p. 3.

222. Mueller, B.A., Scott, M.K., Sowinski, K.M., Prag, K.A., Noni Juice (Merinda Citrifolia): Hidden potential for hyperkalaemia. Amer. J. Kidney Dis., 2000. 35:310-12.

223. Crop M.J., Hoorn, E.J., Lindermans, J.Z., Hypokalaemia and subsequent hyperkalaemia in hospital patients. Nephrol, Dialysis, Transplantation, 2007. 22:3471-7.

224. Kingston, M., Electrolyte and fluid disturbances in Liberian children. M.D., 1978. Thesis submitted for Doctorate of Medicine, University of London.

225. Schlesinger, B., Payne, W., Black, J., Potassium metabolism in gastroenteritis. QJM, 1955. 24:33-48.

226. Ransome-Kuti, O., Elebute, O., Augusto-Odutola, T., Ransome-Kuti, S., Intraperitoneal infusion in children with gastroenteritis. BMJ, 1969. 3:500.

227. Darrow, D.C., The Retention of Electrolyte during recovery from Severe Dehydration due to Diarrhoea. J, Pediat., 1946. 28:515

228. Darrow, D.C. et al, Disturbance of Water and Electrolytes in Infantile Diarrhoea. Pediat., 1949. 3:129.

229. Reynolds EW. The use of potassium in the treatment of Heart Disease. Amer Heart J.1965.70:1-5

230. Koypt N; Dalal F; Narins RG; Renal retention of potassium in fruit. New Engl J med.313 582-583.

231. Epstein, M., Aldosterone blockade: an emerging strategy for abrogating progressive renal disease. Amer. Journal of Medicine, 2006. 119(11): p. 912-9.

232. Baker WL; Craig IC; Kluger J. Comparative effectiveness of angiotensin converting enzyme inhibitors and angiotensin 2 –receptor blockers for ischaemic heart disease. Ann Internal Medicine.2009 151:861-871.

233. McMurray, J.J. and O'Meara, E., Treatment of heart failure with spironolactone--trial and tribulations. New England Journal of Medicine, 2004. 351(6): p. 526-8.

234. Palmer, B.F., Renal Dysfunction complicating the treatment of Hypertension. NEJM, 2002. 347:1258-1261.

235. Pannall, P; Rossi, A., Potassium levels in serum and plasma. Clinica Chimica Acta, 1970. 30(1): p. 218-20.

236. Hultman, E. and Bergstrom, J., Plasma potassium determination. Scandinavian Journal of Clinical & Laboratory Investigation, 1962. 64: p. 87-93.

237. Skinner, S., A cause of erroneous potassium levels. Lancet, 1961. 1:478-480

238. Danowski, T.S., The transfer of potassium across human blood cell membranes. Journal of biological chemistry, 1941. 139 693.

239. Owor, R., Serum potassium and sodium in East Africans and potassium changes in blood at room temperature and at 4 degrees C. East African Medical Journal, 1965. 42(10): p. 541-6.

240. Andres, R., et al., Net potassium movement between resting muscle and plasma in man in the basal state and during the night. Journal of Clinical Investigation, 1957. 36(5): p. 723-9.

241. Izquierdo, J.M., et al., Capillary blood potassium, chloride, sodium, calcium, phosphorus and alkaline phosphatase in the newborn. Clinica Chimica Acta, 1970. 30(2): p. 343-6.

242. Stewart, G.W. Corrall RJM, Fyffe JA, et al., Familial pseudohyperkalaemia. A new syndrome. Lancet, 1979. 2(8135): p. 175-7.

243. Wiederkehr, M.R., Moe, O.W., Factitious Hyperkalaemia. Amer. J. Kid. Dis., 2000. 36:1049-1053.

244. Beurain, G., Mathiueu, F., Grootenboer, S. et al., Dehydrated Hereditary Stomatocytosis mimicking familial hyperkalaemic hypertension: Clinical and genetic investigations. European J. Haematol., 2007. 78:253-9.

245. Bruce, L., Mutations in band 3 and cation leaking red cells. Blood cells, molecules and Diseases, 2006. 36:331-336.
246. Laks, M.M. and Elek, S.R., The effect of potassium on the electrocardiogram: clinical and transmembrane correlations. Diseases of the Chest, 1967. 51(6): p. 573-86.
247. Fisch, C., Relation of electrolyte disturbances to cardiac arrhythmias. Circulation, 1973. 47(2): p. 408-19.
248. Burgen, A.S.V, Terroux, K.G., On the negative inotropic effect of the cats auricle. J. Physiol, 1953. 120:449-464.
249. Ettinger, P.O., Regan, T.J., and Oldewurtel, H.A., Hyperkalemia, cardiac conduction, and the electrocardiogram: a review. American Heart Journal, 1974. 88(3): p. 360-71.
250. Surawicz, B. and Gettes, L.S., Two mechanisms of cardiac arrest produced by potassium. Circulation Research, 1963. 12: p. 415-21.
251. Wang, K., Images in clinical medicine. „Pseudoinfarction" pattern due to hyperkalemia. New England Journal of Medicine, 2004. 351(6): p. 5.
252. Rosen, K.M., Editorial: Hyperkalemic conduction disturbances. JAMA, 1974. 230(1): p. 7.
253. Wrenn, K.D., C.M. Slovis, and B.S. Slovis, The ability of physicians to predict hyperkalemia from the ECG. Annals of Emergency Medicine, 1991. 20(11): p. 1229-32.
254. Montague, B.T., Ouellette, J.R., Buller, G.K., Retrospective Review of the Frequency of ECG changes in hyperkalaemia. Clin. J. Amer. Society Nephrology, 2008. 3:324-30.
255. Helfant, R.H., Hypokalaemia and Arrhythmias. Amer. J. Med., 1986. 80(Suppl. 4A):13-21.
256. Frenkel, M., Groen, J., and Willebrands, A.F., Reduction of serum potassium content and general muscular weakness during diabetic coma. American Journal of Medicine, 1947. 135(602).
257. Welt, L.G., Hollander, W. Jr., Blythe, W.B., The consequences of potassium depletion. Journal of Chronic Diseases, 1960. 11: p. 213-54.
258. Gamble, J.L., Marked hypokalaemia in prolonged diarrhoea: possible effect on the heart. Pediat, 1948. 1(58).
259. Keyes J.D., Death in potassium deficiency. Circulation, 1952. 5:76.
260. Kunin, A.S., Surawicz, B., and Sims, E.A., Decrease in serum potassium concentrations and appearance of cardiac arrhythmias during infusion of potassium with glucose in potassium-depleted patients. New England Journal of Medicine, 1962. 266: p. 228-33.
261. Tamura, K., et al., Transient recurrent ventricular fibrillation due to hypopotassemia with a special note on the U wave. Japanese Heart Journal, 1967. 8(6): p. 652-60.

262. Bellet, S., The electrocardiogram in electrolyte imbalance. A.M.A. Archives of Internal Medicine, 1955. 96(5): p. 618-38.

263. Curry, P; Fitchett D; Stubbs W; Krikler D, Ventricular arrhythmias and hypokalaemia. Lancet, 1976. 2(7979): p. 231-3.

264. Surawicz, B., et al., Clinical manifestations of hypopotassemia. American Journal of the Medical Sciences, 1957. 233(6): p. 603-16.

265. Siegel, D; Hulley SB; Black DM et al., Diuretics, serum and intracellular electrolyte levels, and ventricular arrhythmias in hypertensive men. Jama, 1992. 267(8): p. 1083-9.

266. Siscovick D.S; Raghnathan T; Psaty BM et al., Diuretic therapy for hypertension and the risk of primary cardiac arrest. New England Journal of Medicine, 1994. 330(26): p. 1852-7.

267. McLenachan, J.M; Henderson E; Morris KI et al., Ventricular arrhythmias in patients with hypertensive left ventricular hypertrophy. New England Journal of Medicine, 1987. 317(13): p. 787-92.

268. Keyes, J.D., Death in Potassium Deficiency. Circulation, 1952. 5:766.

269. Surawicz, B. Lepeschkin, E., The electrocardiographic pattern of hypopotassemia with and without hypocalcemia. Circulation, 1953. 8(6): p. 801-28.

270. Holzmann, M., Various types of fusion between T and U waves. Circulation, 1957. 15(1): p. 70-6.

271. Surawicz, B., Electrolytes and the electrocardiogram. American Journal of Cardiology, 1963. 12: p. 656-62.

272. Knochel, J.P., Neuromuscular Manifestations of Electrolyte Disorders. Amer. J. Med., 1982. 72:521-534.

273. Dorin, R.I. and Crapo, L.M., Hypokalemic respiratory arrest in diabetic ketoacidosis. JAMA, 1987. 257(11): p. 1517-8.

274. Roussak, N.J., Fatal hypokalaemia with tetany during liquorice and PAS treatment. BMJ, 1952. 1:360.

275. Nicholson, W.M. Branning, W., Potassium deficiency in diabetic acidosis. JAMA, 1947. 134(1292).

276. Holler, J.W., Potassium deficiency occurring during the treatment of diabetic acidosis. JAMA, 1946. 131(1186).

277. Nabarro, J.D., Spencer, A.G., Stowers, J.M., Metabolic studies in severe diabetic ketosis. Quarterly Journal of Medicine, 1952. 21(82): p. 225-48.

278. Logsdon, C.S. McGavack, T.H., Death, probably due to potassium deficiency, following control of diabetic coma. Journal of Clinical Endocrinology, 1948. 8(659).

279. Talbot, J.H., Periodic Paralysis: A clinical syndrome. Medicine, 1941. 20:85.

280. Tuyman, P.E. Wilhem, S.K., Potassium deficiency associated with diabetic acidosis. Annals of Internal Medicine, 1948. 29(356).

281. Gross, E.G., Dexter, J.D., and Roth, R.G., Hypokalemic myopathy with myoglobinuria associated with liquorice ingestion. New England Journal of Medicine, 1966. 274(11): p. 602-6.

282. Brown, M.R., Currens, J., and Marehand, J., Muscular paralysis and electrocardiographic abnormalities. 1944.J Amer Med Assosciation 124 p 545

283. Streeten, D., Ward, J.N., Potassium and Paralytic Ileus. Brit. Med. J., 1952. 2:587.

284. Eliel, L.P., Pearson, O.H., and Rawson, R.W., Postoperative potassium deficit and metabolic alkalosis. New England Journal of Medicine, 1950. 243(13): p. 471-8.

285. Keyes, J.D., Death in Potassium Deficiency. Circul., 1952. 5:766.

286. Perkins, J.G., Petersen, A.B., Riley, J.A., Renal and cardiac lesions in potassium deficiency due to chronic diarrhoea. American Journal of Medicine, 1950. 8(1): p. 115-23.

287. Andersen, M., Fasting electrocardiogram. Acta Medica Scandinavica, 1970. 187(5): p. 385-90.

288. Berl. T; Linas. SL; Aisenbrey. GA; Anderson. RJ. On the Mechanism of Polyuria in Potassium Depletion.The role of Polydipsia. J Clin Invest.1977.60:620-625

289. Alpern, R.J. and Toto, R.D., Hypokalemic nephropathy--a clue to cystogenesis? New England Journal of Medicine, 1990. 322(6): p. 398-9.

290. Allon, M., Takeshian, A., and Shanklin, N., Effect of insulin-plus-glucose infusion with or without epinephrine on fasting hyperkalemia. Kidney International, 1993. 43(1): p. 212-7.

291. Gifford, J.D ;Rutsky EA; Kirk KA; McDaniel HG, et al., Control of serum potassium during fasting in patients with end-stage renal disease. Kidney International, 1989. 35(1): p. 90-4.

292. Landsberg, L., Young, J.B., Fasting, feeding and regulation of the sympathetic nervous system. New England Journal of Medicine, 1978. 298(23): p. 1295-301.

293. Acker, C.G; Johnson JP; Parevsky PM; Greenberg A, Hyperkalemia in hospitalized patients: causes, adequacy of treatment, and results of an attempt to improve physician compliance with published therapy guidelines. Archives of Internal Medicine, 1998. 158(8): p. 917-24.

294. Paice, B., Gray, J.M.B., McBride, D. et al, Hyperkalaemia in patients in hospital. British Medical Journal, 1983. 286(6372): p. 1189-92.

295. May, R.C., Mitche, W.E., The treatment of Hyperkalaemia p453-466 in Potassium in Cardiovascular and Renal Medicine. Eds. Whelton, P.K., Whelton, A., Gordon-Walker, W., Marcel Dekkerioc.1986

296. Chamberlain, M.J., Emergency Treatment of Hyperkalaemia. Lancet, 1964. 464-67.

297. Merrill, J.P;Levine HD; Somerville W, Clinical recognition and treatment of acute potassium intoxication. Annals of Internal Medicine, 1950. 33(4): p. 797-830.

298. Meroney, W.H., Herndon, R.F., The management of Acute Renal Insufficiency. JAMA, 1954. 155:877-883.

299. Mahoney, B.A; Smith WA; Lo DS, et al., Emergency interventions for hyperkalaemia. Cochrane Database of Systematic Reviews, 2005(2): p. CD003235.

300. Turner, R.C., Grayburn, J.A., Newman, et al., Measurement of the insulin delivery rate in man. Journal of Clinical Endocrinology & Metabolism, 1971. 33(2): p. 279-86.

301. Guerra, S.M.O., Kitabchi, A.E. comparison of the Effectiveness of Various Routes of Insulin Injection :Insulin levels and Glucose response in Normal Subjects.J. Clin. Endocrine. Metab., 1976. 42:869-74.

302. Lens, X.M., Montoliu, J., Cases, J.M. et al, Treatment of hyperkalaemia in renal failure: salbutamol v. insulin. Nephrology Dialysis Transplantation, 1989. 4(3): p. 228-32.

303. Allon, M. and Copkney, C., Albuterol and insulin for treatment of hyperkalemia in hemodialysis patients. Kidney International, 1990. 338(5): p. 869-72.

304. Blumberg, A., Weidman, P., Shaw, S., Gradinger, M. et al., Effect of various therapeutic approaches on plasma potassium and major regulating factors in terminal renal failure. American Journal of Medicine, 1988. 85(4): p. 507-12.

305. Alvestrand, A; Wahren J; Smith D; DeFronzo RA, et al., Insulin-mediated potassium uptake is normal in uremic and healthy subjects. American Journal of Physiology, 1984. 246(2 Pt 1): p. E174-80.

306. Ngugi, N.N., McLigeyo, S.O., and Kayima, J.K., Treatment of hyperkalaemia by altering the transcellular gradient in patients with renal failure: effect of various therapeutic approaches. East African Medical Journal, 1997. 74(8): p. 503-9.

307. Neville, A., Palmer, J.B.D., Gaddie, J. et al., Metabolic effects of salbutamol: comparison of aerosol and intravenous administration. BMJ, 1977. 1:413-4.

308. Murdoch, I.A., Dos Anjos, R., and Haycock, G.B., Treatment of hyperkalaemia with intravenous salbutamol. Archives of Disease in Childhood, 1991. 66(4):p. 527-8.

309. Allon, M., Dunlay, R., and Copkney, C., Nebulized albuterol for acute hyperkalemia in patients on hemodialysis. Annals of Internal Medicine, 1989. 110(6): p. 426-9.

310. Singh, B.S ;Sadiq HF; Noguch A, Keenan WJ. Efficacy of albuterol inhalation in treatment of hyperkalemia in premature neonates. Journal of Pediatrics, 2002. 141(1): p. 16-20.

311.   Mandelberg, A; Kupnik Z; Houri S, et al., Salbutamol metered-dose inhaler with spacer for hyperkalemia: how fast? How safe? Chest, 1999. 115(3): p. 617-22.

312.   Du Plooy, W.J., et al., The dose-related hyper-and-hypokalaemic effects of salbutamol and its arrhythmogenic potential. British Journal of Pharmacology, 1994. 111(1): p. 73-6.

313.   Blumberg, A., Weidmann, P., Ferrari, P., Effect of prolonged bicarbonate administration on plasma potassium in terminal renal failure. Kidney International, 1992. 41(2): p. 369-74.

314.   Allon, M. and Shanklin, N., Effect of bicarbonate administration on plasma potassium in dialysis patients: interactions with insulin and albuterol. American Journal of Kidney Diseases, 1996. 28(4): p. 508-14.

315.   Scherr, L., Ogden, D. A., Mead, A. W., et al. Management of hyperkalemia with a cation-exchange resin. 1961 N Engl J Med, 264, 115-119.

316.   Berlyne, G. M., Janabi, K., Shaw, A. B., & Hocken, A. G. (1966). Treatment of hyperkalemia with a calcium-resin. Lancet, 1(7430), 169-172.

317.   Berlyne, G. M., Janabi, K., Shaw, A. B. (1966). Dangers of resonium A in the treatment of hyperkalemia in renal failure. Lancet, 1(7430), 167-169.

318.   Kruse, J. A., Carlson, R. W. (1990). Rapid correction of hypokalemia using concentrated intravenous potassium chloride infusionsArchives of Internal Medicine, 150(3), 613-617.

319.   Kassirer, J. P., Schwartz, W. B. (1966). The response of normal man to selective depletion of hydrochloric acid. Factors in the genesis of persistent gastric alkalosis. American Journal of Medicine, 40(1), 10-18.

320.   Kassirer, J. P., Appleton, F. M., Chazan, J. A., Schwartz, W. B. (1967). Aldosterone in metabolic alkalosis. Journal of Clinical Investigation, 46(10), 1558-1571.

321.   Relman, A. S., Schwartz, W. B. The effect of DOCA on electrolyte balance in normal man and its relation to sodium chloride intake. Yale Journal of Biology and Medicine, 1952. 540-558.

322.   Black, D. A., Milne, M. D. Experimental potassium depletion in man. Clinical Science, 1952 11(4), 397-415.

323.   Kaess, H., Schliert, G., Ehlers, W et al. The carbohydrate metabolism of normal subjects during potassium depletion. Diabetologia, 1971 7(2), 82-86.

324.   Pullen, H., Doig, A., & Lambie, A. T. (1967). Intensive intravenous potassium replacement therapy. Lancet, 2(7520), 809-811.

325.   Abramson, E., & Arky, R. (1966). Diabetic acidosis with initial hypokalemia. Therapeutic implications. Jama, 401-403.

326.   Clementsen, H. J. (1962). Potassium therapy. A break with tradition. Lancet, 2, 175-177.

327. Stephens, F. I. (1949). Paralysis due to reduced serum potassium during treatment of diabetic acidosis: Report of case treated with 33 grams of potassium chloride intravenously. Annals of Internal Medicine, 30, 1272-1286.

328. Seftel, H. C., Kew, M. C. (). Early and intensive potassium replacement in diabetic acidosis. Diabetes 1966, 15(9), 694-696.

329. Packer, M., Gottlieb, S. S., & Kessler, P. D. (1986). Hormone-electrolyte interactions in the pathogenesis of lethal cardiac arrhythmias in patients with congestive heart failure. Basis of a new physiologic approach to control of arrhythmia. American Journal of Medicine, 80(4A), 23-29.

330. Hollifield, J. W. (1986). Thiazide treatment of hypertension. Effects of thiazide diuretics on serum potassium, magnesium, and ventricular ectopy. American Journal of Medicine, 80(4A), 8-12.

331. Kaplan, N. M., Carnegie, A., Raskin, P et al,. Potassium supplementation in hypertensive patients with diuretic-induced hypokalemia. New England Journal of Medicine1985, 312(12), 746-749.

332. Kassirer, J. P., & Harrington, J. T. (1985). Fending off the potassium pushers. New England Journal of Medicine, 312(12), 785-787.

333. Wahr, J. A., Parks, R., Boisvert, D; et al (1999). Preoperative serum potassium levels and perioperative outcomes in cardiac surgery patients. Multicenter Study of Perioperative Ischemia Research Group. Jama, 281(23), 2203-2210.

334. Nordrehaug, J. E., & von der Lippe, G. (1983). Hypokalaemia and ventricular fibrillation in acute myocardial infarction. British Heart Journal, 50(6), 525-529.

335. Vitez, T. S., Soper, L. E., Wong, K. C.; Soper, P. (1985). Chronic hypokalemia and intraoperative dysrhythmias. Anesthesiology, 63(2), 130-133.

336. Wong, K. C., Schafer, P. G., Schultz, J. R. (1993). Hypokalemia and anesthetic implications. Anaesthesia & Analgesia, 77(6), 1238-1260.

337. Kruse, J. A., Clark, V. L., Carlson, R. W., Geheb, M. A. (1994). Concentrated potassium chloride infusions in critically ill patients with hypokalemia. Journal of Clinical Pharmacology, 34(11), 1077-1082.

338. Rapp, R. P. (1987). Therapy consultation. Clinical Pharmacy, 6(98).

339. Hamill, R. J., Robinson, L. M., Wexler, H. R., Moote, C. (1991). Efficacy and safety of potassium infusion therapy in hypokalemic critically ill patients. Critical Care Medicine, 19: 694-699.

340. Weiss, S. M., Rutenberg, H. L., Paskin, D. L., et al.Gut Lesions Due To Slow-Release KCl tablets. (1977). New England Journal of Medicine, 296, 111-112.

341. Fournier, G., Pfaff-Poulard, Methani, K., Rapid Correction of Hypokalaemia via the Oral Route. Lancet, 1987

MAGNESIUM (Mg)

ATOMIC WEIGHT 24 Valence 2 (1mmol = 2mEq). [1-6]

The greatest deception men suffer from is their own opinion. Leonardo da Vinci.

Total body Mg.	1000mmol. 50% Bone, 50% Soft tissue.
Exchangeable Mg	150mmol (2mmol/kg) in 24hours; 3mmol/kg in 3 days. Bone surface crystal is exchangeable and correlates with Mg^{2+} deficiency.
Plasma Mg^{2+}	0.8mmol/l; 20-30% albumin bound, 15% complexed to phosphate and other anions. Therefore correct serum magnesium for hypoalbuminemia.
Ionised Mg^{2+}	~0.5-0.6mmol/L
	Changes in ionised Mg^{2+} and total magnesium concentration correlate [7] except in seriously ill patients. [8, 9]
Cellular Mg^{2+}	20mmol/l. >95% is bound to organic phosphate, proteins and other molecules. Eg; ATP 5.0mmol/L. Cytosolic ionised Mg^{2+} is 0.5mmol/L and similar to the extracellular ionised level. Therefore a transmembrane concentration gradient is absent and movement of Mg^{2+} into cells depends on electrical rather than concentration gradient.
Bone Mg^{2+}	The major part of magnesium is complexed to apatite crystal rather than bone matrix. Approximately 30% is freely exchangeable.

Importance in physiology.

Magnesium is the second most abundant cation in cells and fourth most abundant cation in the body. Magnesium has a unique ability to bind to organic compounds such as organic phosphates in ATPases. It is a cofactor required for function of Na^+: K^+ pumps. Magnesium is important in cellular energy metabolism, especially in enzymes involved in phosphate transfers;

in nerve conduction; membrane stabilisation; ion transport; Ca^{2+} channel activity; and potassium transport. Mg^{2+} is important in the function of DNA and formation of RNA.

<u>Control of cellular—extracellular Mg^{2+} flux.</u> [10-14]

The mechanism of cellular control of Mg^{2+} and exchange with extracellular fluid is uncertain. Na^+/Mg^{2+} exchangers participate in cellular efflux of Mg^{2+} and two ion channels TRPM6 (Transient receptor potential melastin) and TRPM7 regulate Mg^{2+} influx. TRPM7 is vital for cell viability: gene deletion leads to intracellular magnesium depletion, arrest of growth and death. It is suppressed by cellular ionised Mg^{2+} and is crucial for cellular Mg^{2+} homeostasis. It may be necessary for effective trafficking of TRPM6 from cytosol to its site of action on plasma membranes. [12-14] Insulin and β agonists alter Mg^{2+} influx and efflux into cells.

The relationship between serum and cellular magnesium is highly variable and not understood. <u>Bone</u> magnesium correlates with hypomagnesaemia rather than magnesium concentration in muscle or other tissues.

<u>Magnesium balance.</u>

The following figure (1) shows a simplified model of magnesium homeostasis.

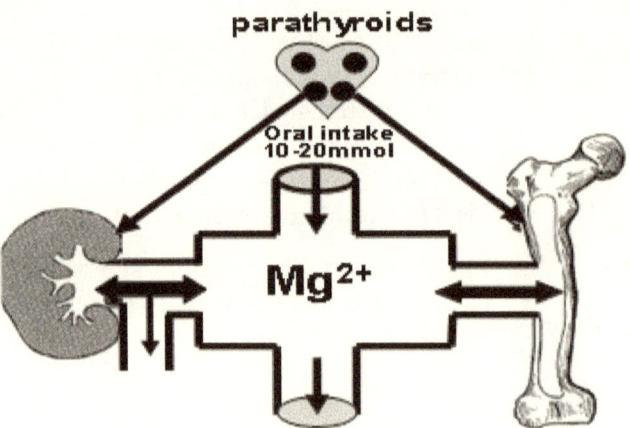

Figure 1: *The amount of magnesium reabsorbed by kidney tubules and intestine depends on dietary magnesium and whether depletion is present. During deficiency bone magnesium maintains extracellular Mg^{2+}. Parathyroid hormone (PTH) is stimulated by a Ca^{2+} Mg^{2+} sensing receptor(CaSR) and increases renal and gastrointestinal reabsorption of magnesium when total Mg^{2+} + Ca^{2+} decrease.*

CASR (Ca^{2+} Mg^{2+} sensing receptor). [15, 16]

The CASR, a G protein coupled receptor, responds to the extracellular concentration of both Ca^{2+} and Mg^{2+}. Calcium is more effective in stimulating the receptor than magnesium. The CASR is located on apical membranes of parathyroids, basolateral membranes of cells of thick ascending loop of Henle (TALH) and distal convoluted tubule (DCT). Decrease in extracellular Ca^{2+} or Mg^{2+} increases parathyroid hormone (PTH) secretion and stimulates the thick ascending loops of Henle (TALH) and distal convoluted tubules (DCT) to increase reabsorption of Ca^{2+} and Mg^{2+} ; whereas increase in serum Ca^{2+} or Mg^{2+} has the opposite effect.

Average intake ~10mmol/day. Magnesium is present in most foods but especially in green vegetables, grains, fruit, nuts, meat and legumes.

Gastrointestinal absorption. [11, 14]occurs in jejunum and ileum and varies with intake. Magnesium deficiency is rarely due to inadequate intake because magnesium is present in most foods; is more efficiently absorbed when dietary intake is low; and can be efficiently conserved by the kidney (< 0.5mmol day).

Renal excretion. [1-4, 10, 11, 13, 17-19]

All magnesium except the bound fraction is filtered.($\approx$ 100mmol daily) Proximal tubules, which are relatively impermeable to Mg$^+$, reabsorb only 15%-20%; thick ascending limbs loop Henle (TAL) 70%; and distal convoluted tubules (DCT) ~10%.

Transport mechanisms.

Magnesium is reabsorbed in both small bowel and kidney by two different transport systems:

- Passive paracellular (between cells): reabsorption is mediated by a strongly negative pore forming protein in tight junctions between cells called paracellin 1 (or Claudin 16). [10-12, 17-19]
- Active transcellular: reabsorption occurs through specific Mg^{2+} selective ion channels in luminal membranes- TRPM6 and TRPM 7 (transient receptor potential melastin). [11, 13, 19,]

Fine tuning of magnesium reabsorption occurs by the transcellular route which is saturable at high luminal magnesium levels. [11, 19] Defective transcellular function can be compensated by reabsorption by the paracellular route provided intake of magnesium is sufficient. [11]

Gastrointestinal Reabsorption: the two transport systems in small bowel are the same as in the kidney but are arranged at random rather than in specific anatomical segments. [14]

Renal Reabsorption. [1-4, 10, 11, 13, 16-19]

The two transport systems are arranged in different parts of the nephron:

> Paracellular reabsorption in the TAL (thick ascending limbs loops of Henle).
> Transcellular reabsorption in the DCT (distal convoluted tubule).

Most Mg^{2+} is reabsorbed in the TAL through tight junctions mediated by paracellin 1 (Claudin 16). Both Ca^{2+} and Mg^{2+} are reabsorbed passively by this route, facilitated by the positive lumen potential in the TAL, produced by recycling of cellular K^+ into the lumen via K^+ channels. Figure 2

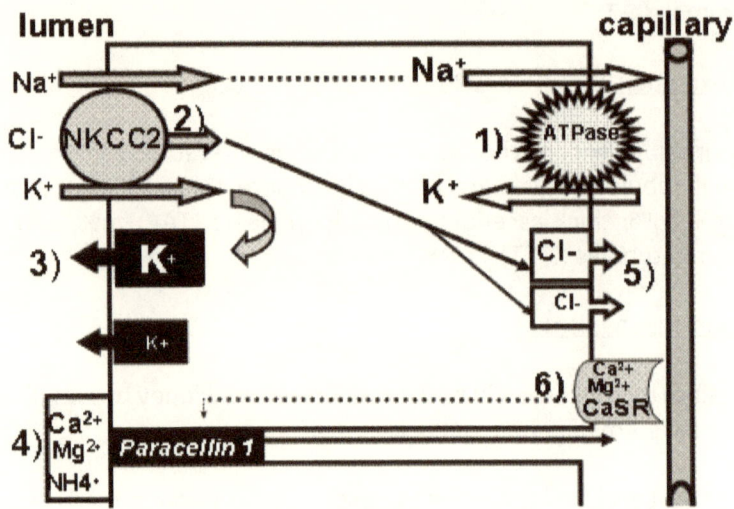

Figure 2: *Transcellular Mg^{2+} reabsorption in thick ascending limb loop of Henle. Numbers correspond to explanation below.*

1. *$Na^+:K^+$ pumps create low sodium concentration and negative intracellular potential.*
2. *This drives NKCC2 cotransporters to reabsorb Na^+, K^+ and Cl^-.*
3. *K^+, of low concentration in the tubular lumen, is recycled by K^+ channels to provide K^+ for NKCC2 cotransporters to function.*

4. Recycling K^+ produces a positive lumen which promotes passive reabsorption of Ca^{2+} and Mg^{2+} by the paracellular route (between cells) facilitated by Paracellin 1.
5. Cl^- exits through Cl channels on basolateral membranes and Na^+ via $Na^+:K^+$ pumps.
6. The CaSR ($Ca^{2+}: Mg^{2+}$ sensing receptor) controls paracellin related reabsorption of Ca^{2+} and Mg^{2+} by decreasing activity of K^+ channels which decrease lumen positivity.

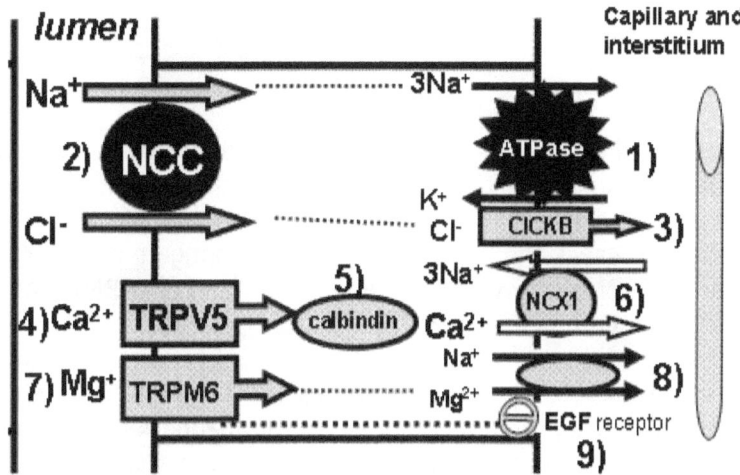

Figure 3: Mg^{2+} reabsorption in bowel and distal convoluted tubule. Numbers correspond to text below. EGF =epidermal growth factor. TRPV5=Transient receptor potential vanilloid 5. TRPM6 =Transient receptor protein melastin 6.

1. $Na^+:K^+$ ATPase pumps create low Na^+ concentration and negative intracellular potential.,
2. This promotes reabsorption of sodium and chloride by Na^+ Cl^- transporters (NCC).
3. Cl^- exists by Cl^- channels (ClCKβ) and Na^+ via Na^+ K^+ pumps (1).
4. Ca^{2+} enters cell via calcium channels, TRPV5, (transient receptor protein vanilloid 5).
5. Ca^{2+} is transported across cell by calbindin, a Ca^{2+} binding protein.
6. Ca^{2+} exits the basolateral membrane on $Ca^{2+}: 3$ Na^+ exchangers (NCX1).
7. Mg^{2+} enters cell by TRPM6 (transient receptor protein melastin 6) channel.
8. Magnesium exits the basolateral membrane on $Na^+:Mg^{2+}$ exchangers.
9. Stimulation by epidermal growth factor (EGFR) receptor is important for optimum function of TRPM6.

A Ca^{2+}: Mg^{2+} sensing cell surface receptor (CaSR), located on the capillary side of the TAL and DCT, control both Ca^{2+} and Mg^{2+} reabsorption. [15,16] Hypercalcaemia, acting on CaSR, inhibits both Ca^{2+} and Mg^{2+} reabsorption in the TAL whereas hypocalcaemia and hypomagnesaemia stimulate Mg^{2+} and Ca^{2+} reabsorption. PTH (parathyroid hormone), acting on CaSR, increases paracellular Mg^{2+} and Ca^{2+} reabsorption by stimulating Na^+:K^+:$2Cl^-$ cotransporters and K^+ channels to increase K^+ secretion. This increases the positive lumen potential.

Fine tuning of Mg $^{2+}$reabsorption (10%) or secretion occurs in distal convoluted tubules.

The lumen in the DCT has a negative rather than positive potential. Mg^{2+} requires a source of energy for transport and is actively reabsorbed by TRPM6 transporters (Transient receptor potential melastin 6). Mg^{2+} probably leaves the cell via Mg^{2+}: Na^+ exchangers on basolateral membranes. TRPM7 may be essential for trafficking of TRPM6 from the cytosol to cell membranes. [11-14, 19]

Epidermal growth factor (EGF), synthesised from proEGF, acts on basolateral EGF receptors to stimulate TRPM6 magnesium transporters to increase Mg^{2+} reabsorption. [11, 13, 20] Defective action of EGF causes Mg^{2+} wasting. [13, 20] Cetumixab, an EGF analogue, used for treatment of cancer causes hypomagnesaemia.

PTH, aldosterone, glucagon, oestrogen and calcitonin enhance Mg^{2+} reabsorption in the DCT by acting on TRPM6 channels [13]. Chronic metabolic acidosis increases and chronic metabolic alkalosis decreases magnesuria. [13, 17]

The major regulator of reabsorption is the extracellular Mg^{2+} level: this acts on CASR and inhibits transport regardless of whether overall magnesium depletion is present. Nearly all intravenously administered Mg^{2+} is excreted once a normal serum Mg^{2+} level is reached [21] despite the presence of severe magnesium depletion. Thus parenteral Mg^{2+} must be given continuously or by repeated injections to correct magnesium depletion. Magnesium depletion cannot be corrected by a single bolus or brief infusion of magnesium.

CAUSES OF SERUM MAGNESIUM DISORDERS. [1-6]

Hypermagnesaemia.

Given the capacity of small bowel to decrease Mg^{2+} reabsorption and the kidney to excrete Mg^{2+} when extracellular levels increase, hypermagnesaemia only occurs in advanced renal failure when oral magnesium intake is excessive. Antacids or laxatives containing magnesium may contribute. Iatrogenic hypermagnesemia may occur unintentionally or intentionally when Eclampsia or other disorders are treated with magnesium.

Hypomagnesaemia. [1-6, 19, 21]

GASTROINTESTINAL	URINE	COMPLEXING
Diarrhoea	Alcoholism.	Pancreatitis.
small bowel resection and fistulae.	Diuretics.	Rhabdomyolysis. Citrated blood.
*Proton pump inhibitors.	Other drugs. Gentamycin. Calcineurin. Cyclosporin Cisplatin, Amphotericin B. EGF analogues used in cancer. Cetuximab *Proton pump inhibitors.	other Subarachnoid haemorrhage. treated with Mg.
Malabsorption. Laxatives. Isolated Mg++ channel mutations.	Metabolic acidosis. Diabetic ketoacidosis Hyperaldosteronism Alkalosis –. Disorders. PTH. Hypercalcaemia.	ACUTE SHIFTS Glucose infusion Refeeding.
Vomiting. Nasogastric suction.	Gitelman's. Barrter's syndrome. Hereditary tubular diseases. Post-obstructive diuresis.	Insulin. Metabolic acidosis. Hungry bone syndrome.

Table 1: Causes of hypomagnesaemia. The most common disorders are underlined. (* = Cause of Mg loss is uncertain)

Hypomagnesaemia is usually due to increased losses from gastrointestinal tract or kidney. (Table 1) Gastrointestinal losses are distinguished from urinary losses by measurement of urine Mg^{2+}: this decreases to <0.5mmol/L when non-urinary losses are responsible. [1-5] Uncommon causes are complexing and acute shifts of Mg^{2+} into cells following glucose-insulin infusion, refeeding and metabolic acidosis.

Hypomagnesaemia is common in hospitalised patients [5, 21, 22] varying from 6.9-11%. The incidence is higher in Intensive Care Units. [21, 22] Hypomagnesaemia is associated with hypokalaemia (42%), hypophosphataemia 29%, hypocalcaemia 22% and hyponatraemia 23 %. [21, 22] Gastrointestinal disorders cause losses of both K^+ and Mg^{2+} but potassium usually exceeds magnesium losses. However Mg^{2+} exceeds K^+ losses in ileostomies, jejunoileal bypass, and biliary fistulas because Mg^{2+} concentration is relatively higher than K^+ in small intestinal fluid; and colonic Na^+: K^+ exchange is absent or decreased.

Magnesium depletion, contrary to some reports, [22-25] is not "characteristic" of malnutrition but depends on the balance between intake and diarrhoeal losses. [26]

Renal Losses of Mg.

Drugs, especially diuretics [1-4, 5, 22-25] and alcoholism are the commonest causes. The pathogenesis of hypomagnesaemia in alcoholism is uncertain and is only partly explained by magnesuria. [21] Decreased intake, vomiting and diarrhoea may contribute.

Diuretics are a common cause of magnesium depletion. [1-6, 22-25] However hypomagnesaemia is less common than low cellular or skeletal magnesium levels [22-24] which are of uncertain clinical importance. Loop diuretics cause Mg^{2+} loss by blocking Na^+: K^+:$2Cl^-$ transporters in the TAL because decreased recycling of K^+ into the tubular lumen decreases the positive lumen potential. This in turn decreases the electrical driving force for Mg^{2+} reabsorption by the paracellular route. Thiazide diuretics or hereditary defects of NaCl cotransporters decrease tubular intracellular Na^+ by acting on NaCl cotransporters in the DCT. The mechanism by which Mg^{2+} reabsorption is decreased is uncertain. The diuretic amiloride spares magnesium as well as potassium.

Drugs other than Diuretics.

Proton pump inhibitors are a rare cause of hypomagnesaemia, but given their extensive use, are important. Hypomagnesaemia usually develops after prolonged use. [27] The mechanism has not been established, but acid may be required for Mg^{2+} absorption in small intestine; or proton pump inhibitors may inhibit renal reabsorption.

Cisplatinum is a common cause of hypomagnesaemia. [28] Hypomagnesaemia due to magnesuria and increased urinary losses of Na^+ and K^+ occur in patients treated with gentamycin, [29, 30] aminoglycosides, amphotericin, foscarnet or cyclosporin. [11, 13] Calcineurin (tacrolimus) and cyclosporin cause down regulation of TRPV5, TRPM6 channels and calbindin.This results in hypercalciuria and hypermagnesuria. [11]

Cetuximab, an EGF receptor monoclonal antibody, used in treatment of colon cancer, causes severe losses of urine magnesium because optimum activity of TRMP6 depends on stimulation by EGF. This may cause severe hypomagnesaemia. [13]

Diabetic Ketoacidosis.

This may cause severe hypomagnesaemia but usually following fluid, potassium and insulin therapy, but treatment is uncommonly required.

Hypercalcaemia and Hyperparathyroidism.

Hypercalcaemia acts on the CaSR receptor and inhibits tubular Mg^{2+} reabsorption. [13, 15, 16] Thus hyperparathyroidism may cause hypomagnesaemia.

Gastrointestinal losses of magnesium.

Diarrhoea causes both K^+ and Mg^{2+} losses. However diarrhoea due to small bowel resection, from ileostomy and intestinal fistulae, may cause Mg^+ without K^+ losses because of the low potassium and relatively greater magnesium concentration in intestinal fluid and absence of colonic $Na^+ K^+$ exchange.

HEREDITARY HYPOMAGNESAEMIA: table 2 [11, 13 19, 31, 32].

Familial Hypomagnesaemia with Hypercalciuria and Nephrocalcinosis [11, 13, 19 31, 32]

This is due to mutations in CLDN16 which is responsible for activity of Paracellin 1 in the TALH. Urinary Mg^{2+} and Ca^{2+} losses increase. Nephrocalcinosis and progressive renal failure result. Large doses of magnesium supplements and thiazide diuretics, to decrease calcium excretion, are effective for treatment.

	Serum		Urine		Defective Action	Other
	Ca^{2+}	K^+	Ca^{2+}	Mg^{2+}		
Familial hypomagnesaemia with hypercalciuria/ nephrocalcinosis	N	N	↑++	↑++	Paracellin 1 (Claudin 16)	Nephrocalcinosis
Hypomagnesaemia with secondary hypocalcaemia	↓	N	↑↓	↑	TRPM6	
Isolated dominant hypomagnesaemia with hypocalciuria	↓	N	↓	↑	Υ subunit of $Na^+ K^+$ ATPase in DCT	
Isolated recessive Hypomagnesaemia with normocalciuria	N	N	N	↑	Mutation of ProEGF	
Autosomal dominant Hypocalcaemia	↓	N	↑	↑	Activating mutations of CASR receptor	Nephrocalcinosis
Gitelman Syndrome	N	↓	↓	↑	NCC ($Na^+ Cl^-$) cotransporter	Alkalosis,Na depletion hypokalaemia
Bartters (classical)	N	↓	↑	N-↑	TAL :several causes	Alkalosis Hypercalciuria
ATP sensitive inward rectifier dysfunction	↓	↓	↓	↓	Kir 4.1	alkalosis

Table 2: Hereditary disorders causing magnesium wasting and hypomagnesaemia (several sources) [13, 19, 31, 32]. N = normal, ↓ = decreased, ↑ = increased. TAL = Thick ascending loop of Henle. DCT=distal convoluted tubule

Familial Hypomagnesaemia with Secondary Hypocalcaemia.

Familial hypomagnesaemia with secondary hypocalcaemia, [11, 13, 19, 31, 33, 35] an autosomal recessive disorder, is due to mutations of the gene controlling TRPM6, the magnesium channel. Both hypomagnesaemia and hypocalcaemia, but normal urinary calcium excretion result. Both intestinal and renal malabsorption of magnesium occurs but the renal leak may result in low rather than high urine Mg^{2+} during severe hypomagnesaemia because the paracellular route compensates and increases reabsorption. This results in low urine magnesium and may cause misdiagnosis. Very low serum Mg^{2+} decreases PTH secretion; increases resistance to its action; and results in severe hypocalcaemia. This causes tetany and seizures. Very high magnesium supplements are effective because paracellular reabsorption can compensate for defective TRPM6 activity. However large amounts of magnesium aspartate or other supplements (16-20 tablets each containing 1.5 mmol of magnesium) are required for treatment. Despite this serum magnesium uncommonly rises above 0.6mmol/L and diarrhoea often results. However children, given sufficient magnesium, grow and develop normally. [28-32]

Isolated Dominant Hypomagnesaemia with Hypocalcaemia. [11, 14, 16,28, 34]

Hypomagnesaemia develops from increased urine losses of Mg^{2+} due to a genetic defect of the FXYD2 gene which encodes the Υ subunit of $Na^+ K^+$ pumps on basolateral membranes of DCT. This decreases the affinity of ATP for Na^+ and K^+ and compromises Na^+: Mg^{2+} exchange on basolateral membranes which uses the Na^+ gradient developed by Na^+: K^+ ATPase pumps to reabsorb Mg^{2+}. Tetany and seizures are due to hypocalcaemia secondary to hypomagnesaemia.

Isolated Recessive Hypomagnesaemia with Normocalcaemia. [11, 13, 19, 20, 31]

A mutation of ProEGF impairs release of EGF on the basolateral membrane of the DCT which in turn decreases activity of TRPM6 on tubular luminal membranes of the DCT.

Hypomagnesaemia and magnesuria are the sole abnormalities. Excretion of calcium and other electrolytes are normal.

$Ca^{2+} Mg^{2+}$ Sensing Receptor Abnormalities (CASR) Mutations of the CASR. [19, 16, 31]

CASR is located in the apical membrane of PTH secreting cells and basolateral membrane of the TAL and DCT cells. The CASR responds to the extracellular concentration of both Ca^{2+} and Mg^{2+}.

Inactivating mutations: increase sensitivity of the CASR receptor causing hypercalaemia, hypocalciuria and hypermagnesemia.

Activating mutations: (autosomal dominant) decreased sensitivity of CASR in the kidney and parathyroid causes hypocalcaemia. Hypomagnesaemia occurs in approximately 50 %.of cases.

Familial Hypomagnesaemia due to defective intestinal absorption [31] is rare.

Barrters Syndrome. [31, 36]—(chapter 14)

This is due to decreased function of Na^+ :K^+ :$2Cl^-$ transporters in the TAL due to several disorders involving the transporter itself, K^+ channels on luminal membranes, Cl^- channels on the basolateral membranes or paracellular protein Barrtin, which is required for paracellular Cl^- reabsorption. The various forms of Bartter's Syndrome usually present in neonates or early childhood.

Gitelman syndrome. [19, 31, 36-41] (chapter 14)

This is due to defective function of Na^+ Cl^- cotransporters in the DCT. This often presents in older children or adults, usually as an autosomal recessive disorder due to mutations of the gene SLC12 A3 on chromosome 16q 13, which codes for Na^+: Cl^- cotransporters. This may involve defective routing of transporters to luminal membranes rather than defective function. [37]

Decrease in reabsorption of Na^+ Cl^- in the DCT leads to hypovolaemia which causes an increase in renin and aldosterone secretion. Aldosterone acts on collecting duct Principal cells to stimulate Na^+ channels, Na^+: K^+ pumps, K^+ channels and H^+ ATPase pumps. Na^+ is preferentially reabsorbed in exchange for K^+ and H^+ and results in hypokalaemic alkalosis.

The cause of hypomagnesaemia is uncertain but may be due to decrease in Mg^{2+} reabsorption in the DCT because its reabsorption depends on normal action of Na^+:Cl^- cotransporters: a decrease in tubular cell Na^+ decreases Mg^{2+} reabsorption by Na^+:Mg^{2+} cotransporters on basolateral membranes.

Hypomagnesaemia stimulates PTH secretion which contributes to Ca^{2+} reabsorption. Volume depletion increases calcium reabsorption in proximal tubules in both Gitelmans syndrome and treatment with thiazide diuretics and contributes to hypocalciuria.

The most common causes of Hypomagnesaemia are due to ileostomy or ileal fistulas, drugs, alcoholism, diarrhoea, pancreatitis, diabetic ketoacidosis and critical illness.

The most common drugs involved are Diuretics, Proton Pump inhibitors, gentamycin, drugs used for cancer treatment-Cisplatinum, EGF analogues (Cetuximab) and immune modulators (Calcineurin, Cyclosporin).

PHYSIOLOGICAL EFFECTS OF MAGNESIUM.

Hypomagnesaemia has two important physiological actions which cause clinical manifestations. Figure 4.

<u>Hypocalcaemia</u>: from decrease in secretion and or action of Parathormone (PTH)

<u>Decrease in cellular potassium</u>: including resistance to full repletion of K^+ deficiency.

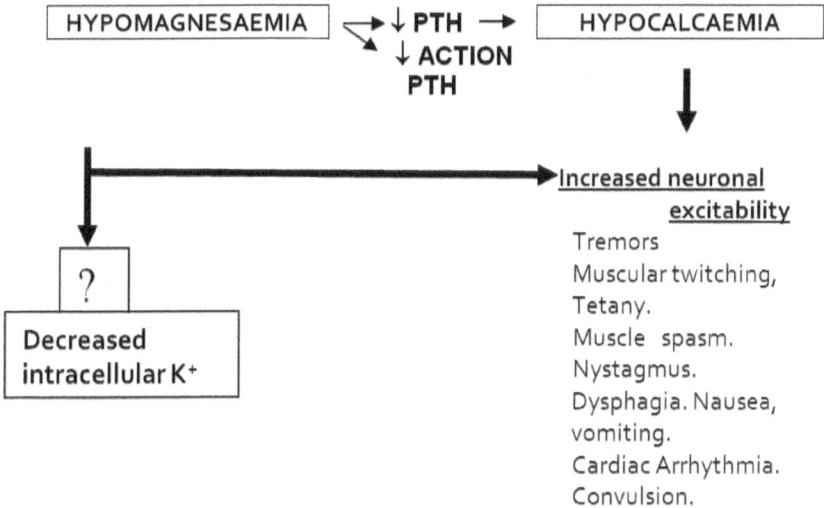

Figure 4. Physiological effects of Hypomagnesaemia.

Hypocalcaemia:

Hypocalcaemia is the most important effect of hypomagnesaemia: both hypermagnesemia and <u>severe</u> hypomagnesaemia cause hypocalcaemia.

PTH secretion depends on the <u>total divalent cation</u> concentration acting on the CASR receptor [16] and therefore responds to changes in both serum Ca^{2+} and Mg^{2+}.Targovnik [40] considered that Ca^{2+} and Mg^{2+} were equivalent in blocking PTH secretion above plasma Mg^{2+} concentration of 0.3 mmol/L, but others consider that Ca^{2+} is more potent in inhibiting PTH secretion than Mg^{2+}. [15, 16,41] Increase in serum Mg^{2+} from infusion of magnesium decreases secretion of PTH in volunteers; [42] pregnant females given Mg^{2+} to suppress premature delivery; [43] in patients with subarachnoid haemorrhage; [44] in other diseases and animal models. [45] This causes hypocalcaemia.

Paradoxically very low serum Mg^{2+} also causes <u>hypocalcaemia</u> by decreasing secretion of PTH and increasing resistance to its action. [46-48] The level at which this occurs, based on limited data in 3 studies, [46-48] is serum Mg^{2+} between 0.3-0.45mmol/L.

Mean serum Mg^{2+} of 0.62 (±.08) mmol/L was associated with normal mean serum calcium of 2.4(±0.11) mmol/L in 23 episodes of hypomagnesaemia in a patient managed by the author with Gitelman's syndrome. Only one level was slightly below normal (unpublished observations). Symptoms suggestive of hypomagnesaemia were absent on all occasions.

Mean serum magnesium was 0.475 (±0.09) mmol/L and mean serum calcium was normal, 2.4mmol/L (±0.8), in subjects with autosomal dominant renal magnesium wasting. Symptoms such as tetany, ataxia, and vertigo were absent and Trousseaus and Chvostek's signs could not be elicited. [34]

Figure 5 below shows 67 serum Mg^{2+} and Ca^{2+} levels of hypomagnesaemia in a patient with Familial Hypomagnesaemia with secondary hypocalcaemia (defective function of TRPM6) managed by the author.

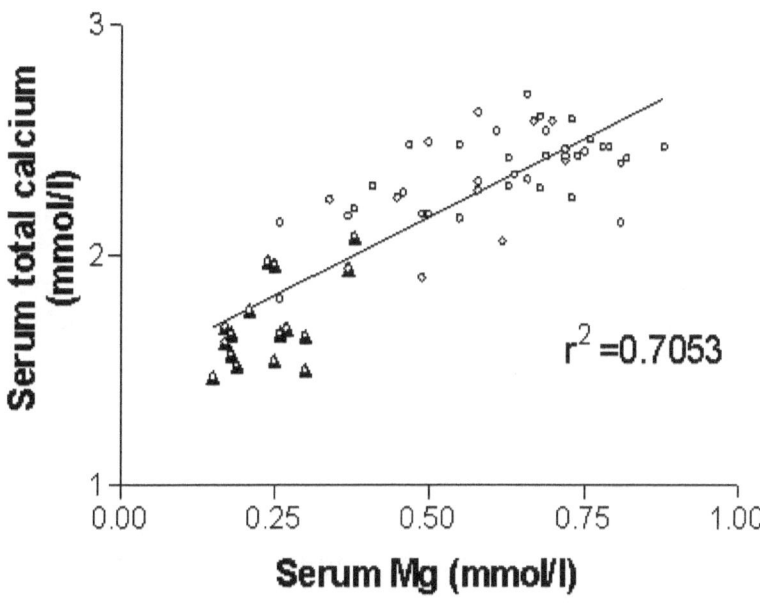

Figure 5: *67 occasions of hypomagnesaemia in a patient with Familial Hypomagnesaemia with Hypocalcaemia. Underlined circles show occasions when neuromuscular manifestations occurred.*

All occasions of severe hypocalcaemia (serum Ca^{2+} ≤ 2.0mmol/L were associated with serum magnesium <0.40mmol/L.The mean serum Mg^{2+} and Ca^{2+} associated with tetany or seizures was 0.24 mmol/L and 1.68 mmol/L respectively.

Serum Ca^{2+} and serum Mg^{2+} are correlated in figure 4. It appears likely that serum Mg concentration below 0.45mmol/L is required to cause hypocalcaemia due to hypomagnesaemia; and that tetany associated with hypomagnesaemia is due to hypocalcaemia.

Serum PTH levels were either undetectable or inappropriately low in the presence of hypocalcaemia in the majority of reports of hypomagnesaemia causing hypocalcaemia.

An intravenous bolus of magnesium sulfate, during hypomagnesaemia, causes an immediate secretion of PTH[46-48] (within one minute).This suggests that secretion from adequate stores rather than synthesis is defective in severe hypomagnesaemia. Some studies have shown an increase in phosphaturia and urine c.AMP in response to either endogenous increase in PTH secretion or exogenous injection; others have not. This suggests that the renal response to PTH is normal -at least in some cases. [46]

However, despite increase in PTH secretion, serum calcium does not increase for several hours and may take 24 hours to normalise. [47, 48] The mobilisation of calcium by bone is clearly resistant to the action of PTH. Indeed serum Ca^{2+} may initially decrease following magnesium infusion.

Mean serum Mg^{2}+increased from a mean of 0.28mmol/L to 1.11mmol/L on 5 occasions during treatment in the case shown in figure 4 but had no effect on increasing serum Ca^{2+} for a mean of four hours (serum calcium 1.84mmol/L rose to 1.88mmol/L). On 2 occasions, when mean serum magnesium increased from 0.26 to 0.82mmol/L, serum Ca^{2+} of 1.9 mmol/L did not increase for 9½ hours following magnesium infusion. Thus when hypomagnesaemia is sufficiently severe to cause hypocalcaemia: there is both defective secretion of PTH and resistance to its action. Hypocalcaemia may take up to 24 hours to normalise following correction of hypomagnesaemia.

In conclusion hypermagnesemia causes hypocalcaemia by acting on the CaSR. Severe hypomagnesemia also causes hypocalcaemia if serum Mg^{2+} is sufficiently low. (<0.45 mmol/L approximately).This decreases secretion of PTH from preformed stores and increases resistance to its action. Hypocalcaemia takes several hours to increase and 24 hours to become normal despite administration of sufficient magnesium to normalise serum Mg^{2+}.

Decrease in Cellular Potassium.

Low serum Mg^{2+} is associated with low intracellular K^+. Magnesium, a cofactor for Na^+: K^+ pump function, may decrease cellular K^+ entry and inhibit full cellular K^+ replacement when deficiency occurs. [49-51] Thus some consider correction of magnesium depletion is necessary before cellular K^+ can be fully replaced. [49-51] Magnesium deficiency decreases the number of Na^+: K^+ pumps. [52] However hypokalaemia, rather than low cellular K^+ levels, has rarely been reported from hypomagnesaemia and when it occurs is probably due to associated K^+ depletion. [53] Potassium depletion and resistance to its full correction is due to an increase in renal tubular K^+ wasting from decrease in inhibition of (ROMK) potassium channels. [53]

Magnesium deficiency does not cause hypokalaemia. [53]

The clinical importance of low cellular potassium associated with hypomagnesaemia has not been established despite considerable speculation. Moreover there is a poor correlation between serum and muscle magnesium [54].

Other effects of Magnesium:

Cardiac: Decrease in extracellular Mg^{2+} has no consistent effects on the single cardiac cell in vitro or electrocardiogram in animal models or humans. [55] Infusion of Mg^{2+} in human subjects did not change the PR, QRS or QT interval. [56] Isolated reports linking hypomagnesaemia with arrhythmias are circumstantial and confounded by associated electrolyte abnormalities and comorbid disease affecting the myocardium. [55, 57] The effects of Mg^{2+} appear to be due to extracellular K^+ and Ca^{2+} concentrations.

Bronchial Muscle.

Mg^{2+} relaxes bronchial smooth muscle in a dose dependent manner and decreases bronchospasm. [58]

Magnesium has a non-specific effect in decreasing seizures [59]. Mg^{2+} affects muscle contraction and relaxation by enhancing actin-myosin interaction, sarcoplasmic reuptake of Ca^{2+} and regulating Ca^{2+} channels [1]. Magnesium has a neuroprotective role in vitro. It can bind to ATP, inhibit the NMDA receptor and causes cerebrovascular dilatation. [60]

Mg^{2+} in vitro and in vivo increases production of prostacyclin and protects against injury by free radicals. [60] It may modify vascular resistance and blood pressure. [1] However Mg^{2+} infusion given to human subjects does not change blood pressure or pulse rate.

Chondrocalcinosis.

Chondrocalcinosis, which complicates Gitelmans syndrome, may be due to hypomagnesaemia. Magnesium may be effective in the prevention of chondrocalcinosis and pseudogout. [37]

CLINICAL MANIFESTATIONS

HYPOMAGNESAEMIA.

Neuromuscular.

Hypomagnesaemia has been reported to cause tremor, muscle twitching, paraesthesia, irritability, nystagmus, convulsions, dysphagia, vertical nystagmus, ataxia, tetany, cardiac arrhythmias and ECG abnormalities. [1] Some consider that hypomagnesemia per se causes neuromuscular manifestations including tetany [60-70] whereas others do not. [71-83].

There are four potential causes of these manifestations:

• Hypocalcaemia secondary to hypomagnesaemia.
• Low intracellular potassium caused by hypomagnesaemia or intracellular Mg^{2+} depletion.
• Low serum ionised Mg^{2+} itself.
• Low intracellular magnesium despite a normal serum Mg^{2+}.
• Other associated diseases.

Hypomagnesaemia, hypokalaemia, metabolic alkalosis and hypocalcaemia were severe and common during both diarrhoea and Protein-Calorie malnutrition (Kwashiorkor) in West Africa: all neuromuscular manifestations and arrhythmias which occurred were explained by conditions other than hypomagnesaemia and rapidly resolved on treatment of these associated conditions before magnesium was given. [82]

In 20 consecutive patients with severe hypomagnesaemia studied prospectively in an Intensive Care Unit (standard observation forms) serum Mg^{2+} <0.5mmol/L, mean serum Mg^{2+} 0.33mmol/L, only three patients, all hypocalcaemic, showed tremor and muscle twitching; and none showed tetany, positive Trousseau sign, arrhythmias or electrocardiographic abnormalities. [71]

A computer generated list of 27 consecutive publications on hypomagnesaemia was critically appraised: tetany was reported in 44 of 225 hypomagnesaemic patients. [71] Hypocalcaemia was present in all but 10: serum Mg^{2+} was normal in 7; high fever present in five; epilepsy in four; vomiting or nasogastric aspiration, which are likely to lead to metabolic alkalosis, in 3; and osmolality disorders in two of these. [71]

In a report of 22 instances of severe hypomagnesaemia (mean serum Mg^{2+} 0.475 mmol/L) from renal magnesium wasting, but normal serum Ca^{2+} levels, none showed tetany or neuromuscular manifestations. [34]

All instances of neuromuscular manifestations in the subject with hereditary hypomagnesaemia with hypocalcaemia, illustrated in figure 4, occurred when serum Ca^{2+} was equal to or less than 2.0 mmol/L. Neuromuscular and cardiac manifestations did not occur in the previously described subject with Gitelmans syndrome.

To establish that hypomagnesemia is the cause of tetany, serum magnesium, corrected for albumin which binds 25% to 30% of magnesium, [1] should be unequivocally low; and metabolic alkalosis, respiratory alkalosis, and hypocalcaemia should be excluded at the time tetany is manifest. Tetany should only be diagnosed if frank or provoked carpopedal spasm is present. Chvostek's sign by itself is an inadequate diagnostic sign because it may be positive in normal persons. [71, 76] Improvement of neuromuscular irritability following magnesium therapy is an inadequate reason for attributing its cause to hypomagnesaemia because magnesium has a non-specific action on neuronal excitability. It may even abolish tetany due to hypocalcaemia. [77]

Hypomagnesaemia does not cause unique or consistent ECG changes. [71, 79, 84] Hypomagnesaemia in man has only rarely been reported to cause ECG changes, and other causes, such as hypokalaemia, alkalosis, hypocalcaemia or cardiomyopathy [71], which cause ST-T segment abnormalities, were not excluded. Thus, ST-T segment changes attributed to hypomagnesaemia in malnourished West African children [85] may have been due to hypokalaemia which was more severe. In another report attributing ECG changes to hypomagnesaemia, serum magnesium levels were normal [86]. My observations failed to show changes in the ECG after parenteral correction of hypomagnesaemia. [71] Infusion of magnesium over a period of six hours had no effect on the QT interval, PR interval or QRS duration in another study. Hypomagnesaemia does not cause major changes of the action potential and its effects on the heart are often confounded by other associated electrolyte disturbances.

Cardiac arrhythmias have also been attributed to hypomagnesaemia on inadequate grounds: [87-90] in individual case reports of patients with alcoholism [88-90] or congestive cardiac failure, [91] both of which predispose patients to cardiac arrhythmias. Moreover respiratory alkalosis, which causes severe arrhythmias; [92] treatment with digitalis or other drugs;

cardiac failure; hypokalaemia; glucose infusion, which predisposes patients with mild hypokalaemia to arrhythmias; [93] alcoholic cardiomyopathy; and other electrolyte aberrations were common among these patients and may have been responsible. In several of these reports serum magnesium levels were normal or near-normal. Abolition of arrhythmias by magnesium infusion is inadequate evidence for attributing the cause to hypomagnesaemia because magnesium has a non-specific anti-arrhythmic effect. [94- 96] Two cases of Torsades were attributed to hypomagnesaemia by Ramee et al: [87] however the patients were malnourished, critically ill, had underlying heart disease and prolonged QT intervals, presumably due to causes other than hypomagnesaemia, because hypomagnesaemia per se does not prolong QT intervals.

Magnesium deficiency has been considered to cause cardiac arrhythmias in the setting of myocardial infarction on the basis of low muscle magnesium levels and response to intravenous magnesium.[97] This has not been confirmed in recent trials.

Several publications suggest that a low intracellular Mg^{2+}, despite normal serum Mg^{2+}, may cause adverse clinical manifestations. [54, 97-101] However the clinical importance of low intracellular Mg^{2+} or K^+ has not been established. Correlation between overall magnesium depletion or cellular magnesium and serum Mg^{2+} levels is poor. Low cellular magnesium may be secondary to more important metabolic aberrations; low muscle Mg^{2+} may be due to a decrease in muscle compared to collagen; cellular water excess; or metabolic factors. [82] Ionised Mg^{2+}, the relevant component, is a small fraction of cellular magnesium concentration.

The extent to which hypomagnesaemia without hypocalcaemia causes symptoms is uncertain. Striking improvement in well being was reported following normalisation of hypomagnesaemia due to proton pump inhibitors [27] although this may have been due to resolution of hypocalcaemia. A patient with serum Mg of only 0.13 mmol/L but with normal serum Ca, (2.5 mmol/L)measured on the same sample, managed by the author, reported striking improvement on normalisation of serum Mg^{2+} when the proton pump inhibitor was discontinued.(Unpublished observation.)

Hypomagnesaemia has been reported to be associated with an increase in mortality but this may be a marker of disease severity or associated electrolyte abnormalities.

The <u>most important clinical manifestations due to hypomagnesaemia are neuromuscular secondary to low extracellular ionised calcium.</u> Hypomagnesaemia, per se has not been established as a cause of tetany or cardiac arrhythmias. The importance of other manifestations due to a low intracellular K^+ secondary to hypomagnesaemia, or to a low cellular Mg^{2+} ion itself, remains to be established.

DIAGNOSIS

Given the absence of clear cut manifestations due to hypomagnesaemia this should be suspected in the following:

- States of K^+ depletion where Mg depletion often coexists—(especially following K^+ correction).
- Hypocalcaemia or tetany.
- Unexplained hypokalaemia.
- Following admission for alcoholism.
- Therapy with diuretics, aminoglycosides, EGF antagonists, proton pump inhibitors and other drugs causing magnesuria.
- Conditions causing diarrhoea: especially ileostomies, small bowel fistulae and jejunoileal bypass.
- Refeeding without adequate Mg^{2+} supplementation.

Hypokalaemia, hypocalcaemia and hypophosphataemia are common in patients with hypomagnesaemia. All three disturbances accompanied severe hypomagnesaemia in 40% of consecutive cases. [71]

<u>Urine magnesium separates renal from gastrointestinal causes</u>. Urine magnesium should decrease below 0.5mmol/L if hypomagnesaemia is due to a non-renal cause. The fractional excretion of magnesium should decrease below 0.5-1% during hypomagnesaemia and urinary magnesium is virtually absent when the serum level falls below 0.7mmol/L.

<u>HYPERMAGNESAEMIA.</u>

This causes interference with acetyl choline release from motor nerve terminals—curafiform action. The PR and QRS intervals are prolonged. The most common causes are renal failure, iatrogenic and rarely Addisonian crisis

	mmol/L
Normal	0.7-1.2
Therapeutic level for eclampsia	2.0-4.0
Nausea, warm sensation, diplopia, dysarthria somnolence, weakness	3.5-5.0
Loss of knee jerk	3.5-7.0
Respiratory depression	>6.0
Cardiotoxicity—prolonged PR, QRS	>7.5
Respiratory arrest	5-7.5
Cardiac arrest	12.5

Table 3: *Manifestations of magnesium toxicity. Adapted from reference 102 (for mEq multiply by 2).*

Magnesium is used for treatment of eclampsia or preeclampsia. If serum magnesium measurements are unavailable monitoring is based on changes in the knee jerk.

TREATMENT OF SEVERE HYPERMAGNESAEMIA.

5mmol bolus Calcium → 5mmol over 6 hours (=10mEq bolus)

Intravenous Saline if renal function permits

↓

Dialysis

TREATMENT OF HYPOMAGNESAEMIA.

The following are important:

- Intramuscular MgSo₄ is erratically absorbed and painful on injection although it has been used successfully. Magnesium sulphate 5 gram is injected, usually every 4 hours, into alternative buttocks.
- Magnesium depletion cannot be corrected by brief infusions because once the normal plasma Mg concentration is exceeded magnesium

infused is excreted in urine. This is because the total divalent concentration ($Ca^{2+} + Mg^{2+}$) activates the CaSR receptor despite severe cellular or bone magnesium deficiency. Thus extended infusion or frequent doses of oral or intramuscular magnesium should be given. Caution should be exercised in renal failure.

- In severe hypomagnesaemia (serum Mg^{2+} <0.3-0.5 mmol/L) PTH is rapidly secreted in response to magnesium infusion but serum Ca^{2+} does not increase for several hours and may take several days to become normal.

Magnesium infusion has a considerable margin of safety. A dose of 0.27mmol/kg over 20 minutes increased serum magnesium from 0.92 to 2.5mmol/L[103] and a dose of 8mmol given as a bolus increased serum magnesium from 0.9 to 1.55mmol/L after 30 minutes. In treatment of Eclampsia an intravenous bolus of 4 g or intramuscular dose of 10 g magnesium sulphate followed by 5 g given intramuscularly into the buttock 4 hourly was safe and effective provided renal failure was absent. [104]

In treating Torsades de pointes serum magnesium increased to 1.15-2.5mmol/L following a bolus of 2 g magnesium sulphate (8 mmol;16 mEq) given intravenously. [105] Facial flushing and occasionally paraesthesias were the only side effects experienced in these studies.

Theoretically a bolus of $MgSo_4$ initially distributes in extracellular water – approximately 20% of body weight. Thus in a 75kg male (extracellular fluid 15L) a bolus of 8mmol should increase the serum Mg by (8mmol/15L) = approximately 0.5mmol/L.

Practical aspects.($MgSO_4$ 1g=98mg elemental Mg^{2+}=4mmol =8mEq)

Initially give an intravenous bolus of $MgSO_4$ –8mmol elemental Mg^{2+} over 10 minutes, but with extreme care in renal failure.

Compatible fluids: Glucose 5%, Hartmann's solution, Ringers solution, normal saline, saline glucose solutions, calcium gluconate.

Incompatible: $CaCl_2$, sodium bicarbonate, phosphate.

Note: Rapid infusion may cause hypotension and flushing.

Continue infusion at 0.5-1 mmol/hour (care in renal failure).

Intramuscular (49.3% MgSO$_4$)   (5ml = 10mmol Mg^{2+}) 10mmol
                                                  2-3 times daily

Oral Mg aspartate 500 mg   (1.56mmol Mg^{++}) per tablet.

Tolerance and bioavailability vary considerably in different oral Mg formulations and large doses have to be given for gastrointestinal disorders, such as small bowel resection, and Hereditary Mg^{2+} wasting disorders (16-24 tablets daily). Diarrhoea is an important side effect which may decrease compliance. Magnesium oxide may be better absorbed.

Magnesium gluconate   tab 500 mg =32 mg elemental
                                                  Mg^{2+} =1.2mmol

Mylanta Double Strength (Mg (OH)^2 tab = 5mmol Mg^{2+}.

                                                  1 teaspoon = 5mmol Mg^{2+}

Diet high in Mg.   Milk, Avocado, bananas etc.

THERAPEUTIC USES OF MAGNESIUM. [60]

Although there are no established clinical manifestations of magnesium depletion, apart from hypocalcaemia, magnesium has been used in pharmacological amounts in several conditions. Those advocating its use have failed to emphasise that hypermagnesemia from Mg^{2+} infusion causes hypocalcaemia and hypotension. Hypocalcaemia decreases cardiac contractility, the extent depending on severity, [106] and causes muscle spasm. Outcome was worse in those who became hypocalcaemic as a result of therapy with intravenous magnesium in the Magnesium in Aneurysmal Subarachnoid Haemorrhage Trial. [44]

CARDIAC ARRHYTHMIAS

Magnesium has a pharmacological effect in reversing arrhythmias. It has been considered the treatment of choice for reversing Torsade de Pointes; [105] is recommended for refractory ventricular fibrillation; decreases ventricular ectopy following cardiopulmonary bypass; [96] and has been used for treatment of supraventricular tachycardia.[107] Tzivoni et al [105] showed that intravenous magnesium sulfate was effective in reversing

Torsades associated with long but not normal QT intervals An Intravenous bolus of 8 mmol magnesium sulphate followed by o.5-1.ommol/hour is recommended for drug induced Torsades.[108] It was more successful in reverting atrial tachyarrhythmias than amiodarone in one randomised trial. [109]

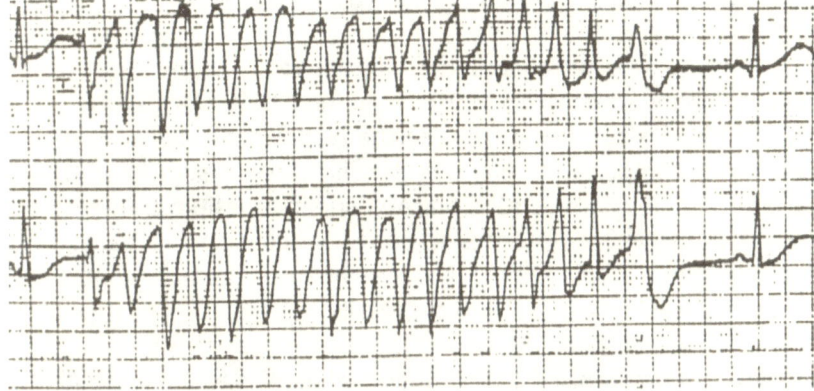

Figure 5. Torsades de Pointes: showing intermittent 180 degree reversal of QRS polarity.

There was no relationship between rhythm conversion and serum magnesium levels. It has also been used successfully in the treatment of digitalis—toxic arrhythmias. [110] A metaanalysis of magnesium therapy for rapid atrial fibrillation showed that it was safe and effective for both rhythm and rate control. [111] However another metaanalysis showed that it was less effective than amiodarone or calcium antagonists in reducing the ventricular response. [112]

ISCHAEMIC HEART DISEASE.

Initial claims of benefit, including improved outcome [113], led to its routine use in many coronary care units. This has been abandoned following the ISIS4 trial which showed no benefit for Mg^{2+} use and a small, but significant increase in heart failure, cardiogenic shock and sinus bradycardia. [114]

ECLAMPSIA.

Magnesium is considered the treatment of choice for preventing eclamptic seizures. Mg^{2+} was superior to phenytoin for preventing seizures in a randomised controlled trial: [104] 10g of a 50% solution of $MgSO_4$, given by intramuscular injection, was followed by 5g in alternative buttocks every four hours with the intention to keep serum Mg^{2+} between 2.0-3.5 mmol/L. In severe cases an initial 4g dose was given intravenously. Alternatively 4-5g is given intravenously followed by 1-2g IV every hour, monitoring symptoms, the knee jerk and serum levels (see Table 3).

ASTHMA AND CHRONIC OBSTRUCTIVE LUNG DISEASE.

A Cochrane review concluded that intravenous magnesium was not beneficial in moderate asthma [115] but 'seemed' to be beneficial in severe asthma. This was surprising because the recommendations were based on only two complete papers, one of which was a subgroup analysis: base line variables between the placebo and magnesium treated groups showed considerable differences in this study. I consider, following critical appraisal of these studies, [116-120] that the evidence does not support use of magnesium in asthma regardless of severity.

A more recent randomised double blind trial showed that magnesium was ineffective for treatment of asthma [121]. A systematic review including metaanalysis concluded that evidence was insufficient to justify use of intravenous magnesium in adults—although it may be beneficial in children. [122]

A randomised trial of intravenous magnesium in Emergency Department admissions for exacerbations of chronic obstructive pulmonary disease showed a statistically significant small increase in FEV in 1 second and a decrease in admissions. [123] However inhaled anticholinergic therapy, which is probably more effective, was not given.

The role of magnesium has not been satisfactorily established for either asthma or chronic obstructive lung disease.

CEREBRAL ISCHAEMIA AND NEUROPROTECTION.

Mg^{2+} causes vasodilation by increasing regional cerebral blood flow and inhibiting calcium influx into cells by blocking calcium at voltage gated channels, possibly blocking NMDA receptors and decreasing apoptosis. [124] It has not been shown to be effective in man, possibly because its entry into cerebrospinal fluid and brain are limited. [125]

Infusion of magnesium in subarachnoid haemorrhage worsened outcome in those who developed hypocalcaemia as a result. [44] However maintenance of high levels of serum magnesium by continuous infusion and monitoring achieved high cerebrospinal fluid Mg^{2+} concentrations and was effective in decreasing vasospasm. Ischaemic events were decreased although mortality was not decreased. [126]

Magnesium is ineffective for improving outcome in brain trauma [127].

Given the potential risk of hypocalcaemia and hypotension magnesium infusion should not be given for conditions for which evidence is questionable.

NEURO PROTECTIVE EFFECT IN PRETERM NEONATES.

In a randomised controlled trial the incidence of severe cerebral palsy in neonatal survivors was less in pregnant woman at risk of imminent preterm delivery, given magnesium, although overall mortality and incidence of overall cerebral palsy was not decreased. [128] In a metanalysis of all randomised controlled trials administration of antepartum $MgSO_4$ decreased the frequency of severe motor dysfunction in the first few years of life but there was no effect on mortality.[129]

Premature Labour.

Magnesium given in pharmacological doses inhibits uterine contraction and has been used to inhibit premature labour. [130]

DIURETICS AND ARRHYTHMIAS.

Although hypomagnesaemia occasionally occurs during diuretic therapy, and low cellular magnesium occurs more commonly, clinical studies have not established a causal relationship between serious arrhythmias or sudden death and so called magnesium depletion. Magnesium has been suggested for decreasing hypertension [131] and the incidence of diabetes [132] but neither use has been established satisfactorily.

Thus magnesium is efficacious in the treatment of Eclampsia, Torsades de pointes and atrial tachyarrhtmias.It may have a role in decreasing the severity of cerebral palsy in woman at risk of preterm delivery.

REFERENCES

General References

1. Sutton, R.A. and Dirks, J.H., Disturbances of calcium and magnesium metabolism. p. 1038-1085. in Brenner and Rector's the kidney, Brenner, B.M. and Rector, F.C., Editors. 1996, Saunders: Philadelphia.

2. Levine, B.S., Coburn J W. Magnesium metabolism, p. 362-379. in Massry & Glassock's textbook of Nephrology, S.G. Massry and R.J. Glassock, Editors. 1995, Williams & Wilkins: Philadelphia.

3. Alfrey, A.C., Normal and abnormal magnesium metabolism, p. 278-302 in Renal and electrolyte disorders, R.W. Schrier, Editor. 2003, Lippincott Williams & Wilkins: Philadelphia.

4. Shafik, I.M. and Dirks, J.H., Hypo- and Hypermagnesaemia, p. 1802-1821 in Oxford textbook of clinical nephrology, S. Cameron, et al., Editors. 1992, Oxford University Press: Oxford.

5. Al-Ghamdi, S.M., Cameron, E.C., and Sutton, R.A., Magnesium deficiency: pathophysiologic and clinical overview. Amer J Kidney Diseases, 1994. 24(5): p. 737-52.

6. Dacey, M.J., Hypomagnesemic disorders. Critical Care Clinics, 2001. 17(1): p. 155-73.

Specific references

7. Lanzinger, M.J. Moretti E W, Wilderman R F et al. The relationship between ionized and total serum magnesium concentrations during abdominal surgery. Journal of Clinical Anesthesia, 2003. 15(4): p. 245-9.

8. Johansson M, Whiss PA. Weak relationship between ionised and total magnesium in serum of patients requiring magnesium status. Biological Trace Elements research. 2007 115 :13-21

9. Zaloga, GP, Wilkens, R, Tourville, J. et al, A simple method for determining physiologically active calcium and magnesium concentrations in critically ill patients. Critical Care Medicine, 1987. 15:813-816.

10. Chubanov, V., Gudermann, T., Schlingmann, K.P., Essential role for TRPM6 in epithelial magnesium transport and body magnesium homeostasis. Pflugers Archiv—European Journal of Physiology, 2005. 451(1): p. 228-34.

11. Yu, A.S., Evolving concepts in epithelial magnesium transport. Current Opinion in Nephrology & Hypertension, 2001. 10(5): p. 649-53.

12. Schlingmann KP, Gudermann T. A critical role of TRPM channel-kinase for human magnesium transport. J Physiol. 2005.566:301-308

13. Cao G, Hoenderop JGJ, Bindels RJM. Insight into the molecular regulation of the epithelial magnesium channel TRPM6. Current Opinion Nephrol Hypert. 2008 17:373-378

14. Quamme, G.A., Recent developments in intestinal magnesium absorption. Current Opinion in Gastroenterology, 2008. 24:230-235.

15. Vetter, T. and Lohse, M.J., Magnesium and the parathyroid. Current Opinion in Nephrology & Hypertension, 2002. 11(4): p. 403-10.

16. Hebert, S.C., Extracellular calcium-sensing receptor: implications for calcium and magnesium handling in the kidney. Kidney International, 1996. 50(6): p. 2129-39.

17. Quamme, G.A., Renal magnesium handling: new insights in understanding old problems. Kidney International, 1997. 52(5): p. 1180-95.

18. Blanchard, A., Jeunemaitre X, Coudol P et al., Paracellin-1 is critical for magnesium and calcium reabsorption in the human thick ascending limb of Henle. Kidney International, 2001. 59(6): p. 2206-15.

19. Naderi A.S.A., Reilley, R.F., Hereditary etiologies of hypomagnesemia. Nature Clinical Practice Nephrology, 2008. 4:80-89.

20. Muallem, S, Moe, O.W., When EGF is offside, magnesium is wasted. J. Clin. Invest, 2007. 117:2086-2089.

21. Weisinger JR, Bellorin-Font E. Magnesium and Phosphorus. Lancet.1998.352:391-396

22. Whang, R., Magnesium deficiency: pathogenesis, prevalence, and clinical implications. American Journal of Medicine, 1987. 82(3A): p. 24-9.

23. Dyckner, T. and Wester, P.O., Potassium/magnesium depletion in patients with cardiovascular disease. American Journal of Medicine, 1987. 82(3A) 11-7.

24. Hollifield, J.W., Magnesium depletion, diuretics, and arrhythmias. American Journal of Medicine, 1987. 82(3A): p. 30-7.

25. Ryan, M.P., Diuretics and potassium/magnesium depletion. Directions for treatment. American Journal of Medicine, 1987. 82(3A): p. 38-47.

26. Kingston, M., Electrolyte disturbances in Liberian children with kwashiorkor. Journal of Pediatrics, 1973. 83(5): p. 859-66.

27. Cundy T, Mackay J. Proton Pump Inhibitors and severe hypomagnesaemia. Curr Opin Gastroenterol 2011.27:180-185.

28. Yao, X., Panchpisal, K., Kurtzman, N., Nugent, K., Cisplatin nephrotoxicity: a review. Amer. J. medical Sciences, 2007. 334:115-24.

29. Giapros, V.I., Cholevas, V.I., and Andronikou, S.K., Acute effects of gentamicin on urinary electrolyte excretion in neonates. Pediatric Nephrology, 2004. 19(3): 322-5.

30. Bar, R.S., Wilson, H.E., Mazzaferri, E.L., Hypomagnesaemic Hypocalcemia secondary to Renal magnesium Wasting. Ann. Int. Med., 1975. 82:646-649.

31. Konrad, M. and Weber, S., Recent advances in molecular genetics of hereditary magnesium-losing disorders. Journal of the American Society of Nephrology, 2003. 14(1): 249-60.

32. San-Cristobal P, Dimke H, Hoenderop JGJ Bindels RJM. Novel molecular pathways in renal Mg²⁺ transport: a guided tour along the nephron. Current Opinion in Nephrology Hypertension.2010 19:456-462

33. Stromme, J.H. Steen-Johnsen J, Harnaes K et al., Familial hypomagnesemia--a follow-up examination of three patients after 9 to 12 years of treatment. Pediatric Research, 1981. 15(8): p. 1134-9.

34. Geven, W.B., Monnens, L.A., Willems, W.C., et al, Renal magnesium wasting in two families with autosomal dominant inheritance. Kidney Internat. 1987. 31:1140-1144.

35. Abdulrazzaq, Y.M., Smigura, F.C., and Wettrell, G., Primary infantile hypomagnesaemia; report of two cases and review of literature. European Journal of Pediatrics, 1989. 148(5): p. 459-61.

36. Bhandari, S., The pathophysiological and molecular basis of Bartter's and Gitelman's syndromes. Postgraduate Medical Journal, 1999. 75(885): p. 391-6.

37. NineV.A.M.Knoers, Gitelman syndrome. Advances in chronic kidney disease.2006 13 148-154

38. Cruz, D.N., Shaer AJ, Bia MJ et al., Gitelman's syndrome revisited: an evaluation of symptoms and health-related quality of life. Kidney International, 2001. 59(2): p. 710-7.

39. Colussi, G.,Rombola G, De Ferrari ME et al., Correction of hypokalemia with anti-aldosterone therapy in Gitelman's syndrome. American Journal of Nephrology, 1994. 14(2): p. 127-35.

40. Targovnik J H, Rodman J S, Sherwood L M. Regulation of Parathyroid secretion in Vitro: Quantitative aspects of Calcium and Magnesium Ion Control. Endocrinology1971.88:1477-1482.

41. Habener J F, Potts J T. Relative effectiveness of Magnesium and Calcium on the Secretion of Parathyroid Hormone in Vitro. Endocrinology. 1976.98:197-202.

42. Mountokalakis, T.H., Tsiotras, S., Skopelitis, P., et al, Hypocalcaemia following Magnesium Sulfate Therapy. JAMA, 1972. 221:195.

43. Cholst, I.N., Steinberg, S.F., Tropper, P.J., et al., The influence of hypermagnesemia on serum calcium and parathyroid hormone levels in human subjects. New England Journal of Medicine, 1984. 310(19): p. 1221-5.

44. Van de Water, J.M., Vandenberg, W.M., Hoff, R.G., et al, Hypocalcaemia may reduce the beneficial effect of magnesium treatment on aneurysmal subarachnoid haemorrhage. Magnesium Research, 2007. 20:130-5.

45.   Care AD, Sherwood LM, Potts JD,Aurbach GD. Perfusion of the isolated Parathyroid Gland of the Goat and Sheep.1966. Nature:209 55-57

46.   Anast, C.S., Winnacker, R.L., Forte, L.R., Burns, T.W., Impaired release of Parathyroid Hormone in Magnesium Deficiency. J. Clin Endocrin Metabolism, 1976. 42:707-17.

47.   Rude, R.K., Oldham, S.B., Singer, F.R. Functional Hypoparathyroidism and parathyroid Hormone End-Organ. Resistance in Human magnesium Deficiency. Clin. Endocrinol, 1976. 5:209-224.

48.   Rude, R.K., Oldham, S.B., Sharp, C.F., Parathyroid hormone Secretion in Magnesium Deficiency. J. Clinic. Endocrinol and Metabolism, 1978. 47:800-806.

49.   Ryan, M.P., Interrelationships of magnesium and potassium homeostasis. Mineral & Electrolyte Metabolism, 1993. 19(4-5):. 290-5.

50.   Whang, R., Whang, D.D., and Ryan, M.P., Refractory potassium repletion. A consequence of magnesium deficiency. Archives of Internal Medicine, 1992. 152(1): p. 40-5.

51.   Dyckner T, Wester PO. Ventricular extrasystoles and intracellular electrolytes before and after potassium and magnesium infusions in patients on diuretic treatment. 1979. Amer Heart Journal:97:12-18

52.   Dorup, I., Skajaa, K, Clausen, T, Kjeldsen, K., Reduced concentrations of potassium magnesium and sodium-potassium pumps in human skeletal muscle during treatment with diuretics. BMJ, 1988. 296:455-458.

53.   Huang, C.L., Kuo, E., Mechanisms of hypokalaemia in Magnesium Deficiency. J. Amer. Soc. Nephrology, 2007. 18:2649-52.

54.   Fiaccadori, E., Del Canale, S., Coffrini, E., et al, Muscle and serum magnesium in pulmonary intensive care unit patients. Crit. Care Medicine, 1988. 16:751-760.

55.   Gettes, L.S., Electrolyte abnormalities underlying lethal and ventricular arrhythmias. Circulation, 1992. 85(1 Suppl).

56.   Rogiers, P ;Vermeier,W ;Kesteloot H; Stroobandt R., Effect of the infusion of magnesium sulfate during atrial pacing on ECG intervals, serum electrolytes, and blood pressure. American Heart Journal, 1989. 117(6):. 1278-83.

57.   Roden, D.M., Iansmith, D.H.S., Effects of low Potassium or Magnesium concentration on isolated cardiac tissue. 1987. 82(suppl3A):18-23.

58.   Spivey, W.H., Skobeloff, E.M., and Levin, R.M., Effect of magnesium chloride on rabbit bronchial smooth muscle. Annals of Emergency Medicine, 1990. 19(10): 1107-12.

59.   Roberts, J.M., Magnesium for preeclampsia and eclampsia. New England Journal of Medicine, 1995. 333(4): 250-1.

60.   McLean, R.M., Magnesium and its therapeutic uses: A review. Amer. J. Medicine, 1994. 96:63-76.

61. Anast, C.S., Gardner, D.W., Magnesium metabolism. pp 424-82 In: Disorders of mineral metabolism. Pathophysiology of calcium, phosphorus and magnesium. Bronner, F., Coburn, J.W., (Eds). New York, Academic Pres, 1981.

62. Balin, J.A., Hirschowitz, B.J., Hypomagnesemia with tetany in nontropical sprue. N Engl J Med, 1961. 265:631.

63. Dooling, E.C. and Stern, L., Hypomagnesemia with convulsions in a newbon infant. Report of a case associated with maternal hypophosphatemia. Canadian Medical Association Journal, 1967. 97(14):. 827-31.

64. Engle, F.L., Martin, S.P., Taylor, H. On the relation of potassium to the neurological manifestations of hypocalcaemic tetany. Bull Johns Hopkins Hosp, 1949. 84:285

65. Freidman, M., Hatcher, G., Watson, L., Primary hypomagnesemia with secondary hypocalcemia in an infant. Lancet, 1967. 1:703.

66. Randall, R.E., Jr., Rossmeisl, E.C., Bleifer, K.H., Magnesium depletion in man. Annals of Internal Medicine, 1959. 50(2):. 257-87.

67. Miller, J.F., Tetany due to deficiency in magnesium. Amer J Dis Child, 1944. 67:117.

68. Vallee, B.L., Wacker, W.E., and Ulmer, D.D., The magnesium-deficiency tetany syndrome in man. New England Journal of Medicine, 1960. 262: 155-61.

69. Wong, H.B. and The, Y.F., An association between serum-magnesium and tremor and convulsions in infants and children. Lancet, 1968. 2(7558): 18-21.

70. Caddell, J.L. and Goddard, D.R., Studies in protein-calorie malnutrition. I. Chemical evidence for magnesium deficiency. New England Journal of Medicine, 1967. 276(10):. 533-5.

71. Kingston, M.E., Al-Siba'i, M.B., Skooge, W.C., Clinical manifestations of hypomagnesemia. Critical Care Medicine, 1986. 14(11): 950-4.

72. Booth, C.C., Barbouris, N., Hanna, S., et al: Incidence of hypomagnesaemia in intestinal malabsorption. Br Med J, 1963. 2:141.

73. Zimmet, P., Breidahl, H.D., Nayler, W.G., Plasma ionized calcium in hypomagnesaemia. British Medical Journal, 1968. 1(5592):. 622-3.

74. Gerst, P.H., Porter, M.R., Fishman, R.A., Symptomatic magnesium deficiency in surgical patients. Annals of Surgery, 1964. 159:. 402-6.

75. Hanna, S Harrison M; MacIntyre I Fraser R., The syndrome of magnesium deficiency in man. Lancet, 1960. 2:. 172-6.

76. Macintyre, I., Hanna S; Booth CC; Read AE. Intracellular magnesium deficiency in man. Clinical Science, 1961. 20:. 297-305.

77. Smith, W.O., J.F. Hammarsten, and L.P. Eliel, The clinical expression of magnesium deficiency. JAMA, 1960. 174: 77-8.

78. Baron, D.N., Magnesium deficiency after gastrointestinal surgery and loss of secretions. Br J Surg, 1960. 48:344.

79. Shils, M.E., Experimental human magnesium depletion. Medicine, 1969. 48(1): 61-85.

80. Martin, H.E., Mehl, J., Wertman, M., Symposium on recent advances in medicine. Medical Clinics of North America, 1952:. 1157-71.

81. MacIntyre, L., Discussion on magnesium metabolism in man and animals. Proceedings of the Royal Society of Medicine, 1960. 53: 1037-9.

82. Kingston, M., M.D. University London 1974. Electrolyte and Fluid disturbances in Liberian Children.

83. Eliel, L.P., Smith, W.O., Thomsen, C., Magnesium and calcium interrelationships. Journal Oklahoma State Medical Association, 1960. 53: 359-67.

84. Diercks, D.B., Shumaik, G.M., Harrigan, R.A., et al, Electrocardiographic manifestations: Electrolyte Abnormalities. Journal Emergency Medicine. 2004 27:153-160.

85. Cadell, J.L., Studies in protein-calorie malnutrition. II. A double-blind clinical trial to assess magnesium therapy. New England Journal of Medicine, 1967. 276(10). 535-40.

86. Chen, W.C., Wan-Chun, C., Xin-Xiara, F, Zhen-Jia, P., ECG changes in early stage of magnesium deficiency. American Heart Journal, 1982. 104 :1115-6.

87. Ramee, S.R., White, C.J., Svinarten JT, Torsades de pointes and magnesium deficiency. Amer. Heart J., 1985. 109:164-167.

88. Iseri, L.T., Freed, J., Bures, A.R., Magnesium deficiency and cardiac disorders. American Journal of Medicine, 1975. 58(6):. 837-46.

89. Fisher, J. and Abrams, J., Life-threatening ventricular tachyarrhythmias in delirium tremens. Archives of Internal Medicine, 1977. 137(9):. 1238-41.

90. Loeb, H.S., Pietras, R.J., Gunnar, R.M., et al: Paroxysmal ventricular fibrillation in two patients with hypomagnesemia. Treatment by transvenous pacing. Circulation, 1968. 37:210-214.

91. Cohen, L. and Kitzes, R., Magnesium sulfate and digitalis-toxic arrhythmias. JAMA, 1983. 249(20):. 2808-10.

92. Mazzara, J.T., Ayres, S.M., and Grace, W.J., Extreme hypocapnia in the critically ill patient. American Journal of Medicine, 1974. 56(4):. 450-6.

93. Kunin, A.S., Surawicz, B., and Sims, E.A., Decrease in serum potassium concentrations and appearance of cardiac arrhythmias during infusion of potassium with glucose in potassium-depleted patients. New England Journal of Medicine, 1962. 266:. 228-33.

94. Ghani, M.F. Rabah, M., Effect of magnesium chloride on electrical stability of the heart. American Heart Journal, 1977. 94(5): 600-2.

95. Boyd, L.J., Sherf, D., Magnesium sulphate in paroxysmal tachycardia. Am J Med Sci, 1943. 206:43.

96. England, M.R., Gordon G Salem M; Chernow B Magnesium administration and dysrhythmias after cardiac surgery. A placebo-controlled, double-blind, randomized trial JAMA 1992. 268(17):. 2395-402.

97. Rasmussen H; Norregard P; Lindeneg O et al.Intravenous magnesium in acute myocardial infarction. Lancet 1:234-235.1986

98. Packer, M., Gottlieb, S.S., Blum, M.A. Immediate and Long-Term Pathophysiologic Mechanisms Underlying the Genesis of Sudden Cardiac Death in Patients with Congestive Heart Failure. Amer. J. Medicine, 1983. 82(Suppl3A):4-8.

99. Rubeizg, J., Thill-Baharozian, M., Hardie, D. et al, Association of hypomagnesaemia and mortality in acutely ill medical patients. Crit. Care Med., 1993. 21:203-209.

100. Hamill-Ruth, R.J. McGory, R., Magnesium repletion and its effect on potassium homeostasis in critically ill adults: results of a double-blind, randomized, controlled trial. Critical Care Medicine, 1996. 24(1): 38-45.

101. Lim P, Jacob, E., Magnesium Deficiency in Patients on Long-Term Diuretic Therapy for heart Failure. BMJ, 1972. 3:620-622.

102. Hughes, M., Hypertensive Disorders of Pregnancy. Emergency Medicine Reports, 2004. 25(No.24):293-305.

103. Miyagi, H., Yasue, H, Okumura, K., et al, Effect of Magnesium on Anginal Attack Induced by Hyperventilation in Patients with Variant Angina. Circulation, 1989. 79:597-602.

104. Lucas, M.J., Leveno, K.J., Cunningham, F.G., A comparison of magnesium sulfate with phenytoin for the prevention of eclampsia.[see comment]. New England Journal of Medicine, 1995. 333(4): 201-5.

105. Tzivoni, D., Banai, S., Schuger, C., et al, Treatment of Torsades de pointes with magnesium sulfate. Circulation, 1988. 77:392-397.

106. Lang, R.M., Fellner, S.M., Neumann, A., et al, Left Ventricular contractility varies directly with blood calcium. Ann. Int. Med., 1988. 108:525-529.

107. Wesley, R.C., Haines, D.E., Lerman, B.B., et al, Effect of intravenous magnesium sulfate on Supraventricular tachycardia. Amer. J. Cardiol., 1989. 63:1129-31.

108. Gupta, A., Lawrence, A.T., Krishnan, K., Current concepts in the mechanisms and management of drug-induced QT prolongation and torsades de pointes. Amer. Heart J., 2007. 153:891-899.

109. Moran, J.L., Gallagher, J., Peakes, et al., Parenteral magnesium sulfate versus amiodarone in the therapy of atrial tachyarrhythmias: a prospective, randomized study. Critical Care Medicine, 1995. 23(11): 1816-24.

110. Cohen, L. and Kitzes, R., Magnesium sulfate and digitalis-toxic arrhythmias. JAMA, 1983. 249(20):. 2808-10.

111. Onalan, O., Crystal, E., Daoulah, A., et al, Meta-analysis of Magnesium Therapy for the Acute Management of Rapid Atrial Fibrillation. Am. J. Cardiol., 2007. 99:1726-32.

112. Ho KM, Sheridan DJ ;Paterson T. Use of intravenous magnesium to treat acute onset atrial fibrillation: a meta-analysis.Heart 2007.93:1433-40

113. Rasmussen, H.S., Norregard P ;Linden EG et al., Intravenous magnesium in acute myocardial infarction. Lancet, 1986. 1(8475):. 234-6.

114. ISIS-4: a randomised factorial trial assessing early oral captopril, oral mononitrate, and intravenous magnesium sulphate in 58,050 patients with suspected acute myocardial infarction. ISIS-4 (Fourth International Study of Infarct Survival) Collaborative Group.[see comment]. Lancet, 1995. 345(8951): p. 669-85.

115. Rowe, B.H., Bretzlaff, J.A., Bourdon, C., et al, Magnesium sulfate for treating exacerbation of acute asthma in the emergency department. The Cochrane Database of Systematic Reviews. 2007. 2.(D001490)

116. Bloch, H., Silverman, R., Mancierje, N., et al Intravenous magnesium sulfate as an adjunct in the treatment of acute asthma. Chest, 1995. 107:1576-81.

117. Green, S.M., Bothrock, S.G., Intravenous magnesium for acute asthma: Failure to decrease emergency treatment duration or need for hospitalisation. Annals of Emergency Medicine, 1992. 21(3):260-5.

118. Silverman, R., Osborne, H., Runge, J., Feldman, J., Scharf, S., Mancherie, N., et al, Magnesium sulfate as an adjunct to standard therapy in acute severe asthma [abstract]. Academic Emergency Medicine, 1996. 3:467-8.

119. Skobeloff, E.M., Spivey, W.H., McNamara, R.M., Greenspoon, L., Intravenous magnesium sulfate for the treatment of acute asthma in the emergency department. JAMA, 1989. 262:1210-3.

120. Tiffany, B.R., Berk, W.A., Todd, I.K., White, S.R., Magnesium bolus or infusion fails to improve expiratory flow in acute asthma exacerbations. Chest, 1993. 104:831-4.

121. Bradshaw, T.A., Matusiewicz, S.P., Crompton, G.K., et al. Intravenous magnesium sulfate provides no additive benefit to standard management in acute asthma. Resp Medicine, 2008. 102:143-9

122. Mohammad, S., Goodacre, S., Intravenous and nebulised magnesium sulfate for acute asthma: systematic review and meta-analysis. Emerg Med. J., 2007. 24:823-830.

123. Skorodin, M.S.,Tenholder MF;Yetter B et al., Magnesium sulfate in exacerbations of chronic obstructive pulmonary disease. Archives of Internal Medicine, 1995. 155(5): p. 496-500.

124. Dohi, K., Otaki H; Seiji S; Tohru A., Magnesium sulfate therapy in patients with acute neuronal damage: The problem of intravenous administration Critical Care Medicine, 2005. 33(3): 698-9.

125. McKee, J.A., Brewer R; Macy GE et al., Analysis of the brain bioavailability of peripherally administered magnesium sulfate: A study in humans with acute brain injury undergoing prolonged induced hypermagnesemia. [see comment]. Critical Care Medicine, 2005. 33(3): p. 661-6.

126. Westermaier TW, Stetter C, Vince GH et al. Prophylactic intravenous magnesium sulfate for treatment of aneurysmal subarachnoid Hemhorrhage randomised, placebo-controlled, clinical study. Crit Care medicine 2010 38:1284-1290

127. Arango, M.F., Mejia-Mantilla, J.H., Magnesium for acute traumatic brain injury. Cochrane Database of Systematic Reviews. (4):CD005400, 2006.

128. Rouse DJ, Hirz DG, Thom E et al. A Randomised, Controlled Trial of Magnesium Sulfate for the Prevention of Cerebral Palsy. New Eng J Med.2008:359: 895-905.

129. Antenatal $MgSO_4$ and Neurologic outcome in Preterm infants: A Systematic Review. Obstetrics and Gynecology. 2009 113:1327-1333.

130. FominVP, Gibbs SG, Vanam R et al. Effect of magnesium sulfate on contractile force and intracellular concentration in pregnant human myometrium. Obstetrics Gynecology.2006 194.:1384-90

131. Touyz, R.M., Magnesium and hypertension. Current Opinion in Nephrology & Hypertension, 2006. 15(2):. 141-4.

132. Schulze, M.B.,Schulz M;Heidmann C et al., Fiber and magnesium intake and incidence of type 2 diabetes: a prospective study and meta-analysis. Archives of Internal Medicine, 2007. 167(9). 956-65.

PHOSPHORUS (P) [1-9] (AW 31).

Phosphorus is unstable, does not exist in free form and is combined with oxygen as phosphate in the body.

Total Body Phosphorus

500gm-800g (20,000-25,000mmol), 80% bone, 9% skeletal muscle, 11% other tissue.

Extracellular fluid 0.1%.

Cell Phosphate

100mmol/L – mainly organic; inorganic= ≈1.0 mmol/L

Serum Phosphate

0.8-1.5mmol/L- 12% protein bound, 5% complexed.

Average intra-extracellular phosphorus ratio ~100-1

Phosphate   Ingestion   1 gm (~30mmol)

Absorption   90% small intestine, 10% loss in stool

Excretion   Glomerular filtration followed by proximal tubular reabsorption— inhibited by parathyroid hormone and FGF23

About 80% of extracellular phosphorus is contained in bone mineral. It is the main intracellular anion. Most cellular phosphorus is organic. Only a minute amount is ionic. This is vital because of its incorporation into ADP to form ATP.(= ≈ 1.0 mmol/L).

Phosphorus is important:

- As the main cellular anion.
- In the structure and strength of bone combined with Ca^{2+}, as hydroxyappatite.

- In energy metabolism involving ATP, NAD^+ (nicotine adenine dinucleotide) and in phosphorylation of glucose, glycogen and other intermediates which require phosphorylation for activity.
- In cell signalling involving cAMP and cGMP (guanosine monophosphate).
- In the structure of DNA and RNA bound to sugars.
- In phosphoproteins and phospholipids, including membrane composition.
- As part of 2:3 disphosphoglycerate in red cells (5mmol/L)—a critical regulator of oxygen disosciation from haemoglobin.
- As a buffer for cell, plasma and urinary acid –base balance.

Inorganic phosphorus has a valence between 1 and 2 depending on arterial blood pH (average 1.8). At arterial blood pH 7.4 the ratio HPO_4^{2-} - $H_2PO_4^-$ is 4:1. [1] Phosphorus should therefore be reported in mmol rather mEq. [10] 1 mmol of phosphate contains 31mg elemental phosphorus; serum phosphorus1 mmol/L=3.1mg phosphorus/dL. [7, 10] Normal serum phosphate is 0.8-1.5mmol/L.

Serum phosphate is composed of organic and inorganic phosphorus. [1] Laboratory tests measure <u>total elemental phosphorus</u>. Inorganic phosphate is composed of 85% free inorganic ions – HPO_4^{2-}, $H_2PO_4^-$ and H_3PO_4 ; approximately 10%-15% is protein bound [7,10] ;and 5% complexed with calcium, magnesium and sodium (Table 1). Serum phosphate, compared to other electrolytes, shows marked fluctuation with age and time during the day. Serum phosphate peaks at night and is lowest at ~ 1100 hours. [1]

Free HPO_4	=0.5 mmol/L	43%
$NaH PO_4$	= 0.33 mmol/L	29%
Free H_2PO_4	= 0.11 mmol/L	10%
Protein bound	= 0.14 mmol/L	12%
$CaHPO_4$	= 0.04 mmol/L	3%
$MgHPO_4$	= 0.03 mmol/L	3%
	————————	
Total	1.15 mmol/ℓ.	

Table 1: Components of plasma phosphate

Phosphorus enters several pools at different rates: injection of radio labelled phosphorus takes several days to transfer to organic phosphate; and there is a several fold variation in the apparent volume of distribution of phosphorus in hypophosphataemic patients.

Ionic calcium and phosphorus exceed their solubility product. [11] Calcification in tissues is prevented by several processes which include matrix Gla protein, gamma carboxyglutamic acid residues [11] and fetuins. [12] These bind calcium and inhibit Ca^{2+} phosphate precipitation. Increase in Ca^{2+} X phosphate product, or hyperphosphataemia itself, are implicated in adverse cardiovascular outcomes, [13, 14] vascular calcification [12, 15, 16] and even aging. [17]

Fetuin-A, (serum 0.4-1.0g/L.), a major component of α_2 globulin, is the most important in preventing Ca^{2+} phosphate‾ precipitation. This is synthesised by hepatocytes, is a powerful inhibitor of hydroxy apatite crystal formation in vitro, stabilises Ca^{2+} phosphate‾ particles, and may be involved in their clearance from tissues. [12]

Alkaline phosphatase promotes mineral deposition in bone [11] by releasing phosphate from bone mineral in the vicinity of bone forming cells; and may control the number and differentiation of osteoclasts.

Phosphorus is tightly regulated by several Na-phosphate cotransporters expressed in microsomal membranes of cells in kidney, intestine and liver. The key transporters in phosphate homeostasis are type 2 – NPT2a, NPT2b and NPT2c. [11, 16- 19] NPT2b is mainly expressed in lungs and small intestine. Type 3 phosphate transporters, which transport phosphate into cells, are widely expressed in tissues and are probably important in bone mineralisation and control of intracellular phosphate concentration. [11, 16, 18]

Phosphorus is essential to meet the demands of bone mineralisation but must be efficiently eliminated during a change in bone mineralisation, diet or Vitamin D excess. Phosphate excretion is vital to prevent vascular and other calcification. Extracellular phosphate is maintained through integration of intestinal absorption, exchange with cells and bone and renal tubular absorption. (Fig 1)

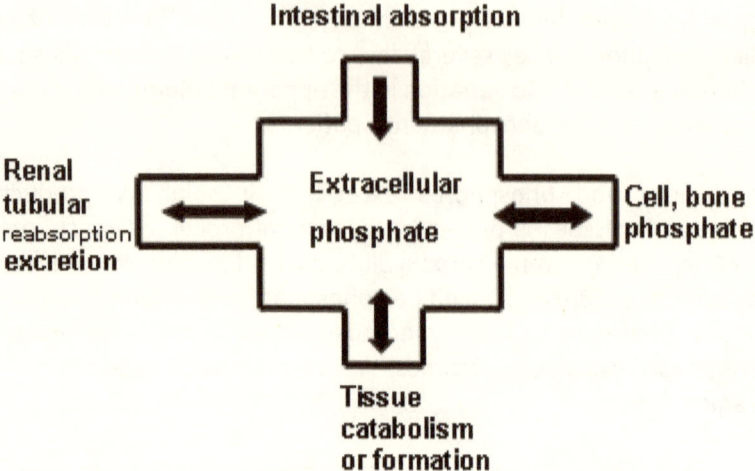

Figure 1. Model of maintenance of extracellular phosphate.

However the main focus of phosphorus homeostasis is to prevent phosphate excess by decreasing renal and intestinal reabsorption.

INTESTINAL ABSORPTION.

The majority of foods contain phosphorus, especially milk, milk products, meat and cereals. Therefore dietary depletion is rare. Dietary phosphorus occurs in both inorganic and organic forms. Most phosphorus in milk is inorganic, as calcium phosphate, whereas most phosphorus in non-dairy sources is organic in the form of phosphoproteins, phospholipids and others.

The small intestine reabsorbs 70-80% of the normal dietary intake of 20-40mmol by the paracellular route or through cells by Na phosphate cotransporters (NPT2b). This is expressed on luminal (apical) membranes of enterocytes. [18, 19] Phosphorus depletion, low dietary intake of phosphorus, [19] $1,25 (OH)_2 D_3$ and low extracellular Ca^{++} increase phosphate absorption whereas hyperphosphataemia decreases absorption. Signals generated in the intestine during phosphorus ingestion signal the kidney to prepare to excrete phosphate: there is an enteric—renal signalling system. [20] Dietary phosphate regulates FGF23 secretion, which alters phosphaturia, and influences I, $25 (OH)_2 D_3$ synthesis. [18, 21]

RENAL PHOSPHATE REABSORPTION. [11, 16, 18, 22, 23]

The unbound fraction, 90% phosphate, is filtered. 80-85% of filtered phosphate is reabsorbed in proximal tubules by sodium phosphate cotransporters, NPT2a [11], the most common, and to a lesser extent

NPT2b and NPT2c. Sodium phosphate cotransporters, normally located in the cytosol, move to cell membranes to carry phosphate with sodium utilising the sodium gradient created by Na^+:K^+ ATPase pumps.

This process requires glycosylsation of NPT2a transporters, proton exchanger regulator factor 1(NHERF1) [18] and suppression of FGF23 to move NPT2a transporters from cytosol to luminal (apical) membranes of proximal tubular cells. [19] NPT2a transporters shift from intracellular vesicles to cell membranes in phosphorus deficiency—or if the dietary phosphate decreases, to enable phosphorus reabsorption. [11, 16, 18 22] Following reabsorption phosphate moves to basolateral membranes and then to circulation down its electro-chemical gradient. (Figure 2)

On the other hand, during a high phosphate diet or hyperphosphatemia, PTH and FGF23 facilitate phosphate excretion by transporting NPT2a transporters from luminal membranes of proximal tubule cells into vesicles in the cytosol for lysosomal destruction. Several other phosphaturic factors, called phosphatonins, are also involved. (Figure 2)

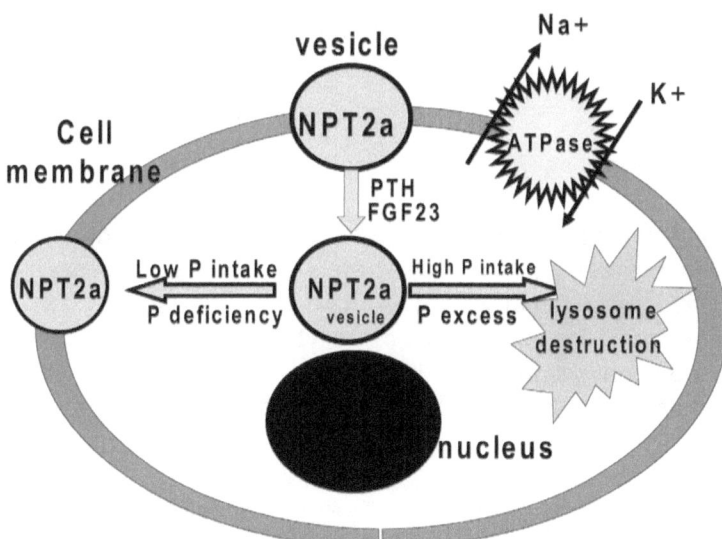

Figure 2: Phosphorus is carried by NPT2a cotransporters from the cell membrane. The transporters are normally contained in vesicles within the cell. A low phosphate diet or phosphate deficiency results in transport of NPT2a vesicles to cell membranes where they increase phosphate reabsorption. PTH and FGF23 cause internalisation of NPT2a transporters by transferring them into vesicles in the cytosol for lysosomal destruction. Thus PTH and FGF23 decrease phosphate reabsorption and enhance phosphaturia.

BONE MODULATION OF SERUM PHOSPHATE LEVELS. [17, 22-25]

Despite the large amount of phosphorous in bone and cells, only a small amount is immediately available to regulate serum phosphate: the small amount of inorganic cell phosphate, 1-2 mmol/L, and that released by osteocytic osteolysis from new bone—a small fraction (1%) of skeletal mass. A bone-renal- parathyroid hormone axis regulates phosphate, calcium and vitamin D homeostasis. Osteocytes pass long dendritic processes within canaliculi which interconnect with one another and form a network with other osteocytes This enables osteocytes to coordinate their response in mineral homeostasis and mineralisation. [22, 24] Osteocytes increase secretion of FGF23 in response to hyperphosphataemia [17,25].Osteocytes and osteoblasts also secrete PHEX (phosphate regulating gene with homology to endopeptidase on X chromosome),Sibling proteins (Small Integrin-Binding Ligand, N-linked Glycoproteins), Dentine Matrix Protein1 (DMP1) and MEPE. These may be involved in the control of mineralisation at the interface of bone surfaces [22-24] and clearance of FGF23.

REGULATION OF PHOSPHATE HOMEOSTASIS (AND CALCIUM) BY GUT, KIDNEY AND BONE IS INTEGRATED BY THREE MAIN HORMONES: PTH, FGF23 AND 1, 25(OH)$_2$D$_3$.

Parathyroid hormone (PTH) binds to PTH-PTHrp receptors to:

- Stimulate osteolysis which increases extracellular Ca^{2+} and phosphate$^-$. PTH activates osteoblasts to secrete RANKL which increases numbers and activity of osteoclasts.
- Stimulate FGF23 synthesis by osteocytes and osteoblasts.
- Increase conversion of 25OHD$_3$ to 1,25(OH)$_2$D$_3$ (calcitriol) by increasing synthesis of 1α hydroxylase in the cortex of renal proximal tubules. 1, 25(OH)$_2$D$_3$ increases both intestinal calcium and phosphate reabsorption.
- Increase Ca^{2+} reabsorption by TRPV5 channels (transient receptor potential vanilloid 5) in distal convoluted tubules.
- Promote phosphaturia by inhibiting transfer of NTPT2a transporters to cell membranes and by regulating Klotho.
- Inhibit intestinal absorption of phosphorus.

The principal action of PTH is to maintain normal extracellular ionised Ca^{2+} concentration in conjunction with 1,25(OH)$_2$D$_3$. Phosphaturia is a secondary process which enables excretion of phosphate released from osteolysis. This prevents increase in the Ca^{2+} x phosphate⁻ product which would otherwise occur.

FGF23 (fibroblast growth factor 23). [17, 18, 22- 25]

FGF23 is the main phosphaturic hormone whereas the phosphaturic action of PTH is secondary to defence of normal extracellular Ca^{2+}. This is crucial to prevent adverse effects of hyperphosphataemia which causes vascular and tissue calcification and even increase in mortality [16-18, 22].

FGF23 is secreted by osteocytes and osteoblasts [17, 18, 22, 24, 25]. Dietary phosphate and extracellular phosphate concentration regulate extracellular FGF23 concentration. [18, 19,21 25] Recall of the actions of FGF23 is facilitated by considering those actions which decrease extracellular phosphate. These are:

1.   Phosphaturia. [17, 18, 22, 23, 25]

2.   Inhibition of 1α hydroxylase. This decreases calcitriol (1:25 (OH)$_2$ D$_3$) synthesis in proximal tubules; and increases synthesis of 24 hydroxylase, an enzyme responsible for calcitriol degradation. This decreases intestinal reabsorption of phosphate and calcium. [17, 18, 22, 23, 24]

3.   Inhibition of parathyroid hormone secretion. [25] This decreases intestinal reabsorption of phosphate and decreases osteolysis.

FGF23 acts on FGF receptor (FGFR1$_C$) in combination with a protein (cofactor) called Klotho. FGF receptor- Klotho complexes form in the kidney, parathyroids, choroid plexus and pituitary. FGF23 binds with higher affinity to the Klotho-FGFR complex than to FGFR or Klotho alone. [25] Therefore disorders of Klotho decrease action of FGF 23.

Paradoxically phosphaturia is induced by FGF23 linking to FGF- Klotho receptor in distal rather than proximal tubules: this signals NaPT2A cotransporters in proximal tubule cells to move from the luminal membrane to the cytosol for destruction [18] and decreases phosphate reabsorption. Klotho is essential for activation of signalling by FGF23 (figure 3).PTH regulates Klotho expression in the kidney.

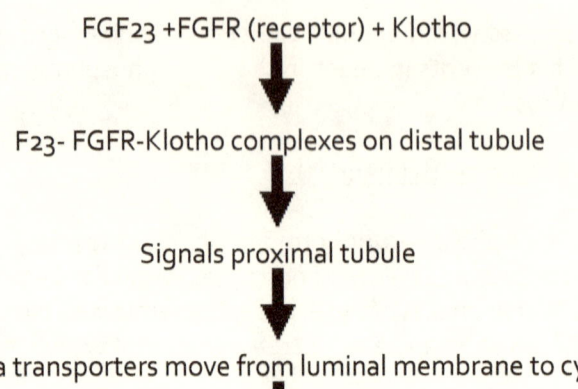

FGF23 +FGFR (receptor) + Klotho

F23- FGFR-Klotho complexes on distal tubule

Signals proximal tubule

NaPT2a transporters move from luminal membrane to cytosol

Decreases renal phosphate absorption

Figure 3. Mechanism of phosphaturia induced by FGF23. PTH regulates Klotho expression in the kidney.

FGF23 acts as a counter regulatory phosphaturic hormone for Vitamin D and coordinates phosphate homeostasis with skeletal mineralisation. Synthesis of FGF23 is stimulated by hyperphosphataemia, dietary phosphate loading and 1, 25$(OH)_2D_3$ and is inhibited by hypophosphataemia.

Vitamin D Metabolites 1, 25$(OH)_2D_3$ (calcitriol).
1, 25$(OH)_2D_3$ acts on Vitamin D receptors (VDR) to:

- Increase intestinal reabsorption of calcium and phosphate.
- Promote mineralisation of bone matrix.
- Inhibit FGF23 and PTH synthesis.
- Increase Ca^{2+} and phosphate mobilisation from bone in conjunction with PTH.
- Augment tubular reabsorption of Ca^{2+} and phosphate.

Synthesis of 1,25$(OH)_2D_3$ by renal cortex is stimulated by both hypocalcaemia and PTH and is inhibited by FGF23.

Calcitonin:

Calcitonin (CT) decreases serum Ca^{2+} slightly by inhibiting bone resorption and increasing excretion of phosphate and calcium independently of PTH.

CONTROL OF PHOSPHATE.

Extracellular phosphate is tightly regulated by bone, kidney and intestine. These are acted on by PTH, calcitriol (1,25 (OH)$_2$ D$_3$ and FGF23 which interact as classical feedback loops.[25] (Figure 4)

Prevention of hyperphosphataemia is crucial for survival.

Raised serum phosphate stimulates secretion of both PTH and FGF23. Both cause phosphaturia by moving NPT2a transporters from membranes of proximal tubule cells into the cytosol for lysosomal destruction. FGF23 suppresses synthesis of 1, 25(OH)$_2$D$_3$ in proximal tubules by inhibiting 1 α hydroxylase.This and PTH decrease intestinal phosphate absorption.

Several other hormones, apart from FGF23, called phosphatonins, lower serum phosphate by decreasing intestinal and renal-tubular phosphate reabsorption. This may be crucial for decreasing calcium phosphate precipitation in tissues.

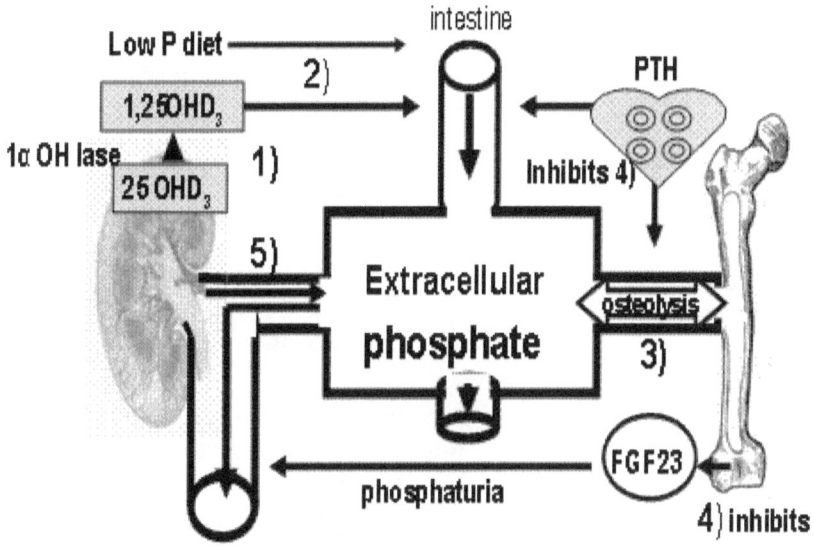

Figure 4: Mechanisms which maintain normal serum phosphate homeostasis. Numbers correspond to text below.

1. Low extracellular phosphate and PTH stimulates synthesis of 1, 25(OH)$_2$D$_3$ from 25OHD$_3$ in renal cortex.

$$25OHD3 \xrightarrow{\text{1αHydroxylase}} 1,25\,(OH)_2D_3$$

2. <u>1,25(OH)2D3</u> and low extracellular phosphate increase intestinal and renal phosphate reabsorption by transferring NPT2 transporters to cell membranes.
3. <u>Osteolysis</u> is stimulated by PTH, hypophosphataemia and $1,25(OH)_2D_3$. This increases serum phosphate.
4. Low serum phosphate inhibits PTH and FGF23 secretion.
5. PTH and FGF23 increase phosphate reabsorption in proximal tubules by moving NPT2a transporters from the cytosol to cell membranes.

HYPOPHOSPHATAEMIA.

Hypophosphataemia may be acute or chronic. The causes of acute hypophosphataemia are shown in table 2.

Intracellular shift.	Alkalosis, especially respiratory. Insulin and glucose infusion. Familial Periodic Paralysis.
Diminished intake.	Alimentation without phosphate. Breast milk feeding.
Diminished absorption.	Phosphate binders, diarrhoea,
Increased Renal Excretion.	Alcoholism, Diabetic Ketoacidosis Diuretics Metabolic acidosis
Increased requirements.	Nutritional recovery syndrome Rapid reformation of tissue e.g. rhabdomyolysis. Rapid formation of bone.
Seriously ill.	Unknown : probably due to several causes; especially gram negative sepsis. Toxic shock syndrome.
Complexing.	Pancreatitis,

Table 2:   *Causes of Acute Hypophosphataemia.*

ACUTE HYPOPHOSPHATAEMIA.

Intracellular phosphate shift (internal shifts).

There is a poor correlation between acute hypophosphataemia and phosphate depletion because of transcellular fluxes of phosphate. Therefore hypophosphataemia does not necessarily indicate that phosphate depletion is present or if present severe. [1, 3, 5, 6, 8].

The most important causes of transfer of phosphorus from the extracellular to intracellular compartment are alkalosis, especially respiratory alkalosis,[1-6, 26] glucose infusion or treatment with insulin. [1-6] The extent to which insulin shifts glucose into cells depends on the amount of glycolysis: 1 mole of glucose binds 4 moles of potassium phosphate during phosphorylation. [27] Alkalosis, especially respiratory alkalosis, activates intracellular glycolysis: the phosphorylation of carbohydrate shifts extracellular phosphate into cells.

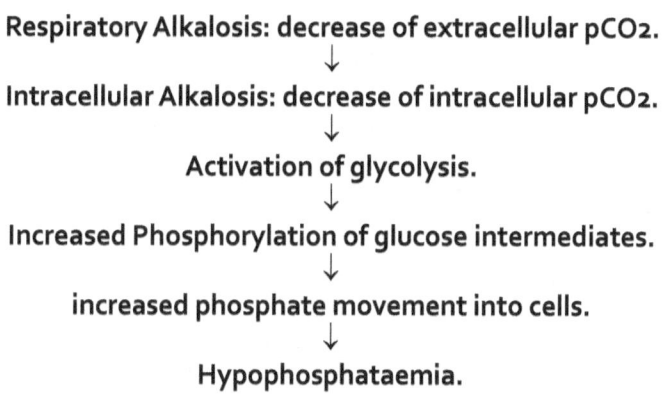

Respiratory Alkalosis: decrease of extracellular pCO2.
↓
Intracellular Alkalosis: decrease of intracellular pCO2.
↓
Activation of glycolysis.
↓
Increased Phosphorylation of glucose intermediates.
↓
increased phosphate movement into cells.
↓
Hypophosphataemia.

Figure 5. Mechanism of Hypophosphataemia during alkalosis.

A more pronounced fall follows fructose infusion because phosphate is trapped within hepatocytes following phosphorylation, as fructose 1 phosphate. This is clinically significant in Congenital Fructose intolerance and intravenous fructose infusion. High dietary fructose increases loss of phosphate in urine.

Moderate hypophosphataemia is common in hospitalised patients [28-31] but its importance is uncertain. Moderate and severe hypophosphataemia are more common in seriously ill patients, including those in Intensive Care Units [29, 32] and seriously ill patients in Emergency Departments. [33]

The most common causes of severe acute hypophosphataemia are alcoholism, rapid reformation of tissue, the recovery phase of diabetic ketoacidosis, severe burns and in seriously ill patients from several causes.

Seriously ill patients.

Seriously ill patients, especially in Emergency Departments [33] and Intensive care units, [32] frequently develop both severe hypophosphatemia and hypocalcaemia. The clinical importance and causes are uncertain but may include phosphaturia from cell breakdown, metabolic acidosis, and hyperparathyroidism secondary to hypocalcaemia, glucose administration and respiratory alkalosis. Acute pancreatitis causes hypocalcaemia and hypophosphataemia due to complexing of Ca^+ and phosphate with fatty acids.

Diabetic ketoacidosis. [34, 35]

Normal or raised serum phosphate levels usually occur on presentation. [34] Following treatment hypophosphataemia often develops [35] but uncommonly requires treatment. Hypophosphataemia is due to previous phosphate depletion from phosphaturia secondary to acid excretion with titratable buffers; phosphorylation of glucose from glycolysis; glycogen reformation; the action of insulin; and rapid reformation of tissue.

Rapid reformation of tissue

Cellular concentrations of phosphate and potassium are 100 and 150mmol/L respectively. Rhabdomyolysis [8, 36-39] initially causes loss of muscle K^+, Mg^{2+} and phosphate which may cause hyperphosphatemia and hyperkalaemia. Phosphate, potassium and magnesium are then excreted. Hypophosphatemia and hypokalemia may develop in the recovery phase when muscle is repaired or reformed [36-39]. Common causes are alcoholism, seizures, and muscle compression.

Refeeding without phosphate in malnourished subjects, [1-6, 40], including those with Anorexia nervosa, [41] has caused severe hypophosphataemia and even death. Rapid formation of cells, following blast crisis in leukaemia or lymphoma, and reformation of skin following severe burns [8] may cause hypophosphataemia.

Bone formation

The rapid reformation of bone, following removal of a parathyroid adenoma and the initial treatment of Ricketts or Osteomalacia with Vitamin D or Calcitriol, can cause both hypocalcaemia and hypophosphataemia. An unusual cause of hypophosphataemia, due to rapid formation of tissue, occurs in breast fed premature infants because breast milk contains a low phosphorus concentration. [42]

Alcoholism. [1-6, 8, 9, 43]

Hypophosphataemia is common in hospitalised alcoholics in 29% in one observational study [43]. Multiple causes are considered responsible: phosphaturia, respiratory alkalosis, diarrhoea and vomiting, glucose infusions, poor intake and antacids. [43]

Multiple rather than a single cause are responsible for acute hypophosphataemia in most cases: malnutrition, inadequate phosphate intake, rapid formation of tissue, glucose infusions, respiratory alkalosis, starvation ketoacidosis causing phosphaturia, increased catecholamine secretion and high PTH levels secondary to hypocalcaemia.

Hypophosphataemia is frequently accompanied by hypocalcaemia, hypokalaemia and hypomagnesaemia.

In conclusion severe hypophosphataemia occurs in refeeding malnourished subjects without phosphorus supplementation; the recovery phase of ketoacidosis and burns; in alcoholics; in severely ill patients from multiple causes; in severe respiratory alkalosis; and in those taking phosphate binding agents.

CHRONIC HYPOPHOSPHATAEMIA (table 3).

Decreased Phosphate Absorption. [1-6, 44,]

Aluminium [1, 5, 44] and magnesium containing antacids form insoluble salts with phosphate causing its malabsorption. [44] Indeed Lotz [9] used aluminium antacids to produce experimental hypophosphataemia. This occurs in those taking antacids for acid neutralisation or for chronic renal disease. Conditions causing malabsorption and diarrhoea cause increased losses of Na^+, K^+, HCO_3^-, Ca^{2+} and phosphate. Hypophosphataemia becomes apparent following rehydration and repletion of K^+. This is common when Protein –calorie malnutrition (Kwashiorkor) is associated.

DECREASED PHOSPHATE ABSORPTION.
Aluminium containing antacids, calcium carbonate, other phosphate binders.
Malabsorption, diarrhoea.

RENAL CAUSES:
Primary hyperparathyroidism.
Secondary hyperparathyroidism -Vitamin D disorders.
Tertiary hyperparathyroidism. Post renal transplant hypophosphataemia.
Increased secretion of PTHrP.
Increased extracellular FGF23 levels.
Defective NPT2 transporters—rare.
Diuretics, proximal tubular disorders.

Table 3: *Causes of chronic hypophosphataemia.*

Primary hyperparathyroidism causes hypercalcaemia and hypophosphataemia secondary to phosphaturia

Secondary hyperparathyroidism This is due to vitamin D disorders. The dominant disturbance initially is low serum phosphate but low normal or slightly low serum Ca^+ because secondary hyperparathyroidism increases serum Ca^{2+} and decreases serum phosphate. The causes are shown in Table 4. (chapter 10)

Vitamin D deficiency	-	Decreased sunlight
	-	Nutritional rickets
Low 25(OH) D3	-	Liver disease
Decreased renal conversion of 25(OH)D$_3$ to 1,25(OH)D$_3$	-	renal disease,
	-	1α hydroxylase deficiency
Resistance to 1, 25(OH) D3)	-	receptor defect

Table 4: Vitamin D disorders causing Hypophosphataemia

DISORDERS OF FGF23 [18, 22, 23, 45-50] (Figure 6)

Disorders of FGF23 are due to increased secretion of FGF23 by osteocytes or decreased destruction.

Increased FGF23 levels cause hypophosphataemia by the following process (figure 6):

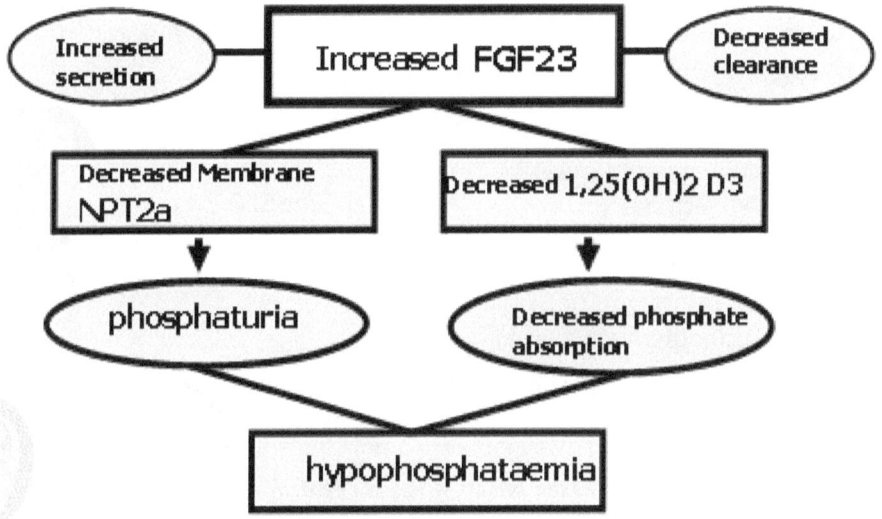

Figure 6. *Hypophosphataemia resulting from increased FGF23*

Decreased Destruction. [18, 22- 24, 45]

Several ligands play a role in clearance of FGF23.Mutations involving some of these may decrease clearance and cause elevated serum FGF23 levels. PHEX is a phosphorus regulating gene (Phosphate with Homology for Endopeptidase on X chromosome), expressed predominantly in osteoblasts, osteocytes and odontoblasts. Mutations are associated with an increase in serum levels of FGF23.

SIBLING (Small Integrin Binding Ligand N Linked Glycoproteins), DMPM1 (Dentin matrix protein 1), MPE, DSPP and osteopontin play key roles in mineralisation of bone and dentition.

Loss of function mutations of PHEX and DMPM1 are associated with decrease in destruction of FGF23 and cause increased serum levels of FGF23.Disorders causing increased serum levels of FGF23 are shown in the following table. [18, 22, 23]

<u>Tumour induced Osteomalacia.</u>	Overproduction of FGF 23 by tumour
<u>Rickets, osteomalacia.</u>	
X-Linked Hypophosphatemic.	Mutation of PHEX gene impairs clearance of FGF23.
Autosomal Dominant Hypophosphataemic Ricketts.	Mutation of FGF23 causing impaired clearance.
Autosomal Recessive Hypophosphatemic Ricketts.	Increased production of FGF23 due to a Mutation of DMPI.
Hereditary Hypophosphataemic Ricketts with hypercalciuria.	Abnormal Gene SLC34A3.
<u>Chronic Kidney Disease.</u>	
<u>Post Renal Transplantation</u> Hypophosphataemia. [47]	
McClure Albright Syndrome and fibrous dysplasia.	? ↑ FGF3 synthesis from fibrous dysplasia tissue.

Table 5: Disorders of increased serum FGF23 concentration. [18, 22-24, 45, 50]

Low FGF23 levels, due to increased destruction, from a mutation of FGF23 binding protein or GALNT3, probably cause tumoral calcinosis.

<u>Tumour induced osteomalacia.</u> [45, 46]

There are 2 main causes of hypophosphatemia resulting from tumours.

<u>PTHrP (PTH related protein)</u> stimulates the PTH receptor in a similar manner to PTH. It is normally secreted by many tissues, including the placenta, and during lactation. Several tumours, especially sqamous cell carcinoma, also secrete PTHrP. This causes hypercalcemia and hypophosphatemia.

<u>Tumour (Oncogenic) Osteomalacia.</u> [45 46,]

FGF23 is considered to be the main cause although other phosphaturic factors have been implicated less commonly. High levels of the FGF23 gene are expressed in tumour tissue. The most common are slowly growing mesenchymal tumours, especially haemangiopericytomas,

(70-80%). Surgical removal cures hypophosphataemia.Serum phosphate is characteristically very low but serum calcium normal. FGF23 decreases reabsorption of phosphate and hydroxylation of 25(OH) D_3 by inhibiting synthesis of 1α hydroxylase. This causes osteomalacia. [45] 1, 25 (OH$_2$) D_3 is inappropriately normal or low and PTH normal. Profound muscle weakness, bone pain and fatigue result. This may be mistaken for adult onset autosomal dominant Hypophosphataemic Ricketts. A previously normal serum phosphate helps exclude Hypophosphataemic Ricketts.

Several other phosphatonins besides FGF23 are associated with oncogenic osteomalacia. Other proximal tubular defects such as glucosuria and amino-aciduria may accompany phosphaturia.

Chronic kidney disease and post transplant patients. [45, 47-49]

The cause of post transplantation hypophosphataemia is uncertain but an increase in FGF23 has been suggested as a cause of both hypophosphataemia and bone disorders. Serum FGF23 commonly increases over 100 times in dialysis patients. [48] This decreases synthesis of 1, 25(OH)$_2$ D_3 and increases PTH secretion which causes phosphaturia. Mortality in chronic kidney disease is linearly correlated with serum FGF23 levels. [48]

Hypophosphatemic rickets due to increased FGF23 [18, 23, 45]

X Linked Hypophosphataemic Rickets. [18, 23, 45]

This is probably due to inactivating mutations of PHEX gene (phosphate regulating gene) and results in increased FGF23 levels either from increased synthesis or decreased clearance. PHEX is predominantly expressed in osteoblasts, osteocytes and odontoblasts and probably normally inactivates FGF23. [45]

An increase in FGF23 increases phosphaturia and causes hypophosphataemia.

Affected children are of short stature, suffer bone pain, fractures, lower extremity deformity, tooth abscesses, and calcification of tendinous insertions, ligaments and joint capsules [45]. Diagnosis is established by genetic testing of PHEX and FGF23 genes. This is treated by phosphate 1g 4 times daily and calcitriol 1-3µg/day. [45]

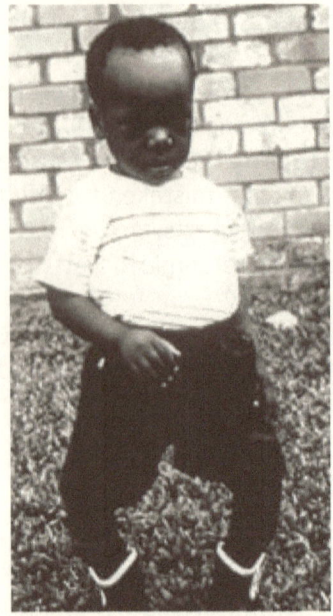

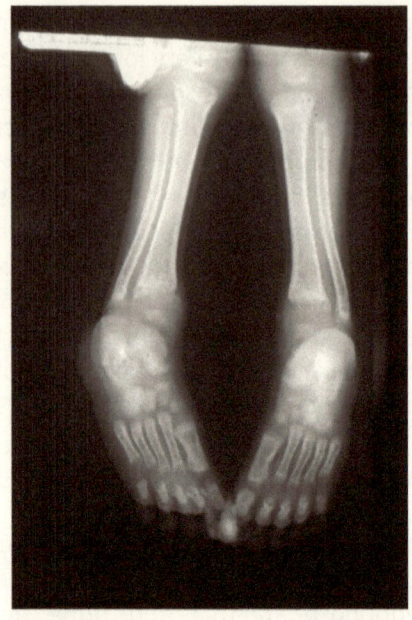

Note: Frontal bossing of skull, Genu valgum and Coxa vara; relative upper limb sparing and normal nutrition.

Note: Demineralization, wide zone of provisional calcification and wide metaphysis

Figure 7: X-linked Hypophosphataemic Ricketts.

<u>Autosomal dominant Hypophosphatemic Ricketts</u>– This is similar to X linked Ricketts in clinical expression but is due to activating mutations of the FGF23 gene. [45].Mutations involve the cleavage site- RXR region of FGF23 which causes resistance to proteolytic cleavage.

<u>Autosomal recessive Hypophosphatemic Ricketts</u> Mutations of the gene controlling Dentin Matrix Protein1 (DMP1) are characterised by increased levels of defective FGF23 and cause hypophosphataemia and bone demineralisation.

Increase in FGF23 is implicated in the pathogenesis of <u>Fibrous Dysplasia</u> and <u>McCune-Albright syndrome</u> [45]. FGF23 is expressed in fibrous dysplasia tissue. [45]

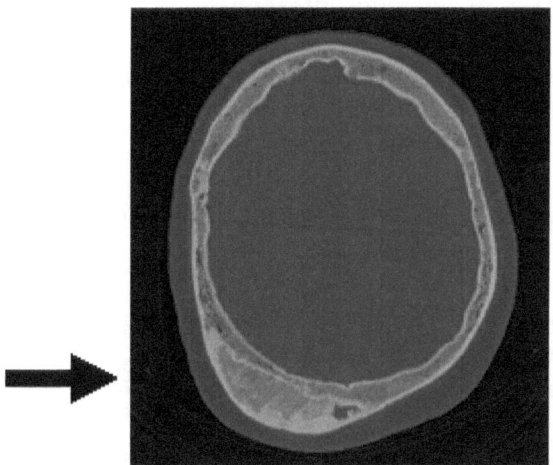

Figure 8. Skull showing Fibrous Dysplasia.

Disorders of sodium phosphate- NPT2 cotransporters.

Renal stones are promoted if function of sodium-phosphate cotransporters is impaired. Water reabsorption in descending loops of Henle increases tubular phosphate and Ca^+ concentration. Phosphate precipitation is promoted if phosphate reabsorption is decreased from disorders of NaPT2 cotransporters. This is facilitated by the abundance of mucopolysaccharides in descending loops which promotes crystallisation. [50]

NaPT2a sodium-phosphate cotransporters. [50,51]

Heterozygous mutations in the gene controlling NPT2a may be responsible for urinary phosphate wasting, urolithiasis and hypophosphataemia.

NaPT2c cotransporter. Hereditary Hypophosphataemic Ricketts with Hypercalciuria. (45, 50)

This is similar to X-linked Hypophosphataemic Ricketts but affected persons show hypercalciuria due to increased levels of $1, 25 (OH)_2 D_3$ and renal stones. The condition was first described in Bedouin families in Saudi Arabia and is probably due to a mutation of the gene, SLC34A3, controlling NaPT2c phosphate transporters. This causes phosphaturia, calcium stones and bone demineralisation. [45, 50] Administration of phosphate results in complete remission.

NPT2b. loss of function causes pulmonary microlithiasis.

Other rare causes of hypophosphataemia.

NHERF1. (Na:H exchanger) regulation factor: loss of function causes similar manifestations to defective function of NPT2a transporters and causes hypophosphataemia, nephrolithiasis and bone demineralisation.

Hyperaldosteronism, Idiopathic hypercalciuria and Wilson's disease are rare causes of phosphaturia.

Proximal tubular abnormalities such as in Fanconi's syndrome or rarely Multiple Myeloma [52] may cause chronic phosphate depletion due to phosphaturia.

ACUTE MANIFESTATIONS OF HYPOPHOSPHATAEMIA.

There is consensus that moderate hypophosphataemia and some cases of severe hypophosphataemia, due to transcellular flux, are often asymptomatic and that there is a poor correlation between serum phosphate levels and symptoms. Lotz [9] reported that symptoms such as fatigue, muscle weakness, bone pain and anorexia only developed when serum phosphate levels decreased below 0.3mmol/L in normal subjects made hypophosphatemic with low phosphate diets plus antacids. Severe hypophosphataemia has been reported to cause the following manifestations (table 6):

Heart Failure, decreased myocardial function, arrhythmias. [1, 53-56]

Respiratory failure or failure of ventilator weaning. [1, 58-63]. Decreased oxygen delivery secondary to low 2:3 DPG. [1, 64, 65]

Muscle weakness and proximal myopathy. [1, 66-70]

Neurological dysfunction—coma, seizures, confusion, tremors, dysphagia. [1, 8, 9, 35, 66-70]

Decreased white cell, platelet function and haemolysis. [1, 71, 72]

Table 6: *Common manifestations due to hypophosphataemia.*

However evidence for reported manifestations is of variable quality, usually based on one or few case reports, which may have been due to comorbid diseases or other electrolyte abnormalities which were often present. Thus both the incidence and importance of reported manifestations have not been established.

Myocardial dysfunction. [1, 53-56]

The best evidence for myocardial dysfunction resulting from hypophosphataemia is the improvement in ventricular stroke work and pulmonary wedge pressure which occurs in severely hypophosphataemic subjects following phosphate infusion. [53]

Improvement in haemodynamic variables occurred in association with rapid correction of hypophosphataemia in 3 studies. [53-56] However low ionised calcium and metabolic alkalosis, which cause low ionised calcium, were not excluded in these and other reports. Treatment of diseases associated with hypophosphataemia may have been responsible for improvement rather than phosphorus replacement. In several reports low ionised Ca^{2+}, either from hypocalcaemia or metabolic alkalosis which decreases cardiac contractility, [57] was not excluded. Left ventricular contractibility varies directly with serum ionised calcium [57] and decreases from hypocalcaemia.

Respiratory manifestations. [1, 58-63]

Hypophosphataemia impairs diaphragm contractility [60] and decreases red blood cell 2.3 DPG (disphosphoglycerate) concentration [8, 64, 65]. This decreases offloading of oxygen to tissues, and in combination with muscular weakness from hypophosphataemia, may cause respiratory failure. Respiratory failure, which improved following phosphate infusion, and failure of weaning [63] have been attributed to hypophosphataemia.

Neurological manifestations. [1, 5, 8,9,35, 66-70]

These include coma [1, 3, 66], seizures, [1, 67] peripheral neuropathy, [35] myopathy, [1,5, 8, 70] rhabdomyolysis, [1,5,9] tremor, confusion, hallucinations [68,69] and manifestations mimicking Wernicke's encephalopathy.[9,68] Underlying disease, such as alcoholism, alkalosis, or low ionised Ca^{2+} may have been responsible rather than hypophosphataemia in several reports.

Haematological manifestations. [71, 72]

Acute haemolytic anaemia [71], due to increased rigidity of red cells, acquired phagocytic [72] and platelet dysfunction, have been reported but their clinical importance has not been established.

Glucose intolerance.[73] due to insulin resistance, which improved following phosphorus repletion, has been reported.

CHRONIC HYPOPHOSPHATAEMIA.

The main manifestations are Ricketts or osteomalacia, bone pain, muscle weakness[74, 75] and fatigue. In chronic hypophosphatemia proximal muscle weakness and bone pain may be due to hypophosphatemia, increased PTH secretion, changes in extracellular calcium or $1,25 (OH)_2 D_3$.

HYPERPHOSPHATAEMIA

Hypoparathyroidism : genetic and acquired.

Pseudohypoparathyroidism.

Renal Failure.

Iatrogenic: intravenous or oral phosphate, cow's milk in neonatal tetany, phosphate enemas, intravenous bisphosphonates, milk alkali syndrome.

Suicidal phosphorus ingestion.

Vitamin D intoxication

Bisphosphonates.

Cell Lysis in the initial phase of Rhabdomyolysis and other massive cell breakdown eg: leukaemia, malignant hyperthermia, severe acidosis, severe haemolysis and burns.

Respiratory Acidosis—malignant hyperthermia. Acromegaly.

Rare genetic disorders.

Loss of function of FGF23:.	familial Tumoral Calcinosis (rare).
Loss of function of Klotho:	hyperphosphataemia, ectopic calcification.
Loss of function of GALNT3:	Familial Tumoral Calcinosis.

Table 7: *Causes of Hyperphosphataemia.*

Pseudohyperphosphataemia [76] from serum monoclonal immunoglobulin occurs in multiple myeloma and in vitro haemolysis.

Physiological Hyperphosphataemia [77]. At the end of exercise plasma phosphate, K^+ and H^+ increase.

The most common causes (Table 7) are decreased renal function and hypoparathyroidism which are differentiated by the serum creatinine and clinical features (chapter 10).

Endocrine causes.

A decrease in phosphorus excretion and hyperphosphataemia rarely occurs in Acromegaly and bisphosphonate therapy.

Massive cell lysis [36-40] from rhabdomyolysis, tumour cell lysis following chemotherapy, hyperthermia and overwhelming infection, liberates phosphorus from cells (cellular phosphate 100mmol/L) and may cause hyperphosphataemia prior to excretion, especially if renal failure is present.

Renal failure. (chapter 10)

Familial Tumoral Calcinosis is a rare condition due to mutations causing decreased secretion of FGF23. Mutations involve the FGF23 gene or GALNT3 which control glycosylation and the effectiveness of FGF23. [45] Affected patients develop hyperphosphataemia, vascular calcification, lobulated periarticular calcification and increased serum $1, 25(OH)_2 D_3$ levels despite low serum PTH levels. [18, 45]

IATROGENIC.

Oral Sodium Phosphate for Bowel Endoscopy Preparation. [78, 79]

Oral sodium phosphate solution is used for bowel preparation for endoscopy: 90mL contains 43.2g monobasic sodium phosphate and 16.2g dibasic sodium phosphate giving a total of 11.52g of elemental phosphate. This can cause hyperphosphataemia, acute and chronic renal failure [78, 79] and may be as nephrotoxic as intravenous contrast media. [79] Acute renal failure is especially common in those with underlying renal disease.

Intravenous phosphate infusion.

This was more common in the past when excessive amounts of phosphate were used in treatment of hypophosphataemia. A precipitous fall in serum calcium can occur from phosphate infusion. [80]

Bisphosphonates.

Probably cause hyperphosphataemia by increasing tubular reabsorption of phosphate. This is most marked from therapy with etidronate [81] and may cause hypocalcaemia.

MANIFESTATIONS OF HYPERPHOSPHATEMIA:

Hypocalcaemia is the most important. However there is increasing recognition of the potential for other adverse effects. Chronic elevation of extracellular phosphate increases Ca^{2+} x phosphate product and promotes vascular and tissue calcification. [12, 13, 15, 16, 18, 82] Phosphorus has been implicated in vascular calcification and mortality in end stage renal failure, [13-16, 81] diabetes and cardiovascular disease. [13-16, 18] Phosphorus is the major factor in mineralisation of extracellular matrix. [22]

Phosphorus uptake occurs in vascular smooth muscle cells by Pit1, type 3 NaPT transporters. [12, 15-18] Mortality in end stage renal disease is linearly correlated with serum phosphate levels. [82] Cardiovascular mortality is 10-20 times higher than in the general population and is related to serum phosphorus levels. [18, 82] Serum phosphorus is tightly controlled by a large number of phosphatonins (which cause phosphaturia) including FGF23, the most important, PTH and several others.

Klotho, named after the Greek goddess who spun the web of life, is an important cofactor for FGF23 which binds to its receptor in renal distal tubules. The effectiveness of FGF23 in causing phosphaturia is decreased in its absence. [17] This results in hyperphosphataemia, an increase in the Ca^{2+} x phosphate product[17] and an increase in concentration of $1, 25(OH)_2 D_3$. Mice with a genetic defect in Klotho develop vascular calcification, premature ageing and death.

APPROACH TO SERUM PHOSPHATE ABNORMALITIES.

In the majority the cause is apparent from the history.

Blood sampling variation: Serum phosphate increases when tourniquets are applied and following a meal.

Circadian variation: serum phosphate shows marked variations during the time of day that blood is sampled: it is lowest in the morning and maximum at night.

HYPERPHOSPHATAEMIA.

Spurious hyperphosphataemia occurs from exercise during blood sampling; following high phosphorus containing meals ; or from serum monoclonal immunoglobulin's. [76]

The serum creatinine differentiates the 2 most common causes: renal failure and hypoparathyroidism. The serum creatinine is raised in acute renal failure, rhabdomyolysis and occasionally in tumour lysis.

HYPOPHOSPHATAEMIA.

- Look at serum calcium A high level suggests the diagnosis of hyperparathyroidism or PTHrp secreting tumour. Consider Measurement of serum PTHrp if the serum PTH level is inappropriately low and diagnosis uncertain.
- If serum Ca^{2+} is low or low normal consider the diagnosis of secondary hyperparathyroidism due to $1,25(OH_2)D_3$ deficiency, in any part of the synthetic pathway from Vitamin D_3 to $1, 25 (OH)_2 D_3$. Consider measurement of serum $25 (OH) D_3$ in elderly patients. (chapter 10)
- If serum Ca^{2+} is normal and serum phosphate severely decreased on several occasions consider measuring serum FGF23 to diagnose tumoral hypophosphataemia (oncogenic osteomalacia), hypophosphatemic Ricketts or osteomalacia.

Urine phosphate is low in gastrointestinal losses, inadequate diet and internal redistribution. High urine phosphate is present before treatment of diabetic ketoacidosis, Fanconi's syndrome and in recovery from renal failure. Suspect Hypophosphataemia during:

- Rhabdomyolysis, the recovery phase of diabetic ketoacidosis, burns, during respiratory alkalosis, seriously ill patients and recovery from malnutrition.
- Patients with hypokalaemia, hypocalcaemia and hypomagnesaemia.

TREATMENT OF HYPOPHOSPHATAEMIA

Hypophosphataemia may not be associated with phosphate depletion. Moderate hypophosphataemia rarely requires treatment with intravenous phosphate except in the setting of rapid reformation of tissue during parenteral nutrition. Intravenous treatment with phosphorus presents a dilemma for 3 reasons:

- Only a small fraction of the total body phosphate is inorganic—approximately 35-40mmol; phosphorus enters several pools at highly variable rates; takes several days to transform to organic phosphate; and moderate hypophosphataemia may occur transiently due to transcellular flux.
- The precise risk from hypophosphataemia is uncertain. It is often difficult to attribute symptoms to hypophosphataemia in seriously ill patients.
- Phosphorus infusion may cause complications.

The risk versus benefit of phosphate infusion is uncertain. Although the clinical importance of severe hypophosphataemia has not been established it seems reasonable to treat patients with serum phosphate <0.3mmol/L or who show symptoms compatible with phosphate depletion.

There are several hazards which result from intravenous infusion:

- Hyperphosphataemia and rarely hyperkalaemia may develop from potassium phosphate infusion. [81, 83]
- Hypocalcaemia, secondary to hyperphosphataemia from phosphate infusion, [81, 83, 84] may cause hypotension, cardiac dysfunction and neuromuscular irritability.
- Precipitation of calcium and phosphate [83-85] may cause metastatic calcification.
- Renal dysfunction. [85]

Large amounts of phosphate were inappropriately infused in the past due to misleading published information and caused the manifestations described above.

Vannatta [86] evaluated intravenous infusion of 9 mmol potassium phosphate given over 12 hours in severely hypophosphataemic patients. However serum phosphate levels remained below 0.42mmol/L in fifty percent of their patients.

Kingston and Al Sibai [87] infused 10-15mmol phosphate intravenously with an infusion pump over 4 hours to 31 consecutive patients with severe hypophosphataemia. (Figure 8)

The initial serum phosphorus rose from a mean of 0.28mmol/L to 0.74mmol/L at the end of the infusion. Individual results are shown in figure 8. Initial serum phosphorus at end of infusion and 8-12 hours following infusion are shown. There was no significant change in mean serum calcium, potassium or blood pressure during the infusion. One patient showed transient deterioration of renal function.

On average 0.25mmol/kg of phosphorus infused increased the serum phosphorus by 0.38mmol/L. No patients showed neuromuscular irritability or hypotension during the infusion.

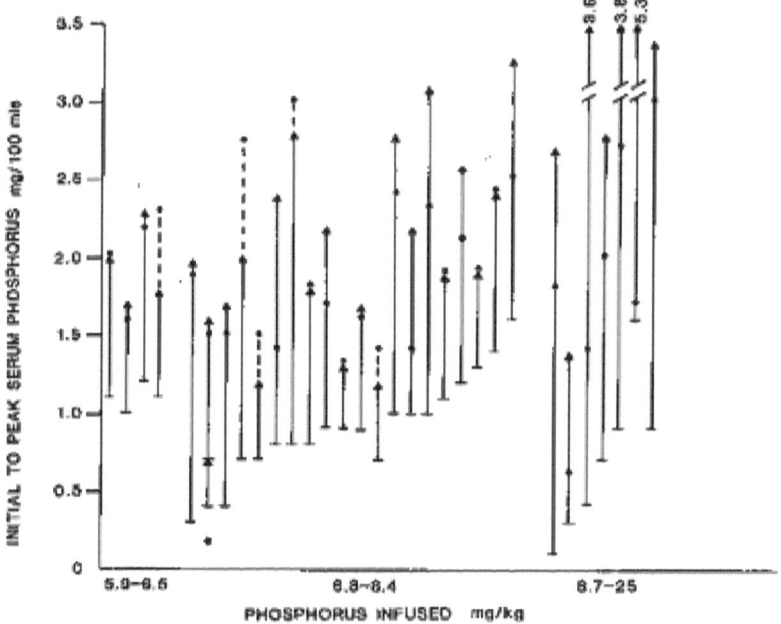

Figure.8 Showing the initial and peak (arrow heads) serum phosphate (mg/dL) 8-12 hours following infusion of phosphorus [87]. (Copyright Wolters Kluwer /Lippincott,Williams & Wilkins. By permission.)

Rosen et al [88] infused 15mmol sodium phosphate in 0.9% sodium chloride over 2 rather than 4 hours in 11 patients with serum phosphorus levels between 0.51-0.61mmol/L. Serum phosphorus increased between 0.74-1.7mmol/L. Thus they infused the same amount of phosphorus in only 2 hours but in less severely hypophosphatemic patients. Phosphorus infusion was repeated if serum phosphorus remained less than 0.65mmol/L six hours following the infusion. Although hypocalcaemia, on average, was absent ionised calcium levels and individual serum calcium results were not reported.

Ionised calcium, often low in severely ill patients, may decrease further following infusion of phosphate and cause adverse effects.

The amount of phosphorus required for correction of hypophosphataemia is highly variable and is probably greater when hypophosphataemia is of long compared to short duration and when multiple causes are responsible, rather than a single cause, such as from glucose infusion.

Based on published information and subsequent experience, I recommend an infusion of 10-15mmol of sodium or potassium phosphate, depending on patient size, over 4-6 hours, to seriously ill patients with serum phosphorus levels of 0.3mmol/L or less. This can be repeated based on remeasurement of serum phosphorus. However caution should be exercised in patients with ionised hypocalcaemia. If possible phosphate should be administered orally. It is essential to prescribe phosphorus in mmol/L because of the variation of mEq with pH. [9]

Oral phosphate.

Phosphorus should be prescribed orally, if practical, in milk (=1g 33mmol /L; or as tablets. Oral phosphate (Sandoz) contains 500 mg (16.1 mmol) phosphate, 20.4 mmol Na and 3.1 mmol K per tablet.

TREATMENT of HYPERPHOSPHATEMIA.(Chapter 10).

REFERENCES

General

1. Knochel JP, Agarwal R. Hypophosphatemia and hyperphosphatemia. p1086-1132. In: Brenner BM, ed. Brenner and Rector's the kidney. 5th ed. Philadelphia: WB Saunders, 1996:
2. Popovtzer MM. Disorders of calcium, phosphorus, vitamin D and parathyroid hormone activity.p 216-277. In: Schrier RW, ed. Renal and electrolyte disorders. 6th ed. Philadelphia: Lippincott Williams & Wilkins, 2003:

3. Kayne LH, Pham P-CT, Pham P-TT, Lee DB. Phosphate metabolism. p355-379 In: Massry & Glassock's Textbook of Nephrology. Massry SG, Glassock RJ, eds. 4th ed. Philadelphia: Lippincott Williams & Wilkins, 2001.

4. Bringhurst FR, Demay MB, Kronenberg HM. Hormones and disorders of mineral metabolism 1192-1195. Bringhurst FR, Demay MB, Kronenberg HM. Disorders of phosphate metabolism. p1155-1210. In: William's textbook of endocrinology. Wilson JD, Foster DW, Kronenberg HM, Larsen PR, Eds. 9th ed. Philadelphia: WB Saunders. 1998:

5. Knochel JP. The pathophysiology and clinical characteristics of severe hypophosphatemia. *Archives of Internal Medicine* 1977; **137**(2):203-20.

6. Gaasbeek A, Meinders AE. Hypophosphatemia: an update on its etiology and treatment. *American Journal of Medicine* 2005; **118**(10):1094-101.

7. Lentz RD, Brown DM, Kjellstrand CM. Treatment of severe hypophosphatemia. *Annals of Internal Medicine* 1978; **89**(6):941-4.

8. Subramanian R, Khardori R. Severe hypophosphataemia. *Medicine* **79**:1-8, 2000.

9. Lotz M, Zisman E, Bartter FC. Evidence for a phosphorus-depletion syndrome in man. *New England Journal of Medicine* 1968; **278**(8):409-15.

Specific

10. Turco SJ, Burke AW. Methods of ordering and use of intravenous phosphate. *Hospital Pharmacy* 1975; **10**(8):320-326.

11. Kronenberg HM. NPT2a—The Key to Phosphate Homeostasis. *NEJM* 2002; **347**:1022-1024.

12. Ketteler M. Fetuin-A and extraosseous calcification in uraemia. *Current Opinion in Nephrology and Hypertension* 2005; **14**:337-342.

13. Foley RN. Phosphorus comes of age as a cardiovascular risk factor. [comment]. *Archives of Internal Medicine* 2007; **167**(9):873-874.

14. Dhingra R, Sullivan LM, Fox CS et al. Relations of Serum Phosphorus and Calcium Levels to the Incidence of Cardiovascular Disease in the Community. *Arch Int Med.* 2007; **167**:879-885.

15. Giachelli CM. Vascular calcification mechanisms. *J. Amer Soc Nephrol* 2004; **15**:2959-2964.

16. Xianwu Li, Giachelli CM. Sodium-Dependent phosphate cotransporters and vascular calcification. *Current Opinion in Nephrology and Hypertension* 2007; **16**:325-328.

17. Lanske B, Razzaque MS. Mineral metabolism and aging: the fibroblast growth factor 23 enigma. *Current Opinion in Nephrology and Hypertension* 2007; **16**:311-318.

18. Prie D, Beck L, Urena P, Friedlander G. Recent findings in phosphate homeostasis. *Current Opinion in Nephrology & Hypertension* 2005; **14**(4):318-24.

19. Miyamoto KI, Itho M. Transcriptional regulation of the NPT2 gene by dietary phosphate. *Kidney International* 2001; **60**(2):412-5.

20. Kumar R. Phosphate sensing. *Current Opinion in Nephrology & Hypertension 2009-18:281-284*

21. Antoniucci DM, Yamashita T, Portale AA. Dietary Phosphorus Regulates Serum Fibroblast Growth Factor-23 Concentrations in Healthy Men.2006.J Clin Endocrinol Metab.**91**:3144-3149

22. Liu S, Gupta A, Quarles LD. Emerging role of fibroblast growth factor 23 in a bone-kidney axis regulating systemic phosphate homeostasis and extracellular matrix mineralisation. *Current Opinion in Nephrology & Hypertension* 2007; **16**(4):329-335.

23. Strom T, Juppner H PHEX, FGF23, DMP1 and beyond. *Current Opinion in Nephrology and Hypertension* 2008; **17**:357-362.

24. Feng JQ, Ling Y, Schiavi S. Do osteocytes contribute to phosphate homeostasis. *Current Opinion in Nephrology & Hypertension.2009.18:000-000:1862-4821*

25. Urena Torres PA, De Brauwere SP. Three Feedback loops precisely regulating serum phosphate concentration. Kidney International 2011. **80**:443-445.

26. Laaban JP, Grateau G, Psychoyos I et al. Hypophosphatemia induced by mechanical ventilation in patients with chronic obstructive pulmonary disease. *Crit. Care Med.* 1989; **17**:1115-1119.

27. Phosphate Metabolic Control of Potassium Movement—its effect on osmotic pressure of the cell. Bessman SP, Pal N p175-186 in Phosphate and Minerals in health and Disease. Eds Massry SG, Ritz E, Jahn H. Plenum Press New York and London.

28. Ritz E. Acute hypophosphataemia. *Kidney International* 1982; **22**:84-94.

29. Halevy J, Bulvik S. Severe hypophosphatemia in hospitalized patients. *Archives of Internal Medicine* 1988; **148**(1):153-5.

30. Betro MG, Pain RW. Hypophosphataemia and hyperphosphataemia in a hospital population. *British Medical Journal* 1972; **1**(5795):273-6.

31. Juan D, Elrazak MA. Hypophosphataemia in hospitalized patients. *JAMA* 1979; **242**(2):163-4.

32. Bugg NC, Jones JA. Hypophosphataemia. Pathophysiology, effects and management on the intensive care unit. *Anaesthesia* 1998; **53**(9):895-902.

33. Shiber JR, Mattu A. Serum phosphate abnormalities in the emergency department. *Journal of Emergency Medicine* 2002; **23**(4):395-400.

34. Kebler R, McDonald FD, Cadnapaphornchai P. Dynamic changes in serum phosphorus levels in diabetic ketoacidosis. *American Journal of Medicine* 1985. **79**(5):571-6.

35. Megarbane B, Guerrier G, Blancher A et al. A possible hypophosphataemia— induced Life-threatening Encephalopathy in Diabetic Ketoacidosis: A case report. *Amer J. Medical Science* 2007; **333**:384-386.

36. Van Holder R, Severs MS, Erek E, Lamiere N. Rhabdomyolysis. *J. Amer. Soc. Nephrol.* 2000; **11**:1153-1561.

37. Knochel JP. Catastrophic medical events with exhaustive exercise: "white collar rhabdomyolysis". *Kidney International* 1990; **38**(4):709-19.

38. Singhal PC, Kumara A, DesRoches L et al. Prevalence and Predictors of Rhabdomyolysis in Patients with Hypophosphataemia. *Amer. J. Med.* 1992; **92**:458-64.

39. Bosch X, Poch E, Grau JM. Rhabdomyolysis and Acute Kidney Injury. New Engl J Med. **361**:62-72 2009

40. Marinella MA. Refeeding syndrome and hypophosphatemia. *Journal of Intensive Care Medicine* 2005; **20**(3):155-9.

41. Haglin L. Hypophosphataemia in anorexia nervosa. *Postgraduate Medical Journal* 2001; **77**(907):305-11.

42. Rowe JC, Wood DH, Rowe DW, Raisz LG. Nutritional hypophosphatemic rickets in a premature infant fed breast milk. *New England Journal of Medicine* 1979; **300**(6):293-6.

43. Elisaf MS, Siamopoulos KC. Mechanisms of hypophosphataemia in alcoholic patients. *International Journal of Clinical Practice* 1997;**51**(8):501-3.

44. Dent CE, Winter C. Osteomalacia due to Phosphate Depletion from Excessive Aluminium Hydroxide Ingestion. *BMJ* 1974; **1**:551-552.

45. Levi M, Blaine J, Breusegem S, et al. Renal Phosphate—Wasting Disorders. *Advances in Chronic. Kidney Dis.* 2006; **13**:155-165.

46. Jan de Beur SM. Tumour-induced osteomalacia. *JAMA* 2005; **294**:1260-7.

47. Emmett M. What does serum fibroblast factor 23 do in hemodialysis patients? *Kidney International* 2008; **73**:3-5.

48. Guiterrez OM, Maunstadt M, Isakov AT, et al. Fibroblast Growth Factor 23 and mortality among patients undergoing Haemodialysis. *NEJM* 2008; **359**:584-92.

49. Ghanekar H, Welch BJ, Moe OW, Sakhaee K. Post-renal transplantation hypophosphatemia: a review and novel insights. *Current Opinion in Nephrology & Hypertension* 2006; **15**(2):97-104.

50. Prie D, Friedlander G. Genetic disorders of Renal Phosphate Transport. Engl J Med 2010. **362**:2399-2409

51. Prie D, Huart V, Bakouh N, et al. Nephrolithiasis and osteoporosis associated with hypophosphataemia caused by mutations in the type 2a sodium-phosphate cotransporter. *N. Engl J Med.* 2002; **347**:983-91.

52. Dash T, Parker MG, Lafayette RA. Profound hypophosphatemia and isolated hyperphosphaturia in two cases of multiple myeloma. *American Journal of Kidney Diseases* 1997; **29**(3):445-8.

53. O'Connor LR, Wheeler WS, Bethune JE. Effect of hypophosphatemia on myocardial performance in man. *New England Journal of Medicine* 1977; **297**(17):901-3.

54. Darsee JR, Nutter DO. Reversible severe congestive cardiomyopathy in three cases of hypophosphatemia. *Annals of Internal Medicine* 1978; **89**(6):867-70.

55. Zazzo JF, Troche G, Ruel P. High Incidence of Hypophosphataemia in Surgical Intensive Care Patients: efficacy of phosphorus therapy on myocardial function. *Intensive Care Medicine* 1995; **21**:826-831.

56. Bollaert PE, Levy B, Nace L, Laterre PF, Larcan A. Hemodynamic and metabolic effects of rapid correction of hypophosphatemia in patients with septic shock. *Chest* 1995; **107**(6):1698-701.

57. Lang RM, Fellner SM, Neumann A et al. Left Ventricular contractility varies Directly with Blood Ionised Calcium. *Ann Int Med.* 1988; **108**:524-529.

58. Newman JH, Neff TA, Ziporin P. Acute respiratory failure associated with hypophosphatemia. *New England Journal of Medicine* 1977; **296**(19):1101-3.

59. Lewis JF, Hodsman AB, Driedger AA, Thompson RT, McFadden RG. Hypophosphatemia and respiratory failure: prolonged abnormal energy metabolism demonstrated by nuclear magnetic resonance spectroscopy. *American Journal of Medicine* 1987;**83**(6):1139-43.

60. Aubier M, Murciano D, Lecocguic Y, et al. Effect of hypophosphatemia on diaphragmatic contractility in patients with acute respiratory failure. *New England Journal of Medicine* 1985; **313**(7):420-4.

61. Gustavsson CG, Eriksson L. Acute respiratory failure in anorexia nervosa with hypophosphataemia. *Journal of Internal Medicine* 1989; **225**(1):63-4.

62. Gravelin TR, Broiphy N, Sieger TC, Peters, Golden M. Hypophosphataemia-associated respiratory muscle weakness in a general inpatient population. *Amer. J. Medicine* 1988; **84**:870-6.

63. Agusti AGN, Torres A, Estopa R, Augusti-Vidal A. Hypophosphataemia as a cause of failed weaning: The importance of metabolic factors. Crit Care Med.**12** :142-143 1984

64. Travis SF, Sugerman HJ, Ruberg RL et al. Alterations of Red-cell Glycolytic intermediates and oxygen transport as a consequence of Hypophosphataemia in Patients receiving intravenous Hyperalimentation. *NEJM* 1971; **285**:763-768.

65. Clerbaux T, Detry B, Reynaert M, Kreuzer F, Frans A. Re-estimation of the effects of inorganic phosphates on the equilibrium between oxygen and haemoglobin. *Intensive Care Medicine* 1992; **18**(4):222-5.

66. Prins JG, Schrijver H, Staghouwer JH. Hyperalimentation, hypophosphataemia, and coma. *Lancet* 1973; **1**(7814):1253-4.

67. Laaban JP, Marsal L, Waked M, Vuong TK, Rochemaure J. Seizures related to severe hypophosphataemia induced by mechanical ventilation. *Intensive Care Medicine* 1990; **16**(2):135-6.

68. Vanneste J, Hage J. Acute severe hypophosphataemia mimicking Wernicke's encephalopathy. *Lancet* 1986; 1(8471):44.

69. Treloar A ;Crook M; Parker I; Doig R.Hypophosphatemia hallucinations, and delirium tremens. Lancet 338:1407-8 1991.

70. Ravid M, Robson M. Proximal myopathy caused by Iatrogenic phosphate depletion. *JAMA* 1976; **236**(12):1380-1.

71. Jacob HS, Amsden T. Acute haemolytic anaemia with rigid red cells in hypophosphatemia. *New England Journal of Medicine* 1971; **285**(26):1446-50.

72. Craddock PR, Yawata Y, VanSanten L, Gilberstadt S, Silvis S, Jacob HS. Acquired phagocyte dysfunction. A complication of the hypophosphatemia of parenteral hyperalimentation. *New England Journal of Medicine* 1974; **290**(25):1403-7.

73. DeFronzo RA, Lang R. Hypophosphatemia and glucose intolerance: evidence for tissue insensitivity to insulin. *New England Journal of Medicine* 1980; **303**(22):1259-63.

74. Moser CR, Fessel WJ. Rheumatic manifestations of hypophosphatemia. *Archives of Internal Medicine* 1974; **134**(4):674-8.

75. Baker LR, Ackrill P, Cattell WR, Stamp TC, Watson L. Iatrogenic osteomalacia and myopathy due to phosphate depletion. *British Medical Journal* 1974;**3**(5924):150-2.

76. Weisbord SD, Chaudhuri A, Blauth K, DeRubertis FR. Monoclonal gammopathy and spurious hypophosphatemia. *American Journal of the Medical Sciences* 2003; **325**(2):98-100.

77. Coester N, Elliott JC, Luft UC. Plasma electrolytes, pH and ECG during and after exhaustive exercise. *J. Applied Physiol.* 1973; **34**:677.

78. Fine A, Patterson J. Severe hyperphosphataemia following phosphate administration for bowel preparation in patients with renal failure: two cases and a review of the literature. *Amer J. Kidney Dis.* 1997; **29**; 103-105.

79. Khurana A, McLean L, Atkinson S, Foulks CJ. The effect of oral phosphate drug products on Renal Function in Adults Undergoing Bowel Endoscopy. *Arch Int Med.* 2008; **168:593**-597.

80. Shackney S, Hasson J. Precipitous fall in serum calcium, hypotension, and acute renal failure after intravenous phosphate therapy for hypercalcemia. Report of two cases. *Annals of Internal Medicine* 1967; **66**(5):906-16.

81. McCloskey, EV, Yates AJP, Gray RES, et al Diphosphonates and Phosphate homeostasis in man. Clinical Science.1988.**74**:607-612.

82. Friedman EA. Consequences and management of hyperphosphatemia in patients with renal insufficiency. *Kidney International—Supplement* 2005(95):S1-7.

83. Chernow B, Rainey TG, Georges LP, O'Brian JT. Iatrogenic hyperphosphatemia: a metabolic consideration in critical care medicine. *Critical Care Medicine* 1981; **9**(11):772-4.

84. Hebert LA, Lemann J, Jr., Petersen JR, Lennon EJ. Studies of the mechanism by which phosphate infusion lowers serum calcium concentration. *Journal of Clinical Investigation* 1966; **45**(12):1886-94.

85. Thomas G. Iatrogenic hyperphosphatemia: a metabolic consideration in critical care medicine. *Critical Care Medicine* 1981;**9**(11):772-4.

86. Vannatta JB, Whang R, Papper S. Efficacy of intravenous phosphorus therapy in the severely hypophosphatemic patient. *Archives of Internal Medicine* 1981; **141**(7):885-7.

87. Kingston M, Al-Siba'i MB. Treatment of severe hypophosphatemia. *Critical Care Medicine* 1985;**13**(1):16-18.

88. Rosen GH, Boullata JI, O'Rangers EA, Enow NB, Shin B. Intravenous phosphate repletion regimen for critically ill patients with moderate hypophosphatemia. *Critical Care Medicine* 1995; **23**(7):1204-10.

Calcium (Ca). [1-5]

AW = 40. Valence = 2. Conversion factor mg/dL to mmol/L = 0.25. mEq=2x mmol/L.

Total body calcium	1000g (25,000 mmol). Skeleton 99 %, soft tissues and body fluids 25mmol.
Exchangeable calcium	100 mmol
Intracellular concentration	0.5mmol/L. Ionised Ca^{2+} ~ 100 nmol/L
Plasma calcium+	2.0-2.6 mmol/L, 50% ionised, 40% protein bound, 10% complexed to citrate, phosphate and HCO_3
Ionised Plasma calcium	1-1.25 mmol/L. [4]
Albumin binding	1g/dL binds 0.2 mmol calcium/L. [4]
Alkalaemia	increases albumin binding and reduces ionised Ca^{2+} but not total calcium.
Acidaemia	decreases binding and increases ionised Ca^{2+}: Each 0.1 unit decrease pH increases ionised Ca^{2+} by .05 mmol/L. Lactate may bind Ca^{2+}.
Dietary calcium	1000 mg (25 mmol).

Mg^{2+} and K^+ antagonize the action of calcium.

Calcium is the fifth most common element in the body. It imparts strength to the skeleton. Extracellular Ca^{2+} is important in coagulation, membrane excitability and electrical properties.

Hypocalcaemia increases and hypercalcaemia decreases membrane permeability. Intracellular Ca^{2+} acts as a signal for neuronal activation, hormone secretion, and muscle contraction. It is important in the coupling of excitation and contraction in all forms of muscle—cardiac, skeletal and smooth. Depolarization of cells and microsomal membranes release calcium which then activates the contractile process. It is important in the myogenic response which causes vascular vasoconstriction. [6] Calcium is an important regulator of cell function. It plays a direct role as coupler between stimulus and secretion in many tissues: for example catecholamine and HCl secretion; adrenocorticotrophic hormone stimulation of adrenal steroidogenesis; and vasopressin action on kidney tubules. It is important in numerous enzyme reactions, especially those involving transfer of organic ions across cell membranes. Calcium exists in three main pools:

- Skeleton—contains 99% of total body calcium but less than 1% of this interacts with extracellular fluid. The turnover of skeletal calcium is ~ 5.0mmol/day.
- Extracellular calcium pool contains 0.1% total body calcium at a concentration of 1-1.25 mmol/L. This serves as a conduit for Ca^{2+} transport and is crucial in blood coagulation, neuromuscular function and signalling.
- Intracellular pool 0.5mmol/L. The majority of calcium is sequestered in endoplasmic reticulum, mitochondria or bound to cytoplasmic proteins. Only 100nmol/L (0.1 micromol/L) is ionised [4,7]. Thus the ratio of extracellular: cellular ionised Ca^{2+} is over 1000. Intracellular sequestration and active Ca^{2+} extrusion are crucial ancient mechanisms, present even in protozoa, which maintain low intracellular Ca^{2+} because of its importance in signalling and cellular function. [7]

Calcium enters cells by 2 different channels: voltage and ligand gated. Voltage channels, called transient receptor potential vanilloid (TRPV), are activated by cell membrane depolarisation [6]; whereas ligand gated channels are activated by several different neurotransmitters and hormones. On entry into cells Ca^{2+} regulates various reactions, is extruded or transferred to mitochondria, endoplasmic reticulum or sarcoplasmic reticulum in muscle [7]-so that cellular concentration remains at only 100 nmol/L.

Plasma calcium exists in three forms:

- Ionised ~ 1-1.25 mmol/L ~ 50%.
- Bound to albumin ~ 40%.
- Complexed with citrate, phosphate and HCO_3 (~ 9%).

Extracellular ionised Ca^{2+}, but not total calcium, is strenuously regulated. Total calcium should be corrected for binding to albumin if it is used for assessment: approximately 0.2mmol should be added to serum calcium for every 1 g/L of albumin below normal. Alkalaemia increases protein binding. Thus in severe alkalaemia total serum calcium may be normal despite low ionised Ca^{2+}. This may cause neuromuscular manifestations such as Tetany.

Acidaemia decreases protein binding so that low total serum calcium may occur despite a normal ionised Ca^{2+}: Each decrease in arterial blood pH 0.1 unit increases ionised Ca^{2+} by approximately 0.05mmol/L. Hyponatraemia increases and hypernatraemia causes a slight decrease in protein binding to calcium.

The factor for correction of calcium for abnormal serum albumin concentration has been challenged.[8] Although total serum calcium correlates with serum ionised Ca^{2+}, the correlation is unreliable in critically ill patients [9-11] and those with renal failure. [12] In seriously ill patients the poor correlation between ionised and total serum calcium is due to the effects of pH, free fatty acids, other organic acids and osmolality. [1, 9, 10] For example 1mmol of lactic acid binds ~ 0.05mmol calcium. [11]

The product of ionised calcium and phosphorus are close to the concentration at which precipitation as calcium phosphate occurs. This is prevented by several inhibitors such as pyrophosphate and Fetuin. The concept that the Ca^{2+} phosphate product is important as a risk factor for mortality or ectopic calcification has been challenged. [13]

Maintenance of normal extracellular Ca^{2+} is crucial to enable skeletal mineralisation to proceed; for the coagulation cascade; and stability of plasma membranes. Change in extracellular Ca^{2+} alters permeability of cell membranes to Na^+: decrease in extracellular Ca^{2+} increases permeability to Na^+ and promotes initiation of action potentials; increase decreases initiation of action potentials. When extracellular Ca^{2+} decreases by 50% of normal peripheral nerves may discharge spontaneously causing tetany and promoting seizures. Thus maintenance of normal extracellular Ca^{2+} is strenuously defended. This is achieved by a:

Sensing system: calcium sensing receptor (CaSR) which senses change in extracellular ionised divalent cations, Ca^{2+} and Mg^{2+}.

Response system: hormone secretion, predominantly PTH and 1,25 (OH)$_2$ D$_3$, in response to signalling from CaSR. These act on an.

Effector system: bone, kidney and intestine.

CALCIUM SENSING RECEPTOR (CASR). [14, -17]

CaSR in the Parathyroids, kidney and intestine, a G protein coupled receptor, functions like a thermostat by sensing and regulating extracellular Ca^{2+} flux from bone mineral and reabsorption of Ca^{2+} by intestine and kidney. [14, 15]

CaSR responds to the combination of Ca^{2+} and Mg^{2+} ions although magnesium is less effective in stimulating receptors. [4] CaSR is exquisitely sensitive to extracellular ionised Ca^{2+}: the set point for PTH secretion is extracellular ionised calcium of approximately 1.0 mmol/L. [4] When Ca^{2+} decreases below this level PTH is secreted within seconds.

CaSR is also located on basolateral membranes of the medullary thick ascending limbs loops of Henle (TALH) of the kidney. Activation of CaSR from increase in extracellular Ca^{2+} decreases calcium reabsorption through paracellular pathways [15]. The mechanism is as follows: the signal from the CaSR decreases activity of K$^+$ channels on luminal membranes of TALH; decrease in transfer of K$^+$ into the tubular lumen decreases the positive potential in the lumen. This normally drives Ca^{2+} reabsorption through the paracellular route. [15]

Inhibition of K$^+$ transfer into the lumen also inhibits action of Na$^+$:K$^+$:2Cl$^-$ transporters (NKCC2) because K$^+$ is one of 3 ions transported together. Thus hypercalcaemia causes natriuresis. This dilutes tubular Ca^{2+} concentration and decreases nephrocalcinosis and stones which are promoted by hypercalciuria. Indeed the CaSR is a carry over in evolution from fish where it acts as a salinity sensor. [14] Activation of CaSR also increases H$^+$ secretion which acidifies urine and decreases calcium precipitation. A mutated gain of function of CaSR causes autosomal dominant hypocalcaemia with hypercalciuria, sodium, chloride and potassium wasting—a cause of Barrters syndrome. [15]

The function of CaSR in the DCT is uncertain but probably acts by inhibiting basolateral inwardly rectifying K$^+$ channels (Kir$_{4.1}$). This inhibits transcellular Ca^{2+} reabsorption by TRPV and inhibits Na$^+$: Cl$^-$ transporters. This protects the kidney by diluting tubular Ca^{2+} concentration.

Ca^{2+} transport is at the mercy of sodium homeostasis. A consequence of the present day high sodium diet is that a smaller percentage of sodium filtered is reabsorbed. This results in higher proximal tubular sodium concentration which decreases tubular Ca^{2+} concentration and the force for reabsorption. This results in a high load of Ca^{2+} delivered to distal tubules and promotes hypercalciuria [7]. CaSR, acting on both TALH and DCT, protects man from hypercalcaemia and the kidney from hypercalciuria by inhibiting NaCl reabsorption distally, which dilutes Ca^{2+} in distal tubular fluid, and by acidifying urine. [14, 15]

EFFECTOR SYSTEM. Three systems are involved in maintaining normal serum calcium:

Dietary Intake and absorption of calcium

Renal filtration, reabsorption and excretion of calcium

Bone osteolysis and formation

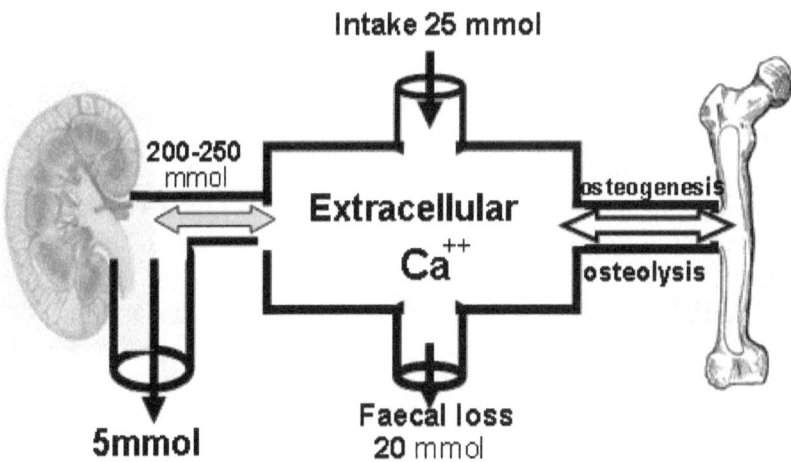

Figure 1: Effector system for calcium homeostasis.

Turnover of skeletal calcium and renal excretion are both approximately 5 mmol/day.

| Calcium absorption and excretion |

Approximately 1g (25 mmol) of calcium, the amount contained in 1L of cow's milk, is consumed in a normal diet, chiefly in the form of milk and milk products. Approximately 200mg (5mmol) are additionally secreted into gastro-intestinal fluids each day and mix with ingested calcium in small intestine. The small intestine, mainly duodenum, reabsorbs 98- 99% of ingested calcium. Absorption is impaired by bile salt deficiency, fatty acids, high dietary fibre and achlorhydria.

Renal Filtration and Reabsorption [1-3, 18-22]

All unbound serum calcium is filtered daily. In a female with a GFR of 100mL/minute (0.1L/minute) and serum Ca^{2+} 2.5mmol/L. (60% ionised) filtered Ca^{2+} per day =

$$0.1(L) \times 60(mins) \times 24(hours) \times 0.6 \times 2.5 = 216 \text{ mmol/day.}$$

Approximately 5.0mmol, the amount excreted, must be reabsorbed daily without disturbing the low tubular intracellular ionic concentration of only ~ 0.1 µmol/L (100 nmol/L). [7]

60 to 70% of Ca^{2+} is reabsorbed passively through the paracellular pathway in proximal tubules, linked to sodium: The gradient for calcium reabsorption is generated by sodium-anion reabsorption which increases calcium concentration in proximal tubular fluid. [7]

Approximately 20% is reabsorbed in medullary thick ascending limbs (TALH), by the paracellular route, using the driving force of the positive lumen potential created by K^+ recycling from tubular cell to lumen.

5-10% of Ca^{2+} is reabsorbed through cells of distal convoluted tubules (DCT) and connecting tubules (CNT). Although a small percentage, fine tuning of calcium reabsorption and excretion is carried out here.

Cellular Mechanisms

Reabsorption of Ca^{2+}, from both intestine and kidney, in mmol amounts, must be accomplished without disturbing the low cellular ionic concentration of Ca^{2+} of only 0.1micromol/L (100 nmol/L). Absorption of Ca^{2+} requires movement through luminal (apical) membrane channels ; binding to Ca^{2+} binding proteins for transport across the cell; and a process for exit into the interstitial fluid and circulation by energy dependent Ca^{2+} transporters (Ca^{2+} ATPase) or Na^+: Ca^{2+} exchangers. [18]

	Intestinal absorption	Renal reabsorption in distal tubule
Luminal membrane	**TRPV6** Ca²⁺ channel	**TRPV5** Ca²⁺ channel
Intracellular transport	Calbindin	Calbindin
Exit from cell	3Na⁺ / Ca²⁺ exchangers (NCXI) and Ca²⁺ ATPase (PMCA1b) pumps	

Table 1. Cellular mechanisms for calcium reabsorption in intestine and kidney.

Intestinal Calcium Reabsorption. [18]

Ca^{2+} enters cells through TRPV6 channels (transient receptor potential vanilloid 6). Ca^{2+} binds to Calbindin for transfer to the membrane and exits the cell either by 3Na⁺:Ca²⁺ exchangers or by active transport using Ca^{2+} :ATPase pumps.

Renal Calcium Reabsorption. [15, 18-22]

Calcium is reabsorbed passively in proximal tubules through the paracellular route in response to its increasing concentration as Na^+ and accompanying anions are reabsorbed isotonically. Proximal tubule reabsorption is not modulated by PTH or 1, $25(OH)_2D_3$. Less is reabsorbed when the diet is high in sodium. Hypercalciuria results as the capacity of distal tubules to reabsorb calcium is overwhelmed. This predisposes to stone formation.

Approximately 20% of Ca^{2+} is reabsorbed in the TAL through the paracellular route (between cells) in response to the positive lumen potential created by K^+ recycling (figure 2).

The CaSR (Ca^{2+}: Mg^{2+} sensing receptor) controls Paracellin related reabsorption of Ca^{2+} and Mg^{2+} by increasing activity of K^+ channels. Hypercalcaemia stimulates the CaSR to decrease the number or activity of K^+ channels. This decreases the lumen positive potential which in turn decreases paracellular Ca^{2+} reabsorption.

Decrease in luminal K^+ also decreases Na^+ reabsorption by interfering with action of NKCC2 transporters. Thus hypercalcaemia, or mutations causing a decrease in function of the CaSR, causes natriuresis.

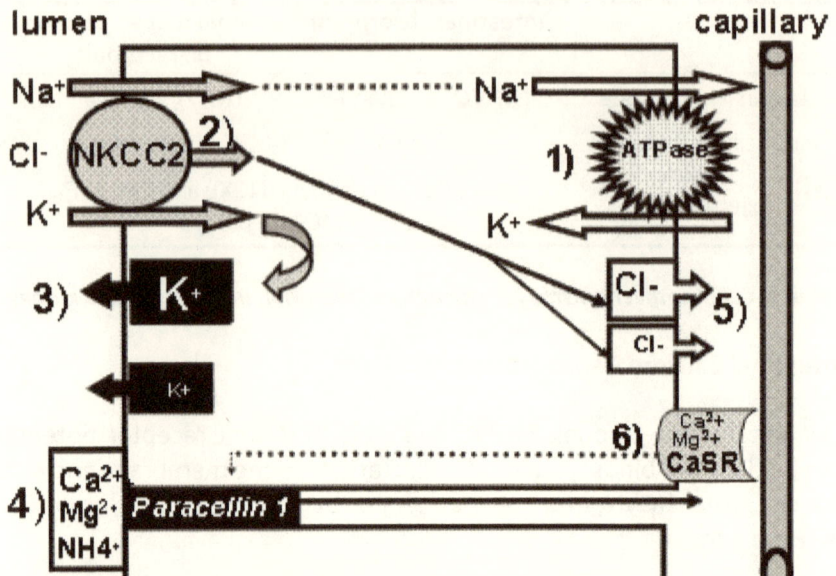

Figure 2: Calcium reabsorption in thick ascending loop Henle (TALH). Numbers corresponds to text below.

1) *Na⁺: K⁺ pumps create low sodium concentration and negative intracellular potential*
2). *Drives NKCC2 cotransporters to reabsorb Na, K⁺ and Cl⁻.*
3) *K⁺ (low concentration in the lumen) is recycled into tubular lumen by K⁺ channels to provide K⁺ for operation of NKCC2.*
4) *The positive lumen potential produced by recycled K⁺ promotes passive reabsorption of Ca²⁺ and Mg²⁺ by the paracellular route (between cells). This is facilitated by Paracellin 1.*
5) *Cl⁻ exits through Cl⁻ channels on basolateral membrane.*
6) *Paracellin 1 is activated by CaSR.*

Approximately 5-10% of filtered calcium is reabsorbed actively through tubular cells of distal convoluted tubules (DCT) and connecting tubule (CNT) as shown in Figure 3. Ca^{2+} enters the cell through TRPV5 (calcium) channels In the DCT.

Reabsorption is regulated by PTH 1, 25(OH) D_3 and calcitonin. A protein called Klotho, originally considered an antiageing hormone, [20-22] regulates Ca^{2+} reabsorption by glycosylating TRPV5 channels. This traps channels on cell membranes and promotes calcium reabsorption. [20-22] Urinary pH alters expression of TRPV channels so that less calcium is excreted in alkaline urine.

This is important in preventing stone formation [20].Inhibition of NaCl uptake in the DCT by thiazide diuretics or tubular disorders of NaCl cotransporters (NCC) leads to hypercalciuria [20]. Volume contraction, due to treatment with thiazides, increases reabsorption of calcium in proximal tubules [20] and decreases calcium transport proteins, messenger RNA expression of TRPV5 and Calbindin. [23]

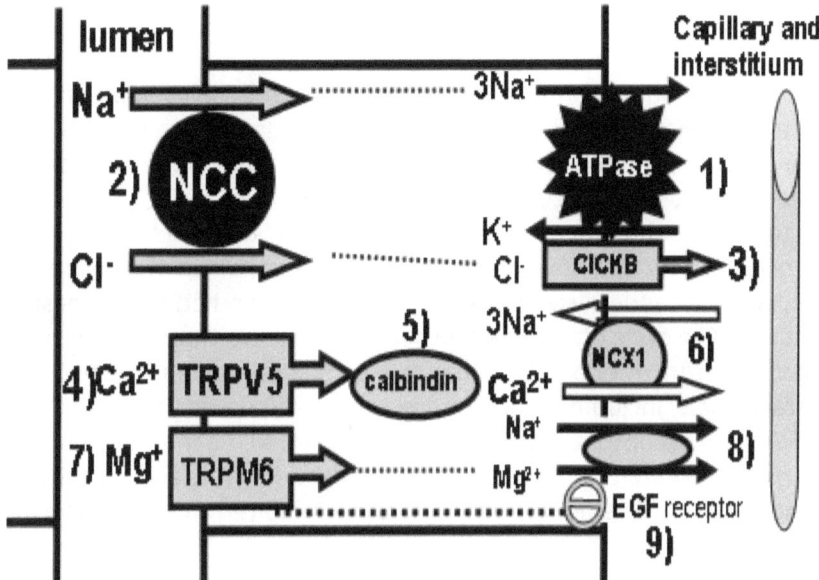

Figure 3: Model of calcium reabsorption in Distal Convoluted Tubule. Numbers correspond to explanation in text.

1. *Na⁺:K⁺ ATPase pumps create low cellular Na⁺ concentration and negative intracellular potential by exporting 3 Na⁺out for 2 K⁺ into cells.*
2. *This promotes sodium and chloride reabsorption by Na⁺ Cl⁻ transporters (NCC).*
3. *Cl⁻ exists via Cl⁻ channels (CLCKβ) and Na⁺ exits via Na⁺:K⁺ pumps (1). Na⁺ and Cl⁻ are reabsorbed without water thus diluting tubular fluid.*
4. *Ca²⁺ enters the cell through TRPV5 (transient receptor potential vanilloid) calcium channels in response to the cellular negative potential.*
5. *Ca²⁺ is transported across the cell by calbindin, a Ca²⁺ binding protein.*
6. *Ca²⁺ exits the basolateral membrane on Ca²⁺:3 Na⁺ exchangers (NCX1).*

BONE CALCIUM EXCHANGE. [24-27]

Two systems in bone influence extracellular Ca²⁺:

Bone remodelling system—balances bone resorption and formation
Calcium mobilising system –maintains extracellular Ca²⁺ concentration.

Bone remodelling.

Bone remodelling continues throughout life and helps maintain the structure and integrity of bone in a continual cycle of bone renewal. Five –10% of existing bone is replaced at any one time. Bone remodelling replaces micro fractures and bone subject to mechanical stress with structurally sound bone and participates in calcium homeostasis. Osteoclasts, which remove bone, and osteoblasts, which synthesise new bone, work in tandem so that removed bone is matched by synthesis of new bone. The cycle of remodelling begins with recruitment of osteoclast precursors from monocytes lining the endosteal sinus in response to several signals, including macrophage colony stimulating factor (M-CSF) and RANKL (Receptor activator of nuclear factor kb ligand). They mature into multinucleated osteoclasts stimulated by RANKL and parathyroid hormone (PTH). The actions of RANKL are inhibited by Osteoprotegrin (OPG) (Figure 4)

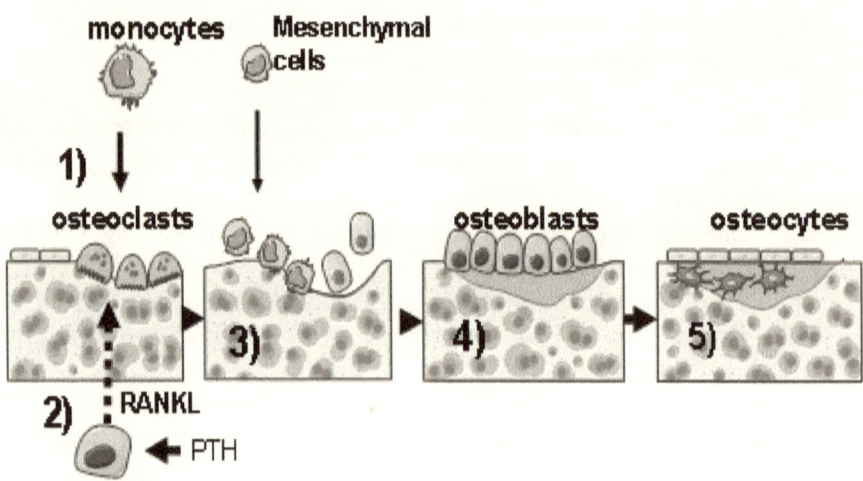

Figure 4. *The process of bone remodelling. (Produced using Servier medical art.)*

1) Recruitment of osteoclast precursors from monocytes lining endosteal sinus which mature into multinucleated osteoclasts stimulated by PTH and RANKL.

2) Osteoclasts reabsorb bone stimulated by RANKL secreted by osteoblasts.

3) Mesechymal cells change into osteoblasts which move into eroded bone (pits).

4) Osteoblasts secret osteoid. Hydroxyappatite is deposited in osteoid and hardens it.

5) Osteoblasts mature into osteocytes as they embed in bony matrix and interconnect with one another by canaliculae.

Osteoclasts develop villi (called lamellapodia) and form a ruffled membrane at the interface with bone. This is sealed (insulated from extracellular fluid) by integrins. Osteoclasts solubilise bone minerals by secreting HCl. H^+ is secreted by H^+ ATPase pumps and Cl^- by chloride channels and in combination with proteolytic enzymes digest organic bone matrix. In the process of acidifying bone osteoclasts must transport HCO_3^-, left over from the formation of H^+ from H_2CO_3, through the basolateral membrane. Alkalinisation may activate osteoblasts. [26]

Osteoclastic reabsorption of bone is stimulated by PTH (parathyroid hormone) acting on PTH receptors on osteoblasts (not osteoclasts): and stimulates osteoblasts to produce a signalling ligand called RANKL (receptor activator of nuclear factor kappa B ligand). RANKL acts on RANK receptors present on osteoclasts. In this way osteoblasts induce osteoclast differentiation. Osteoprotegrin (OPG) antagonises RANKL and inhibits bone resorption. Genetic defects in RANKL or in the production of acid cause Osteopetrosis, The absence of OPG causes osteoporosis in mice.

Osteoblasts, which are specialised fibroblasts derived from mesenchymal cells, move into eroded bone pits and secrete organic matrix composed of collagen fibres and mucopolysaccharides, called osteoid, in response to stimulation by several cytokines.

Calcium phosphate crystals, as hydroxyappatite, are deposited in osteoid and harden it. Osteoblasts mature into osteocytes as they become embedded in bony matrix and interconnect with other osteocytes in lacunae by a network of canaliculi. (Osteons).

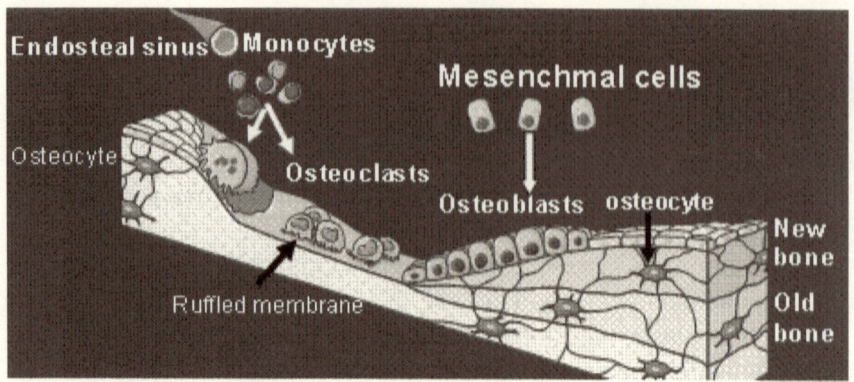

Figure 5. Bone remodelling. (Produced using Servier medical art)

Receptors for vitamin D metabolite and PTH are present on osteoblasts, but not osteoclasts. Vitamin D receptors (VDR) play an important role in normal bone formation and mineralisation by enhancing differentiation of osteoblasts and stimulating new bone formation. [27]

Osteoblasts have <u>Megalin</u> receptors which incorporate circulating $25OHD_3$ and synthesise 1; 25 $(OH)_2 D_3$ by local production of 1 α hydroxylase. Low $1,25(OH)_2 D_3$ increases PTH levels and decreases VDR expression on osteoblasts. Both $1,25(OH)_2 D_3$ (calcitriol) and PTH are required for bone formation. The group of osteoclasts and osteoblasts which interact during bone remodelling is referred to as a basic multicellular unit (BMU) and the site of bone resorption and formation as a bone remodelling compartment (BRC).

Intermittent PTH injections increase bone mass and formation whereas continuous infusion causes bone loss [23]. Bisphosphonates, which inhibit the action of osteoclasts, are used for treatment of osteoporosis. Strontium both inhibits the action of osteoclasts and stimulates osteoblasts. Recently RANKL antagonists, which inhibit activation of osteoclasts, have been used for treatment of osteoporosis. Thus there are two processes which regulate extracellular Ca^{2+}:

<u>Ca^{2+} exchange with mineral crystal</u> (orchestrated by osteocytes)

<u>Bone resorption</u>

Calcium Mobilising System. [24-26]

A bone-renal- parathyroid hormone axis regulates phosphate, calcium and calcitriol1 $(,25(OH)_2 D_3)$ homeostasis. Communication between osteocytes and osteoblasts is essential for bone remodelling. Osteocytes communicate with each other through long dendritic processes within canaliculi which interconnect and form a network with other osteocytes. This enables coordination of their responses for mineral homeostasis, osteoid formation and mineralisation. [24, 26]

Only 0.5-1% of bone calcium is exchangeable. Osteocytes in bone lacunae and on the surface of bone regulate movement of Ca^{2+} between bone and extracellular fluid. A hydration shell, which contains Mg^{2+}, Na^+, H^+, carbonate and K^+ ions surrounds bone crystal and provide a buffer for Ca^{2+}, phosphate, Mg^{2+}, H^+ and other ions.

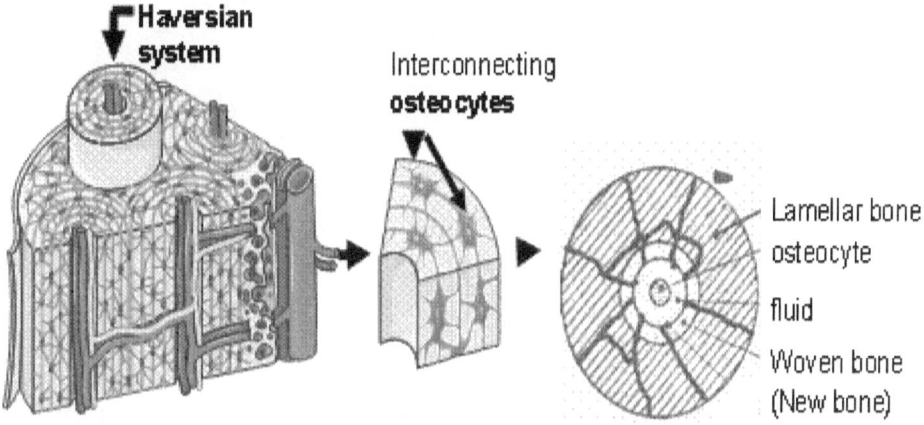

Figure 6. Model of the Haversian system of bone showing canalicular interconnections of osteocytes, fluid and new bone surrounding osteocyte. (Produced using Servier medical art).

Stimulation and integration of gastrointestinal, renal reabsorption and calcium transfer from bone, in order to achieve normal extracellular ionised Ca^{2+}, is achieved by a sensing mechanism—the CaSR (Calcium Sensing Receptor) and a response process which stimulates the secretion of PTH, $1,25(OH)_2D_3$ and calcitonin.

RESPONSE SYSTEM

The effector system—bone, kidneys and gastrointestinal tract are acted on by 3 main hormones which regulate extracellular Ca^{2+} and the bone remodelling process:

- <u>PTH—the most important for regulating extracellular Ca^{2+}.</u>
- <u>Metabolites of Vitamin D.</u>
- <u>Calcitonin (CT)—the least important.</u>

PARATHYROID HORMONE (PTH) [1-4, 16, 17,]

The **Parathyroids** are small 5 x 5 x 3mm reddish brown glands, usually 4 in number, situated close to the posterior surface of the thyroid on the upper and lower lobes of each side. PTH (parathyroid hormone) is formed from a larger precursor ProPTH in parathyroids. PTH acts on PTH receptors by non genomic (fast) and genomic (slow) action on target cell surface receptors by releasing adenyl cyclase. This enhances calcium entry into cells.

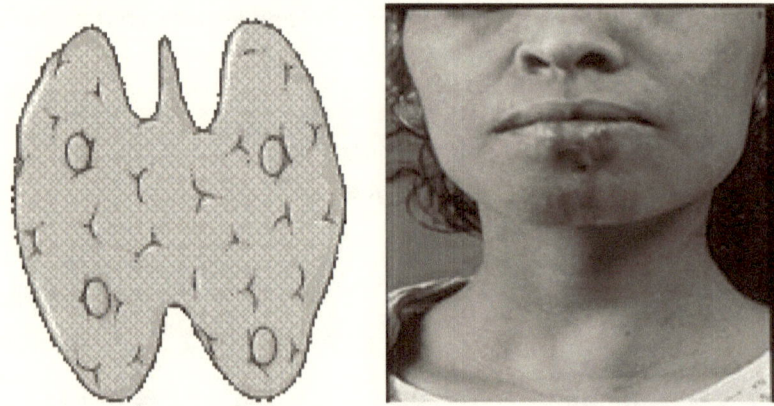

Figure 7.Parathyyroid glands and parathyroid adenoma

The main action of PTH is to maintain normal extracellular Ca^{2+}. Receptors also bind PTH related protein (PTHrp).

The main stimulus for PTH secretion is low ionised Ca^2 acting on CASR. Mg^{2+}, also acts on CASR but stimulates PTH secretion less than does Ca^{2+}.

<u>Paradoxically very low serum Mg2+ inhibits PTH secretion and causes hypocalcaemia.</u>

Mutations involving the receptor alter the set point for PTH secretion in response to Ca^{2+} and cause either hypo or hypercalcaemia. Calcimimetics such as Cinacalet bind to the CaSR, increase its sensitivity to calcium and decrease secretion of PTH.

The Parathyroid response occurs in 3 phases: [4]

1) **Release of PTH** from preformed stores within seconds.
2) **Synthesis of PTH** if ionised hypocalcaemia persists.
3) **Parathyroid cell hyperplasia** if hypocalcaemia is prolonged.

Recall of the actions of PTH is facilitated by considering the physiological processes which defend extracellular Ca^{2+}.(Figure 8)

1. Phosphaturia.
2. Osteolysis (bone resorption).
3. Stimulation of renal synthesis of $1, 25(OH)_2D_3$ in renal cortex
4. Increase in renal calcium reabsorption.
5. Increase intestinal calcium reabsorption in conjunction with $1, 25(OH)_2D_3$.

Phosphaturia is an important part of the process in that phosphate, released from osteolysis, must be excreted to decrease the calcium phosphate product and prevent calcification. PTH acts within minutes to decrease phosphorus reabsorption and increase Ca^{2+} reabsorption by kidney but takes 1-3 hours to mobilise calcium from bone.

PTH may cause mild metabolic acidosis by decreasing reabsorption of HCo_3^- in proximal tubules ($\downarrow$Tm HCo_3^-) and increases Mg^{2+} reabsorption.

Action on Bone. [1-5, 16, 17, 24, 25]

PTH increases bone resorption by activating osteoclasts but in conjunction with $1, 25(OH)_2D_3$ also increases bone formation. PTH is thus crucial for bone remodelling: it acts on both osteoblasts and osteoclasts to increase bone laid down in each remodelling cycle.

Paradoxically however PTH receptors are present on osteoblasts not osteoclasts. The resorptive effect of PTH is mediated through cell signalling molecules from osteoblasts which regulate osteoclast differentiation: The principal ligand, RANKL, (Rank ligand) secreted by osteoblast precursors, binds to RANK receptors on osteoclasts. PTH and oestrogens up regulate RANKL production.

The RANK ligand system (RANKL) is important as a new target for treatment of bone disorders such as osteoporosis.

Chronic PTH administration causes resorption of cortical bone, while low doses given intermittently, act on osteoblasts to increase trabecular bone [1,25] in conjunction with $1,25(OH)_2D_3$ and other cytokines: insulin like growth factor (IGFI) and transforming growth factor (TGFβ) released from bone during osteoclastic bone resorption. [1]

PTH activates 1 α hydroxylase in renal cortex to synthesise $1,25(OH)_2D_3$ (calcitriol) and in turn $1,25(OH)_2D_3$ inhibits PTH secretion in a classical feed back loop.

PTH related peptide (PTHrP). [28, 29]

PTH related peptide (PTHrP) mimics the action of PTH by acting on PTH receptors. PTHrp is produced by several tissues, including placenta, proliferating chondrocytes and breast. It plays a crucial role in endochondral bone development and coordination of chondrocytes in the foetus. PTHrp probably plays an important role in lactation by mobilising Ca^{2+} for breast milk production. [29] PTHrP and Indian Hedgehog interact in this process. [28]

PTHrP is important because it is produced by several tumours and causes hypercalcaemia by its action on PTH receptors.

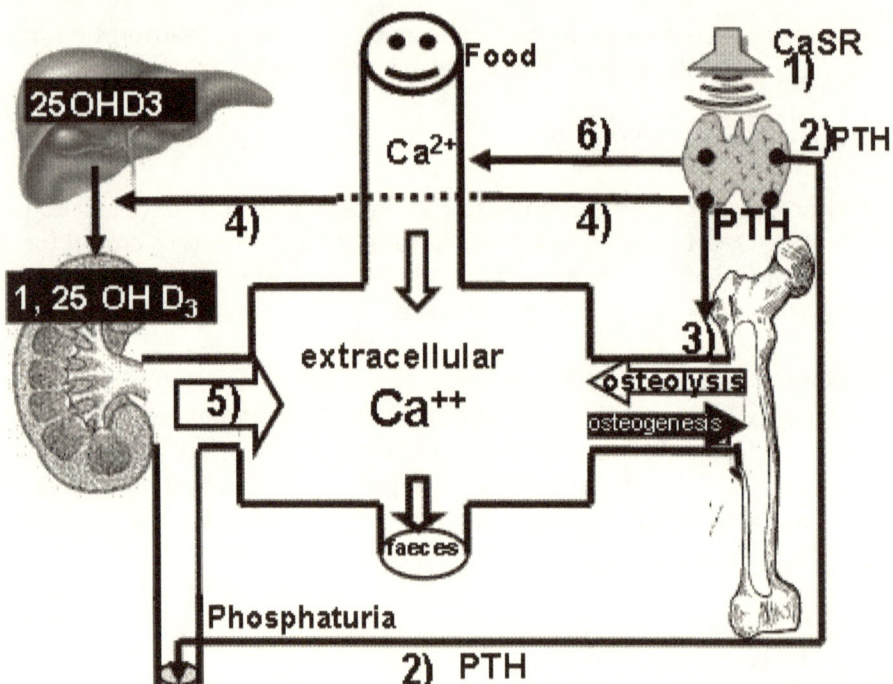

Figure 8. Actions of PTH. Numbers correspond to numbers below. (*Produced with use of Servier medical art*).

1) **CaSR stimulates PTH secretion in response to low extracellular Ca $^{2+}$ and Mg^{2+}**

PTH stimulates:

2) **Phosphaturia.**
3) **Osteolysis.**
4) **Synthesis of 1,25 (OH)$_2$D$_3$ in kidney cortex from 25(OH)D$_3$.**
5) **Renal reabsorption of Ca^{2+}.**
6) **Intestinal reabsorption of Ca$^+$.**

1, 25 (OH)$_2$D$_3$ (1, 25 DIHYDROXYCHOLECALCIFEROL). [1-5, 30-32]

The precursor of the active metabolite, Vitamin D$_3$ (Cholecalciferol), is present in several foods which have been fortified with D$_3$: for example milk products and bread and is naturally present in large quantities in fish oils and egg yolk. The daily requirement is 400-800 units. Other less active Vitamin D compounds are ergocalciferol (D$_2$), produced by irradiation of ergosterol, or derived from ingested plant products and dihydrotachysterol produced by longer irradiation of ergosterol. Although the latter's antirachitic action is much less that D$_2$ or D$_3$ it has weak PTH—like activity and is more potent in elevating plasma calcium in hypoparathyroid subjects.

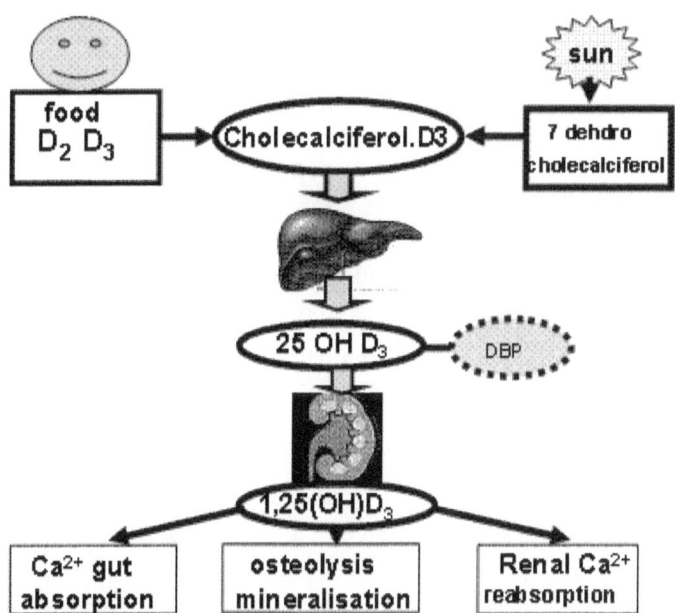

Figure 9: Simplified Model of synthesis of 1, 25(OH)$_2$D$_3$ from precursors and main actions. (Produced using Servier medical art)

Cholecalciferol, (D3), is ingested in food or synthesised in skin from irradiation of 7 dehydrocholecalciferol by sunlight. D_3 is hydroxylated to 25 (OH) D_3 in liver and circulates combined with DBP (vitamin D binding protein) .25(OH) D_3 is hydroxylated in renal cortex to 1,25 (OH)$_2D_3$ (calcitriol).The main actions are shown.

Cholecalciferol (D_3) is also produced in skin by the action of ultraviolet light on 7-dehydrocholesterol. Vitamin D_3, which requires fat for solubility, is absorbed in jejunum and ileum and passes into lymphatics with chylomicrons. Cholecalciferol (D_3) is hydroxylated to 25 (OH) D_3 in microsomes and mitochondria in liver cells.

25 (OH) D_3 is bound to vitamin D binding protein (DBP), an $\propto$ globulin, and circulates in blood. Low DBP in the nephrotic syndrome decreases the concentration of 25(OH) D3.

25, (OH) D3 undergoes further hydroxylation to 1, 25 (OH) $_2D_3$ by 1 α hydroxylase in proximal tubules of the renal cortex.

The complex vitamin D-DBP is filtered by the glomerulus, transferred from the lumen to the renal proximal tubule where it is taken up by Megalin, a multifunctional clearance receptor, on luminal (apical) cell membranes of proximal tubules.

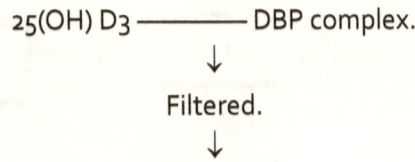

25(OH) D3 ———— DBP complex.
↓
Filtered.
↓
Megalin mediated endocytosis in proximal tubule.
↓
Lysosomal degradation of 25(OH)D_3-DPB in renal proximal tubule cells.
↓
Cytosolic free 25(OH) D_3
↓
Mitochondrial conversion to 1, 25(OH)$_2$ D_3

Thus, proximal tubules regulate synthesis of 1, 25(OH)$_2$ D_3. Other vitamin D metabolites of uncertain importance are 24, 25 (OH)$_2D_3$; 1, 24, 25(OH)$_2$ D_3 and 25, 26(OH)$_2$ D_3.

Synthesis of $1 \propto$ hydroxylase is stimulated by low plasma Ca^{2+}, low serum phosphate and PTH. Inactive 24, 25 $(OH)_2 D_3$ is produced instead of 1, 25$(OH)_2 D_3$ if serum Ca^{2+} is elevated. PTH controls plasma calcium and 1, 25$(OH)_2 D_3$ and these operate as feedback inhibitors of its secretion.

1, 25$(OH)_2 D_3$ (calcitriol) acts by binding to a receptor called VDR. 1, 25(OH)$_2 D_3$: VDR complex translocates to the nucleus and forms a heterodimer with RXR (Retinoid X receptor) to produce its effect on target tissues [31]. Vitamin D negative response elements, which repress activated VDR, are involved in the fine tuning of the effects of Vitamin D metabolites. [32]

There are several metabolites of vitamin D, in addition to 1.25$(OH)_2 D_3$, which have different quantitative and qualitative effects on bone and calcium regulation. For example 24,25 OHD_3 may directly antagonise the Ca^{2+} mobilising effect of 1, 25$(OH)_2 D_3$.

<u>1, 25$(OH)_2 D_3$ has the following actions:</u>

- Intestinal reabsorption of calcium by promoting synthesis of TRPV6 and calcium binding proteins in intestinal mucosa.
- Increase in renal Ca^{2+} reabsorption by acting on TRPV5 calcium channels in the DCT.
- Mineralization of osteoid by direct action on osteoblasts or osteocytes—probably by increasing their permeability to calcium.
- Stimulation of bone resorption in conjunction with PTH.
- Inhibition of PTH secretion.

Vitamin D metabolites, including 1, 25$(OH)_2 D_3$, have several other actions: this includes differentiation of a wide variety of cells and interaction with the immune system.

CALCITONIN. (CT) [1-5]

Calcitonin, secreted by thyroid chief cells, inhibits osteoclastic bone resorption and causes mild hypocalcaemia. Calcitonin increases urinary excretion of sodium and calcium. It is secreted by several endocrine malignancies including thyroid medullary carcinoma.

FGF23. (chapter 9)

causes phosphaturia and decreases synthesis of 1α hydroxylase—

INTERRELATIONSHIP OF CA^{2+}, PHOSPHATE, PTH, D$_3$ AND CT IN MAINTAINING NORMAL EXTRACELLULAR IONIC CALCIUM CONCENTRATION (FIGURE 8).

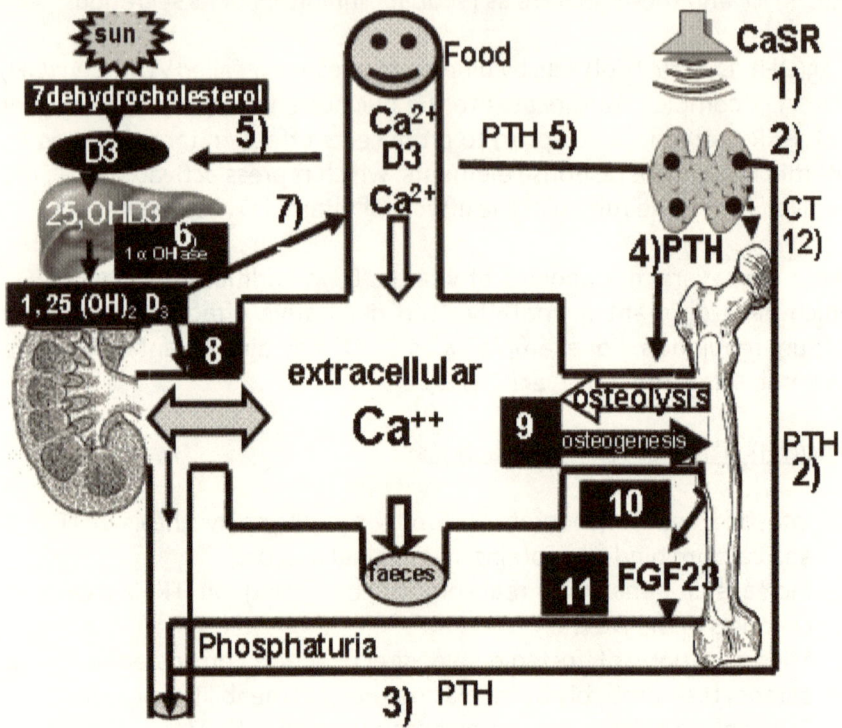

Figure 10 : Maintenance of normal serum Ca^2 comprises the 3 main effector systems: gastrointestinal tract, bone and kidney which change the input and output of Ca^{2+} to ECF; CaSR which senses extracellular Ca^{2+};and response system-PTH, 1,25(OH)$_2$D$_3$, CT(calcitonin) and FGF23. Actions of) 1, 25(OH)$_2$ D$_3$ and FGF23 are shown in black boxes. Production of 1, 25(OH)$_2$ D$_3$ from precursors is shown on the left hand side of the figure. (Produced by using Servier medical art)

1) *CaSR senses extracellular ionised Ca^{2+}.*
2) *Stimulates secretion of PTH if ionised Ca^{2+}is low.*
3   *PTH causes phosphaturia.*
4) *PTH increases osteolysis.*
5) *PTH Increases absorption of D$_3$ and conversion to 25OHD$_3$.*
6) *PTH converts 25OHD$_3$ to 1,25 (OH$_2$)D$_3$ by 1αOHlase in cortex.*
7) *1,25 (OH)$_2$ D$_3$ increases intestinal reabsorption of Ca^{2+}.*
8) *1, 25(OH)$_2$ D$_3$ increases renal reabsorption of Ca^{2+}.*

9) 1, 25(OH)$_2$D$_3$ increases osteogenesis (and osteolysis in conjunction with PTH).

10) FGF23 is secreted by osteocytes in bone.

11) FGF23 causes phosphaturia.

12) CT (calcitonin)n increases osteogenesis.

Given its many important actions extracellular ionic Ca²⁺ is tightly regulated. A small reduction in plasma Ca²⁺ is sensed by CaSR which stimulates PTH secretion. This immediately increases phosphaturia and acts on osteoblasts to activate osteoclasts to cause osteolysis.

More prolonged hypocalcaemia and stimulation of PTH secretion converts 25(OH) D$_3$ to 1, 25 (OH)$_2$D$_3$ in renal cortex, a process however, which takes several hours.

1,25(OH)$_2$D$_3$ enhances calcium absorption by enterocytes (TRPV6) and distal convoluted tubules by increasing calcium binding protein and calcium channels (TRPV5). PTH also acts with 1, 25 (OH)$_2$D$_3$ to increase renal and intestinal calcium absorption.

FGF23, produced by osteocytes in response to hyperphosphataemia, causes phosphaturia, activates PTH and suppresses synthesis of 1 α hydroxylase.

High extracellular Ca²⁺ turns PTH off and increases CT secretion, both of which decrease osteolysis and promote new bone formation. Decreased PTH secretion and hyperphosphataemia inhibit conversion of 25(OH) D$_3$ to 1, 25(OH)$_2$D$_3$.

HYPERCALCAEMIA AND HYPOCALCAEMIA. (table 1).

Serum ionised calcium may increase or decrease, despite a normal total serum calcium, from changes in pH or complexing. The causes of both low and high serum total calcium, shown in Table 1, can be rationalised by considering:

The two main sources of calcium—bone and gut

The main hormones acting on them—PTH, 1;25(OH)$_2$D$_3$.

Neoplasia, drugs and complexing (Table 1).

	Hypercalcaemia	Hypocalcaemia
PARATHYROID DISORDERS	1° Hyperparathyroidism PTH secreting tumours 3° Hyperparathyroidism	Acquired hypoparathyroidism Post parathyroidectomy. Thyroidectomy Hereditary hypoparathyroid Pseudo hypoparathyroidism Neonatal hypoparathyroidism
CaSR abnormality	**Decreased sensitivity** Familial Hypocalciuric Hypercalcaemia. Lithium	**Increased sensitivity** Autosomal dominant Hypercalciuric hypocalcaemia
Magnesium		Hypo and hypermagnesaemia
NEOPLASTIC	Osteolysis PTHrp secreting tumours PTH secreting tumours $1,25(OH)_2D_3$ secreting tumours	Calcitonin secretion from Thyroid Medullary Carcinoma -
VIT. D DISORDERS D3 ingestion skin synthesis of D3 absorption of D3	Vit. D or Calcitriol excess	Inadequate Vitamin D intake Lack of Sunlight Malabsorption of Vit. D
Liver Hydroxylation		Severe Liver Disease Phenytoin, rifampicin
1,25(OH)2D3	Oral Calcitriol excess Increased synthesis, granulomatous disorders	Increased loss— Nephrotic syndrome ↓ synthesis Hered: 1α Hydroxylase Receptor– VIT D dependent. Hungry bone syndrome
COMPLEXING Albumin Globulin	Hyperalbuminaemia (Addison's) Multiple Myeloma (Cationic protein) Rhabdomyolysis (rare)	Hypoalbuminaemia
Phosphate		Recovery Rhabdomyolysis. Renal failure. Phosphate infusion. Neonatal cow's milk Tetany.
Fatty Acids Oxalate Citrate		Pancreatitis, Fat emboli Ethylene Glycol Poisoning Multiple blood transfusions
DRUGS	Vitamin A excess Vitamin D excess Thiazide Diuretics Lithium Milk—Alkali syndrome Calcitriol Treatment Sex hormones	Phosphate—rectal, oral, IV. Foscarnet. Phenytoin. Citrate—blood transfusions. Calcitonin. Bisphosphonates. Drugs causing hypomagnesaemia.
OTHER	Immobilisation—relative cause Endocrine—Thyrotoxicosis, Acromegaly Vipomas, Addison's Disease Renal failure—Multiple causes	**Critically ill—sepsis,** Toxic Shock Syndrome Trauma, Tumour Lysis Syndrome Renal failure

TABLE 1: Causes of Hypercalcaemia and Hypocalcaemia. Some conditions are tabled in more than one category. vit=vitamin; 1 =primary; 3=tertiary.

HYPERCALCAEMIA

The most common causes of hypercalcaemia are primary hyperparathyroidism and cancer. The cause is usually Hyperparathyroidism in those who are relatively well or in whom hypercalcaemia is discovered on routine testing. Hypercalcaemia is also common in patients with advanced chronic renal disease or on dialysis.

Hypercalcaemia associated with cancer. [33-35] There are several mechanisms which cause hypercalcaemia:

- Bone breakdown—due to local osteolysis and actions of various cytokines, especially in breast, prostate cancer, and multiple myeloma.

- Tumoral hypercalcaemia of malignancy. This is characterised by high serum Ca^{2+}, low serum phosphate and raised urine cAMP without an increase in serum PTH.

  PTHrp, which mimics the actions of PTH, is considered to be responsible for many cases based on high levels in patients and animal models. Squamous cell, renal cell, bladder and breast carcinoma; T cell lymphoma and benign tumours, such as carcinoids, phaeochromocytoma and islet cell tumours secrete PTHrp. [33] PTH secreting tumours are rare and 1, 25(OH)$_2$D$_3$ is rarely secreted by lymphomas. [33, 34]

Serum PTH should be measured if the diagnosis is in doubt. This is suppressed in hypercalcaemia due to malignancy. However primary hyperparathyroidism may coexist with malignancy [33].

Hyperparathyroidism. [1-4, 35]

Primary: Adenoma 80%, hyperplasia, carcinoma, ectopic PTH secretion.

               Familial Hyperparathyroidism: MEN1, MEN2, isolated familial hyperparathyroidism.

Secondary: increased PTH secretion due to Hypocalcaemia.

Tertiary: increased PTH secretion due to parathyroid hyperplasia from a previous stimulus which is no longer present. Eg: renal failure which has been treated. Discussed at end of this section.

Manifestations of hyperparathyroidism result from osteolysis, hypercalciuria and hypercalcaemia. Histologically bone mass, cortical more than trabecular, decreases, fibrosis is excessive and osteoclasts increased.

Bone shows generalised osteopenia, osteoporosis and patchy rarefaction, most characteristically as subperiosteal erosions in the phalanges, especially on the radial side (figure 10). Serum Ca^{2+} is increased, serum phosphorus decreased and alkaline phosphatase increased. Osteitis fibrosa cystica, figure 9, and pseudoclubbing are rare manifestations. Stone formation results from hypercalciuria.

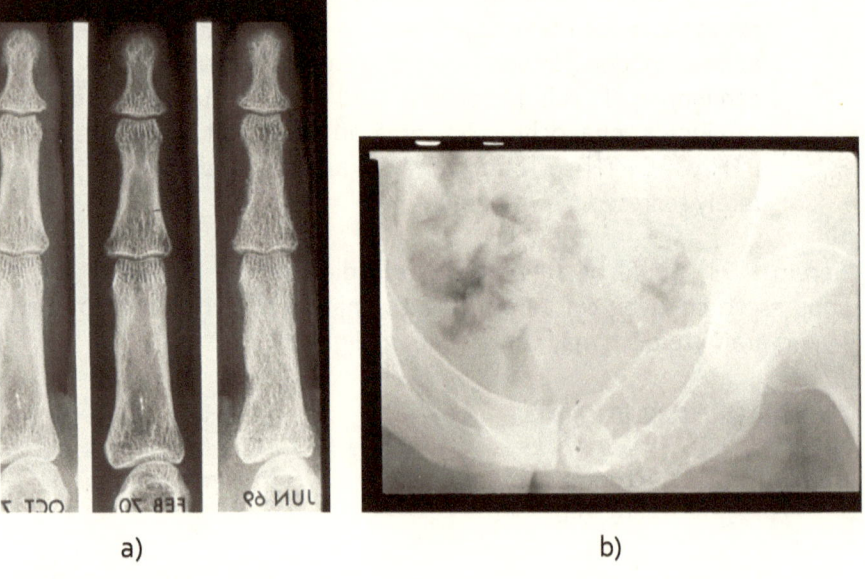

a)   b)

Figure 10.a) subperiosteal erosions: most marked on the radial side of phalanges. b) Osteitis fibrosa cystica in pelvis.

Symptoms of Hypercalcaemia (see following section).

Increased incidence of peptic ulcer and pancreatitis may be due to hypercalcaemia or to hyperparathyroidism itself.

Nephrocalcinosis, symptoms of hypercalcaemia, manifestations of arthritis—pseudogout, involvement of the skull, clavicle and long bones occur but are uncommon.

Recall of the manifestations of hyperparathyroidism is aided by the aphorism: Bones, moans,(psychiatric) stones and abdominal groans –due to pain from duodenal ulcer, pancreatitis, renal stones, or constipation. However, most patients are discovered during routine screening or less commonly investigation of renal stones, fatigue or fracture.

Indications for removal of a Parathyroid adenoma are controversial. The following have been suggested: Bone mineral densitometry of 2Z scores below normal, serum calcium between 2.8-3.0mmol/L, raised serum creatinine, age <50 years, urine calcium >10mmol/day and an episode of life threatening hypercalcaemia or renal stones.

Familial Hypocalciuric Hypercalcaemia. [1, 2, 5 14]

Autosomal dominant mutation of genes controlling CaSR decrease sensitivity of the calcium receptor in parathyroids, kidney and other organs. Higher levels of Ca^{2+} than normal are needed to suppress PTH secretion. Serum PTH is normal or relatively increased despite hypercalcaemia and urinary Ca^{2+} excretion is low because of abnormal calcium sensor (CaSR) function in the thick ascending loop of Henle. Plasma calcium is usually only slightly elevated (<3.0mmol/L). Diagnosis may be difficult because serum calcium levels overlap with primary hyperparathyroidism. Acquired mutations rarely occur. Severe Neonatal Hyperparathyroidism is caused by two defective CaSR genes.

Hypercalcaemia of Lithium resembles Familial Hypocalciuric Hypercalcaemia and may be due to decreased sensitivity of CaSR to Ca^{2+}, but is unproven.

Immobilisation, usually in conjunction with bone disease or thyrotoxicosis may cause hypercalcaemia.

Granulomatous Disorders. [36]

Hypercalcaemia associated with granulomatous disease, such as Sarcoidosis, Eosinophilic granuloma, Berylliosis, Wegener's granulomatosis and Breast implants[36] is considered to be due to increased synthesis of $1,25(OH)_2D_3$ from $25(OH)D_3$ by macrophages in lung or other tissues. Serum calcitriol and ACE (angiotensin converting enzyme) are usually increased whereas $25OHD_3$ is normal. Glucocorticoids, which suppress 1 α hydroxylase, are effective for treatment.

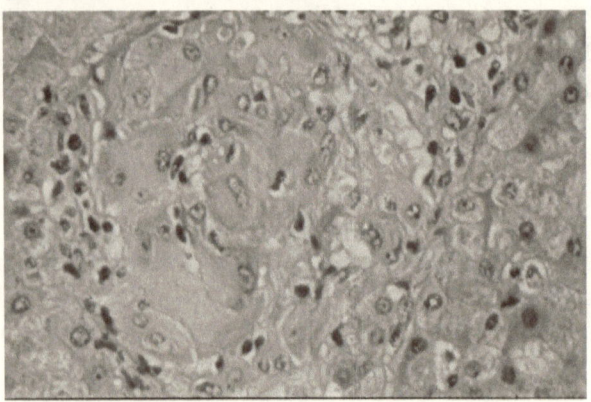

Figure11. *Granuloma in liver.* **Serum Ca 3,9 mmol/L.**

Other Endocrine Disease.

Hypercalcaemia is rarely caused by adrenal insufficiency, probably due to haemoconcentration, thyrotoxicosis in combination with immobilisation, acromegaly, hypophosphatasia and Vipoma.

Drugs and Intoxications.

- Vitamin A: Excessive consumption causes skin erythema, desquamation and hair loss. Increased bone resorption leads to osteoporosis, fractures, hypercalcaemia, hyperostosis and hepatomegaly which results from steatosis and fibrosis. [1-4, 35]

- Vitamin D. [1-3,35,37-39] Unintentional Vitamin D_3 intoxication is uncommon. Dietary supplements of Vitamin D cause occult vitamin D intoxication and hypercalciuria but rarely cause hypercalcaemia. Milk, fortified with Vitamin D3, has caused hypercalcaemia [39]. Treatment of patients with Hypoparathyroidism [40] and Pseudohypoparathyroidism [41] with calcitriol may cause hypercalcaemia, especially in breast feeding woman because decreased requirements occur. [40]. A more common cause is treatment of chronic renal failure with calcitriol. [42] Based on a metaanalysis Palmer et al [42] questioned the usefulness of calcitriol in chronic kidney disease and warned of its risks.

- Thiazide Diuretics. [1-3, 35] may cause mild hypercalcaemia or exacerbate hypercalcaemia in those with undiagnosed hyperparathyroidism or immobility. Hypovolaemia and a decrease in urinary calcium excretion probably contribute.

- Milk—Alkali Syndrome [1-5, 43] results from absorption of large amounts of calcium in milk or calcium carbonate and alkali. Renal failure is usually present. Alkalosis increases renal reabsorption of calcium. This has become uncommon since more effective treatment of ulcer disease has become available. Symptoms are due to both hypercalcaemia and alkalosis. Natriuresis, due to activation of CaSR in the TALH, causes volume depletion and a decrease in GFR. Low GFR increases hypercalcaemia and alkalosis increases calcium reabsorption and precipitation. [43]

- Lithium. Hypercalcaemia is a common side effect of lithium. The mechanism is uncertain [1-3,35] but may be due to decreased sensitivity of the CaSR from lithium.

- Oestrogen [1-3] may cause mild hypercalcaemia or increase serum Ca^{2+} in association with primary hyperparathyroidism, immobility, thiazide diuretics or breast cancer.

Chronic Kidney Disease. End of chapter.

Rhabdomyolysis. [44]

Muscle damage causes release of protein, organic acids and ions in muscle: K^+, Mg^{2+}, and phosphate. In the early stages hypocalcaemia may occur as calcium enters damaged muscle and precipitates as calcium phosphate. During recovery calcium is released and in conjunction with hyperparathyroidism may cause hypercalcaemia. [44]

APPROACH TO HYPERCALCAEMIA.

- Check serum albumin (increased by hypovolaemia). Estimate ionised calcium by subtraction of 0.2mmol of the serum calcium for each gram of albumin above or below normal. Check plasma globulin: raised in multiple myeloma.
- Check serum phosphate.
    - o Raised in renal failure and vitamin D toxicity.
    - o Normal in sarcoidosis and neoplastic replacement of bone.
    - o Low in primary hyperparathyroidism.
    - o Low or normal in hypercalcaemia of malignancy due to PTHrP.
- Check serum creatinine to exclude renal failure.
- Exclude drugs as the cause.
- Are systemic manifestations which suggest underlying cancer present—weight loss, anaemia of chronic disease, high serum CRP?
- Review chest imaging for sarcoidosis, lymphoma and Cancer.
- Measure plasma PSA (prostate surface antigen) and ACE.
- Consider statistical probability in a particular patient. Primary hyperparathyroidism is the cause in over 90% of asymptomatic patients; carcinoma is the second most common cause.

If the diagnosis is uncertain consider ordering a bone scan and measure serum calcium, phosphorus, PTH and serum PTHrp on the same blood sample.

- Consider measurement of 24 hour urine calcium.
- If Lymphoma or granuloma is suspected measure 1, $25(OH)_2D_3$ and $25(OH)D_3$ and ACE.
- If Vitamin D excess is suspected measure $25(OH) D_3$.

HYPOCALCAEMIA (table 1).

Hypoalbuminaemia is probably the commonest cause of mild hypocalcaemia.

Common causes of low ionised Ca^{2+} are Vitamin D deficiency, critical illness, in which causes are multiple and uncertain, renal failure, pancreatitis, hypoparathyroidism secondary to neck surgery, hypomagnesaemia and hypermagnesaemia.

DECREASED ACTION OF VITAMIN D METABOLITES (Table 3).

- **Decreased intake or synthesis of cholecocalciferol—** nutritional Rickett's or Osteomalacia and limited sun exposure.
- **Malabsorption of cholecalciferol—**Malabsorption disorders.
- **Defective conversion to 25OHD$_3$—**Liver disease, Phenytoin.
- **Decreased synthesis of 1, 25(OH)$_2$D$_3$ in renal cortex.**
  Acquired kidney disorders
  Hereditary 1 α hydroxylase deficiency.
- **Resistance to 1,25(OH)$_2$D$_3$.** Defective action of Vitamin D receptor (VDR).

Table 3: *Abnormalities of Vitamin D action.*

Nutritional Rickets' and osteomalacia.

These occur in undeveloped countries from inadequate vitamin D in the diet or decreased sun exposure (Figure 15). Malnutrition may be associated. Synthesis of cholecalciferol is less efficient in pigmented skin, in northern latitudes in winter, in aging skin and in those whose body is covered by clothes. Paradoxically nutritional osteomalacia in women occurs in some countries with high levels of sunlight due to cultural—religious practices of covering the entire body, for example Saudi Arabia (personal observations) (figure 15)

Vitamin D deficiency evolves through 3 stages : initially serum Ca^{2+} and phosphorus are normal; serum phosphorus then becomes low but serum Ca^{2+} remains normal due to secondary hyperparathyroidism; finally both serum Ca^{2+} and phosphorus decrease. Vitamin D deficiency is diagnosed by measuring 25OH D$_3$, which best reflects overall vitamin D status: 25OHD$_3$ is less than 50 nmol/L and less than 15-20 nmol/L in severe deficiency.

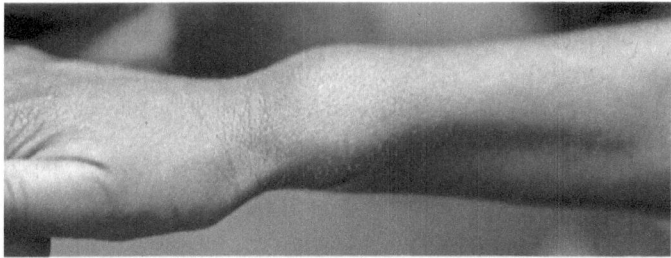

Figure 12. Showing characteristic swelling at the end of the radius and ulna due to enlargement of cartilage at end of bones from nutritional ricketts in a child.

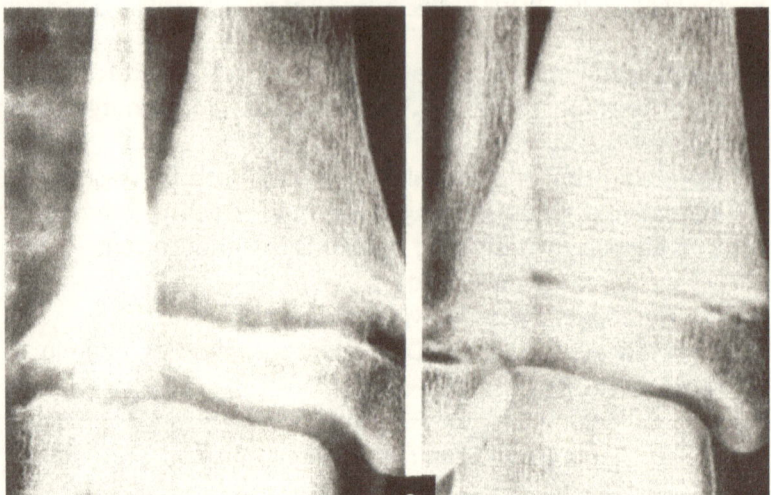

Figure 13: Nutritional Ricketts in the distal tibia and fibula before and after treatment.

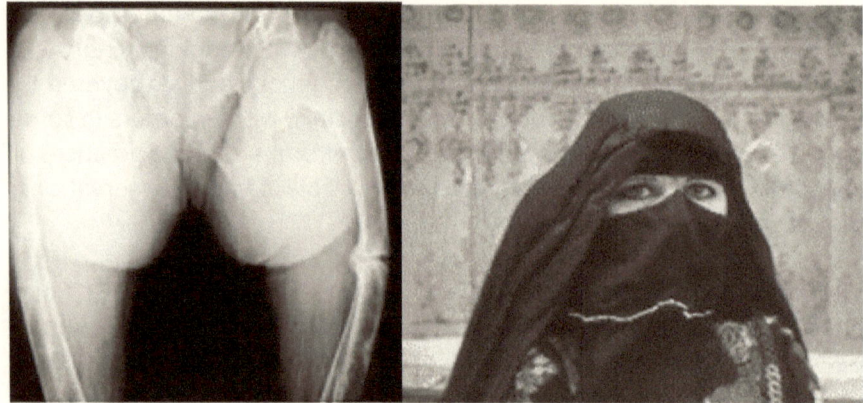

Figure 14 Looser zone due to osteomalacia Figure 15. Vitamin D deficiency due to decreased exposure to the sun is common in Saudi-Arabian woman

Vitamin D deficiency causes osteomalacia in adults and Ricketts in children. Osteomalacia leads to accumulation of poorly mineralised osteoid in both cortex and trabecular bone.(Figure 13) Fibrous tissue replaces normal bone in osteitis fibrosa. Bones show osteopenia, bowing, are prone to low trauma fractures and spontaneous pseudofractures- looser zones, especially in long bones, ribs, pubic rami and scapula.Subpereosteal erosions are due to secondary hyperparathyroidism. Severe bone pain, worse on weight bearing and sudden movement, may be present but are often vague and non specific.This may lead to delayed diagnosis. Muscles are weak and proximal myopathy occurs in severe cases and may cause a waddling gait.

Mineralisation of cartilage and primary spongiosa is deficient in Rickets (Figure 13). Before epiphyseal closure the provisional zones of cartilage at end plates are increased causing enlarged bone ends (Figure 12) and costochondral junctions of ribs—Rickety Rosary. (Figure 17)

Vitamin D deficiency in the elderly. [45-49]

Vitamin D deficiency is common in the elderly. In one observational study 50% of those with low impact trauma fractures had serum $25(OH)D_3$ levels below 30nmol/L and 32% showed secondary hyperparathyroidism[47].

There are several causes of Vitamin D deficiency in elderly:

- Decreased exposure to sunlight, especially in those in nursing homes and hospitals. [46]
- Decreased synthesis of Vitamin D in ageing skin. [48]
- Decreased synthesis of Vitamin D by skin in winter. [46]
- Decreased dietary Vitamin D content.

Vitamin D deficiency decreases muscle strength which contributes to falls. [48]The evidence for benefit of Vitamin D supplementation is mixed. A recent Cochrane review suggested that Vitamin D alone did not prevent fractures in the elderly, [49] although a small decrease in fractures resulted when combined with calcium.

However Vitamin D supplements increase hypercalciuria, which has the potential to increase renal stones, [38, 42] and could theoretically increase vascular calcification. [42]

In view of its low toxicity Vitamin D supplements of 800 -1000 U day plus calcium should be considered for those who are housebound or have risk factors for falls.

Malabsorption of Cholecalciferol.

Various disorders of malabsorption cause decreased absorption of cholecalciferol and sometimes calcium. An increased dose of cholecalciferol—25,000-100,000 IU and calcium supplements can be used in treatment. Calcitriol should not be used chronically because Vitamin

D metabolites, other than $1,25(OH)_2D_3$, such as $24,25(OH)_2D_3$, may be important in bone metabolism

Liver Conversion of Cholecalciferol to 25(OH) D3.

Advanced liver disease and some drugs, for example, Phenytoin decreases synthesis of $25(OH)D_3$.

Decreased synthesis of $1,25(OH)_2D_3$ from $25(OH)D_3$.

- Hereditary 1 α hydroxylase deficiency is a rare cause of Vitamin D dependent Rickett's which is reversed by treatment with calcitriol (1 α OH D_3). Diagnosis is suggested by normal or raised serum $25(OH)D_3$.
- Resistance to $1,25(OH)_2D_3$ Vitamin D dependent Rickett's Type II is a rare hereditary condition due to mutations leading to decreased sensitivity of the Vitamin D receptor (VDR). [50]

HUNGRY BONE SYNDROME.

Demineralised bone may take up calcium avidly when the cause is corrected: For example following removal of a parathyroid adenoma; and on initial treatment of Nutritional Rickett's with Vitamin D. (personal observations)

CRITICALLY ILL PATIENTS. [9-11, 51-55]

20– 80% of critically ill, septic patients, those with toxic shock syndrome or trauma are reported to have low ionised Ca^{2+} often with hypophosphataemia. Over 70% of severely ill trauma patients had low ionised Ca^{2+} on arrival in an Emergency Department. [55] Severe ionised hypocalcaemia (<0.7mmol/L) was present in 10%. Predictors of hypocalcaemia were low arterial blood pH, treatment with colloid (but not crystalloid), low initial blood pressure and low Glasgow Coma Score. Prognosis was worse in those with hypocalcaemia. [9]

The causes of low ionised Ca^{2+} are uncertain. The following have been suggested: inadequate PTH response to hypocalcaemia; increased complexing with citrate, fatty acids, other organic acids; haemodilution; failure of the underperfused kidney to synthesise $1,25(OH)_2D_{3i}$ hypomagnesaemia; and intracellular hypercalcaemia. [9]

The prognosis of patients with hypocalcaemia due to critical illness is worse than those without, [9, 10, 55] but there is no evidence that treatment with

Ca^{2+} is beneficial.[56] On the contrary calcium infusion to normocalcaemic animals and man is detrimental:[57, 58] this may be due to alterations in left ventricular contractility which varies directly with blood ionised calcium.[58]

RHABDOMYOLYSIS. [44]

Muscle damage initially releases protein, organic acids and cellular ions. Hypocalcaemia may occur secondary to hyperphosphataemia and sequestration of calcium in damaged muscle.

MAGNESIUM. (chapter 8)

Magnesium acts on CaSR to suppress PTH secretion. Hypermagnesaemia causes hypocalcaemia but acts with approximately one third the effect of calcium [59]. For example hypocalcaemia occurred when magnesium was infused therapeutically to treat eclampsia, premature labour [60] and subarachnoid haemorrhage. [61]

Paradoxically severe hypomagnesaemia also causes hypocalcaemia by inhibiting both secretion and action of PTH [62]. The magnesium level, which causes hypocalcaemia, is 0.3-0.45mmol/L. Despite correction of hypomagnesaemia serum calcium takes 24-48 hours to normalise. [62] (Chapter 8)

Although hypomagnesaemia is reported to be a common cause of hypocalcaemia in hospitalised patients this is probably due to causes other than hypomagnesaemia because serum magnesium levels rarely fall below 0.45mmol/L—the level at which hypocalcaemia occurs.

HYPOPARATHYROIDISM: ACUTE OR CHRONIC. [1-3, 63, 64] (table 4).

Post Thyroidectomy and Neck surgery Hypocalcaemia. [63-65]

Previous neck surgery is a common cause of parathyroid damage and hypocalcaemia.

Hypoparathyroidism causes hypocalcaemia because of decreased mobilisation of Ca^{2+} from bone and inadequate synthesis of $1, 25(OH)_2 D_3$ which is normally stimulated by PTH. Inadequate $1,25 (OH)_2 D_3$ causes decreased Ca^{2+} reabsorption from intestine and distal tubules. The most common cause is damage to or inadvertent removal of parathyroid glands during thyroidectomy, parathyroidectomy or radical neck dissection.

Transient hypocalcaemia occurs in a substantial minority of patients after partial thyroidectomy, (7-25%) in one review) [64] but depends on the level of surgical expertise. Serum Ca^{2+}, phosphorus and Mg^{2+} should be measured preoperatively and 12 and 24 hours postoperatively. [64]

- Post thyroidectomy, Parathyroidectomy or trauma.
- Genetic mutations involved in the development of parathyroids, PreproPTH or PTH genes.
- Idiopathic—autoimmune, sporadic, part of a polyglandular autoimmune disturbance.
- Parathyroid gland infiltration by amyloid, copper or iron (haemochromatosis).
- Severe hypomagnesaemia: extracellular Mg^{2+} <0.4mmol/L; Hypermagnesaemia.
- Chemotherapy: Doxorubicin, Cytosine arabinoside. Post irradiation.
- Transient neonatal hypoparathyroidism due to maternal hyperparathyroidism.
- Autosomal dominant hypoparathyroidism—activating mutations of the gene encoding the extracellular CaSR (calcium sensor).

Table 4: Causes of Hypoparathyroidism [1-3, 63, 64]

Factors predictive of post operative hypocalcaemia are thyroid cancer, substernal goitre, revision thyroid surgery and thyrotoxicosis [65].On average the lowest serum Ca^{2+} occurs 48 hours following surgery. The absence of symptoms of hypocalcaemia at 20 hours and an upward trend in serum Ca^{2+} predict that significant hypocalcaemia will not occur. Damage to the parathyroids rarely results from infiltration by amyloid, copper (Wilson's disease) or iron (Haemochromatosis).

Genetic disorders. [1-3, 63]

Numerous genetic disorders involved in development of the parathyroids, PreproPTH, PTH or interference with the PTH secretory process cause hypoparathyroidism. For example the DiGeorge syndrome, an autosomal dominant mutation of the 22q 11.2 chromosome, is due to failure of the third and fourth pharyngeal pouches, and therefore parathyroids, to develop normally.

<u>Familial Isolated Hypoparathyroidism</u> is inherited as dominant, recessive or X linked disorders. The sporadic form usually occurs in childhood but can occur at any age.

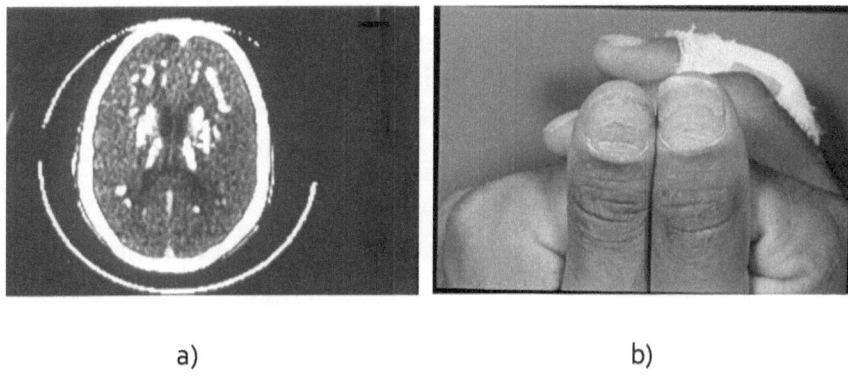

a)   b)

Figure 11. Idiopathic Hypoparathyroidism showing a) cerebral calcification and b) characteristic nail changes.

Clinical manifestations are due to hypocalcaemia and/or hyperphosphataemia (Figure 16): metastatic calcification, unexplained ectodermal defects—cataracts, dry scaly skin, sparse hair, brittle nails, chronic Candida infections and underdeveloped teeth. Frank tetany is uncommon whereas muscular rigidity, laryngospasm and generalised convulsions are more common. Hypoparathyroidism is a component of various mitochondrial genetic disorders. These include: MELAS (mitochondrial encephalopathy, lactic acidosis, and stroke), Kearns Sayer syndrome and MPDS.

<u>Autoimmune Hypoparathyroidism.</u>

This occurs as an isolated deficiency or as part of an autoimmune polyglandular disorder.

<u>Transient neonatal hypoparathyroidism.</u>

There are two varieties: hypocalcaemia may develop soon after birth in neonates of mothers with hyperparathyroidism due to deficient PTH secretion. Hypocalcaemia occurs 4-6 days after birth in infants with immature parathyroids who are fed high phosphorus containing cow's milk.

Pseudohypoparathyroidism. [63]

This is due to peripheral unresponsiveness to PTH and causes hypocalcaemia, hyperphosphataemia and elevated PTH. Some patients show round faces, short stature, obesity, brachydactyly (short metacarpals and metatarsals), subcutaneous ossification, bone exostoses and mental retardation.

PseudoPseudohypoparathyroidism. [63]

This shows similar physical manifestations as above but without evidence of resistance to the actions of PTH.

Autosomal dominant hypocalcaemia with hypercalciuria. [66]

Mutations causing overactivity of the CaSR (lower serum calcium inhibits the receptor) cause hypocalcaemia and hypercalciuria. This resembles and needs to be distinguished from hypoparathyroidism because treatment with Vitamin D may increase hypercalciuria and cause nephrocalcinosis.

Complexing.

- Albumin: hypoalbuminaemia is a common cause of mild hypocalcaemia but ionised Ca^{2+} is normal. Respiratory and metabolic alkalosis increase binding of calcium to albumin thus decreasing the ionised component of calcium while leaving total calcium normal.

- Phosphate. Hypocalcaemia is an important complication of phosphorus infusions in the treatment of hypophosphataemia [9, 67, 68]. This has become less common since use of excessive phosphate administration has decreased. [69] Severe hypophosphataemia and hypocalcaemia may follow bowel preparation. [70] Liberation of cellular phosphate from necrosed cells in the initial phase of acute tumour lysis or rhabdomyolysis [44] can cause hypocalcaemia.

- Fatty Acids: Hypocalcaemia is an important complication of pancreatitis [71, 72] and worsens prognosis. It is due to soap formation—a complex of calcium with fatty acids. [71] The parathyroid response to hypocalcaemia is inappropriately low [72].

- The fat emboli syndrome is due to complexing of calcium with fatty acids.

- <u>Ethylene glycol intoxication</u>: complexing of calcium with oxalic and hippuric acids.

- <u>Citrate</u>: Citrate causes hypocalcaemia following massive blood transfusions due to citrate complexing with Ca^{2+} (whole blood contains 7 mmol/L; packed cells 17 mmol/L citrate per unit infused).

<u>Renal failure</u>. Causes of hypocalcaemia are multiple and include hyperphosphataemia due to low glomerular filtration rate; decreased synthesis of 1, 25(OH)$_2$ D$_3$ by the kidney and acidosis. Secondary hyperparathyroidism occurs due to increase serum Ca^{2+}. This is discussed at the end of this chapter.

<u>Drugs.</u>

Phosphate, calcitonin, EDTA, seldom used at present, and Bisphosphonates cause hypocalcaemia. Phosphate, used for bowel preparation for endoscopy, causes hyperphosphataemia and hypocalcaemia (see chapter 9 on Phosphorus). Hypocalcaemia occurs in approximately 10% following an infusion of 4 mg of Zolendronate used for treatment of osteoporosis [73] but can be minimised by ensuring the patient is vitamin D replete beforehand. Loop diuretics rarely cause hypocalcaemia due to hypercalciuria.

<u>Malignant associated hypocalcaemia.</u>

Secretion of calcitonin by thyroid medullary carcinoma may occur sporadically or as an autosomal dominant familial disorder. [1-3]

<u>DIAGNOSIS OF HYPOCALCAEMIA.</u>

Consider if ionised Ca^{2+} is low, from alkalosis, when the total calcium is normal but symptoms are suggestive. Associated alkalaemia, which is common, exacerbates manifestations due to hypocalcaemia.

<u>Correct for hypoalbuminemia</u>. Correct for hypoalbuminemia by adding 0.2 mmol/L for each 1g albumin below normal. However binding with albumin shows considerable variation due to changes in pH, free fatty acids, lactic acid, osmolality and unknown factors. Consider measuring ionised Ca^{2+} if corrected Ca $^{2+}$ is low, especially in critically ill patients.

Total serum calcium, as an indication of ionised Ca^{2+}, is especially unreliable in renal failure and critically ill patients. [9-11] Marked differences between calculated and measured ionised calcium occurred in over 15% of those with severe trauma, despite taking arterial blood pH, binding to lactate and colloids, into account. [11] Multiple myeloma may cause raised serum total calcium but ionised calcium is normal. If in doubt ionised calcium should be measured.

Look at serum creatinine: to exclude renal failure.

Look at the serum phosphorus: A low level suggests secondary hyperparathyroidism is present. If raised either renal failure or hypoparathyroidism is suggested.

Is serum Mg low: the level should be less than 0.40-0.50 mmol/L in order to cause hypocalcaemia. If low, correct and see if hypocalcaemia normalises.

Important features in the history:

- Neck surgery suggests hypoparathyroidism.
- Family history suggests a genetic cause.
- Candidiasis or other autoimmune disorders suggest autoimmune hypoparathyroidism may be present.
- Characteristic physical appearance—round faces, short stature, brachydactyly, short metacarpals and metatarsals suggest the diagnosis of hypoparathyroidism.
- Pseudohypoparathyroidism. Other defects and immune deficiency suggest the diagnosis of DiGeorge's Syndrome.

Is the patient seriously ill or has gram negative sepsis. Hypocalcaemia is common and of multiple or unknown causes. Hypophosphataemia often coexists.

Consider rhabdomyolysis—Measure serum CPK. Is there previous coma, alcoholism, seizures?

In seriously ill patients consider the following: Complexing from pancreatitis, fat emboli, multiple blood transfusions, ethylene glycol intoxication. Measure serum lipase and observe for oxalic acid crystals if indicated.

When serum phosphorus is low, consider deficiency of 1, 25 (OH)$_2$D$_3$ or its precursors in non-acutely ill patients.

Especially consider Vitamin D deficiency in elderly or nursing home patients and measure 25(OH) D$_3$ levels.

ManifestationS of Hypocalcaemia. [1-3, 37, 74]

These are due to both the level of extracellular ionised Ca^{2+} and the rate of its fall. Low ionised Ca^{2+} causes increased neuromuscular excitability, proximal and distal limb paraesthesia, restlessness and painful muscle cramps. Tetany shows generalized muscle spasm, especially of facial muscles, and carpopedal spasm. The hand adopts a characteristic position of flexion of the wrist and metacarpophalangeal joints, extension of the interphalangeal joints, adduction of the thumb and extreme pronation.

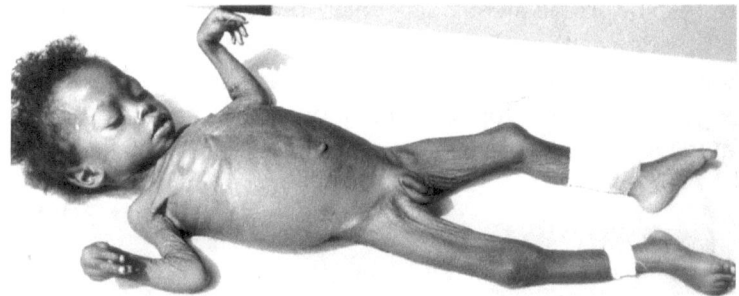

Figure 17 Carpopedal spasm and dorsiflexion due to tetany in a child with Nutritional Ricketts. Note malnutrition, abdominal protruberance, Rickety rosary, frontal bossing.

In less severe cases twitching may only involve the lateral angles on the eye or lip at the corner of the mouth. Spasm of one facial muscle may be mistaken for stroke (Personal observations). Spasm of the frontalis muscle may be the sole manifestation. Nystagmus, both vertical and horizontal or both may occur. Laryngospasm, which may be life threatening, dysphagia and hypersalivation from spasm of the muscles of swallowing, paraesthesias, fasciculations, severely symptomatic muscle cramps, generalized convulsions and a raised serum CPK from rhabdomyolysis may also occur. The development of tetany is related to the rapidity of onset of ionised hypocalcaemia.

Tetany rarely occurs from hypocalcaemia of long duration, as in chronic idiopathic hypoparathyroidism, whereas grand mal epilepsy and muscle rigidity, which may simulate Parkinsonism, is relatively common. It may be possible to provoke tetany in hypocalcaemic subjects by tapping on the facial nerve—Chovstek's Sign; or decreasing the blood supply to the limbs by inflating a cuff 10mm above the systolic pressure for 3 to 5 minutes (Trousseau's Sign). This causes tetany due to spasm of the median and ulnar nerves. The specificity of Chovstek's Sign is low however [74]. The only established cause of tetany is a low level of extracellular ionized calcium—usually resulting from acute rather than chronic reduction.

Tetany May Therefore be Due to:

Hypocalcaemia—low total plasma calcium.

Alkalaemia—respiratory or metabolic.(figure 18) Total plasma Ca^{2+} may be normal or slightly low but ionized Ca is very low due to increased binding of Ca^{2+} with albumin which is pH dependant. A relatively common cause is acute respiratory alkalemia secondary to panic attacks or functional hyperventilation, although paraesthesias, syncope, chest pain, muscle rigidity and cramps are more common.Tetany is more likely to occur following rather than before correction of hypokalemia during alkalosis associated with hypokalemia. (K^+ is a physiologic antagonist of Ca^{2+}.

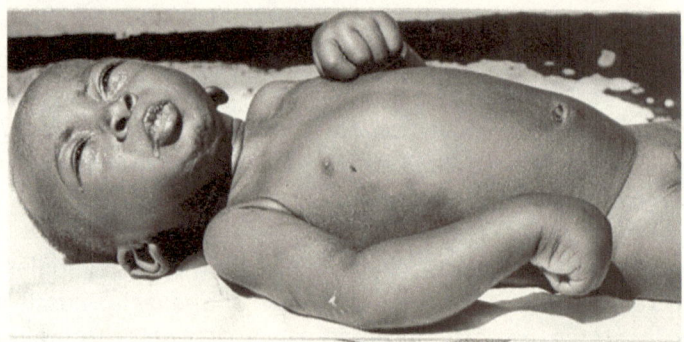

Figure 18: Tetany in an infant due to metabolic alkalosis. This followed recovery from severe Na+ and K+ depletion. Plasma HCO_3^- 45 mmol/L, Ca^{2+} 2.0mmol/L.Note facial spasm, hypersalivation and typical spasm (main d'accoucher).

Many texts report that hypomagnesaemia causes tetany. Critical review of individual papers does not support this. (chapter 8)

Hypocalcaemia may also cause muscle weakness, which is a common and important sign in osteomalacia, and decreased cardiac contractility. Cardiac contractility has been reported to decrease in several case reports [56] but only one observational study has shown that the severity of hypocalcaemia correlates with changes in myocardial contractility. [58] Calcium chloride administration in normocalcaemic subjects does not improve the cardiac index. [56] Arrhythmias are rare: a Medline search by the author revealed only two case reports in children; [75, 76] other causes may have been responsible in both these cases.

Hypocalcaemia prolongs the repolarization phase of heart muscle and Q-T interval (figure 19) but only in a minority of cases. [77, 78] Hypercalcaemia has the opposite effect and shortens the Q-T interval. (Figure 20) However the QT interval has poor sensitivity for diagnosis of both hypocalcaemia and hypercalcaemia. [77, 78]

Longstanding hypocalcaemia [63] may be responsible for many of the manifestations of hypoparathyroidism: dystrophic nail changes with a predisposition to chronic Candida infection, underdeveloped teeth, sparse hair, cataracts, choreoathetosis and extrapyramidal manifestations.

Blood coagulability decreases when plasma ionised Ca^{2+} falls below 0.6-0.7mmol/L. Some of the manifestations associated with hypocalcaemia may be due to hyperphosphataemia or an increase in the calcium x phosphate product. In chronic hypoparathyroidism basal ganglia and cerebral calcification, organic brain syndrome, mental retardation in children, cataracts, brittle nails and dry skin may be due to this or associated genetic traits rather than hypocalcaemia alone.

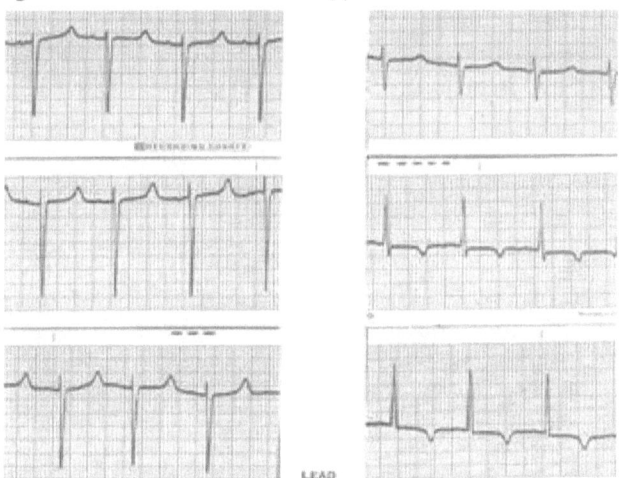

Figure 19. ECG (leads V1-V4) showing prolonged QT interval, slight tenting of T waves and left ventricular hypertrophy in a patient with hypocalcaemia, hyperkalaemia and hypertension due to renal failure.

MANIFESTATIONS OF HYPERCALCAEMIA. [1-4 35]

Hypercalcaemia affects the heart, kidney, neurological and gastrointestinal systems. The severity of manifestations is due to both the severity and rate of increase in serum calcium.

Mild hypercalcaemia is usually asymptomatic. Recall of symptoms is facilitated by the adage: bones, moans, stones and abdominal groans.

Moans or Psychogenic Like Symptoms.

- Fatigue.
- Decreased memory, concentration and depression.
- Confusion, coma in severe cases.

Abdominal Groans.

Constipation, nausea and vomiting; increased frequency of peptic ulcer (questionable), pancreatitis and renal colic.

Stones, Renal Manifestations, Nephrocalcinosis.

Tubular dysfunction. A characteristic tubular dysfunction causes defective urinary concentration and sodium reabsorption which results in polyuria, nocturia, natriuresis volume depletion and eventually renal failure. A high extracellular Ca^{2+} causes natriuresis by acting on the calcium sensing receptor (CaSR) in thick ascending limbs loops of Henle: stimulation increases both hypercalciuria and sodium excretion. [14, 15]

Bones and Musculoskeletal manifestations. Chondrocalcinosis, pseudogout, proximal muscle weakness.

Cardiovascular.

The ECG shows QT shortening but only in a minority of cases. [77, 78] Impaired cardiac contractility, which varies with the level of ionised calcium, has been reported. [58] Other manifestations are probably due to the cause of hypercalcaemia rather than hypercalcaemia.

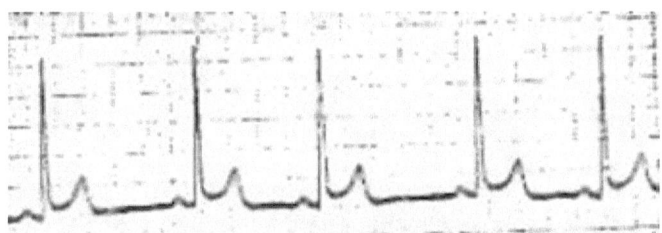

Figure 20: ECG shows a shortened QT interval. Serum calcium *3.1mmol/L.*Serum calcium 4.0 mmol/L

Subperiosteal erosions, osteofibrosa, conjunctivitis and band keratopathy occur in hyperparathyroidism.

In longstanding hypercalcaemia nephrocalcinosis and renal failure may occur. A band of calcium in the cornea and keratopathy may occur in end stage renal disease: It resembles the arcus senilis; but is usually present on the sides rather than the superior and inferior limbus.

Confusion occurs in severe cases.

Severe hypercalcaemia, especially developing rapidly, is a medical emergency which may cause severe saline depletion, coma, renal failure, cardiac failure, and may terminate in asystole.

TREATMENT

HYPERCALCAEMIA. [1-3, 79, 80]

Urgency of treatment is dependent on both the serum level, the rate of rise of serum Ca^{2+} and severity of symptoms. The mode of treatment depends on assessment of volume status.

Stop drugs which increase serum calcium: Thiazides, Vitamin D metabolites and Lithium. Increase mobilisation.

Hypovolaemia and euvolaemia—with or without prerenal failure occurs in the majority. Infuse normal saline to maintain urine output of 100mL/ hour. When volume depletion is corrected frusemide is added but not before hypovolaemia is corrected. Saline increases renal calcium excretion because it decreases proximal tubule reabsorption of calcium and increases action of Na^+: K^+: $2Cl^-$ transporters in thick ascending limbs loops of Henle (TALH) which increases the positive lumen potential which stimulates Ca^{2+} reabsorption.

Cardiac Failure.

Give a loop diuretic (intravenous Furosemide, 40mg) from the beginning if cardiac failure is present rather than saline. Monitor SO_2 (saturation oxygen) and neck veins. However saline infusion and frusemide therapy for hypercalcaemia due to cancer is not based on randomised controlled trials. [80]

Intravenous Bisphosphonates.

These decrease osteoclastic bone resorption. Pamidronate 90mg given in 4 hours reduces serum Ca^{2+} in 2-3 days. Response lasts for several weeks in most but not all cases.

Zolendronate, 4mg in 15-30 minutes, is slightly more effective and can be given more rapidly. Transient fever, lymphopenia hypophosphataemia, hypocalcaemia, myalgia and slight decrease in renal function may occur during treatment with bisphosphonates.

Glucocorticoids.

High doses are effective in Vitamin D intoxication, Sarcoidosis and haematological malignancies such as multiple myeloma.

Calcimimetics.

The CaSR receptor is activated by Ca^{2+}, other divalent cations such as Mg^{2+} and several other agents. Medications which increase the sensitivity of the CaSR which decreases PTH secretion and the serum Ca^{2+} level, have been developed. [81]. Cinacalcet, a calcium receptor antagonist, which inhibits PTH secretion, has been shown to be effective for treatment of hypercalcaemia in primary' [82] secondary hyperparathyroidism and hypercalcaemia due to lithium therapy. [83]

Calcitonin.

4-8 IU/kg sub cutis every 12 hours. Calcitonin acts within 12 hours but results in only slight and transient decrease in serum calcium. This is rarely indicated but may be considered if renal failure is present.

TREATMENT OF HYPOCALCAEMIA. [1-3, 9, 54, 84-86]

Symptoms occur when total calcium is < 1.8mmol/L or ionised Ca^{2+} less than1.0 mol/L. Treatment of critically ill patients with hypocalcaemia has not been shown to improve outcome.

Treat the cause.

Hypomagnesaemia.

Give a bolus of Mg^{2+} 8.0mmol, if the serum magnesium is less than 0.5 mmol/L, followed by 0.5-1.0mmol/hour or oral magnesium (see Mg^{2+} section). Serum Ca^{2+} does not increase for 12-24 hours.

Vitamin D disorders.

Calcitriol 0.25-1.0μg acts faster than Vitamin D but should usually be changed to cholecalciferol for chronic treatment of vitamin D deficiency apart from renal disease. Daily requirements of Vitamin D are 800-10000 U/day.Cholecalciferol 1000 U (25microgm) is a popular formulation. For the first 6 weeks a larger dose - 3000-5000 U is given to replenish stores.

Intravenous Calcium.

There are no controlled observational data on intravenous treatment. Theoretically 7.5 mmol (15 mEq) infused as a bolus in an average man should immediately raise the serum Ca^{2+} by 0.5 mmol/L (15 L (extracellular volume) ÷ 7.5). Calcium should be continuously infused within hours following a bolus.

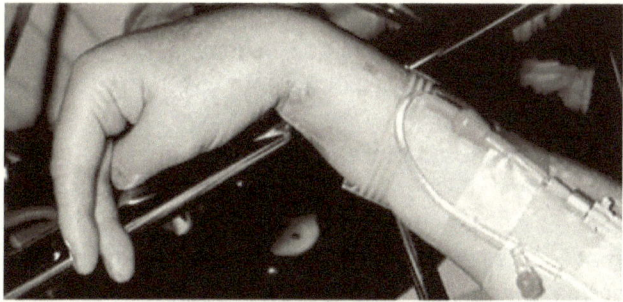

Figure 21.Initiation of intravenous calcium in a patient with tetany due to hypocalcaemia causing severe laryngospasm and respiratory failure.

Two preparations for intravenous use are available.

<u>Calcium gluconate</u>: elemental Ca^{2+} 93 mg (2.5mmol) in 10mls.

<u>Calcium chloride</u>. (Ca Cl_2) elemental Ca^{2+} 272mg (4.8 mmol) in 10 mL is more venotoxic and should be avoided in favour of calcium gluconate.

11 ampoules of calcium gluconate in 900mls 5% dextrose water (to make 1L) given at 50mls/hour delivers 45mg (1.1 mmol) Ca^{2+}/hour.

Unfortunately movement of extracellular Ca^{2+} to bone varies considerably depending on the cause of hypocalcaemia. Therefore frequent monitoring of serum calcium during infusion is essential. Various recommendations for intravenous correction of hypocalcaemia have been made. [85]

Zaloga [9] recommended an initial bolus of 2.5-.5.0mmol followed by 1-2mg/kg/hour. (0.025-.05mmol/kg/hour) to adults with frequent monitoring (1-2mg/kg/hour is equivalent to 1.75 mmol-3.5 mmol hour to a 70kg person). When serum calcium normalises the rate should be decreased to 0.3-0.5mg/kg/hour of elemental calcium (.0075-.0125mmol/kg hour) equivalent to 0.13-0.875 mmol/hour in a 70kg person.

Prendiville [64] recommended 1-1.5mg/kg/hour elemental Ca^{2+} per hour in post thyroidectomy patients with hypocalcaemia.

The author's unpublished observations suggest that a 2.5-5.0 mmol bolus of elemental calcium over 10-15 minutes in adults followed by infusion at 0.5-1.0mmol/hour, with frequent monitoring, is effective.

CHRONIC TREATMENT.

Supplemental cholecalciferol (~8000IU/day) is given for long term treatment of nutritional deficiency; 50-100,000 IU/day for malabsorption; and calcitriol for other disorders, with or without, calcium supplementation.

Hypoparathyroidism should be treated with calcium supplementation and calcitriol only added if the response is inadequate. However hypercalciuria should be avoided. Calcitriol requirements for hypoparathyroidism vary and may decrease as pregnancy advances and during lactation. Hypercalcaemia can result if the dose is not decreased. [88]

Synthetic PTH, given by subcutaneous injection twice daily, is as effective as Calcitriol but causes less hypercalciuria. [87]

	Tab	Elemental Calcium (mmol)
Calcium carbonate	500mg	5
Calcium lactate	325mg	~10
Calcium gluconate	500mg	~10
OSCAL	1250mg	12.5
Calcium citrate	950mg	5
Cow's milk per litre	1200 mg	~ 30

Table 5: *Commonly used calcium preparations.*

Vitamin D preparations

	Physiological Dose	Pharmacological Dose	ONSET(days)	DURATION
D_2 or D_3	5-10µg	1-10mg	10-14	4-12 weeks
25OHD (Calciferol)	1-5µg	20-200	7-10	2-6 weeks
$1,25(OH)_2D_3$ (Calcitriol)	0.25-0.5µg	0.5-2.0µg	1-2 days	2-5 days

Table 6: *Vitamin D preparations, dose, onset of action and duration. Modified from Refer & Heath.* [85]

CALCIUM, PHOSPHATE AND BONE DISEASE IN CHRONIC RENAL FAILURE. (89,90)

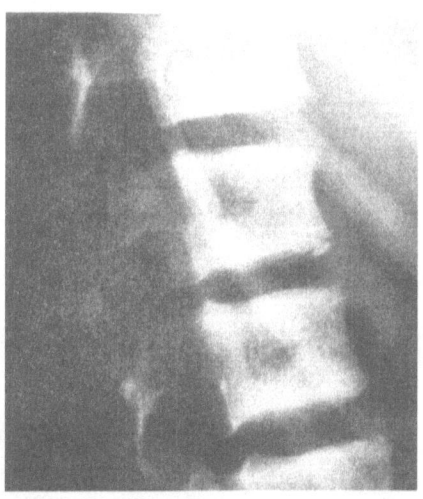

Figure 22. Renal osteodystrophy of the spine.

This highly controversial and complicated subject is characterised by the following changes in mineral metabolism (Table 7):

- Hyperphosphataemia and hypocalcaemia.
- Secondary hyperparathyroidism.
- Tissue resistance to PTH and accumulation of PTH metabolites.
- Decrease in VDR and CaSR receptors in Parathyroids.
- Increased serum FGF23.
- Decreased $1,25(OH)_2D_3$ synthesis
- Decreased intestinal calcium reabsorption due to decreased $1,25(OH)_2D_3$.
- Abnormal renal excretion of calcium and phosphorus.
- Bone disease: skeletal resistance to PTH, decreased synthesis of $1,25(OH)_2D_3$.
- Ectopic calcification: vascular, skin and other tissues.
- Hypercalcaemia from calcium carbonate, high Ca^{2+} in dialysis solutions, autonomous hyperparathyroidism and Calcitriol.

Table 7: Changes in mineral metabolism in chronic renal failure.

Extracellular phosphate increases progressively as GFR decreases. Synthesis of $1,25(OH)_2D3$ by renal cortex decreases and leads to decrease in intestinal and renal reabsorption of calcium. Hypocalcaemia develops due to this and hyperphosphataemia. Hyperphosphataemia, hypocalcaemia and decreased $1,25(OH)_2D_3$ cause secondary hyperparathyroidism. Autonomous hyperparathyroidism, a clonal proliferation of parathyroid cells, develops after prolonged stimulation.

Hyperparathyroidism, secondary to hypocalcaemia, stimulates bone resorption and increases serum Ca^{2+} levels. This increases the Ca^{2+} x phosphate product, promotes vascular and ectopic calcification [90-92] and is associated with an increase in mortality. [92,93]

Secretion of FGF23 is markedly increased secondary to hyperphosphataemia.

Fetuin-A, a glycoprotein, inhibits calcification, but is decreased in dialysis patients. [93]

The three main hormones involved are: PTH, $1,25(OH)_2D_3$ and FGF23. PTH and FGF23 increase and $1,25(OH)_2D_3$ decreases in renal failure.

PT.H. [89, 94]

PTH increases early in renal failure in response to hyperphosphataemia, hypocalcaemia and deficiency of 1, $25(OH)_2D_3$ which normally suppresses PTH secretion [89,94].This causes phosphaturia and an increase in serum Ca^{2+}, stimulates synthesis of $1,25(OH)_2D_3$ but increases resorption of bone. The increase in extracellular Ca^{2+} may increase the Ca^{2+} phosphate product and promote vascular and ectopic calcification.

Parathyroid hyperplasia is highly variable and may become autonomous from adenoma formation. When PTH secretion is high (> 50 pmol/L) osteitis fibrosa is a risk; while if it is low adynamic bone disease is a risk. When renal disease progresses resistance to parathyroid stimulation develops due to a decrease in sensitivity to the calcium sensing receptor CaSR), a decrease in Vitamin D receptors (VDR) and resistance to action of PTH on bone.

1, $25(OH)_2D_3$. [89]

Decrease renal synthesis of 1, $25(OH)_2D_3$ and later resistance to its action occurs both as a result of renal disease and increased levels of FGF23 which suppress synthesis.

Decreased intestinal reabsorption of Ca^{2+} and phosphate results and PTH secretion increases in response to hypocalcaemia. This causes defective osteoid formation, mineralisation and muscle weakness.

FGF23. [17-19, 95, 96]

FGF23 Is markedly increased in renal failure and following renal transplantation. In dialysis patients serum FGF23 is between 10 and 600 times the normal range [96]. The main actions are to increase phosphaturia and decrease synthesis of 1, $25(OH)_2 D_3$. [93, 96] This decreases bone mineralisation. FGF23 regulates 1 α hydroxylase which converts 25(OH) D3 to the active metabolite 1, $25(OH)_2 D_3$. FGF23 acts on a receptor (Klotho FGF receptor) in distal tubules to inhibit sodium phosphate cotransporter (NaP2a) activity in proximal tubules. FGF23, in combination with Klotho also stimulates TRPV5 calcium channels in distal tubules to increase reabsorption of calcium. [19, 95]

Phosphate retention.

This is a key factor in renal osteodystrophy and ectopic calcification. Phosphate retention increases as GFR decreases and causes secondary hyperparathyroidism, increased secretion of FGF23, skeletal resistance to PTH, vascular and other tissue calcification.

Factors affecting the serum phosphorus in chronic renal disease are:

- Dietary phosphorus intake.
- Ingestion of phosphate binders including calcium.
- The extent of secondary hyperparathyroidism and skeletal response to PTH.
- The extent of $1,25 (OH)_2 D_3$ deficiency.
- The balance between catabolism and anabolism of protein: cellular phosphate is 100mmol/L.

Bone Disease.

A relative or absolute deficiency of Vitamin D metabolites causes:

- Defective collagen synthesis and maturation.
- Defective mineralisation of osteoid. Osteitis fibrosa results.

Aluminium toxicity may contribute if aluminium is used as a phosphate binder. Acidosis causes loss of $CaCo_3$ from bone and retention of H^+ but does not play a major role in bone disease. Hypophosphataemia contributes to bone disease in post transplant patients. [97]

High levels of PTH (>50 pmol/L) predispose to osteitis fibrosa.

Adynamic Bone Disease.

This occurs in 15-60% of dialysis patients due to decreased levels of PTH. PTH levels 2-3 times normal are required to maintain a normal rate of bone formation. Adynamic bone disease is characterised by defective bone matrix formation and mineralisation, increased osteoid thickness, and both decreased osteoblasts and osteoclasts on bone surfaces. Osteosclerosis and osteoporosis mainly occur in trabecular bone in vertebrae, ribs, clavicles and metaphysis of long bones and may cause painful micro fractures.

Ectopic calcification. [89, 93, 94, 98]

Soft tissue calcification results from hyperphosphataemia, increased Ca^{2+} X phosphate product, local tissue injury, rise in local pH, high calcium intake, removal of calcification inhibitors by dialysis and unknown factors. Ectopic calcification increases when the calcium X phosphate product exceeds 70 (in mg/dl). A target in chronic renal failure is to keep the product less than 55.

Vascular calcification, related to an increase in the calcium-phosphate product, is an important cause of death or cardiovascular disease in those with chronic renal failure. Increasing attention is being focused on this problem. Vascular calcification of intimal plaque of large arteries and media of small arteries and arterioles causes rigidity and characteristic pipe stem appearance on imaging. Arterial rigidity causes systolic hypertension with a narrow pulse pressure. Periarticular calcification causes attacks of tenosynovitis and pseudogout due to microcrystals of Hydroxyappatite.

Increase in pH at exposed surfaces predisposes to conjunctival and corneal calcification at the medial lateral limbus (band keratopathy) due to loss of CO_2 which increases pH. Soft tissue calcification occurs in arteries, eyes, visceral organs, periarticular areas and skin. Calcification in skin (calciphylaxis) is rare but causes considerable morbidity and mortality. [98] Painful necrotic skin ulceration is due to calcification in small blood vessels which undergo intimal proliferation, endovascular fibrosis and thrombosis. Intravenous thiosulphate has been reported to be effective in treatment [98] Large tumoral masses containing chalky fluid may occur adjacent to joints of dialysis patients. Visceral calcification due to amorphous calcium magnesium phosphate may contribute to cardiac failure, a decrease in vital capacity of the lungs and arrhythmias.

TREATMENT. [99-103]

The following is a brief simplified account of a rapidly evolving subject.

The most important component of treatment is reduction of raised serum phosphate: to decrease ectopic calcification from raised calcium-phosphate product and to limit secondary hyperparathyroidism.

Traditionally calcium carbonate has been used but non calcium phosphate binders such as Sevelamer and lanthanum, a rare earth, are being advocated to avoid an increase in calcium reabsorption. [99] However there is controversy on their use, based on the high cost of Sevelamer, inadequate well designed trials and potential for acidosis. [102] Use of Sevelamer carbonate, rather than Sevelamer hydrochloride, may decrease acidosis. [101] Sevelamer also increases serum Fetuin-A which binds phosphate, may decrease the Ca^{2+} X phosphate product and vascular calcification. [102] Although promising, there is inadequate evidence at present to justify use of the much more expensive newer agents. [103] Dietary phosphate should be decreased.

Vitamin D Analogues

Calcitriol has been given in the past to prevent bone disease and improve calcium reabsorption. However this increases the Ca^{2+} X phosphate product and may oversuppress PTH secretion. Vitamin D analogues, for example Paricalcitol (19 nor 1, 25$(OH)_2$ D_2, cause less intestinal absorption of calcium and phosphate and less resorption of bone. [91,104] A significant survival advantage occurred in those receiving paracalcitol compared to Calcitriol. [103]

Treatment of Secondary and Tertiary Hyperparathyroidism

Prolonged secondary hyperparathyroidism leads to clonal proliferation of parathyroid cells which express less CaSR and Vitamin D receptors. This leads to decreased responsiveness to extracellular Ca^{2+} especially in patients on haemodialysis.

Calcimimetics, such as Cinacalcet, are useful because they mimic the effects of calcium by increasing the sensitivity of CaSR. [91]

Calcylytics decrease sensitivity of CaSR to Ca^{2+} and causes hyperparathyroidism. Their intermittent use by, increasing PTH secretion, may be useful in the treatment of a dynamic bone disease

Suggested Targets at time of publication.

Serum phosphate and calcium in normal reference range.
Calcium/phosphate product <4.0 mmol/L.
PTH: (GFR<15 mL/min) 2-3 times upper limit of normal.
Decrease acidosis to prevent loss of bone in buffering.

References

General references

1. Bringhurst FR, Demay MB, Kronenberg HM. Hormones and Disorders of Mineral Metabolism. p1155-1209 In William's textbook of Endocrinology. Wilson JD, Foster DW, Kronenberg HM, Larsen PR, Eds. 8th ed. Philadelphia: WB Saunders., 1998.
2. Popovtzer MM. Disorders of calcium, phosphorus, vitamin D and parathyroid hormone activity.p216-277. In Renal and Electrolyte disorders. Schrier RW, ed. 6th ed. Philadelphia: Lippincott Williams & Wilkins., 2003:
3. Sutton RAL, Dirks J. Disturbances of calcium and magnesium metabolism. p 1038-1085. In: Brenner BM, Rector FC, The Kidney eds. Brenner and Rector's. 5th ed. Philadelphia: WB Saunders., 1996.
4. Brown EM Physiology of Calcium metabolism.Ch48.p 437-447 in Principles and Practice of Endocrinology and Metabolism. Second edition. Becker KI ed.JB Lipincott Company Philadelphia 1995
5. Shoback D, Marcus R, Bile D. Metabolic Bone Disease p 295-361. In: Basic & Clinical Endocrinology. Greenspan FS, Gardner DG, eds. 7th Ed. New York: McGraw-Hill., 2004.

Specific references

6. Inoue R, Hai L, Honda A. Pathophysiological implications of transient receptor potential channels in vascular function. Current opinion in Nephrology Hypertension. 17:193-198, 2008.
7. Moe OW, Preisig PA. Hypothesizing on the evolutionary origins of salt-induced hypercalciuria. *Current Opinion in Nephrology & Hypertension* 2005:14(4):368-72.
8. Pain RW, Rowland KM, Phillips PJ, Duncan BM. Current "corrected" calcium concept challenged. *British Medical Journal* 1975:4(5997):617-9.
9. Zaloga, GP, Hypocalcaemia in critically ill patients. *Critical Care Medicine,* 1992. 20(2):251-62.
10. Carlstedt F, Lind L. Hypocalcaemic syndromes. *Critical Care Clinics,* 2001. 17(1):139-53.
11. Benoit V, Langeron O, Morell E et al. Early hypocalcaemia in severe trauma. *Critical Care Medicine,* 2005. 33:1946-1952.
12. Conceicao SC, Wightman D, Smith PA, et al. Serum ionized calcium concentration: measurement versus calculation. *British Medical Journal* 1978, 1(6120):1103-5.

13. O'Neill WC. The fallacy of the calcium-phosphorus product. *Kidney Int.* **72**:792-756, 2007.

14. Hebert SC. Calcium and salinity sensing by the thick ascending limb: a journey from mammals to fish and back again. *Kidney Int.—Supplement.* 2004 **91**:S28-33.

15. Huang C, Miller RT. Novel Ca receptor signaling pathways for control of renal ion transport. *Current Opinion in Nephrology & Hypertension* **19**:106-112, 2010.

16. Van Abel M, Hoenderop JG, van der Kemp AW, Friedlaender MM, van Leeuwen JP, Bindels RJ. Coordinated control of renal Ca (2+) transport proteins by parathyroid hormone. *Kidney Int.* 2005:**68**(4):1708-21.

17. Green DE, Epstein S. Parathyroids, bone and mineral metabolism. *Current Opinion in Endocrinology & Diabetes* 2006:**13**(6):503-508.

18. Lambers TT, Bindels RJ, Hoenderop JG. Coordinated control of renal Ca^2+ handling. *Kidney Int.* 2006, **69**(4):650-4.

19. Rouse D, Suki WN. Renal control of extracellular calcium. *Kidney Int.* 1990:**38**(4):700-8.

20. Mensenkamp AR, Hoenderop JG, Bindels RJ. Recent advances in renal tubular calcium reabsorption.*Current Opinion in Nephrology &Hypertension* 2006:**15**(5):524-9.

21. Topala CN, Bindels RJM, Hoenderop JG. Regulation of the epithelial calcium channel TRPV5 by extracellular factors. *Current Opinion in Nephrology & Hypertension* 2007:**16**(4):319-324.

22. Makato Kuro O. Klotho as a regulator of fibroblast growth factor signaling and phosphate/calcium metabolism. *Current Opinion in Nephrology & Hypertension* **15**:437-441, 2006.

23. Nijenhuis T, Hoenderop JGJ, Loffing A et al. Thiazide—induced hypercalciuria is accompanied by a decreased expression of Calcium transport proteins in kidney. *Kidney Int.* **64**:555-564, 2003.

24. Rosenberg AE. Bones p1273-1278. In Robbins and Cotran Pathologic Basis of Disease. 7th ed. Kumar V, Abbas AK, Fausto N, RS, eds. Philadelphia: Saunders, 2005:

25. Rang HP, Dale MM, Ritter JM, Moore PK. Bone metabolism p. 461-470 in *Rang and Dale's Pharmacology.* 2007, Churchill Livingstone/Elsevier: London

26. Matsuo K. Cross –talk among bone cells. Current Opinion Nephrol and Hypert.**18**:292-297 2009

27. Andress D.L. Adynamic bone in patients with chronic kidney disease. Kidney International. 2008 **73** 1345-1354

28. Chung U, Kronenberg HM. Parathyroid hormone-related peptide and Indian hedgehog. *Current Opinion in Nephrology & Hypertension* 2009:**9**(4):357-62.

29. Sowers MF, Hollis BW, Shapiro B, et al. Elevated parathyroid hormone-related peptide associated with lactation and bone density loss. *JAMA* 1996:**276**(7):549-54.

30. Friedman PA. Calcium transport in the kidney. *Current Opinion in Nephrology & Hypertension* 1999:**8**(5):589-95.

31. Goodman WG. The flavors of Vitamin D: tasting the molecular mechanisms *Kidney Int.* 2004:**66**(3):1286-7.

32. Kato S, Kim M, Yamaoka K, Fujiki R. Mechanisms of transcriptional repression by 1, 25(OH)$_2$ vitamin D. *Current Opinion in Nephrology & Hypertension* 2007:**16**(4):297-304.

33. Stewart AF. Hypercalcaemia associated with cancer.NEJM:**352** 373-379, 2005.

34. Ludmerer KH, Kissane JM. Hypercalcaemia in a man with Non-Hodgkin's Lymphoma. *American Journal of Medicine* **72**:451-458, 1982.

35. Manolagas SC, Olefsky JM. Metabolic Bone and Mineral Disorders: Contemporary issues in Endocrinology and Metabolism.**5**:63-981988.

36. Koethe J, Kulesza P. Hypercalcaemia and Lymphadenopathy. American Journal of Medicine: **119**(11):902-2. 2006

37. Clemens TM, O'Riordan, JL. Vitamin D: p 417-423. in Principles and Practice of Endocrinology and Metabolism. Becker KL. Ed Philadelphia. Lippincott 1990.

38. Adams JS, Lee G. Gains in Bone Mineral density with Resolution of Vitamin D Intoxication. *Annals Int. Med.* 1997:**127**:203-206.

39. Jacobus CH, Holick MF, Shao Q et al. Hypervitaminosis D associated with Drinking Milk. *NEJM* 1992:**326**:1173-7.

40. Caplan RH, Beguin EA. Hypercalcaemia in a Calcitriol-treated hypoparathyroid woman during lactation. *Obstetrics & Gynaecology* 1990:**76**(3 Pt 2):485-9.

41. Bell NH, Stern PH. Hypercalcaemia and increases in serum hormone value during prolonged administration of 1alpha,25-dihydroxyvitamin D. *New England Journal of Medicine* 1978, **298**(22):1241-3.

42. Palmer SC, McGregor DO, Macaskill P et al. Meta-analysis: Vitamin D Compounds in Chronic Kidney Disease. *Ann. Intern. Med.* 2007, **147**:840-853.

43. Felsenfeld AJ, Levine BS. Milk alkali syndrome and the dynamics of Calcium Homeostasis. Clin J American society Nephrology 2006 **1** 641-654

44. Bosch X, Poch MD, Grau JM.Rhabdomyolysis and Acute Kidney Injury New Engl J Med 2009 361:62-72.

45. Reginster JY. The high prevalence of inadequate serum vitamin D: levels and implications for bone health. *Current Medical Research & Opinion* 2005, **21**(404:579-86

46. Chatfield SM, Brand C, Ebeling PR, Russell DM. Vitamin D deficiency in general medical inpatients in summer and winter. *Internal Medicine Journal* 2007, **37**(6):377-382.

47. Hii S, Scherer S. Vitamin D deficiency and secondary hyperparathyroidism in older people with low trauma fractures. *Australian Journal on Ageing* 2004, **23**(1):45-47.

48. Venning G. Recent developments in vitamin D deficiency and muscle weakness among elderly people. *BMJ* 2005, **330**(7490):524-6.

49. Avenell A, Gillespie WJ, Gillespie LD, O'Connell DL. Vitamin D and Vitamin D analogues for preventing fractures associated with involutional and post-menopausal osteoporosis Cochrane Database of Systematic Reviews 2008. Issue 3 Art No:CD000227.D01:10.1002/14651858CD000227.pub 2.

50. Portale AA, Miller WL. Hereditary rickets revealed. *Kidney International* 1998, **54**(5):1762-4.

51. Zaloga GP, Chernow B. The multifactorial basis for hypocalcaemia during sepsis. Studies of the parathyroid hormone-vitamin D axis. *Annuls of Internal Medicine* 1987, **107**(1):36-41.

52. Chernow B, Zaloga G, McFadden E, et al. Hypocalcaemia in critically ill patients. *Critical Care Medicine* 1982, **10**(12):848-51.

53. Steendijk P. Sepsis and intracellular calcium homeostasis, a sparkling story *Critical Care Medicine* 2005, **33**(3):688-90.

54. Zaloga GP, Chernow B. Hypocalcaemia in critical illness. *JAMA* 1986, **256**:1924-1929.

55. Spahn DR. Hypocalcaemia in trauma: frequent but frequently undetected and underestimated *Critical Care Medicine* 2005, **33**(9):2124-5.

56. Carlon GC, Howland WS, Kahn RC, Schweizer O. Calcium chloride administration in normocalcaemic critically ill patients. *Critical Care Medicine* 1980, **8**:209.

57. Mathru M, Rooney MW, Goldberg SA, Hirsch LJ. Separation of Myocardial Versus Peripheral Effects of Calcium Administration in Normocalcaemic and Hypocalcaemic States Using Press-Volume (Conductance) Relationships. *Anesth. Analgesia.* 1993, **77**:250-255.

58. Lang RM, Fellner SK, Neumann A, et al. Left Ventricular Contractility varies directly with Blood Ionized Calcium. *Annals of Internal Medicine.* 1988, **108**:524-529.

59. Targovnik JH, Rodman JS, Sherwood LM. Regulation of parathyroid hormone secretion Invitro: quantitative aspects of calcium and magnesium ion control. *Endocrinology.* 1971, **88**:1477-1482.

60. Cholst IN, Steinberg SF, Tropper PJ, et al. The influence of hypermagnesaemia on serum calcium and parathyroid hormone levels in human subjects. *New Eng J Med* 1984, **310**(19):1221-1225.

61. VandeWater JM, Van den Berg WM, Hoff RG, et al. Hypocalcaemia may reduce the beneficial effect of magnesium treatment in aneurismal subarachnoid haemorrhage. *Magnesium Research*. 2007, **20**:130-5.

62. Rude RK, Oldham SB, Sharp CF, Singer FR. Parathyroid Hormone secretion in Magnesium Deficiency. *Clin. Endocrinol. Metab.* 1978, **47**:800-806.

63. Shoback D. Hypoparathyroidism. *New Eng J Med* 2008 **359** 391-403

64. Prendiville S, Burman KD, Wartofsky L, et al. Evaluation and Treatment of Post-thyroidectomy Hypocalcaemia. *The Endocrinologist.* 1998, **8**:34-40.

65. McHenry CR, Speroff T, Wentworth D, Murphy T. Risk factors for post-thyroidectomy hypocalcaemia. *Surgery*. 1994, **116**(4):641-7.

66. Pearce SH, Williamson C, Kifor O, et al. A familial syndrome of hypocalcaemia with hypercalciuria due to mutations in the calcium-sensing receptor. *New England Journal of Medicine.* 1996, **335**(15):1115-22.

67. Chernow B, Rainey TG, Georges LP, O'Brien JT. Iatrogenic hyperphosphataemia : a metabolic consideration in critical care medicine. *Critical Care Medicine. 1981,9:772-774.*

68. Hebert LA, Lemann J. Jr., Petersen JR, Lennon EJ. Studies of the mechanism by which phosphate infusion lowers serum calcium concentration. *J Clin Invest.* 1996, **45**:1886-94.

69. Kingston M, Al-Sibai MB. Treatment of severe hypophosphataemia. *Critical Care Medicine.* 1985, **13**:16-18.

70. Fine A, Patterson J. Severe hyperphosphataemia following phosphate administration for bowel preparation in patients with renal failure: two cases and a review of the literature. *Amer. J. Kidney Disease.* 1997, **29**:103-105.

71. Stewart AF, Longo W, Kruetter D, et al. Hypocalcaemia due to calcium soap formation in a patient with pancreatic fistula. *New Eng J Med.* 1986, **315**:496.

72. Robertson GM, Moore EW, Switz DM, et al. Inadequate parathyroid response in acute pancreatitis. *New Eng J Med.* 1976, **294**:512.

73. Chennuru S; KoduriJ; Baumann MA.Risk factors for symptomatic hypocalcaemia complicating treatment with Zoledronic acid. Internal medicine J **38**:635-637 2008

74. Urbano FL.Signs of Hypocalcaemia: Chvostek's and Trousseau's signs. Hospital Physician 2000 (March) 43-45.

75. Johnson JD.Jennings R.Hypocalcemia and Cardiac Arrhythmias. Amer J Diseases Child.1968 **115**:373-376.

76. Fishbein JT, Hebert LJ, Shadravan IJ. An unusual cardiac arrhythmia caused by hypocalcemia. Amer J Dis Child.1982.**136**:372-373.

77. Rumancik WM, Denlinger JK, Nahrwold ML, Falk RB. The QT Internal and Serum Ionized Calcium. *JAMA*. 1978, **240**:366-368.

78. Ellman H, Dembin H, Seriff N. The rarity of shortening of the Q-T Interval in patients with hypercalcaemia. *Critical Care Medicine*. 1982, **10**:320.

79. Edelson, GW and Kleerekoper M. Hypercalcaemic crisis. *Medical Clinics of North America*. 1995, **79**(1):79-92.

80. LeGrand SB,Lekuski DZ. Narrative review:Furosemide for Hypercalcemia:an unproven but common practice.Ann Int Med 2008 **149** 259-263

81. Steddon SG; Cunningham MJ. Calcimimetics and Calcylytics –fooling the calcium receptor.Lancet 2005 **365** 2237-2239

82. Peacock M, Bilzekian JP, Klassen P S et al Cinalcet hydrochloride maintains long-term normocalcemia in patients with hyperparathyroidism.J Clin Endocrinol Metab 2005 **90** 135-141

83. Sloand JA, Shelley MA, Normalisation of Lithium-induced Hypercalcemia and Hyperparathyroidism with Cinaclet. Amer J Kidney Disease 2006 **48** 832-837

84. Tohme JF, Bilezikian JP. Hypocalcaemia emergencies. *Endocrinology & Metabolism Clinics of North America*. 1993, **22**(2):363-75.

85. Reber PM, Heath H. Hypocalcaemic emergencies. *Medical Clinics of North America*. 1995, **79**(1):93-106.

86. Tohme JF and Bilezikian JP. Diagnosis and treatment of hypocalcaemia emergencies. *The Endocrinologist*. 1996, **6**(1):10-18.

87. Winer KK, Ko CW, Reynolds JC, et al. Long-term treatment of hypoparathyroidism: a randomized controlled study comparing parathyroid hormone-(1-34) versus Calcitriol and calcium. *Journal of Clinical Endocrinology & Metabolism*. 2003, **88**(9):4214-20.

88. Callies F, Arlt W, Scholz JT, et al. Management of hypoparathyroidism during pregnancy—report of twelve cases. *Eur. J. Endocrinol*. 1998, **139**:284-289.

89. K/DOQ1 Clinical Practice Guidelines for Bone Metabolism and Disease in Chronic Kidney Disease. Background. *American Journal Kidney Disease*. 2003, **42**(Suppl 3):S29-S44.

90. Bushinsky DA, Silver J. Risks in dysregulation of the divalents. *Current Opinion in Nephrology and Hypertension*. 2005, **14**:315-317.

91. Goodman WG,Goldin J,Kuizon BD, et al Coronary-Artery Calcification In Young Adults With End –Stage Renal Disease Who Are Undergoing Dialysis. *New Eng J Med*.2000 :**342**:1478-83.

92. Shanahan CM. Vascular Calcification. *Current Opinion in Nephrology and Hypertension*. 2005, **14**:361-367.

93. Li X, Giachelli CM. Sodium-dependent phosphate cotransporters and vascular calcification. *Current Opinion in Nephrology and Hypertension.* 2007, **16**:325-328.

94. Goodman WG. Recent developments in the management of secondary hyperparathyroidism. *Kidney International.* 2001, **59**:1187-1201.

95. Fukagawa M, Tomoko NK, Junichiro K. Role of fibroblast growth factor 23 in health and in chronic kidney disease. *Current Opinion in Nephrology and Hypertension.* 2005, **14**:325-329.

96. Emmet M. What does serum fibroblast growth factor 23 do in hemodialysis patients. Kidney International.2008.**73**:3-5

97. Levi M. Post-transplant hypophosphataemia. *Kidney International.* 2001, **59**:2377-2387.

98. Rogers NM, Coates PTH.Calcific uraemic arteriolopathy.Current Opinion Nephrol Hypertens.2008.**17**:629-634.

99. Bushinsky DA. Phosphate Binders: Hold the Calcium? *Clin J. Am. Soc. Nephrol.* 2006, **1**:695-696.

100. Friedman EA. Calcium-Based Phosphate Binders are appropriate in Chronic Renal Failure. *Clin. J. Amer. Soc. Nephrol.* 2006, **1**:704-709.

101. Ketteler M, Rix M, Fan S, et al. Efficacy and Tolerability of Sevelamer Carbonate in Hyperphosphataemic Patients who have Chronic Kidney Disease and are not on Dialysis. *Clin. J. Am. Soc. Nephrol.* 2008, **3**:1125-1130.

102. Caglar K, Illker-Yilmaz M, Saglam M, et al. Short-Term Treatment with Sevelamer Increases Serum Fetuin-A concentration and improves Endothelial dysfunction in Chronic Kidney Disease Stage 4 Patients. *Clin. J. Am. Soc. Nephrol.* 2008, **3**:61-68.

103. Tonelli M, Pannu N, Manns B.Oral Phosphate Binders in Patients with Kidney Failure. New Engl J Med. **362**:1312-24.

104. Teng M, Wolf M, Lowrie E, et al. Survival of Patients Undergoing Haemodialysis with Paricalcitol or Calcitriol Therapy. *New Eng J Med.* 2003, **349**:446-55.

Oliguria, renal failure, hyponatraemia, hypotension or Low Cardiac Output

"If it were done when tis done
Then twere well it were done quickly" Macbeth. W. Shakespeare.

These conditions, singly or in combination, are common in those presenting to the Emergency Department or in postoperative patients. Oliguria or renal failure was the commonest postoperative reason for medical consultation in an orthopaedic ward [1] and in a nephrological consultation service [2]. Inadequate fluid administration was an important underlying factor.

In patients presenting to Emergency Departments low cardiac output (CO), due to effective hypovolaemia or cardiac failure, can be differentiated in most cases because there is either a source of fluid loss or cause for cardiac failure. The decision whether to infuse fluids, especially the amount, is more difficult in sepsis or in patients with renal failure. This review is not intended for patients managed in an Intensive Care Unit where more sophisticated monitoring is available.

The most common cause of the conditions described above is low cardiac output resulting from effective hypovolaemia or cardiac failure; less commonly intrinsic renal failure; and in those with hyponatraemia unsuppressed ADH secretion. Differentiating hypovolaemia from euvolaemia and cardiac failure can be difficult because volume depletion cannot be measured accurately.

However differentiation is important because delay in volume replacement in hypovolaemic patients may lead to renal failure or acute tubular necrosis, [2-6] irreversible shock; and multiple organ dysfunction. [7] Hypoperfusion of the heart, even without hypotension, is a component of endotoxic related myocardial dysfunction. [7] Adequate early fluid replacement improves outcome in septic [7-11] and hypovolaemic shock; [12-16] decreases the incidence of renal failure; [2-6, 17] and decreases risk of infection in patients with trauma. [16]

Persistent oliguria (>6 hours), even in the absence of raised serum creatinine, considerably increases the incidence of acute kidney injury and death in critically ill patients. (Kidney International 80 p760 2011). Early fluid resuscitation and duration of profound hypotension was considered the main reason for improved survival and decreased incidence of renal failure in the Vietnam compared to the Korean War. [12] Indeed early treatment of hypovolaemia is considered to be the most effective means of renal protection and for preventing renal failure. [3] Optimisation of vascular volume may decrease length of stay. [18, 19]

On the other hand inappropriate volume replacement can cause pulmonary oedema in those with heart failure or intrinsic renal failure with euvolaemia. Aggressive fluid resuscitation, with the goal to preserve renal function, has been questioned in severe sepsis [20-24]—especially use of colloids. [20] Once adult respiratory distress syndrome develops conservative, rather than aggressive fluid management, may improve outcome. [23-25]

Some advise caution in fluid administration in elderly or in those with heart disease. This often leads to delayed or inadequate volume repletion. Those with underlying heart disease are more dependent on optimum cardiac filling than are those without. Although formal studies have not been done—and are very unlikely ever to be done, the elderly, often with narrowed coronary, renal or cerebral arteries are theoretically more likely to develop cardiac infarction, stroke, irreversible shock and renal failure if effective treatment of hypotension or hypovolaemia is delayed. Patients with diastolic dysfunction, especially if atrial fibrillation is present, are critically dependent on adequate venous return.

Elderly subjects often have extensive comorbidity and take drugs which compromise vasoconstriction, decrease cardiac contractility, inhibit heart rate and cause hypovolaemia. Senescense of the microcirculation probably compromises flow to tissues.

Acute renal injury is more common in elderly compared to young patients in septic shock. [20]

The goal is to maximise preload but minimise risk of pulmonary oedema.

Cardiac failure, hypovolaemia and renal failure are differentiated clinically by a combination of the following:

• A cause for hypovolaemia, cardiac failure or renal failure is present or likely.

- <u>Supine and erect blood pressure and pulse</u>. An increase in pulse or decrease in blood pressure on standing are important clues to hypovolaemia.
- <u>Examination of the jugular venous pulse (JVP) and its response to elevation of the lower limbs, inspiration and abdominal compression (hepatojugular reflex).</u>
- <u>Other signs and symptoms of heart failure.</u>
- <u>Chest imaging.</u>
- <u>Saturation oxygen (SO$_2$) on room air (RA).</u>
- <u>Laboratory tests</u>—serum creatinine, serum urea, serum urea / creatinine ratio, serum uric acid, serum HCO$_3^-$ and anion gap.
- <u>Urine Na$^+$, Cl$^-$ ± K$^+$.</u>

Hypovolaemia (or effective vascular under filling) is diagnosed based on the following:

- <u>A cause of external fluid loss or sepsis is present and a cause for cardiac failure is absent. Common causes of fluid losses are:</u>
  * blood loss
  * diuretic use
  * diarrhoea and/or vomiting
  * excessive sweating, especially in patients with cystic fibrosis
  * chronic renal salt loss—especially in disease involving the medulla
  * diabetic ketoacidosis
  * third space fluid loss
- <u>Analysis suggests that insufficient fluid has been given</u> to treat trauma, peri operative losses of blood or other fluids, internal bleeding or third space losses.
- <u>Sepsis is present,</u> suggesting that there is inadequate vascular filling. This is especially likely in patients who are taking diuretic or vasodilator drugs who develop an infection.
- <u>Signs and symptoms support a diagnosis of effective hypovolaemia.</u> Manifestations which support a diagnosis of effective hypovolaemia are discussed further in the chapter 5 but are summarised below:
  * <u>Orthostatic hypotension and tachycardia</u>
  * An increase in pulse of ≥ 20 or fall in systolic blood pressure on standing suggests hypovolaemia, ineffective arterial filling or both are present. Unfortunately many patients are unable to stand.
  * <u>Elevated JVP is absent and jugular veins appear under filled on lying flat.</u>
  * <u>Diminished skin turgor and sunken eyes suggest saline depletion.</u>
  * <u>Absence of clinical and imaging signs of heart failure.</u>

* <u>Laboratory tests are compatible</u>
* <u>Signs of volume depletion.</u> (chapter 6)

The most useful are an increase in pulse on standing and for more severe hypovolaemia orthostatic hypotension or inability to stand. [26] Observational studies in general have failed to establish whether skin, turgor, sunken eyes, dry mucous membranes or capillary refill are useful for diagnosing hypovolaemia. In the authors experience skin inelasticity and enophthalmos are useful in diagnosing sodium depletion in children; dry mucous membranes are not [27].

Cardiac failure is the probable cause.

* <u>A cause for cardiac failure is present</u>.
* Clinical data, ECG and serum troponin suggest cardiac infarction, pulmonary embolism or cardiac arrhythmia have occurred. Serum BNP (brain natriuretic peptide) has high sensitivity for the presence of cardiac failure but may not be immediately available.
* <u>Effects of standing on blood pressure and pulse</u>. If venous return is optimal and the heart is on the plateau part of Starlings curve, relating stroke volume (S.V.) to atrial filling, there should be no decrease in blood pressure or increase in heart rate following 1-2 minutes of standing or sitting from the supine position.
* <u>Other signs of heart failure</u>. In a systematic review of 22 studies, [28] from 815 citations, the following were useful in predicting the presence or absence of heart failure in patients presenting to an Emergency Department (Table 1).

Positive Likelihood	Ratio	Negative Likelihood	Ratio
Chest imaging pulmonary vein distension	12.0	Absent cardiomegaly	0.33
Third heart sound	11.0	Absence RALES	0.51
Jugular venous distension (JVD)	5.8	Absent JVD	0.66
Past history of heart failure	5.8	No past history	0.45
Atrial fibrillation on ECG	3.8	Normal ECG	0.64
Paroxysmal nocturnal dyspnoea	2.6	No dyspnoea	0.48

Table 1: *Positive and negative likelihood ratios for diagnosis of congestive cardiac failure from a systematic review. Modified from reference 28.*

Low serum BNP was the best test but added little to Table 1. [29]

In an observational blinded study of patients with dyspnoea BNP levels and chest imaging were complementary and useful in diagnosis of heart failure. [28] A combination rather than individual symptoms and signs were highly predictive.

In another systematic review [30] each of the jugular venous pressure and imaging signs of pulmonary venous hypertension had a sensitivity of over 80% for diagnosing left-sided heart failure, but their absence could not exclude an increase in filling pressure. Dyspnoea, orthopnea, decrease in systolic pulse pressure and third heart sound were reported as 'somewhat' helpful.

In a prospective observational study in 50 patients, raised JVP and pulmonary oedema were absent in 18/43 (40%) but when present were 100% specific. It has been emphasised however that the low incidence of signs of heart failure may be due to a lack of skills in auscultation and estimation of the JVP by clinicians. [32-34]

A third heart sound is highly specific but is only heard in a minority of those with heart failure. [28, 31-33] Various scores utilising a combination of symptoms, physical signs and imaging have been suggested for the clinical diagnosis of congestive heart failure. The Framingham [35] and Boston Criteria [36] are shown in Table 2.

Marantz et al [37] compared the left ventricular ejection fraction with the Boston Criteria for the clinical diagnosis of congestive cardiac failure. There was a poor correlation. This was not surprising because left ventricular function is often normal in diastolic dysfunction. Thus in the absence of an accepted gold standard for the diagnosis of congestive cardiac failure reliability of clinical signs is difficult to establish.

In my experience examination of the jugular veins is the most important examination in differentiating heart failure from hypovolaemia.

FRAMINGHAM CRITERIA[35]	BOSTON CRITERIA[36]	
Major Criteria	**Category I: History**	**Point Value^**
	Rest dyspnea	4
Paroxysmal nocturnal dyspnea or orthopnea		
Neck-vein distension	Orthopnea	4
Rales	Paroxysmal nocturnal dyspnea	3
Cardiomegaly	Dyspnea on walking on level	2
Acute pulmonary oedema	Dyspnea on climbing	1
S_3 gallop		
Increased venous pressure >16cm of water	Maximum 4 points	
Circulation time >25 sec		
Hepatojugular reflux	**Category II: Physical examination**	
	Heart rate abnormality	1-2
Minor criteria	(if 91-110 beats/min, 1 point;	
Ankle oedema	if >110 beats/min, 2 points)	
Night cough	Jugular-venous pressure elevation	
Dyspnea on exertion	(if >6cm H_2O, 2 points; if >6cm	2-3
Hepatomegaly	H_2O plus Hepatomegaly or oedema,	
	3 points)	
Pleural effusion	Lung crackles	1-2
Vital capacity decreased 1/3 from maximum	(if basilar, 1 point; if more than basilar, 2 points)	
Tachycardia (rate of >120/min)	Wheezing	3
Major or minor criterion	Third heart sound	3
Weight loss >4.5kg in 5 days in response to treatment	Maximum 4 points	
	Category III: Chest radiography	
	Alveolar pulmonary oedema	4
	Interstitial pulmonary oedema	3
	Bilateral pleural effusions	3
	Cardiothoracic ratio >0.50 (posteroanterior projection)	3
	Upper zone flow redistribution	2
	Maximum 4 points	
A	**B**	
Definite Diagnosis 2 major or 1 major plus 2 minor criteria	4 maximum points per category giving a maximum score of 12.	

	Heart failure	
	Definite	8-12
	Possible	5-7
	Unlikely	≤4

Table 2: (A) Framingham [35] and (B) Boston Criteria [36] for clinical diagnosis of congestive cardiac failure.

Measurement of the Jugular Venous Pressure [38,]

A wave = atrial contraction V wave =ventricular relaxation and opening of tricuspid valve x descent = atrial relaxation y descent =atrial emptying on opening of tricuspid valve c wave =minor positive deflection from bulging of tricuspid valve into right atrium.	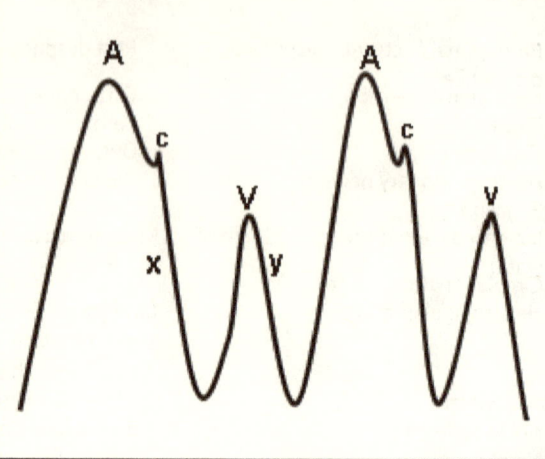

Figure 1. Components of the jugular venous wave formation.

The patient is positioned at 30-45 degrees above the horizontal. The head should be supported to relax neck muscles and the patient positioned to bring the JVP above the clavicle. At 45 degrees the clavicle is 2 cm above the angle of Louis or 7 cm above the right atrium (RA). The level of venous pressure is the highest point of oscillation of the internal or external jugular veins during quiet non forced expiration Regardless of patient position the vertical line 5 cm below the sternal angle roughly approximates the midpoint of the RA which is normally zero. Thus jugular venous distension vertically above the sternal angle + 5 cm approximates central venous pressure. To convert mmHg to cm of water multiply by 1.36.

The jugular venous pressure has two separate waves: a large 'a' wave due to atrial contraction and a smaller v wave due to ventricular relaxation and opening of the tricuspid valve. Each wave is followed by a fall called x and y descent. The x descent is punctuated by a small superimposed 'c' wave which is due to bulging of the tricuspid valve into the right atrium during isovolumetric right ventricular contraction.

The normal CVP is 5cm with an upper limit of 9cm. At 45 degrees the venous pulse should be seen just above the clavicle: this represents a CVP of approximately 7 cms water. A CVP above 30cm results in disappearance of pulsation behind the angle of the mandible and may be misdiagnosed unless the patient sits upright. If hypovolaemia is present the patient may have to lie flat for visualisation. JVP is difficult to assess in agitated patients or those with tachypnoea. Examination following sedation is more reliable. The external and internal jugular veins are both examined for pressure and wave form analysis although the right internal jugular vein is usually better visualised because it is more directly in line with the right atrium.

Confidence in identification of the internal jugular from arterial pulsation is increased by:

* Identification of at least two waves, a and v, (a double flicker) corresponding to atrial contraction and atrial filling during diastole. The carotid pulsation appears as a single deflection.
* Venous pulsation usually shows a slow upward diffuse non-palpable deflection rather than abrupt palpable deflection as in the carotid pulsation.
* Effect of posture—changing the patient's position has a minimal effect on carotid pulsation while the height of venous pulsation changes. When there is a marked increase the venous pulsation may be difficult to locate supine but easy to identify sitting upright.
* Effect of inspiration on the jugular venous pressure or distension. The jugular venous pressure normally falls on inspiration.
* Pressure with the finger at the root of the neck distends the vein and obliterates pulsation.
* Hepatojugular reflux. The JVP should increase and in heart failure remain elevated for longer than 10 seconds when constant pressure is applied to the abdomen.

Elevated JVP is due to increase in RV diastolic pressure, pulmonary hypertension or stenosis, obstruction to RV inflow from tricuspid stenosis, constrictive pericarditis, hypervolaemia or superior vena cava obstruction.

Usefulness of Jugular Venous Pressure

There is controversy about the usefulness of examination of the jugular venous pulse in estimating right sided cardiac filling. Some consider estimation of JVP is inaccurate, insensitive and non-specific as a sign of heart failure in critically ill patients. Specificity is high but sensitivity low. [38] Jugular vein assessment by clinicians has been reported to be poor. [38-40] Clinical assessment of venous pressure showed a poor correlation with catheter measurement of Central Venous Pressure (CVP) in critically ill patients. [39, 40]

This may be due to one or a combination of the lack of expertise of observers; lack of a gold standard for comparison; the failure to consider all important components of the examination; and expectation that observers should be able to predict venous pressure within 2-3 cm of the measured CVP which is both impractical and irrelevant. For example, in one study junior doctors assessed jugular venous pressure: reliability was based on unrealistic clinical predictions which were within the error of estimation of catheter levelling. [39]

Pressure recorded by a CVP catheter also depends on estimation of the location of the right atrium and changes caused by mechanical ventilation. Thus the gold standard for clinical assessment of jugular venous pressure may be flawed

A recent study, in which the central venous pressure was estimated either as low (≤ 5cm of water) or high (≥ 10cm of water), showed that clinical estimation of JVP was reliable and correlated highly with CVP (central venous pressure) measured with an indwelling catheter. Attending physicians determined low and high CVP with areas under the receiver operating curves of 0.95 (0.88-1.0) and 0.97 (0.92-1.0) respectively. [41]

Surprisingly the external jugular vein was easier to visualise and estimation was not more difficult in mechanically ventilated compared to spontaneously breathing patients. The venous pressure measured in the external jugular vein shows high correlation with central venous pressure in the right atrium. [41-43]

The central venous pressure which determines preload is the CVP relative to the transmural pressure (pressure around the heart). [44-46] The heart is surrounded by pleural pressure which varies relative to atmospheric pressure during the respiratory cycle. Breathing with forced expiratory efforts, pursed lip breathing, pneumothorax and mediastinal oedema may increase intrathoracic pressure and JVP in the presence of hypovolaemia. Pericardial effusion, chronic pulmonary hypertension and positive pressure ventilation may require a higher than normal venous pressure for optimum preload.

An important reason for assessing JVP or in using more invasive measurements of fluid status or preload is to determine if patients with oliguria, hyponatraemia, hypotension or shock are likely respond to additional infusion of fluid.

The safest manoevre is to establish fluid responsiveness without giving fluid –to avoid the hazards of fluid infusion.

An important criticism of the usefulness of JVP is that a high pressure does not necessarily indicate that optimum cardiac filling is present—that the heart will not respond to fluid infusion even when central venous pressure appears to be raised.

Single measurements (static indices) of preload do not correlate with fluid responsiveness. [25, 47-58]

The majority of studies and reviews have shown that CVP (central venous pressure) measured by catheter, [25, 45-49, 51, 54] left ventricular end diastolic pressure or left ventricular volumes measured by pulmonary artery occlusion pressure (PAOP); [25, 40, 47, 48, 50 52- 54, 56,] single measurements of cardiac output and stroke volume [53], in both ventilated and spontaneously breathing patients, do not correlate with fluid responsiveness.

For example cardiac output may increase in response to fluid infusion when static (single) measurement of CVP varies between 2mmHg and 18 mmHg. [45] This may be due to variations in right or left ventricular contractility or compliance; afterload; or valvular function (mitral or tricuspid regurgitation).

Dynamic indices, in which the CVP, JVP, pulmonary artery occlusion pressure or other variables are measured before and after bolus fluid infusions are better predictors of fluid responsiveness.

Ventilated Patients:

Minimally invasive indices of fluid responsiveness, which avoid fluid infusion, have been developed in patients receiving ventilatory support. Some of these depend on heart-lung interactions by noting changes in variables over three or more breaths. Positive pressure inspiration induces cyclical increases in right atrial pressure (RAP) which in turn causes inverse changes in right ventricular (RV) filling and ejection and ultimately left ventricular (LV) preload. The greater degree of pressure or volume variations over the course of the respiratory cycle, for a fixed specific tidal volume, the more likely is fluid responsiveness present. Measurements include:

- Arterial or pulse pressure variation in response to ventilation. [49 50- 53, 55 -57]

- Transthoracic or transoesophageal (with Doppler) aortic blood flow variations or stroke volume variations with respiration. [47, 49, 50- 52, 54 57, 58]

- Right atrial pressure variation with respiration. [25, 44, 46, 50]

- Superior or inferior cava vascular diameter in response to ventilation measured by echocardiogram. [47, 52, 55, 60].

- Central venous oxygen saturation: SvO_2 and $ScvO_2$. [47]

Peripheral leg raising (PLR). [49, 51, 52, 56, 59 - 63]

Peripheral leg raising transfers blood towards the thorax, increases venous return and is followed by an increase in LV stroke volume. Peripheral leg raising is carried out by raising both lower limbs from the supine position; or by reversing the semirecumbent position and then raising the limbs as follows:

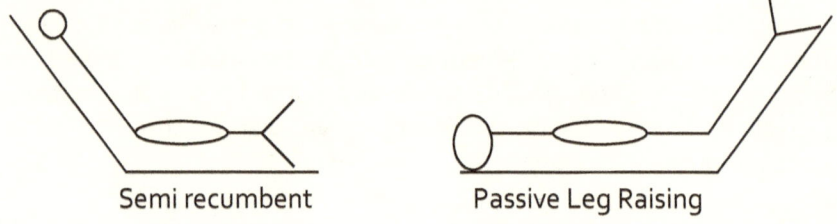

Semi recumbent   Passive Leg Raising

Figure 2: Change from semirecumbent to Passive Leg Raising.

Raising both lower limbs from the semirecumbent position increases preload to a greater extent than from the supine position. [63]

Measurement of CVP, SV by echocardiogram, [51, 56] venous collapsibility, [60] pulse pressure variation, [49, 51, 52] aortic flow [56, 59, 61] or Valsalva manoeuvre should be carried out soon after the manoeuvre. The majority of these measurements however have been validated in mechanically ventilated but not spontaneously breathing patients.

Spontaneously Breathing Patients:

The measurements, described previously, change in the opposite direction during inspiration in spontaneously breathing patients in comparison to ventilated patients because the RAP becomes negative rather than positive on inspiration. Thus preload increases. However these measurements are less reliable and have been inadequately evaluated in spontaneously breathing patients.

A systematic review, which identified only eight robust studies, found that only respiratory variation of RAP (measured by CVP catheter) identified those who responded to a fluid infusion. [25]

Dynamic non-invasive studies in spontaneously breathing patients which can be done include:

- Response of the JVP to inspiration
- Hepatojugular reflux sign.
- Response to the Valsalva manoeuvre.
- Response to peripheral leg elevation.
- Pulse pressure variation measured by echocardiography.

Response of Jugular Venous Pressure to Inspiration:

Failure of venous pressure to decrease on inspiration or continued elevation of venous pressure on abdominal compression suggests that the heart is on the plateau of the cardiac pressure volume curve and that volume infusion will not increase cardiac output. An increase in JVP on inspiration, called Kussmaul's sign, suggests that right ventricular failure, pericardial fluid or constrictive pericarditis is present.

I have found that the response to inspiration and performance of hepatojugular reflux is useful in predicting fluid responsiveness (unpublished observations). However there is limited experimental evidence in support of the reliability of the clinical response of jugular venous pressure to inspiration.[64, 65] The close correlation between measured jugular venous pressure and the right atrial pressure [41-43] and between fluid responsiveness and CVP respiratory variations suggests that the clinical examination of the jugular venous response to inspiration may be useful in assessing fluid responsiveness.

Abdominojugular Reflux. [66-69]

The hepatojugular reflux sign is carried out by gradual abdominal pressure applied for 10-15 seconds: if the jugular venous pressure increases (<4 cm), or falls promptly the heart is considered to be able to increase cardiac output further on volume infusion. A sustained (≥ 10 seconds) elevation (> 4 cm) of the jugular venous pressure or sustained engorgement of jugular veins suggest that the right heart is unable to accommodate an increase in venous return. It is important to avoid producing pain, breath holding and straining.

The hepatojugular reflux sign reflects the inability of the right ventricle to increase output from an increase in venous return. It is therefore positive in both left and right ventricular disorders. It has been found useful in the diagnosis of heart failure [66-69] but has low sensitivity [67] and has not been validated for predicting fluid responsiveness.

Valsalva Manoeuvre. [67, 70-76]

This is carried out by a sustained respiratory effort for at least 10 seconds against a closed glottis. The normal arterial blood pressure response consists of the following in sequence shown in figure 3 and table3.

Phase1: Transient increase of BP with the onset of straining due to effort involved.

Phase 2: BP and pulse pressure decrease and pulse increases as venous return is inhibited.

Phase 3: Transient decrease in BP on initial release of strain.

Phase 4: BP overshoot and reflex bradycardia occurs due to an increase in venous return following release of strain.

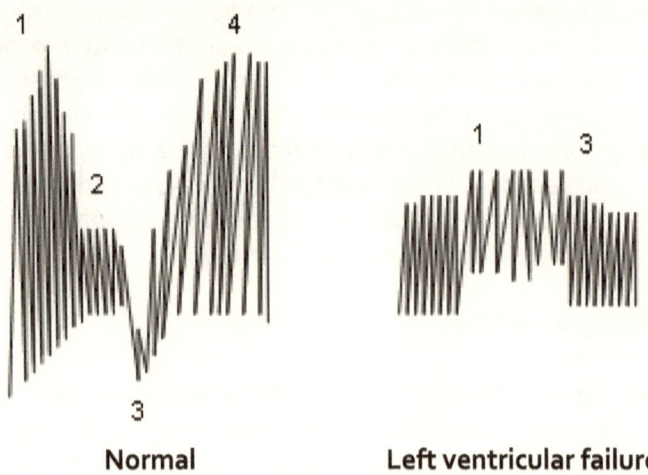

Normal   Left ventricular failure

Figure 3: Intra-arterial pressure during Valsalva manoeuvre.

In patients with heart failure the overshoot response is absent in mild heart failure(figure 3b), and square wave response present in severe heart failure: an initial increase in blood pressure, which remains elevated during the entire effort (strain), with return to resting levels at release of strain. This is because left ventricular filling and SV are maintained despite decrease in venous return. This suggests that fluid responsiveness will be absent. Indeed following diuretic treatment the response normalises. [67]

Strain Initiation	
1. Initial ↑ in BP	Acute increase in intrathoracic pressure,
2. Sharp ↓ in BP below base line HR while effort is maintained.	Decrease in SV due to ↓ venous return and ↑ PVR.
Strain Release	
3. Short decrease in BP	Acute increase in intrathoracic pressure
4. Overshoot increase of BP, reflex bradycardia	Acute ↓ intrathoracic pressure with ↑ SV and ↓ PVR.

Table 3: *Phases of the Valsalva manoeuvre (BP = blood pressure, SV = stroke volume. HR = heart rate, PVR = peripheral vascular resistance.*

The Valsalva manoeuvre responses can be recorded by bedside blood pressure measurement, echocardiography or arterial pressure wave forms. The test using BP measurements has been validated for left ventricular systolic dysfunction [76] and congestive cardiac failure. [67] Using more sophisticated equipment the Valsalva response correlates with pulmonary capillary wedge pressure. [73-75] However the Valsalva manoeuvre is difficult to perform in patients with congestive failure and has poor sensitivity. [67] The validity of the Valsalva manoeuvre in predicting fluid responsiveness in spontaneously breathing patients was shown recently using transthoracic echocardiography for measurement. [77]

Passive Leg Raising

The effects of passive leg raising in predicting fluid responsiveness in spontaneously breathing patients is controversial but is the best validated. [56] However there are few studies and only one which used non invasive assessment.

In mechanically ventilated patients the effect of passive leg rising in assessing fluid responsiveness appears to be highly effective by using a variety of non-invasive measurements, including Doppler transoesophageal echocardiography. [59-61] transthoracic echocardiography [51, 77] and pulse pressure variation. [59]

In the majority of situations, outside of the intensive care or high Dependency Unit, the decision on fluid loading has to be based on clinical assessment without using sophisticated equipment.

In practice there are three diagnostic outcomes following clinical assessment of the venous pressure:

- Venous pressure is raised and does not decrease on inspiration. Further volume replacement would not increase cardiac output.
- The venous pressure is clearly low and volume infusion will raise cardiac output.
- There is uncertainty between the above two so that a trial of fluids is required to differentiate them.

Laboratory Tests.

These give support for low cardiac output as the cause of oliguria, hypotension or hyponatraemia, but does not differentiate between hypovolaemia and heart failure.

An abnormally low serum creatinine, urea and uric acid [78] strongly suggest that unsuppressed (inappropriate) ADH secretion is the cause of hyponatraemia. Serum uric acid may discriminate between hypovolaemia, in which it is high, and SIADH where it is low. [79]

Moderate increase in serum creatinine (≤ 300 µmol/L) in combination with raised urea-creatinine ratio (≥ 60) (urea and creatinine both in µmol/L) suggests that a low cardiac output is present rather than renal failure, especially if the ratio exceeds 100. In intrinsic renal failure the ratio of urea to creatinine is normal (<60).

Urine Electrolytes. (chapter 16)

Low urine Na^+ (≤ 20 mmol/L) or $C\ell^-$ in alkalosis are evidence of low cardiac output. The normal kidney responds immediately to hypovolaemia by decreasing Na^+ excretion. It is useful to measure on presentation and gives an ongoing indication of volume status on treatment. In severe alkalosis urine Na^+ may be paradoxically raised because Na^+ excretion is obligated by HCO_3^- (poorly reabsorbable anion) excretion. However urinary Cl^- concentration is very low. On the other hand urine Cl^- may be raised when acidosis accompanies hypovolaemia.

A low urinary Na^+ suggests:

- A need for Na+ conservation because a low cardiac output or vascular under filling is present.
- Kidney function is relatively normal (exceptions include acute glomerulo-tubular nephritis, contrast nephropathy; bilateral renal artery stenosis).
- Aldosterone secretion is adequate.

High urine Na^+ ($\geq$ 20 mmol/L) is present in:

- Inappropriate ADH secretion (serum creatinine, urea and uric acid are usually low).
- Absence of a need to conserve sodium provided renal function is normal –evidence of normal cardiac output.
- Intrinsic renal failure.
- Diuretic use.
- Renal causes of sodium loss—especially conditions affecting the medulla.
- Aldosterone deficiency (Addison's disease).

Spot urine sodium predicted the presence of hypovolaemia better than clinical signs in one study [80]. The fractional excretion of sodium (FE Na^+) makes assessment of urine sodium less dependent on urine volume. This is normally less than 0.5% if sodium depletion or a low cardiac output. [81]

Fe Na+ = urine Na+ / plasma Na+ X plasma creatinine/urine creatinine X 100(%)

Units should be the same for sodium and creatinine i.e. mmol/L or gm/L

Spot urinary sodium is useful in the differential diagnosis of hyponatraemia: it is low in sodium depletion or hypovolaemia; high in severe renal failure, diuretic use and in the syndrome of inappropriate ADH secretion. (SIADH). A low fractional excretion of sodium plus urea provided a better prediction for hypovolaemia than sodium alone. [81]

Urine sodium should be high in SIADH because hypovolaemia is characteristically absent. In practice there is a considerable overlap between SIADH and sodium depletion. [82] During a low sodium intake, or low urine output, reflected in a high urine creatinine/plasma creatinine ratio, even the $FeNa^+$ may be low (<0.5%) in the SIADH. [82] However during a low urine output (antidiuresis) from sodium depletion, reflected in a urine Cr/plasma Cr ratio more than 140, the FeNa was <0.15 % and the Fe urea <45 %. [82]

If the differential diagnosis between SIADH and sodium depletion is uncertain a trial of saline infusion can be carried out safely provided serum sodium is monitored [83] Musch and Decaux [83] infused 2 L of n.Saline over 24 hours: an increase of the plasma sodium of at least 5 mmol/L combined with a low FeNa identified sodium depletion. Decrease in plasma sodium of up to 4 mmol/L occurred in a minority who had a urinary concentration of $Na^+ + K^+$ of 300 mmol/L or over suggesting that this strategy is safe. [83]

Natriuretic Peptides. (chapter 6)

At present natriuretic peptides may not be immediately available and their role in fluid responsiveness has not been established.

From an analysis of the above signs the diagnosis falls into three main groups which are potentially reversible:

1. Hypovolaemia or vascular under filling is probable.
2. Cardiac failure is probable and treatment with volume replacement will be ineffective.
3. These cannot be differentiated with confidence.

Diagnosis of irreversible renal failure should not be made unless reversible causes are excluded.

<u>The default position should be that hypovolaemia is present. This should lead to a trial of fluids.</u>

For example, normal supine but orthostatic tachycardia or hypotension, low jugular venous pressure, urea: creatinine ratio >100, low urinary Na^+ and fever suggests effective hypovolaemia is present.

Raised jugular venous pressure, unexplained low SO_2, (room air) and pulmonary congestion on imaging strongly suggests the diagnosis of heart failure.

A trial of fluids should be undertaken If the cause of oliguria, hypotension, and signs of low CO, renal failure and hyponatraemia are uncertain.

A trial of fluids should not be withheld solely based on the level of venous pressure alone. The response to dynamic measures such as inspiration, leg raising, posture and abdominal compression, although not validated, should be considered based on biological plausibility.

Infiltrate on chest imaging or an abnormally low SO_2 are not absolute contraindications to a 'trial of fluids'. SO_2 frequently improves in hypovolaemic patients following fluid infusion (personal observations).

A loop diuretic should not be given if oliguria is present and the cause uncertain. It is ineffective and potentially dangerous. [84, 85]

Fluid should be infused rapidly, so that if the heart is unresponsive, fluid will redistribute into a lesser space than if a larger amount is given more slowly. A slow infusion also makes assessment of the response more difficult.

The ongoing controversy on whether crystalloid or colloid should be used continues. [86, 87] However, if the heart is unresponsive, crystalloid will rapidly redistribute to the extracellular space and is potentially safer. Several systematic reviews have failed to establish the superiority of colloid compared to saline. In some of these studies the quantity of crystalloids administered were not equivalent in expanding vascular volume than colloids. Indeed it is surprising that 500 mL colloid, but only 1L crystalloid is recommended in a trial of fluids considering that the ratio of interstitial fluid to plasma volume is 3:1.

If saline depletion is the cause of hypovolaemia saline should be used in treatment—not colloid.

Trial of fluids. I use the following protocol.

500-1000mL (usually 1000mL) normal saline is infused in 15-30 minutes with documentation of the following before and immediately following the challenge:

Urine output and urine Na+.
Blood pressure and pulse and, if possible, response to standing or limb elevation.

SO_2 (on room air) and respiratory rate; patient's perception of both breathlessness and improvement.
Assessment of jugular venous pressure and response to inspiration, leg elevation if appropriate) and hepato-jugular reflux.
± repeat chest imaging.

There are three outcomes:

1. Urine output increases (previous oliguria present), SO_2 (RA) does not decrease or increases and respiratory rate does not increase; the blood pressure or pulse improve; and the patient feels better. Hypovolaemia is diagnosed and saline infusion is continued to maintain a urine output >30-50 mL/hour.

2. Urine output does not increase, the respiratory rate increases, SO_2(RA) decreases, the patient feels more breathless and jugular venous pressure increases. Cardiac failure is diagnosed. This is then treated with a loop diuretic and other measures to improve heart failure.

3. The diagnosis remains uncertain following the fluid challenge.

In this case a further trial of fluids is given. The SO_2 (RA) is especially useful. It often improves in hypovolaemic patients following fluid infusion, presumably because ventilation perfusion mismatch due to hypovolaemia improves. A decrease in SO_2, an increase in respiratory rate, the patients' perception of increased breathlessness and chest imaging are useful indications of increasing pulmonary congestion.

The author's observations in an orthopaedic ward, general medical ward and emergency department, in which data was entered prospectively on specific forms showed that a trial of fluid infusion rarely resulted in cardiac failure. The majority of patients responded suggesting they were effectively hypovolaemic. In 11 consecutive cases, 9 showed improvement of SO_2 on room air following initial or subsequent fluid infusion suggesting that ventilation/perfusion mismatch had improved.

If available, clinical data can be supplemented with non invasive measurement of stroke volume, as discussed previously.

REFERENCES

1. Kingston M: Determining the professional attributes of a hospitalist: experience in one Australian metropolitan hospital. *Intern Med. J.* **35**:305-8, 2005.

2. Davidman M, Olson P, Kohen J, Leither T, Kjellstrand C: Iatrogenic renal disease. *Arch Intern Med.* **151**:1809-12, 1991.

3. Kellum JA, Leblanc M, Gibney RT, Tumlin J, Lieberthal W, Ronco C: Primary prevention of acute renal failure in the critically ill. *Curr. Opin Crit Care.* **11**:537-41, 2005

4. Bennett-Jones DN: Early intervention acute renal failure. *BMJ.* **333**:407-7, 2006.

5. Star RA: Treatment of acute renal failure. *Kidney Int.* **54**:1917-31, 1998.

6. Edwards BF: Postoperative renal insufficiency. *Med Clin North Am.* **85**:1241-54, 2001.

7. Parrillo JE: Pathogenic mechanisms of septic shock. *New Engl J Med.* **328**:1471-7, 1993.

8. Vincent JL, Weil MH: Fluid challenge revisited. *Crit Care Med.* **34**:1333-7, 2006.

9. Rivers E, Nguyen B, Havstad S, Ressler J, Muzzin A, Knoblich B et al: Early goal-directed therapy in the treatment of severe sepsis and septic shock. *New Engl J Med.* **345**:1368-77, 2001.

10. Vincent JL, Gerlach H: fluid resuscitation in sever sepsis and septic shock: an evidence-based review. *Crit Care Med.* **32**:S451-4, 2004.

11. Oleivera CF, Oleivera DS, Gottschald AF, Moura JD et al. ACCM/PALS haemodynamic support guidelines for paediatric septic shock: an outcome comparison with and without monitoring central venous oxygen saturation. Intensive Care Medicine **34**:1065-1075.2008

12. Butkus DE. Post traumatic acute renal failure in combat casualties: A historical review. Military Medicine **149** 117-24 1984

13. Guly, UM, Turney JH. Post traumatic acute renal failure. Clin Nephrol **34** 79-83 1990

14. Carcillo JA, Tasker RC: Fluid resuscitation of hypovolaemic shock: acute medicine's great triumph for children. *Intensive Care Med.* **32**:958-61, 2006.

15. Blow O, Magliore L, Claridge JA, Butler K, Young JS: The golden hour and the silver day: detection and correction of occult hypoperfusion within 24 hours improves outcome from major trauma. *J. Trauma.* **47**:964-9, 1999.

16. Claridge JA, Crabtree TD, Pelletier SJ, Butler K, Sawyer RG, Young JS: Persistent occult hypoperfusion is associated with a significant increase

in infection rate and mortality in major trauma patients. *J. Trauma.* **48**:80-14, 2000.

17. Sladen RN. Anesthesia and renal considerations.Oliguria in the ICU. Anesthesiol Clin North America. **18** 739-752 2000

18. Venn R, Steele A, Richardson P, Poloniecki J, Grounds M, Newman P: Randomised controlled trial to investigate influence of the fluid challenge on duration of hospital stay and perioperative morbidity in patients with hip fractures. *Br. J. Anaesth.* **88**:65-71, 2002.

19. Sinclair S, James S, Singer M: Intraoperative intravascular volume optimization and length of hospital stay after repair of proximal femoral fracture: randomised controlled trial. *BMJ.* **315**:909-12, 1997.

20. Bagshaw SM, Bellomo R: Fluid resuscitation and the septic kidney. *Curr. Opin Crit Care.* **12**:527-30, 2006.

21. Bagshaw SM,BellomoR,Kellum JA Oliguria,volume overload and loop diuretics.Crit Care Medicine **36:** S172-S178, 2008

22. Holte K, Sharrock NE, Kehlet H: Pathophysiology and clinical implications of perioperative fluid excess. *Br. J. Anaesth.* **89**:622-32,2002.

23. Rivers EP: Fluid-management strategies in acute lung injury-liberal, conservative, or both? *New Engl J Med.* **354**:2598-600, 2006.

24. Comparison of two fluid-management strategies in acute lung injury. N, Wiedemann HP, wheeler AP, Bernard GR, Thompson BT, et al: *New Engl J Med.* **354**:2564-75, 2006

25. Coudray A, Romand JA, Treggiari M, Bendjelid K: Fluid responsiveness in spontaneously breathing patients: a review of indexes used in intensive care. *Crit Care Med.* **33**:2757-62, 2005.

26. McGee S, Abernethy WB 3rd, Simel DL: The rational clinical examination. Is this patient hypovolaemic? [see comment]. *JAMA.* **281**:1022-9, 1999.

27. Kingston M: Thesis for Degree of Doctorate of Medicine. 1974.

28. Wang CS, FitzGerald JM, Schulzer M, Mak E, Ayas NT: Does this dypsnoeic patient in the emergency department have congestive heart failure? *JAMA.* **294**:1944-56, 2005.

29. Knudsen CW, Orland T, Clopton P et al: Diagnostic value of B-type natriuretic peptide and chest radiographic findings in patients with acute dyspnoea. *Amer J. Med.* **116**:363-368, 2004.

30. Badgett RG, Lucey CR, Mulrow CD: Can the clinical examination diagnose left-sided heart failure in adults? *JAMA.* **277**:1712-9, 1997.

31. Stevenson LW, Perloff JK: The limited reliability of physical signs for estimating haemodynamics in chronic heart failure. *JAMA.* **261**:884-8, 1989.

32. Drazner MH, Rame JE, Stevenson LW, Dries DL: Prognostic importance of elevated jugular venous pressure and a third heart sound in patients with heart failure. *New Engl J Med.* **345**:574-81, 2001.

33. Perloff JK: The jugular venous pulse and third heart sound in patients with heart failure. *New Engl J Med.* **345**:612-4, 2001.

34. Marcus GM, Vessey J, Jordan MV,et al: Relationship between accurate auscultation of a clinically useful third heart sound and level of experience. *Arch Intern Med.* **166**:617-22, 2006.

35. McKee PA, Castel WP, McNamara PM, Kannel WB: The natural history of congestive heart failure: The Framingham Study. *New Engl J Med.* **285**:1441, 1971.

36. Carlson KJ, Lee DC-S, Goroll AH et al: An analysis of physicians reasons for prescribing long term digitalis therapy in outpatients. *J. Chronic Dis.* **38**:733, 1985.

37. Marantz PR, Tobin JN, Wassertheil-Smollers et al: The relationship between left ventricular systolic function and congestive heart failure diagnosed by clinical criteria. *Circulation.* **77**:607-12, 1988.

38. Cook DJ, Simel DL. Does this patient have abnormal central venous pressure? The Rational Clinical Examination *JAMA.* **275**:630-4, 1996.

39. Cook DJ: Clinical assessment of central venous pressure in the critically ill. *Amer. J. Med Sci.* **299**:175-8, 1990.

40. Eisenberg PR, Jaffe AS, Schuster DP: Clinical evaluation compared to pulmonary artery catheterization in the haemodynamic assessment of critically ill patients. *Crit Care Med.* **12**:549-553, 1984.

41. Vinayak AG, Levitt J, Gehlback B et al. Usefulness of the external jugular vein examination in detecting abnormal central venous pressure in critically ill patients. *Arch Intern Med.* **166**:2132-7, 2006.

42. Parker JL, Flucker CJ, Harvey N et al: Comparison of external jugular and central venous pressure in mechanically ventilated patients. *Anaesthesia.* **57**:596-600, 2002.

43. Stoelting RK: Evaluation of external jugular venous pressure as a reflection of right atrial pressure. *Anaesthesiology.* **38**:291-294, 1973.

44. Magder S: How to use central venous pressure measurements. *Curr. Opin Crit Care.* **11**:264-70, 2005.

45. Magder S: Central venous pressure: A useful but not so simple measurement. *Crit Care Med.* **34**:2224-7, 2006.

46. Magder S: Respiratory Variations in Right Atrial Pressure Predicts Fluid Response in the critically ill. *J. Crit. Care.* **7**:76-85, 1992.

47. Pinsky MR: Assessment of indices of preload and volume responsiveness. *Curr. Opin Crit Care.* **11**:235-9, 2005.

48. Kumar R, Anel R, Bunnell E, Habet K, Zanotti S, Marshall S, et al: Pulmonary artery occlusion pressure and central venous pressure fail to predict ventricular filling volume, cardiac performance, or the response to volume infusion in normal subjects. *Crit Care Med.* **32**:691-699, 2004.

49. Boulain T, Achard JM, Teboul JL, Richard C, Perrotin D, Ginies G: Changes in BP induced by passive leg raising predict response to fluid loading in critically ill patients. *Chest.* **121**:1245-52, 2002.

50. Michard F, Teboul JL: Predicting fluid responsiveness in ICU patients: a critical analysis of the evidence. *Chest.* **121**:2000-8, 2002.

51. De Backer D, Pinsky MR: Can one predict fluid responsiveness in spontaneously breathing patients? *Intensive Care Med.* **33**:1111-1113, 2007.

52. Monnet X, Teboul JL: Volume Responsiveness. *Curr. Opin Crit Care.* **13**:549-553, 2007.

53. Bouchard MJ,Denault A,Couture P,et al. Poor correlation between haemodynamic and echocardiographic indices of left ventricular performance in the operating room and intensive care unit.Crit Care Med.32 :644-648.2004

54. Osman D, Ridel C, Ray P, et al: Cardiac filling pressures are not appropriate to predict haemodynamic response to volume challenge. *Crit Care Med.* **35**:64-68, 2007.

55. Soubrier S, Saulnier F, Hubert H, et al: Usefulness of dynamic indicators to predict fluid responsiveness in spontaneously breathing critically ill patients. *Intensive Care Med.* **33**:1117-1124, 2007.

56. Teboul JL, Monnet X: Prediction of volume responsiveness in critically ill patients with spontaneous breathing activity. *Curr. Opin Crit Care.* **14**:334-339, 2008.

57. Pinsky MR: Using ventilation-induced aortic pressure and flow variation to diagnose preload responsiveness. *Intensive Care Med.* **30**:1008-1010, 2004.

58. McKendry M, McGloin H,Saberi D, et al Randomised controlled trial assessing the impact of a nurse delivered, flow monitored protocol for optimisation of circulatory status after cardiac surgery.BMJ 329:258-265 2004

59. Monnet X, Rienzo M, Osman D, Anguel N, Richard C, Pinsky MR, et al: Passive leg raising predicts fluid responsiveness in the critically ill. *Crit Care Med.* **34**:1402-7, 2006.

60. Caille V, Jabot J, Belliard G et al: Haemodynamic effects of passive leg raising: an Echocardiographic study in patients with shock. *Intensive Care Med.* **34**:1239-1245, 2008.

61. Lafanechére A, Péne F, Goulenok C et al: Changes in aortic blood flow by passive leg raising predict fluid responsiveness in critically ill patients. *Crit Care Med.* **10**:R132, 2006.

62. Monnet X, Teboul JL: passive leg raising. *Intensive Care Med.* **34**:659-664, 2008.

63. Jabot J, Teboul J-L, Richard C, Monnet X. Passive leg raising for predicting fluid responsiveness: importance of the postural change. Intensive Care Medicine.**35** 85-90.

64. Heenen S, De Backer D, Vincent JL: How can the response to volume expansion in patients with spontaneous respiratory movements be predicted. *Critical Care.* **10**:R102, 2006.

65. Magder S: Predicting volume responsiveness in spontaneously breathing patients: still a challenging problem. *Critical Care.* **10**:165, 2006.

66. Wiese J: the abdominojugular reflux sign. *Am J Med.* **109**:59-61, 2000.

67. Marantz PR, Kaplan MD, Alderman MH: Clinical diagnosis of congestive heart failure in patients with acute dyspnoea. *Chest.* **97**:776-81, 1990.

68. Ducas J, Magder s, Gregor M: Validity of the hepatojugular reflux as a clinical test fore congestive heart failure. *Amer J. Cardiol.* **52**:1299-1303, 1983.

69. Ewy, GA: The abdominojugular test: technique and haemodynamic correlates. *Ann Int. Med.* **109**:456-60, 1988.

70. Nishimura RA, Tajik AJ. The Valsalva manoevre and response revisited. Mayo Clinic Proceedings 61 211-217 1986

71. Garcia MIM, Cano AG, Monrove JCD, Arterial pressure changes during the Valsalva manoevre to predict fluid responsiveness in spontaneously breathing patients. Intensive Care Medicine 35:77-84.2009

72. Felker GM, Cuculich PS, Gheorghiade M: The valsalva maneuver: a bedside "biomarker" for heart failure. *Amer J Med.* **119**:117-22, 2006.

73. McIntyre KM, Vita JA, Lambrew CT, Freeman J, Loscalzo J: A non-invasive method of predicting pulmonary-capillary wedge pressure. *New Engl J Med.* **327**:1715-20, 1992.

74. Sharma GVRK, Woods PA, Lambrew CT et al: Evaluation of a non-invasive system for determining left ventricular filling pressure. *Arch Intern Med.* **162**:2084-88, 2002.

75. Weilenmann D, Rickli H, Follath F et al: Non-invasive evaluation of pulmonary capillary wedge pressure by BP response to the Valsalva maneuver. *CHEST.* **122**:140-145, 2002.

76. Zema MJ, Caccavano M, Kligfield B: Detection of left ventricular dysfunction in ambulatory subjects with the bedside Valsalva maneuver. *Amer J. Med.* **75**:241-8, 1983.

77. Lamia B, Ochagavia A, Monnet X et al: Echocardiographic prediction of volume responsiveness in critically ill patients with spontaneous breathing activity. *Intensive Care Med.* **10**:1007/s 00134-007-0545, 2007.

78. Beck LH: Hypouricaemia in the syndrome of inappropriate secretion of Antidiuretic hormone. *NEJM.* **301**:528-30, 1979.

79. Liamis G, Christidis D,Alexandridis G, et al.Uric acid Homeostasis in the evaluation of Diuretic-Induced Hyponatremia Investigative Medicine.**55**:36-44.2007

80. Chung HM, Kluge R, Schrier RW, Anderson RJ: Clinical assessment of extracellular fluid volume in hyponatraemia. *Amer J. Med.* **83**:905-8, 1987.

81. Musch W, Thimpont J, Vandervelde D, Verhaeverbeke I, Berghm`ans T, Decaux G: Combined fractional excretion of sodium and urea better predicts response to saline in hyponatraemia than do usual clinical and biochemical parameters. *Amer. J. Med.* **99**:348-55, 1995.

82. Musch W, Hedeshi A, Decaux G.Low sodium excretion in SIADH patients with low Diuresis. Nephron Physiol **96** 11-18 2004

83. Musch W, Hedeshi A, Decaux G: Treating the syndrome of inappropriate ADH secretion with isotonic saline.QJM **91** 1998 749-753

84. Mehta RL, Pascual MT, Soroko S, Chertow GM, Group PS: Diuretics, mortality, and non-recovery of renal function in acute renal failure. *JAMA.* **288**:2547-53, 2002.

85. Ho KM, Sheridan DJ: Meta-analysis of frusemide to prevent or treat acute renal failure. *BMJ.* **333**:420, 2006.

86. Boluyt N, Bollen CW, Bos AP, Kok JH, Offringa M: Fluid resuscitation in neonatal and pediatric hypovolaemic shock: a Dutch Pediatric Society evidence-based clinical practice guideline. *Intensive Care Med.* **32**:995-1003, 2006.

87. Waikar SS, Chertow GM: Crystalloids versus colloids for resuscitation in shock. *Curr Opin Nephrol Hypertens.* **9**:501-4, 2000.

GASTROINTESTINAL DISORDERS AND ELECTROLYTES.

A few observations and much reasoning leads to error.
Many observations and little reasoning leads to truth. W.Osler.

NORMAL GASTROINTESTINAL FUNCTION.

1-2L of gastric juice, containing an average of 122mmol chloride, 57mmol sodium but only 10mmol potassium are secreted daily (Table 1) [1-6] depending on pH: gastric juice, of low acidity, contains more sodium and less H+. [5-6]

A variable quantity of fat, carbohydrate, protein and water in food progressively mix with approximately 7L of gastrointestinal secretions. Food is rapidly broken down to osmotically active particles in the stomach, reaches isotonicity in the jejunum, and remains isotonic until passed as faeces. Gastric emptying is retarded by duodenal osmoreceptors. [1] The electrolyte concentration of gastrointestinal secretions varies considerably in different reports and in the same individual at different times. The average volume and electrolyte concentrations from six sources are shown below.

	Volume (mL)	Na^+	K^+	Cl^-	HCO_3^-	pH
SALIVA	1 (500-2000)	10 (2-10)	26 (20-30)	10 (8-18)	30	6-7
		(10-50)	(15-26)	(10-40)		
GASTRIC JUICE	1.5 (1-2L)	57 (40-100)	10 (7-15)	122 (100-280)	0	(1-3.5)
BILE	1	155 (131-164)	5.8 (3-12)	113 (90-180)	29	7.8
PANCREATIC	1.5 (1-2)	127 (130-150)	5.5 (5-7)	75 (40-60)	115 (100-120)	115 7.5-8.0
SMALL INTESTINE ILEAL DRAINAGE	1,200 (1000-2000)	(140-150)	(5-10)	(100)		
TOTAL	7	800	100	700		

TABLE 1: Volume and electrolyte concentration of gastrointestinal secretions from various sources [1-6] (Range in parentheses).

Gastric juice contains predominantly H^+, Cl^- and Na^+. Bile, pancreatic juice and small intestinal fluid are isotonic and contain predominantly Na^+ and Cl^- but low concentration of K^+.

Bile and pancreatic juice are alkaline and contain HCO_3^- and less chloride.

Approximately 9L of gastrointestinal secretions and food are reduced to 2L on reaching the colon, and 200mL in formed stool. All segments of the gastrointestinal tract both secrete and absorb water and electrolytes.

Secretion from immature cells occur in crypts and absorption occurs from more mature superficial cells of villi [7-12]. Epithelial enterocyte cells are initially formed in crypts, migrate to the tip of the villus, die and slough off into the lumen. [8-12] As they migrate they mature and their function changes from secretion in crypts to absorption in villi, associated with change in polarity of transporters. [8-12]

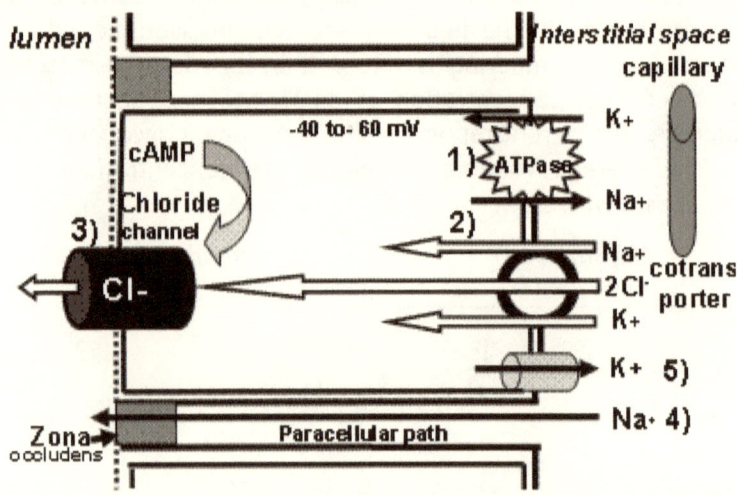

Figure 1: Model of chloride secretion in intestinal epithelial crypt cell. Cl channels are located on the luminal membrane and cotransporters on the basolateral membrane. (Numbers correspond to text below).

1. *Na:K$^+$ pumps generate negative intracellular potential*
2. *Cl$^-$ enters cells from basolateral membranes via Na$^+$:K$^+$:2Cl$^-$ cotransporters.* [10-12]
3. *Cl$^-$ channels on luminal membranes open in response to cAMP and Ca^{2+} and transfer Cl$^-$ into lumen.*
4. *Na$^+$ moves into the lumen between cells (paracellular) route) to maintain electroneutrality.*

5. *K$^+$ channels, on basolateral membranes recycle K$^+$ to make it available for Na$^+$ K$^+$ 2Cl$^-$ cotransporters.*

Villous reabsorption

Fluid in small bowel is isotonic and contains sodium, low potassium concentration, chloride as the main anion, and a variable amount of bicarbonate and magnesium.

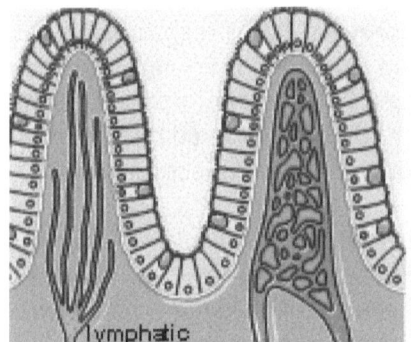

Figure 2. Model of villous (produced using Servier art)

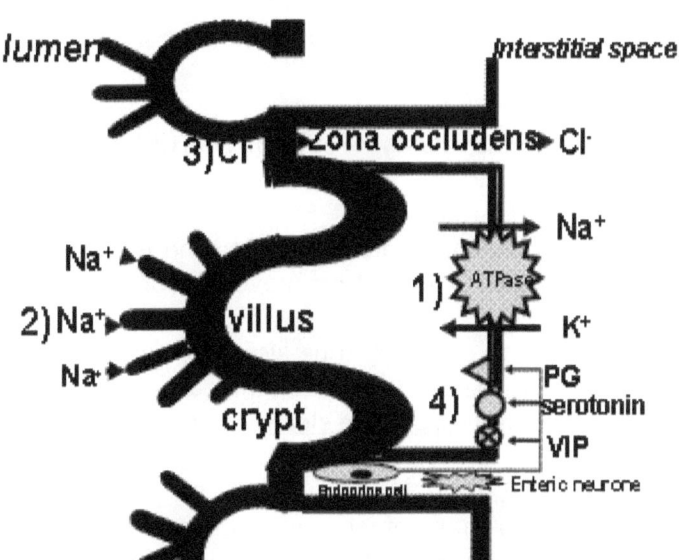

Figure 3. Model of absorption in intestinal mucosa. Numbers correspond to text below.

1. *Na: K$^+$ pumps generate negative cell potential (- 40- -6omV) and low Na$^+$ concentration gradient.*
2. *Na$^+$ is reabsorbed through villus.*

3. *Cl⁻ is reabsorbed through Zona occludens to maintain electroneutrality. Na+ moves out of the cell into interstitiium via Na⁺:K⁺ pumps as in 1).*

4. *Enteroendocrine cells and enteroneural networks coordinate secretion, absorption and motility. Endocrine cells and enteric neurons stimulate production of mediators such as prostaglandin E2 (PG), serotonin, vasointestinal polypeptide (VIP,) substance P and play a role in motility.*

Na⁺: K⁺ pumps in the villus create both a negative potential and sodium gradient which drives sodium absorption. Na⁺ is reabsorbed by sodium channels in villous epithelial cells and is pumped out of cells into interstitial fluid and capillary by Na⁺: K⁺ pumps. Sodium reabsorption is stimulated by aldosterone, low Na⁺ and high K⁺ diet and blocked by amiloride. Cl⁻ is reabsorbed via the paracellular route to maintain electroneutrality.

Water follows solute movement through the paracellular space in response to osmotic gradients. The paracellular route varies in its "leakiness": [13] jejunum has a relatively leaky epithelium and maximum water flow; water movement is lowest in colon; and intermediate in ileum. [13]

The main function of crypts is to secrete Cl⁻ ; Na⁺ follows to maintain electroneutrality.

The main function of the villus is to reabsorb Na⁺; Cl⁻ follows to maintain electroneutrality.

Within a particular region of intestine water and electrolytes may be absorbed, secreted or both without net movement of either. [13]

Sodium reabsorption in small intestine also occurs by cotransport with glucose and amino acids—as in renal proximal tubules. This provides the <u>rationale for effectiveness of glucose electrolyte solutions in treatment of diarrhoea.</u>

Na⁺ reabsorption from lumen of jejunum, ileum and colon is coupled to H⁺ extrusion driven by Na⁺:K⁺ pumps.Acidification of luminal fluid occurs in jejunum as a result of Na⁺:H⁺ exchange. The pH of lumen contents increases in ileum and distal colon as a result of Cl⁻: HCo_3^- exchange and other mechanisms. Chloride is the main anion in the jejunum and its concentration decreases distally by replacing HCO_3^- in ileum and HCO_3^- and organic acids in colon.

Magnesium is reabsorbed in small bowel by two routes: paracellular involving paracellin 1 (Claudin) and transcellularly through magnesium selective channels- transient receptor potential melastin 6 (TRPM6). [14, 15] These 2 processes occur randomly rather than in specific areas of the intestine.

Submucosal neuronal circuits and local paracrine and systemic hormones influence enterocyte function. A large number of neurotransmitters and chemical mediators, for example AMP, GMP, VIP—(vasointestinal polypeptide), substance P, prostaglandins and others activate Cl⁻ channels, inhibit Na⁺ reabsorption and influence motility.

Small intestinal fluid is isotonic and contains mainly sodium and chloride, <u>but only 5.0mmol potassium, on average, and relatively more magnesium.</u>

Colon.

The colon contains crypts but is mainly devoid of villi. Its main function is to decrease the liquid content it receives from the ileum, approximately 1.5-2L; to further reabsorb sodium and chloride ; exchange Na⁺ for K⁺ stimulated by aldosterone; and exchange Cl⁻ for organic anions and HCO_3^-. [11, 16-18]

Short chain fatty acids (>100mmol/L) are the predominant anions in the colonic lumen. They are produced by colonic bacteria from metabolism of unabsorbed carbohydrate, approximately 30-150gm per day, depending on the type of food ingested [19]. Short chain fatty acids (SCFA), especially butyrate, are reabsorbed in exchange for HCO_3^- and enhance colonic Na⁺ and water reabsorption.

Sodium accompanies Cl⁻ reabsorption in proximal colon against high concentration gradients in conjunction with $Cl^-:HCO_3^-$ exchangers; and in distal colon electrogenically by epithelial sodium channels (ENaC). $Cl^-:HCO_3^-$ exchangers reabsorb chloride in exchange for bicarbonate mediated by the DRA gene [18], present in both ileum and proximal colon [11]. A defective gene causes congenital chloride-losing diarrhoea containing a high chloride concentration. [11, 18, 20]

Sodium is progressively reabsorbed and exchanges with K⁺ in colon, modulated by aldosterone. Potassium is usually secreted passively or actively, stimulated by aldosterone, but if potassium depletion occurs or a low potassium diet ingested' K^+ is reabsorbed by K^+: H^+ exchange in distal colon. [11]

In conclusion: <u>All regions of intestine secrete and reabsorb solute. Water follows passively by the paracellular route. Ion transport and motility are coordinated by the enteric nervous system and neuroendocrine cells.</u>

<u>Crypt cells</u> secrete chloride into intestinal lumen. Sodium follows passively by the paracellular route to maintain electroneutrality. Cl^- enters cells via Na^+:K^+:$2Cl^-$ co-transporters in basolateral membranes.

<u>Villous cells,</u> which have matured from migrating crypt cells, reabsorb sodium through Na^+ channels (ENaC). Cl^- is reabsorbed through the zona occludens to maintain electroneutrality. Sodium is then pumped out of cells by Na^+:K^+ pumps on basolateral membranes into interstitiium. Cl^- is reabsorbed in both ileum and colon.

Stool volume normally decreases to 100-200 mL daily, usually contains more K^+ than Na^+, and HCo_3^- and organic anions rather than Cl^-. Given the large volume and electrolyte content of gastrointestinal secretions, diarrhoea can cause large losses of water and electrolytes.

VOMITING AND NASOGASTRIC ASPIRATION. [21-29]

Loss of gastric juice in vomiting, regurgitation or nasogastric aspiration results in sodium depletion, metabolic alkalosis and hypokalaemia. [21] The pathogenesis is as follows:

- Each mmol of H^+ and Cl^- secreted into the stomach results in transfer of 1mmol of HCO_3^- into interstitiium and circulation. This generates mild metabolic alkalosis-the post prandial alkaline tide.
- If vomiting or naso-gastric suction occurs $NaHCO_3$ is generated as HCl is lost.
- The kidney initially excretes Na^+ with HCO_3^- because HCO_3^- is poorly reabsorbed in distal tubules (poorly absorbed anion). Urine is initially alkaline and contains an increase in concentration of sodium and bicarbonate.
- Volume depletion occurs from loss of Na^+ and Cl^- in gastric juice and initially from sodium bicarbonate lost in urine.
- Severe hypovolaemia stimulates the Renin-Angiotensin-Aldosterone-Sympathetic nervous system (RAAS). Glomerular filtration rate (GFR)

falls; proximal tubule reabsorption of sodium increases; and arterial blood pCO_2 rises to compensate for metabolic alkalosis.
- Proximal tubules increase bicarbonate reabsorption beyond the normally set threshold of approximately 24mmol/L ($Tm\,HCO_3^-$)—called <u>Reclamation</u>.
- Extracellular and plasma bicarbonate concentration increase.

Under normal circumstances the kidney has an enormous capacity to excrete bicarbonate when serum and thus filtered HCO_3^- exceeds threshold [22]. If reclamation of bicarbonate did not occur HCO_3^- generated from HCl loss would be excreted. There are several factors which increase <u>reclamation</u> of $NaHCO_3$ by proximal tubules:

* Decrease in filtered HCO_3^- from low GFR. [21, 23].
* Sodium reabsorption from volume depletion. [21, 23]
* Decrease in availability of Cl^- required to accompany Na^+ reabsorption to maintain electroneutrality.
* Raised pCO_2 increases HCO_3^- synthesis in proximal tubule cells. [25]
* Hypokalaemia increases HCO_3^- reabsorption and stimulates synthesis of NH_4^+ and HCO_3^- in proximal tubules.
Angiotensin II stimulates H^+:ATPase pumps (NHE) in proximal tubules to secrete H^+ in exchange for Na^+ and to reabsorb HCO_3^-.

Volume depletion has a marked effect in increasing HCO_3^- reabsorption, so that metabolic alkalosis can be corrected by NaCl alone, even when moderate hypokalaemia is present [23]. Depletion of chloride is an important modulator of HCO_3^- transport [23, 24] and is the most important factor in maintenance of metabolic alkalosis. [26]

Distal tubules.

Principal cells in collecting ducts increase Na^+ reabsorption in exchange for K^+ secretion stimulated by aldosterone (Electrogenic Na^+ reabsorption). Aldosterone increases:

* Activity of basolateral Na^+ :K^+ pumps.
* Activity of number of apical Na^+ channels (ENAC).
* Activity and number of apical K^+ channels.
* Activity of H^+: ATPase pumps which secrete H^+ in exchange for Na^+ reabsorption.

Urine potassium increases as a result.

The cause of hypokalaemia is urinary and not gastric losses of potassium.

α Intercalated cells in collecting ducts increase H^+ secretion, in exchange for sodium, stimulated by aldosterone [27, 28]. Reabsorbed Na^+ is transported across basolateral membranes with HCO_3^- on Na^+:HCO_3^- exchangers. This generates metabolic alkalosis.

If hypokalaemia increases in severity K^+ is reabsorbed in exchange for H^+ by H^+: K^+ ATPase exchangers in α intercalated cells. [21] Urine acidity increases despite presence of metabolic alkalosis.

The usefulness of separating proximal from distal tubular factors in the genesis and maintenance of metabolic alkalosis is questionable because:

* Volume depletion stimulates HCO_3^- reabsorption in both proximal [25] and distal tubules. [29]
* HCO_3^- reabsorption increases in both proximal and distal tubules. [29]
* Angiotensin2 and aldosterone, produced systemically and locally, increases reabsorption of both Na^+ and HCO_3^- in proximal and distal tubules.
* K^+ depletion acts on both proximal and distal tubules.
* Ammonium is generated by proximal tubules but secreted by distal tubules.
* Chloride depletion is essential for development of alkalosis because HCO_3^- must take its place in exchange to satisfy electroneutrality.

Electrolyte composition of urine varies depending on the severity and duration of hydrochloric acid loss: in the initial stages, before RAAS is fully activated, HCO_3^- loss in urine is accompanied by Na^+. The urine is initially alkaline and urine chloride extremely low but urine sodium may not be low.

When sodium depletion increases in severity both urinary Na^+ and Cl^- decrease but urine K^+ increases despite the presence of hypokalaemia. Urine has low concentrations of Na^+, K^+ and Cl^-. When hypokalaemia is severe K^+:H^+ exchange in α intercalated cells decreases excretion of K^+ and urine becomes acid despite metabolic alkalosis.

Ingestion of water may cause hyponatraemia from stimulation of ADH by volume depletion, stress, nausea or vomiting provided vomiting is not sufficiently severe to prevent water intake or is self-induced. Unexpected hypokalaemic metabolic alkalosis is an important clue to Bulimia: in

168 cases metabolic alkalosis and hyperchloraemic were present in approximately one quarter and hypokalaemia in 14 %. [30]

Loss of HCl in vomitus decreases from concomitant use of proton pump inhibitors and leads to volume depletion with less severe alkalosis.

DIARRHOEA

Diarrhoea is decrease in faecal consistency, volume or number of bowel actions and is usually associated with stool volume >200mls/day. Diarrhoea is due to one or a combination of:

- Increase in fluid delivery to colon which exceeds its normal absorptive capacity.
- Decrease in colonic absorption or Increase in colonic secretion.

Increase in delivery of solute and water to colon from small intestinal disease is due to one or a combination of:

- Increase is small bowel secretion (secretory diarrhoea).
- Decrease in small bowel absorption (absorptive diarrhoea).

Increase in small bowel secretion results from:

Action of hormones and paracrine ligands.

Toxins secreted by microorganisms.

Laxatives and drugs.   Secretagogues

Fatty and bile acids.

Immunological mediators.

Decrease in absorption results from:

* Decrease in number or function of villi.
* Osmotic effects of drugs, including laxatives, sugars or short chain fatty acids.
* Motility disorders.

Motility is important in allowing adequate time for mixing, secretion, digestion and absorption, while acting as a defence against pathogenic colonization.

SPECIFIC CAUSES [7]

SMALL INTESTINE.

Several bacteria secrete toxins which stimulate chloride secretion. Vibrio cholera secretes several toxins which cause profuse secretion of fluid of similar electrolyte composition to plasma. [7] The most important mechanism is activation of Cl^- channels in crypts. The toxin enters intestinal cells and stimulates release of adenyl cyclase on basolateral membranes. This increases cAMP secretion which, after several intermediate processes, phosphorylates Cl^- channels. This results in profuse loss of chloride. Cholera toxin also decreases Na^+ reabsorption by villi and stimulates secretion of several locally produced mediators, such as VIP and prostaglandins, which increase motility.

Enterotoxins of Enteropathogenic E.coli are similar to cholera toxin and activate adenyl cyclase or increase cGMP (cyclic guanyl monophosphate). In both cases toxins act in the absence of invasion or inflammation. Salmonella penetrate epithelium and interact with white blood cells in the lamina propria. Rotavirus invades epithelial villous cells, but not crypts, causing villus death or atrophy while leaving crypt cells intact: Secretion remains normal while villous reabsorption decreases. Norovirus and Cryptosporidiosis causes both damage to villi in small bowel and crypt cell hyperplasia: this increase secretion while decreasing absorption.

Gastrointestinal secretion and motility are stimulated by secretagogues other than bacterial toxins: These include stimulant laxatives, fatty and bile acids.

Laxatives.

Laxatives work by several mechanisms. Non-osmotic laxatives stimulate water and electrolyte secretion and increase peristalsis in small intestine and/or colon.

Stimulant laxatives result in fluid loss (average 2L in normal subjects) containing an average of 108mmol sodium and 23mmol of potassium. The volume decreases on fasting. [31] Phenolphthalein and bisacodyl are potent colonic stimulants. Phenolphthalein also increases intestinal chloride secretion. Senna combines with sugars to form glycosides which act on colon. Castor oil forms ricinoleic acid which increases motility in small intestine.

Several tumours produce secretory diarrhoea. [7]

Vipomas [31-36]—secrete vasointestinal polypeptide.
Glucagonomas [36, 37]—islet cell tumours secrete glucagon.
Calcitonin Secreting Tumours- medullary cell carcinoma, rarely Pheochromocytoma.
Histamine Secreting Tumours—Mastocytosis.
Carcinoids [7, 38]—secrete serotonin, bradykinin and substance P.
Gastrinomas secrete HCl which lowers pH in proximal small bowel and inactivates pancreatic enzymes. [39]

Vipoma Syndrome. [19, 31-36] Vasointestinal Polypeptide is released by pancreatic islet cell tumours, tumours of neural crest origin and bronchogenic carcinoma. Stool volume is over 700mL a day and in 70% over 3L. Stool contains an average concentration of sodium of 108mmol/L and potassium 23 mmol/L [31]. Severe hypovolaemia, [32, 34],hypokalaemia and acidosis result from colonic exchange of Na^+ for K^+ and Cl^- exchange for HCo_3^-. Hypomagnesaemia, hypercalcaemia, peripheral vasodilatation, including facial flushing often occur.[34].The cause is controversial: vasointestinal polypeptide is raised in most but not in all cases. [31, 34]

Carcinoid Syndrome. [7, 38] Increase in intestinal secretion and motility result from several mediators including kinins, serotonin, prostaglandin E and substance P produced by gastrointestinal, bronchogenic and other tumours. Facial oedema, flushing, asthma and right-sided heart failure are clues to diagnosis.

Glucagonomas. [36, 37]

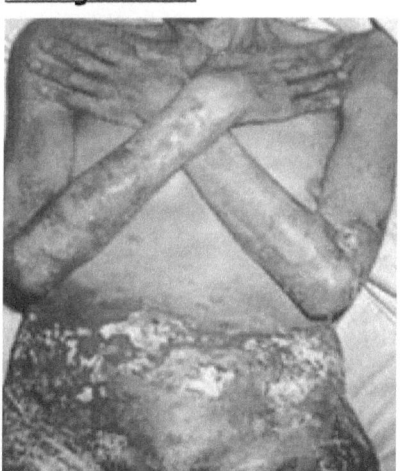

Figure 4. Erythema necrolysis migrans due to pancreatic glucagonoma.

Glucagonomas, tumours of pancreatic α cells, secrete glucagon. This causes a characteristic rash, shown above, mild diabetes mellitus, neuropsychiatric symptoms, severe weight loss and diarrhoea due to secretory effects of glucagon on small bowel.

Gastrinomas: secrete large amounts of HCl which inactivate pancreatic enzymes in small bowel and gastrin causes a net secretion compared to absorption in colon. [39] Profuse diarrhoea results.

Substances which cause or contribute to secretory diarrhoea but which also have osmotic effects are:

- Dihydroxy bile acids.
- Fatty acids.
- Non-osmotic laxatives.
- Unabsorbed sugars such as lactose in lactase deficiency.

Watery diarrhoea from malabsorption is due to increased secretion of fluid due to fatty acids and dihydroxy bile acids. [32]Secretion is often amplified by several systemic and locally produced hormones and mediators.

Small Bowel Malabsorption causing diarrhoea results from three main mechanisms:

- *   Osmotic effects of poorly absorbed substances.
- *   Damage to villous epithelial cells.
- *   Decrease of surface area of bowel.

Several diseases damage mucosa: for example Crohns disease, Whipple's disease, tuberculosis, other infections and infestations by bacteria or parasites.

Bacterial overgrowth in small bowel interferes with absorption of water and electrolytes and, in association with antibiotics, may rarely cause D. lactic acidosis.

Osmotic diarrhoea: Ingestion of osmotic laxatives, such as magnesium, phosphate, lactulose, polyethylene glycol and sorbitol are common causes of diarrhoea. Fatty acids and dihydroxy bile acids exert an osmotic effect and thus decrease absorption in addition to increasing secretion.

Lactase deficiency decreases breakdown of lactose. This is not absorbed in small bowel, but is broken down in colon by bacteria, and has osmotic and stimulatory effects on colon.

Malabsorption decreases absorption by causing damage to intestinal mucosa, osmotic effects and stimulation of secretion. Coeliac disease, chronic pancreatitis and other malabsorptive states cause fluid and electrolyte losses from stimulation of secretion by bile, fatty acids and osmotic effects. Diarrhoea, due to coeliac disease, is due to a combination of the osmotic effects of unabsorbed solutes, villous atrophy, crypt hypertrophy [7] and stimulation of crypt secretion by dihydroxy bile and fatty acids. [7] Bile acids are deconjugated to hydroxy bile acids by ileal and colonic bacteria. Approximately 50% with steatorrhoea have watery rather than 'fatty' diarrhoea.

MOTILITY DISORDERS.

Chemical mediators, hormones, enteric neuronal stimulation, hydroxylated bile acids, fatty acids and laxatives increase motility and stimulate secretion of fluid.

Hypomotility.—as a result of strictures, diverticulae, blind loops, neuromuscular disease and infiltration (e.g. Scleroderma) predisposes to bacterial overgrowth in small bowel. Bacteria deconjugate bile and hydroxy fatty acids which may cause or contribute to diarrhoea. Antibiotic induced diarrhoea may be due to alteration of the normal conversion of carbohydrate to short chain fatty acids.

Diabetes.—the cause of diabetic diarrhoea has not been established but may be due to hypomotility secondary to autonomic dysfunction with or without bacterial overgrowth. It is commonly worse at night.

DECREASE IN SURFACE AREA OF THE SMALL BOWEL.

Considerable resection of small intestine occurs before clinically important effects on fluid and electrolyte losses occur. Considerable adaption occurs with time. Moreover colon has a large capacity to reabsorb sodium and water which escapes absorption in small bowel

Small bowel resection and ileostomies.

Losses of Na+ and water are slight in extensive small bowel resection provided the colon is intact. Small bowel resection results in large Na+ losses which are greater for jejunostomy compared to ileostomy. However, if anastomosis is made to intact colon, diarrhoeal volume and sodium losses decrease considerably and treatment with additional Na$^+$ and water is usually not required. Patients with at least half a normal colon have much less Na$^+$ loss (median 8mmol/24 hours) than those without (median 49mmol/24 hours.

When colon is not intact or is bypassed by jejunostomy or ileostomy considerable losses of fluid and electrolytes occur. Patients with ileostomy, following small bowel resection, have high faecal losses of Na$^+$ (median 149 mmol/day) which causes sodium depletion [40], but low losses of K$^+$. Hypovolaemia stimulates renin [41] and aldosterone [40] secretion. Patients with extensive small bowel resection, with jejunostomy, usually need intravenous saline to avoid severe sodium depletion. [40]

Magnesium losses increase with increasing length of small bowel resection. [42] Extensive small bowel resection, ileostomy and small bowel fistulas result in magnesium without potassium depletion (personal observations).

Patients with continent ileostomies (with pouches) lose as much K$^+$ and chloride as conventional ileostomies if fluid output is high (>1000mL) but less if fluid output is low. [43] Na$^+$ and K$^+$ losses were 78mmol and 10mmol per day in patients with a faecal output of less than 1000gram (mean 650gram) compared to 139mmol and 20mmol for output exceeding 1000gram per 24 hours (mean 1400mL). On average chloride losses were 33 mmol/day for conventional ileostomies and 39mmol/day for continent ileostomies. [43]

COLONIC DISEASE :

Intrinsic colonic disease may be due to hereditary defects in electrolyte transport or acquired local disease.

Extensive resections of ileum and right colon cause diarrhoea due to decrease in absorptive area, decrease in transit time and malabsorption of bile acids which deplete the bile acid pool. Bile acids, unabsorbed in ileum, increase colonic secretion of water and electrolytes.

Mucosal damage decreases electrogenic Na^+ transport. Inflammatory colonic disease and bacterial invasion decreases colonic absorption and causes inflammatory exudate. Chronic Inflammatory colonic disease causes inhibition of salt and water absorption, possibly by increasing local mucosal prostaglandin or cytokines [7, 44] and increases mucosal leakiness to electrolytes. [45]

Microorganisms

Shigella species, Enteropathogenic E.coli (EPEC) and Clostridium difficile produce both colonic inflammation and toxins. [7] Shigella species cause impairment of colonic water absorption but no increase in small intestinal flow rate. [46]Clostridium difficile causes colonic damage including pseudomembranes from toxin.

Villous adenoma. [47] Profuse secretion of water, sodium and water, less commonly marked potassium losses, are stimulated by prostaglandins. Daily fluid losses of 1000-2000 mL, containing high concentrations of Na+ and Cl- but only 15-31mmol/L of K+, occurred in two reported cases. Inhibitors of prostaglandins, for example Indomethacin, decrease fluid loss.

Defective electrolyte transporters

Congenital Chloridorrhoea: [20] is due to a hereditary defect in $Cl^-:HCO_3^-$ exchangers (DRA gene) in ileum and colon. Large losses of Cl^-, which exceed the Na^+ plus K^+ concentration in stool, occur.

Congenital Sodium Diarrhoea: this rare condition is due to a defect in $Na^+: H^+$ exchange in colon [7].

OSMOTIC EFFECTS OF COLONIC LUMINAL FLUID.

Delivery of unabsorbed carbohydrates, which are converted to short chain fatty acids (SCFA) in colon, trap water by osmotic action. Laxatives, such as magnesium hydroxide, polyethylene glycol, sorbitol and lactulose cause diarrhoea by osmotic effects. A high sorbitol containing diet may also cause diarrhoea by this mechanism.

ACUTE DIARRHOEA DUE TO MICROORGANISMS. Various factors, other than the specific cause, influence the extent of volume depletion and electrolyte losses from diarrhoea In the majority of cases.

- Food and fluid intake during the episode.
- Presence or absence of vomiting.
- Severity of gastrointestinal involvement and transit time of intestinal contents.
- Site of involvement.
- Effects of colonic function including action of aldosterone.

The volume and composition of stool is also influenced by food and fluid intake during an episode of diarrhoea. Although continuing fluid and food intake increase diarrhoeal losses a net gain of fluid, electrolytes and nutrients occurs. [48]

Continued breast feeding during infantile diarrhoea is important in maintaining water balance and nutrition. [49, 50] Marked net loss of Na^+ and K^+ losses can be avoided by supplemental provision of these ions. Free water depletion virtually never occurs when demand breast feeding continues during infantile gastroenteritis. Adding glucose or polysaccharide to oral fluid containing electrolytes, in both children and adults, promotes absorption [51-53] and decreases the volume of diarrhoea.

Several oral fluids are available for rehydration. The WHO oral rehydration solution contains a concentration of 90mmol/L Na^+, 20mmo/L K^+, 80mmol/L Cl^-, 30 mmol/L bicarbonate and glucose 111mmol/L. [52]

The composition of diarrhoeal stool also depends on a normal colon and the time available for colon to exchange K^+ for Na^+ and HCO_3^- and organic ions for Cl^-. The severity of fluid losses in small intestine is probably the most important influence. The electrolyte composition of diarrhoeal stool in children shows considerable variation but contains similar or greater amounts of potassium than sodium. Table 2.

Author and Reference		Number Patients	Period (Hours)	Stool Volume	Na	K	Cl
Holt[54]	Severe	7	10	293mls	40	60	28
	Moderate	8	14	133mls	40	57	
Darrow[55,56]		7	15	50mL/Kg	66	34	54
Kooh & Metcoff[57]			10	96mL/Kg	57	35	20
Weil & Wallace[58]		6			46	49	26
Cheung[48]				97mL/Kg	59	27	51
Finberg et al [59]		75			65	45	51
Teree et al [60]		28			36	36	
Bruck et al [61]		10			21.5	50	
Molla et al [62]		13			45	37.5	23
MEAN (mmol/L)					48	43	36

Table 2. Electrolyte content of stool from various sources (*From Darrow 1946 and Darrow et al., 1949: only those periods where stool loss exceeded 100mls daily were selected for determining the mean in references 54-61. In reference (62) cholera is excluded.

The extent of volume depletion, plasma electrolytes and acid base abnormalities depend on the composition and quantity of diarrhoeal losses. This is influenced by:

Specific disease causing diarrhoea.

- Severity of diarrhoea.
- Contact time in the colon.
- Amount and composition of oral intake.

The electrolyte content of stool was much less than that shown in table 2 in infants who continued demand breast feeding during an episode of acute diarrhoea: In 10 consecutive infants the mean stool concentration of sodium was 18.0mmol/L and potassium 20.0mmol/L.[63] This was probably due to the low sodium and potassium concentration in breast milk (5.0 and 10.0mmol/L respectively).

The composition of stool in cholera is very different in containing much less K^+ and HCO_3^- than Na^+. In 8 studies the average stool concentration of Na^+ was 128mmol/L; K^+ 18mmol/L; Cl^- 80mmol/L and HCO_3^- 37mmol/L. [64, 65]. Molla et al [62] reported stool Na^+ concentrations of 88 mmol/L and K^+ of

30mmol/L compared to mean stool Na$^+$ of 45mmol/L and K$^+$ 37.5mmol/L in infants with rotavirus and EPEC (enteropathic E.coli) gastroenteritis.

Fluid losses in cholera are so rapid, colonic transit time low and time for adaption to hypovolaemia so short that patients often present with signs of severe hypovolaemia or shock, pre-renal failure, with relatively normal plasma Na$^+$ and K$^+$ but with severe acidosis. Acidosis is usually associated with high anion gap due to hyperalbuminaemia from haemoconcentration, lactic acid (mean 4.0mmol/L) and hyperphosphataemia.

In contrast infants with less severe diarrhoea, who continue to "demand" breast feed during illness, present with large deficits of Na$^+$ and K$^+$, severe hyponatraemia, severe hypokalaemia, and absence of both acidosis and renal failure. [50]

In most cases of diarrhoea hypernatraemia is uncommon because ADH and thirst are stimulated by volume depletion. The extent to which vomiting occurs and composition and amount of fluid taken orally determines whether free water depletion or excess develops.

APPROACH TO OBSCURE CAUSES OF CHRONIC DIARRHOEA. [32, 66-69] The cause is easily established in the majority of cases of chronic or subacute diarrhoea

<u>**Colonic inflammatory disease**</u> is characterized by small volume diarrhoea, nocturnal diarrhoea, urgency and stools which are brown in colour containing mucous and blood. Stool microscopy shows leucocytes. The serum C.reactive protein is high.

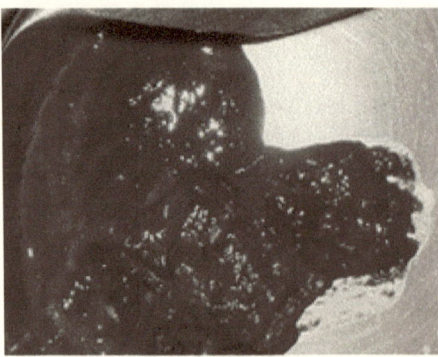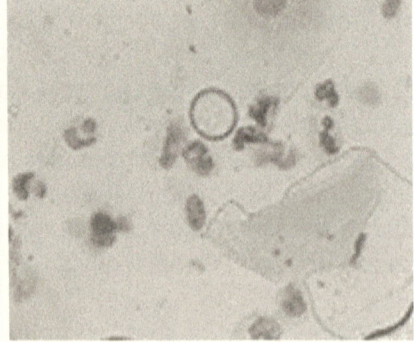

Figure 4. Brown stool mixed with blood and microscopy showing neutrophils due to colonic inflammation.

Diarrhoea due to small bowel disease

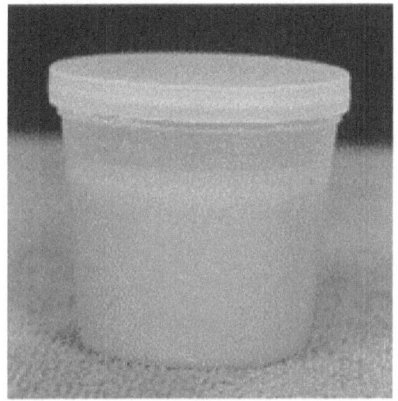

> **Figure 5** *Yellow stool typical of small bowel disease*

This is characterized by watery, yellow or green stool due to unreduced bile and absence of pus cells although mononuclear cells may be present in Salmonella infection. Steatorrhoea gives rise to either yellow or watery diarrhoeal stools or both.

Second line tests include a screening test for coeliac disease, endoscopy with biopsy, faecal fat estimation, small bowel capsule, breath test, stool examination for ova and parasites, stool giardial antigen test and tests to exclude immune deficiency such as immunoglobulin measurement and HIV testing.

Dietary review is important to exclude ingestion of high sorbitol containing foods such as apples, peaches, pears, prunes, fruit juices and some dietetic foods. [19] If the diagnosis is uncertain the following may be useful:

* Stool osmolality [32, 66-69], electrolyte concentration and pH.
* Response to fasting. [32,66]
* Response to lactose free diet, sorbitol free diet and administration of cholestyramine. [19]

Freshly collected stool has an osmolality of 280-330 mOsmol/kg H_2O, mean 290mOsmol/kg H_2O. Osmolality is difficult to measure because it rapidly increases when stool is left at room temperature because macromolecules are broken down to smaller molecules by bacteria. [66-68] Stool pH also decreases due to an increase in short chain fatty acids. [67]

Stool osmolality is sufficiently predictive that measurement is unnecessary. Thus stool osmolality can be assumed to be ~ 290mOsmol/kg H_2O. The stool osmolality can be <u>estimated</u> by measuring concentrations of the two main cations, Na^+ and K^+ and doubling to include unmeasured anions.

The osmolal gap is thus estimated as :

<u>290—estimated stool osmolality.</u>{ $=2 \times Na^+ + K^+$}

Diarrhoeal fluid due to secretory causes, such as from hormone secreting tumours, has a normal stool osmolal gap.

An osmolal gap greater than 50 mosmol/kg H_2O suggests that an abnormal osmotically active substance, which has drawn and held water in the intestinal lumen, is present [32, 69]. Diarrhoea due to magnesium hydroxide, polyethylene glycol, lactulose or sorbitol has an osmotic gap >50mosm/kg [69]. Stool magnesium can be measured if the osmolal gap is greater than 50 mosmol/kg H_2o to establish or exclude intake of magnesium containing laxatives. Normal stool contains less than 4.5 mmol/L or <15 mmol output of magnesium per day. [32, 70]

Lower than normal stool osmolality < 250mosmol/Kg is due to dilution with water or urine and is a clue to factitious diarrhoea.

Low stool pH is characteristic of carbohydrate malabsorption: faecal pH less than 5.6 suggests carbohydrate intolerance is present such as occurs from lactase deficiency, ingestion of excessive sorbitol or lactulose. [32, 69] Causes of diarrhoea other than carbohydrate intolerance rarely cause stool pH less than 5.3. [69]

High volume of stool suggests an endocrine cause: Vipomas cause stool volumes greater than 3L per day in over 70% of cases. High stool K^+ concentration suggests that adequate colonic function and contact time has occurred to allow K^+: Na^+ exchange.

In rare cases of Congenital Chloride Losing Diarrhoea measurement of stool Cl^- suggests the diagnosis.

The response to fasting is useful. Failure to decrease diarrhoeal volume suggests that secretory diarrhoea, especially from hormonal secreting tumours, is present. [32, 66, 68]

RESPONSE TO FASTING

Diarrhoea resolves:

Bile acid diarrhoea.
Steatorrhoea.
Osmotic diarrhoea.
Carbohydrate malabsorption.
Secretogogue. Laxatives.
Food allergy.
Neurogenin-3 mutation.

Diarrhoea only partially resolves:

Neuroendocrine tumours.
Hyperthyroidism.
Congenital chloride diarrhoea.
Bacterial overgrowth.
Inflammatory bowel disease.
Villous adenoma.

Stool volume remains greater than 200g/day after 24-72 hours fasting in secretory diarrhoea. Administration of pancreatic enzymes decreases diarrhoea in chronic pancreatitis and cystic fibrosis.

ASCITES

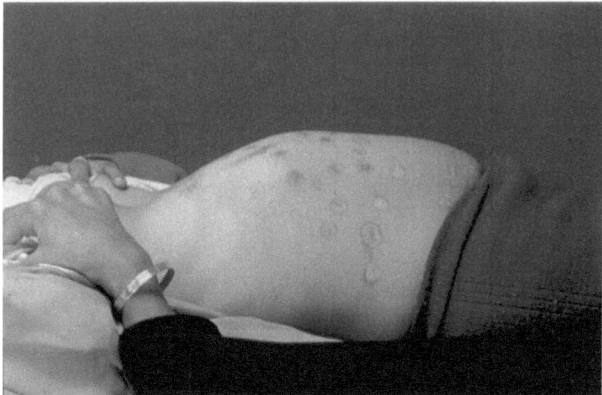

Figure 6. Ascites and traditional West African doctor scarifications on abdomen.

Ascites is caused by cirrhosis in 75%, malignancy in 10% and congestive cardiac failure in 5 %[71] of cases. Portal hypertension develops due to increased sinusoidal resistance to portal flow, from structural distortion -fibrosis, regenerative nodules and increased flow from splanchnic vasodilatation.

Liver cirrhosis leads to:

*   Increasing portal hypertension.
*   Splanchnic and later systemic vasodilation which increases the capacity of the splanchnic circulation. [71-77]
*   Portosystemic shunts increase vascular capacity.

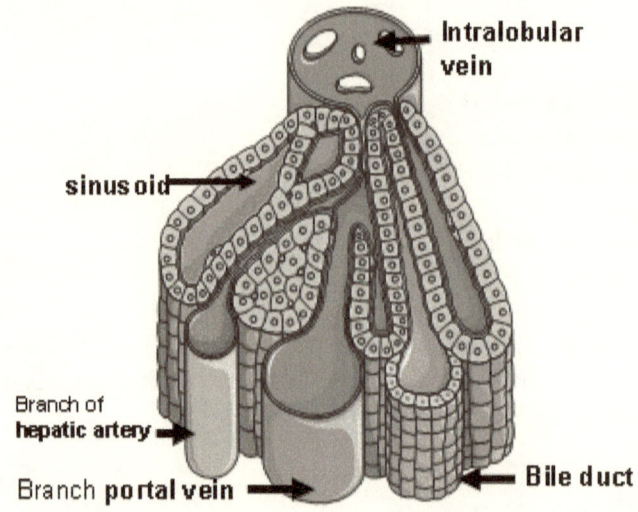

Figure 7. Model of Liver lobule. (produced using Servier medical art)

Splanchnic vasodilation results from either or both an increase in production or reduced clearance of vasodilators such as nitric oxide (NO), prostacyclin, natriuretic peptides, carbon monoxide, endogenous canabinoids and others. [74]

This leads to arterial underfilling. [72-77]Severe splanchnic dilatation correlates with hepatic decompensation. [75]

Activation of the renin angiotensin aldosterone sympathetic system (RAAS), in response to arterial underfilling, causes sodium retention. Increase in plasma volume and cardiac output compensate initially so that effective arterial volume is normal. Peripheral vasodilatation and hyperdynamic circulatory state results. There is controversy whether factors other than arterial underfilling explain intense sodium reabsorption [77]. Natriuretic peptides increase but natriuresis does not occur. [77]

Hepatic and intestinal lymph flow increase with progression—from 800mL-1000mL to as much as 20L day. [75]

Ascites initially responds to low sodium diet, (no added salt = ~ 50-100mmol sodium), and diuretics. Distal tubule diuretics, such as spironolactone, which can be given once daily, are chosen because they act on elevated aldosterone and are potassium sparing.

As liver disease progresses portal hypertension and splanchnic vasodilatation increase. Cardiac contractility decreases due to liver disease itself—reversal follows liver transplantation. [75].

Translocation of bacteria from intestinal lumen to mesenteric lymph glands [74] and from portosystemic shunts to systemic circulation may contribute to splanchnic vasodilation. Refractory ascites is associated with intense proximal tubule reabsorption of sodium which results in less Na^+ delivery to distal nephrons where aldosterone acts.

Ascitic fluid forms relatively easily in the highly capacious peritoneal cavity. High portal pressure and hypoalbuminaemia decrease transfer of fluid to the circulation. Renal excretion of free water is impaired and leads to hyponatraemia.

Vasoconstriction eventually develops in most non-splanchnic beds from intense activation of the RAAS and secretion of AVP (vasopressin). A hepato-renal reflex has been invoked: an increase in hepatic sinusoidal pressure or low flow activates intense renal vasoconstriction. [75]

Renal circulation is extremely sensitive to vasoconstriction: initially renal vasodilators, including prostaglandins, compensate by maintaining renal perfusion and glomerular filtration. Renal excretion of sodium becomes resistant to both spironolactone and atrial natriuretic infusion.

As hypotension and arterial underfilling increase in severity ascites becomes increasingly resistant to paracentesis, even when intravenous albumin is administered. Refractory ascites is defined as lack of response to maximum doses of diuretics (400mg spironolactone + 160mg frusemide) daily or when recurrent hyponatraemia, renal failure or hepatic encephalopathy occur on treatment with lower doses. Treatment options include:

* Repeated paracentesis with albumin administration.
* Provision of transjugular intrahepatic portosystemic shunt.
* Liver transplantation.

Acute renal failure, in association with cirrhosis, is due to prerenal renal failure in 35%, acute tubular necrosis in 32% and Hepatorenal syndrome in 26% of cases. [75]

Renal failure is defined as serum creatinine above133 μmol/L.-a lower level than usual because serum creatinine is misleadingly low due to.

• Decrease in skeletal mass.
• Decrease in liver creatinine synthesis.
• Increase in tubular creatinine secretion.

The processes described above are summarized in the following figure 8.

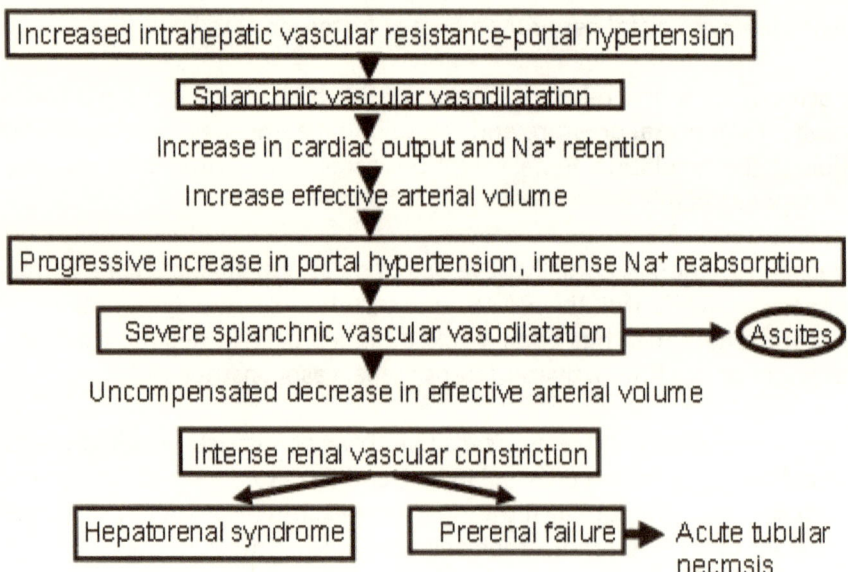

Figure 8. Model showing pathogenesis of changes in liver cirrhosis leading to renal failure.

Hepato-renal syndrome. [75-81]

This is a form of reversible renal failure which develops in those with advanced cirrhosis or fulminant hepatic failure when renal compensatory vasodilators such as NO, prostaglandins, ANP and others are inadequate to maintain renal blood flow.

Unopposed intense renal cortical ischemia, secondary to vasoconstriction and hypotension, lead to cortical hypoperfusion, severe sodium retention and oliguria. Tubular function is preserved and proteinuria absent. Correlation between cardiac output and renal perfusion is poor. [75] An initiating event is often present such as volume depletion, large volume paracentesis, sepsis, haemorrhage, obstructive jaundice or use of nephrotoxic drugs. Diagnosis of Hepato-renal syndrome is based on the following:

* Serum creatinine > 133 μmol.
* Hypovolaemia is absent or has been treated and nephrotoxic drugs are not responsible.
* Resting blood pressure is usually lower than normal.
* Hyponatraemia is usually present.
* Urinary sodium is extremely low despite oliguria.
* Proteinuria is low (< 500 mg / day) and parenchymal renal disease excluded.

Hypovolaemia and prerenal failure are very difficult to exclude: serum creatinine should not decrease following cessation of diuretics and administration of albumin 1.5 g/kg body weight followed by 1.0 g/kg body weight in 48 hours. [74]

Biochemical disturbances in hepato-renal syndrome are similar to those of pre-renal failure due to hypovolaemia. Urine sodium is low. Serum creatinine does not accurately reflect GFR and vasodilatation masks signs of hypovolaemia. Diagnosis is therefore extremely difficult. Administered fluid rapidly moves into the ascitic pool rather than remain in the vascular volume.

The Hepato-renal syndrome occurs in 39% of patients within five years of diagnosis of cirrhotic ascites [78, 81] The probability of occurrence increases if hyponatraemia, high plasma renin and absence of hepatomegaly are present. [81] Hypovolaemia [79] may be an important underlying factor because infusion of fresh frozen plasma to expand plasma volume to supranormal levels, but not angiotensin II, is effective in improving GFR, renal plasma flow and urine output. The ascitic fluid pressure increases. [71] Effective hypovolaemia is common because of:

* Repeated tapping and reaccumulation of Ascites.
* Administration of Diuretics and sodium restriction.
* Sequestration of blood within a dilated splanchnic or systemic circulation.
* Porto-systemic collaterals.
* Recurrent episodes of bacteraemia, variceal bleeding or spontaneous bacterial peritonitis.
* Lower limb oedema which is difficult to mobilize.

Thus hepato-renal syndrome should only be diagnosed if response to standard volume replacement fails.

The problem is the difficulty of ever being certain if sufficient fluid has been given to correct hypovolaemia.

Hepato-renal syndrome has been divided into:

Type 1—progressive oliguria with a doubling of serum creatinine to >221 µmol/L within 2 weeks.

Type 2—a moderate rise in serum creatinine which stabilizes.

The international Ascites Club has defined hepato-renal syndrome as: [81]

• Serum creatinine >130µmol/L or GFR < 40mL/minute.
• Absence of shock, sepsis, fluid loss or nephrotoxic drugs.
• No improvement following withholding diuretics and fluid challenge.
• Proteinuria < 500mg day ; < 50 red cells/hpf and exclusion of obstructive uropathy by ultrasound or other imaging.
• Urine Na^+ < 10mmol/L and urine osmolality >plasma osmolality.
• Serum Na^+ < 130mmol/L.
• Urine volume < 500mL/day.

Mortality in type 1 is 80% within 2 weeks and 90% within 3 months.

Management of Ascites.

Ascitic fluid should be examined initially to rule out spontaneous bacterial peritonitis and on subsequent occasions for unexpected deterioration, fever or an increase in inflammatory markers. The serum albumin: ascites—albumin gradient (serum albumin minus ascitic fluid albumin concentration in (g/L) reliably differentiates portal hypertension from other causes of ascites. [82] A high gradient ≥ 11g/L occurs in portal hypertension. It is not changed by diuretics, paracentesis or by spontaneous bacterial peritonitis. [82]

Severity of cirrhosis, renal failure, electrolytes and volume status should be assessed. Serum creatinine gives a misleading indication of GFR because considerable reduction occurs in the presence of normal serum creatinine during hypovolaemia. [83] Hypovolaemia, sufficiently severe to decrease GFR, is common and has many causes: a sudden increase in ascites; the effects of diuretics; variations in salt intake; bleeding varices; infection, including spontaneous bacterial peritonitis, vomiting and diarrhoea.

Arterial blood gas often shows respiratory alkalosis and mild metabolic alkalosis, secondary to hypoalbuminaemia, in severe cirrhosis. [84] Hyponatraemia is common, with or without reduction in GFR, and is probably due to the non-osmotic release of ADH (AVP) secondary to arterial underfilling. [85] Hypokalaemia commonly occurs due to secondary hyperaldostereonism. Hypokalaemia has been reported to increase encephalopathy.

Spontaneous bacterial peritonitis (SBP) should be treated with a third generation cephalosporin and albumin, 1.5 g/kg body weight and 1.0 g/kg body weight, in 48 hours.

Diuretic Therapy.

Spironolactone (50-200mg/day) or amiloride (5-20mg/day) are diuretics of choice for treatment of ascites. High doses of spironolactone have an anti-testosterone effect and cause gynaecomastia and decreased libido. Furosemide is added if ascites is inadequately controlled but increases the risk of developing effective hypovolaemia and renal dysfunction. Weight should be checked regularly. Diuretics should be used carefully to decrease the risk of renal failure.

Paracentesis.

This is indicated for severe discomfort, interference with activities of daily living or severe respiratory restriction. Paracentesis is more effective and causes fewer complications than "pushing" diuretics. [85] Initially rapid total paracentesis for tense ascites improves cardiac output, decreases right atrial pressure, serum renin and aldosterone levels. [86, 87] However deterioration follows after a variable time. Effective hypovolaemia, recurrence of ascites, increased vasoconstriction, hyponatraemia and renal dysfunction increase the risk of hepato-renal syndrome. [88]

Administration of albumin decreases these complications [89, 90] but has not demonstrated survival advantages in randomised studies, but these may have had inadequate power to detect a statistically significant difference. [76] Albumin is probably superior to other colloids [91]. Intravenous albumin administration has been shown to decrease mortality in patients with cirrhosis and spontaneous bacterial peritonitis. [92]

Refractory Ascites.

This is defined as lack of response of ascites to high doses of spironolactone (400mg/day) plus frusemide 160mg day or recurrent side effects of renal failure, hyponatraemia or hepatic encephalopathy on lower doses. [80]

Recurrent episodes of ascites occur at short intervals (often every two weeks) following paracentesis plus albumin. The risk of the hepato-renal syndrome increases.

Transjugular intrahepatic portosystemic shunting decreases recurrence of ascites and renal failure [93,94], but two recent randomised trials failed to decrease mortality in the absence of liver transplantation. [95, 96]

Hepato-renal Syndrome.

Mortality was previously extremely high. Terlipressin, a vasopressin analogue, improves renal function in conjunction with albumin [97 98] presumably by decreasing vasodilatation in splanchnic circulation. Terlipressin without albumin is much less effective. [99] However randomized controlled trials have not decreased mortality and its superiority over volume expansion has not been established. [75]

Haemodialysis [99] and Transintraperitoneal shunts (TIPS), which decrease the hepatorenal reflex, [75] may also prolong life. However use of haemodialysis and Terlipressin with albumin should only be used to buy time for liver transplantation.

In conclusion the following are important in management of ascites:

* Avoid excessive use of diuretics, large volume paracentesis without infusion of albumin, electrolyte imbalance and use of nephrotoxic drugs. Treat bleeding and infection promptly and adequately. Initially restrict sodium and increase spironolactone from 50 to 400mg daily.
* Avoid nephrotoxins, especially non steroidal inflammatory drugs, gentamycin and dye.

Treat large volume ascites by:

* Adding frusemide to spironolactone.
* Using large volume paracentesis with albumin replacement. Albumin is effective in preventing hypovolaemia, the hepato-renal syndrome and recurrence of ascites, although the impact on long term survival is uncertain.
* Treat underlying causes of deterioration. Effective hypovolaemia is a more common cause of oliguria and hypotension than hepato-renal syndrome and is difficult to differentiate from it.
* Treat spontaneous bacterial peritonitis with third generation cephalosporins and intravenous albumin, 1.5g/kg body weight, followed by 1 g/kg body weight in 48 hours. However an increasing number of cases are due to gram positive organisms.
* Use Norfloxacin or Trimethoprim—sulphamethoxazole for prophylaxis of Bacterial Peritonitis. [101] However quinalone resistance is a serious emerging problem. [100] Use non selective β antagonist to decrease variceal bleeding.
* Avoid hypokalaemia and treat it rapidly because hypokalaemia increases ammonium synthesis and worsens hepatic encephalopathy. [102]
* Hepato-renal syndrome: improve renal perfusion and GFR with :
    ❖ Plasma volume expansion with albumin.
    ❖ Reduction of splanchnic vasodilation with vasopressin analogues and alpha adrenergic agonists.
* Correct electrolyte disorders, especially hypokalaemia.

Vasoconstrictor drugs have been shown to improve renal function and prolong survival in the short term but randomized controlled trials have not shown decrease in mortality. Liver transplantation is the only treatment that improves long term mortality.

METABOLIC COMPLICATIONS OF URINARY DIVERSION. [103-106]

Urinary diversion mainly involves four types of procedures:

- Implantation of ureters into sigmoid colon (ureterosigmoidostomy) to enable passage of urine per rectum.
- Augmentation of the bladder—intestinal cytoplasty.
- Construction of new bladders using a segment of small bowel or colon into which ureters are implanted. The segment of bowel is detubularised to create a spherical reservoir and ureters are implanted at an angle to prevent reflux. The other end of the new reservoir is joined to the abdominal wall to form a stoma. This is emptied intermittently by catheter. [105]
- Ileal ureters may substitute for defective ureters.

The factors which influence secretion and absorption by bowel segments were described in the previous section.

Complications which occur are influenced by:

- Type of bowel and surface area used.
- Contact time of urine with bowel.
- Renal function, pH and osmolality of urine excreted.

Ileal conduits have the least incidence of complications and use of jejunal conduits the highest. The jejunum is a net secretor of fluid and has a high permeability to water. [19,103] Severe volume depletion, hyponatraemia, metabolic acidosis and hyperkalaemia are relatively common [105] and magnesium deficiency may occur because magnesium is normally reabsorbed in small bowel.

In contrast ileum and colon are especially effective in reabsorbing Na^+, water and Cl^- in exchange for bicarbonate. K^+ is reabsorbed by ileum but secreted in exchange for Na^+ in colon.

ELECTROLYTE AND ACID BASE ABNORMALITIES

Hyperchloraemic Acidosis. occurs in ureterosigmoidostomies, colonic and ileal conduits due to reabsorption of Cl^-, NH_4^+ and H^+. It is less common in ileal conduits, occurring from 1.7-15 %[105], probably because Cl^- is less readily reabsorbed.

Hypokalaemia occurs more commonly when the colon is used as a conduit because it is efficient in reabsorbing Na^+ in exchange for K^+.

Magnesium deficiency and hypomagnesaemia. occasionally occur from ileal conduits.

Coma due to Ammonia.

Ammonium (NH_4^+) may be generated by the kidney or NH_3 produced by urea splitting bacteria in the conduit [104,105]. Ammonia is reabsorbed by the ileum and colon and passes to liver because these segments retain their normal vascular connections. When liver's capacity to metabolise NH_3 is exceeded encephalopathy may occur. This rarely occurs when liver function is normal unless infection is coexists. [106] Drainage by rectal tube is highly effective In ureterosigmoidostomies. [105]

Infection. Pyelonephritis and infection of the conduit are common and are usually due to Escherichia coli, Proteus, Pseudomonas, and Enterobacter bacteria. Eighty percent of those with a conduit or continent diversion have bacteriuria. [105]

Bone disease and Urinary Stones.

Rickets, osteomalacia and renal stones occur from chronic metabolic acidosis. This causes loss of calcium and phosphate from bone in buffering and inhibits renal reabsorption of calcium and magnesium. Calcium, phosphate and magnesium are excreted in excess in urine associated with an increase in sulfate excretion. Ammonium enhances intestinal sulphate absorption and renal excretion. Patients with ileal conduits have a 20% incidence of renal stones. Pouch calculi occur in up to one third. [107]

Altered Drug Metabolism. Drugs or metabolites normally excreted in urine can be absorbed into the portal circulation and increase plasma drug levels.

Diarrhoea, B12 Deficiency and Gallstones.

Although complications are less from ileal, compared to colonic conduits, loss of normal ileum can result in B12 deficiency and gallstones from decreased absorption of bile salts. The osmotic effect of unabsorbed bile salts in colon may cause diarrhoea.

Cancer,

The incidence of cancer at the ureterointestinal anastomosis varies between 6-29 %. [104,105] Malignancies are especially common in bladder augmentation and intestinal conduits. Adenocarcinoma is the most common. [104,105]

Treatment

- Sodium bicarbonate is given to maintain normal serum bicarbonate.
- Regular and frequent conduit emptying. [105]
- Surveillance for infection.

Ammoniagenic encephalopathy: Place a rectal tube for drainage of ureterosigmoidostomy and catheter drainage of conduits which may be obstructed. Administer lactulose and treat infection.

REFERENCES

1.   Phillips, SF: (Progress in Gastroenterology) Diarrhoea: A current view of Pathophysiology. *Gastroenterology.* **63**:495-518, 1972.
2.   Shires, GT; Shires III, GT; Lowry, SF: Fluid, Electrolyte and nutritional management of the surgical patient. p.65 in *Principles of Surgery* Eds. Schwartz, SI; Shires, GT and Spencer, FC. McGraw Hill Inc. 6th Edition, 1994.
3.   Daly, JM; Copeland III, EM; Dudrick, SJ: Preparation of the patient. p7 in *Master of Surgery*. Second Edition. Ed Nyhus, LM; Baker, RJ; Little, Brown & Coy 1992.
4.   Black, DAK: *Lancet.*1: 353-360, 1953.
5.   *Manual of Surgical Therapeutics* 9th Ed. Eds Condon, R; Nyhus, L. 1996. Boston: Little Brown.

6.   Humphreys, MH: Fluid and Electrolyte Management. P147 in *Current Surgical Diagnosis andTreatment*. Ed. Way, LW, Doherty, GM, 11th Edition. 2003. Lange Medical Books/McGraw Hill.

7.   Field, M; Rao, MC; Chang, EB: Intestinal electrolyte transport and diarrhoeal disease. *NEJM*. **321**: Part 1, 800-806, 1989; Part 2, p879-883.

8.   Sellin JM: The pathophysiology of diarrhoea. *Clinical Transplantation*. **15(suppl 4)**:2-10, 2001.

9.   Binder, HJ: Causes of chronic diarrhoea. *NEJM*. **355**:236-239, 2006.

10.   Farthing, MJG: Novel targets for the pharmacotherapy of diarrhoea: A view for the millennium. *J. Gastroenterology and Hepatology*. **15**(Suppl):G38-G45, 2000.

11.   Binder, HJ: Intestinal fluid and electrolyte movement, p 931-945 in *Medical Physiology (updated edition)*. Eds. Boron, WF; Boulpaep, EL, 2005. Elsevier Saunders.

12.   Matthews, JB; Hassan, I; Meng, S; et al: Na-K -2Cl cotransporter gene expression and function during enterocyte differentiation: Modulation of Cl⁻ secretory capacity by butyrate. *J Clin Invest*. **101**:2072-2079, 1998.

13.   Bridges, RJ; Rummel, W: Mechanistic Basis of alterations in mucosal water and electrolyte transport. *Clinics in Gastroenterology*. **15**:491-506, 1986.

14.   Chubanov, V; Gudermann, T and Schlingmann, KP: Essential role for TRPM6 in epithelial magnesium transport and body magnesium homeostasis. *Pflugers Archiv—European Journal of Physiology*. **451(1)**:228-234, 2005.

15.   Yu, AS: Evolving concepts in epithelial magnesium transport. *Current Opinion in Nephrology & Hypertension*. **10(5)**:649-653, 2001.

16.   Phillips, SF: Functions of the large bowel: an overview. *Scandinavian J. of Gastroenterology*. **93(Suppl)**:1-12, 1984.

17.   Kunzelmann, K; Mall, M: Electrolyte transport in mammalian colon : mechanisms and implications for disease. *Physiolog. Reviews*. **82**:245-289, 2002.

18.   Binder, HJ; Rajendran, V, Sadasivan, V, Gbel, J: Bicarbonate secretion: a neglected aspect of colonic ion transport. *J. of Clinical Gastroenterology*. 39(suppl) :S53-S58, 2005.

19.   Greenberger, NJ: Diagnostic approach to the patient with a chronic diarrhoeal disorder. *Disease a Month*. **36(3)**:135-179, 1990.

20.   Jenkins, HR; Milla, PJ: Congenital chloride—losing diarrhoea: absence of the anion-exchange mechanisms in the rectum. *Journal of Paediatric Gastroenterology and Nutrition*. **24**:518-521, 1997.

21.   Kassirer, JP; Schwartz, WB: The response of normal man to selective depletion of hydrochloric acid. *Amer. J. Med.***40** : 10-18.1966

22. Van Goidsenhoven, GM-T; Gray OV; Price, AV; Sanderson, PH: The effect of prolonged administration of large doses of sodium bicarbonate in man. *Clin. Sci.* **13**:383-401, 1952.
23. Seldin, Donald W; Floyd C Rector: The generation and maintenance of metabolic alkalosis. *Kidney International.* **1**:306-321, 1972.
24. Levine, David Z: Single-nephron studies: Implications of acid-base regulation. *Kidney International.* **38**:744-761, 1990.
25. Sabatini, Sandra: The cellular basis of metabolic alkalosis. *Kidney International.* **49**:906-917, 1996.
26. Rosen, Randy A; Julian, Bruce A; Dubovsky, Eva V; et al: On the mechanisms by which chloride corrects metabolic alkalosis in man. *Amer. J. Med.* **84**:449, 1988.
27. Stone, DK; Xie, XS: Proton translocating ATPases: Issues in structure and function. *Kidney International.* **33**:767, 1988.
28. Garg, LC; Narang, N: Effects of aldosterone on NEM sensitive ATPase in rabbit nephron segments. *Kidney International.* **34**:13, 1988.
29. Wesson, D: Augmented bicarbonate reabsorption by both the proximal and distal nephron maintains chloride—deplete metabolic alkalosis in Rats. *J. Clin. Invest.* 84:1460, 1989.
30. Mitchell, JE; Pyle, RL; Eckert, ED; et al: Electrolyte and other physiological abnormalities in patients with bulimia. *Psychological Medicine.* **13**:273-8, 1983
31. Krejs, GJ; Walsh, JH; Morawski, SG, Fordtran, JS: Intractable diarrhoea. intestinal perfusion studies and plasma VIP concentrations in patients with pancreatic cholera syndrome and surreptitious ingestion of laxatives and diuretics. *Dig. Diseases.* **22**:280-282, 1977.
32. Donowitz, M; Kokke, FT, Saldi, R: Evaluation of patients with chronic diarrhoea. *NEJM.* **332**:725-731, 1995.
33. Bloom, SR, Polak, JM, Pearce, AGE: Vasoactive intestinal peptide and watery diarrhoea syndrome. *Lancet 2.* 14-16.1973.
34. Krejs, GT: Vipoma Syndrome. *Amer. J. Med.* **82(supple 5B)**:37-46, 1987.
35. Masel, SL, Brennan, BA; Turner, JH et al: Pancreatic vasoactive intestinal polypeptide-oma as a cause of secretory diarrhoea. *Gastroenterology and Hepatology.* **15**:457-460, 2000.
36. Said, SI; Faloona, GR: Elevated plasma and tissue levels of vasoactive intestinal polypeptide in the watery-diarrhoea syndrome due to pancreatic, bronchogenic and other tumours. *NEJM.* **293**:155-160, 1975.
37. Jaffe, BM; Kopen, DF; Deschryver-Kecskemeti, K; et al: Indomethacin-Responsive Pancreatic Cholera. *NEJM.* **297**:817-820, 1977.
38. Cruetzfeldt, W; Stockman, F: Carcinoids and Carcinoid Syndrome. *Amer. J. Med.* **82(Suppl 5B)**:4-12, 1987.

39. El Masri SH; Lewin, MR; Clark, CG: Invitro effects of Gastrin in movement of electrolytes across the human colon. *Scan. J. Gastroent.* **12**:999-1002, 1977.

40. Ladefoged, K; Olgbaard, K: Sodium homeostasis after small-bowel resection. *Gastroenterology.* **20**:361-369, 1985.

41. Moss, S; Gordon, D; Forsling, ML; et al: Water and electrolyte composition of urine and ileal fluid in its relationship to renin and aldosterone during dietary sodium deprivation in patients with ileostomies. *Clinical Science.* **61**:407-415, 1981.

42. Hessov, I; Hasselblad, C, Fasth, C; Hulton, L: Magnesium deficiency after ileal resections for Crohns disease. *Scandinavian J. Gastroenterology.* **18**:643-649, 1983.

43. Kelly, DG; Branon, ME; Phillips, SF; Kelly, KA: Diarrhoea after continent ileostomy. *Gut.* **21**:711-716, 1980.

44. Rampton, DS; Sladen, GE: Relationship between rectal mucosal prostaglandin production and water and electrolyte transport in ulcerative colitis. *Digestion.* **30**:13-22, 1984.

45. Sandle, GI; Higgs, N; Crowe, P et al: Cellular bases for defective electrolyte transport in the inflamed human colon. *Gastroenterology.* **99**:97-105, 1990.

46. Butler, T; Speelman, P; Kabir, I; Branwell, J: Colonic dysfunction during shigellosis. *J. Infect. Diseases.* **154**:817-824, 1986.

47. Older, J; Older, P; Colker, J; Brown, R: Secretory villous adenomas that cause depletion syndrome. *Arch. Int. Med.* **159**:879-880, 1999.

48. Cheung, AW: The effect of oral feeding at different levels on the absorption of food stuffs in infantile diarrhoea. *J. Pediat.* **33**:1.1948

49. Kingston, ME: Continued breast feeding and concentrated diarrhoeal formula (CDF) in the outpatient treatment of Gastroenteritis. *Environmental Child Health (Special Issue), June 168-170, June 1973.*

50. Kingston, ME: Biochemical disturbances in breastfed infants with gastroenteritis and dehydration. *J. Pediatrics.* **82**:1073-1081, 1973.

51. Carpenter, CCJ; Greenough, WB; Pierce, NF: oral-rehydration therapy—the role of polymeric substrates. *NEJM.* **319**:1340-1348, 1988.

52. Balistreri, WF: Oral rehydration in acute infantile diarrhoea. *Amer. J. Med.* **88(suppl 6A)**:305-335, 1990.

53. Alam, NH; Majumder, RN; Fuchs, GJ: Choice Study Group. Efficacy and safety of oral rehydration solution with reduced osmolarity in adults with cholera : a randomised double-blind clinical trial. *Lancet.* **354**:296-299, 1999.

54. Holt, LE; Courtney, AM; Fales, HL: Chemical composition of diarrhoeal as compared with normal stools in infants. *Amer. J. Dis. Child.* **9**:213, 1915.

55. Darrow, DC: The Retention of Electrolyte during recovery from severe dehydration due to diarrhoea. *J. Pediat.* **28**:515, 1946.

56. Darrow, DC et al: Disturbance of water and electrolytes in infantile diarrhoea. *Pediat.* **3**:129, 1949.

57. Kooh, SN, Metcoff, J: Physiological consideration in fluid and electrolyte treatment with particular reference to diarrhoeal dehydration in children. *J. Pediat.* **62**:107, 1963.

58. Weil, WB; Wallace, WM: Hypertonic dehydration in infancy. *Pediat.* **17**:171, 1956

59. Finberg, L; Cheung O, Fleishman E: The significance of the concentration of electrolytes in stool water during infantile diarrhoea. *Amer. J. Dis. Child.* **100**:809.1960

60. Teree, TM et al: Stool losses and acidosis in diarrhoeal disease of infants. *Pediat.* **36**:704.1965

61. Bruck, E; Abal, G; Aceto, T: Pathogenesis and pathophysiology of hypertonic dehydration. *Amer. J. Dis. Child.* **115**:122.1968

62. Molla, AM; Rahman, M; Sarker, SA et al: Stool electrolyte content and purging rates in diarrhoea caused by rotavirus enterotoxigenic E.coli and V. cholerae in children. *J. Pediat.* **98**:835,838, 1981.

63. Kingston, M: Electrolyte and fluid disturbances in Liberian children. A thesis submitted for the Degree of Doctor of Medicine. University of London.1974

64. Mahalanabis, P: Water and electrolyte losses due to cholera in infants. *Pediat.* **45**:374, 1970.

65. Griffiths, LSC et al: Electrolyte replacement in pediatric cholera. *Lancet.* **1**:1197, 1967.

66. Shiau, YF; Feldman, GM; Resnick, MA; Coff, PM: Stool electrolyte and osmolality measurements in the evaluation of diarrhoeal disorders. *Ann. Int. Med.* **102**:773-775 1985.

67. Ladefoged K, Schaffalitzky, DE; Muckadell, OB; Jarnum, S: Faecal osmolality and electrolyte concentrations in chronic diarrhoea: Do they provide diagnostic clues? *Scand. J. Gastroenterol.* **22**:813-820, 1987.

68. Binder, HJ: The Gastroenterologists' osmotic gap: Fact or fiction? *Gastroenterology.* **103**:702-704, 1992.

69. Eherer, AJ, Fordtran, JS: Faecal osmotic gap and pH in experimental diarrhoea of various causes. *Gastroenterology.* **103**:545-551, 1992.

70. Fine, KD, Santa, CA, Fordtran, JS: Diagnosis of magnesium-induced diarrhoea. *NEJM.* **324**:1012-1017, 1991.

71. Krige, JE; Beckingham, I: Portal hypertension-2, ascites, encephalopathy and other conditions. *BMJ.* **322**:416-418, 2001.

72. Schrier, RW: Pathogenesis of sodium and water in high-output and low output cardiac failure, nephritic syndrome, cirrhosis and pregnancy (First of Two Parts). *NEJM.* **319**:1065-1071, 1988.

73. Schrier, RW: Pathogenesis of sodium and water in high-output and low output cardiac failure, nephritic syndrome, cirrhosis and pregnancy (Second of Two Parts). *NEJM.* **319**:1127-1132, 1988.

74. Gines P, Schrier RW.Renal Failure in Cirrhosis. New Engl J Medicine.**361**:1279-90 2009

75. Ley, M: Hepatorenal syndrome. *Kidney Int.* **43**:737-753, 1993.

76. Gines, P; Cardenas, A; Arroyo, V; Rodes, J: Management of cirrhosis and ascites. *NEJM.* **350**:1646-1654, 2004.

77. Wong, F; Girgrah, N; Blendis, L: Review: The controversy over the pathophysiology of ascites formation in cirrhosis. *Gastroenterology and Hepatology.* **12**:437-444, 1997.

78. Barada, K: Hepatorenal syndrome: pathogenesis and novel pharmacological targets. *Current Opinion in Pharmacology.* **4**:189-197, 2004.

79. Cade, R; Wagemaker, H; Vogel, S et al: Hepatorenal syndrome : Studies of the effect of vascular volume and intraperitoneal pressure on renal and hepatic function. *Amer. J. Medicine.* **82**:427-438, 1987.

80. Gines, A; Escorsell, A; Gines, P et al: Incidence, predictive factors and prognosis of Hepatorenal syndrome in cirrhosis with ascites. *Gastroenterology.* **105**:229-236, 1993.

81. Arroyo, V; Gines, P; Gerbes, AL: Definition and diagnostic criteria of refractory ascites and hepatorenal syndrome in cirrhosis. *Hepatology.* **23**:164-176, 1996.

82. Runyon, BA, Montano, AA; Arkiviadis, EA et al: The serum-ascites albumin gradient is superior to the exudate-transudate concept in the differential diagnosis of ascites. *Ann. Int. Med.* **117**:215-220, 1992.

83. Sherman, DS; Fish, DN; Teitelbaum, I: Assessing renal function in cirrhotic patients: problems and pitfalls. *Amer. J. Kid. Dis.* **41**:269-278, 2003.

84. Funk, GC; Doberer, D; Osterreicher C, et al: Equilibrium of acidifying and alkalinizing metabolic acid-base disorders in cirrhosis. *Liver Internat.* **25**:505-512, 2005.

85. Gines, P; Arroyo, V; Quintero, E et al: Comparison of paracentesis and diuretics in the treatment of cirrhosis with tense ascites: Results of a randomised study. *Gastroenterology.* **93**:234-241, 1987.

86. Luca, A; Feu, F; Garcia-Pagan, JC et al: Favourable effects of total paracentesis on splanchnic haemodynamics in cirrhotic patients with tense ascites. *Hepatology.* **20**:30-33, 1994.

87. Pozzi, M; Osculati, G; Boari, G et al: Time course of Circulatory and Humeral effects of rapid total paracentesis in Cirrhotic patients with tense refractory ascites. *Gastroent.* **106**:709-719, 1994.

88. Ruiz-Del-Arbol, L; Monescillo, A, Wladimiro, J et al: Paracentesis-induced circulatorydysfunction:mechanismandeffectonhepatichaemodynamics in cirrhosis. *Gastroenterology.* **113**:579-586, 1997.

89. Luca, A, Garcia-Pagan, JC, Bosch, J et al: Beneficial effects of intravenous albumin infusion on haemodynamic and humeral changes after total paracentesis. *Hepatology.* **22**:753-758, 1995.

90. Gines, P, Tito, L; Arroyo, V et al: Randomised comparative study of therapeutic paracentesis with and without intravenous albumin in cirrhosis. *Gastroenterology.* **94**:493-1502, 1988.

91. Gines, A; Fernandez, Esparrach, G; Monescillo, A et al: Randomised trial comparing albumin dextran 70 and polygeline in cirrhotic patients with ascites treated by paracentesis. *Gastroenterology.* **111**:1002-1010, 1996.

92. Sort, P; Nayasa, M; Arroyo, V et al: Effect of intravenous albumin on renal impairment and mortality in patients with cirrhosis and spontaneous bacterial peritonitis. *NEJM.* **341**:403-409, 1999.

93. Ochs, A; Rossle, M; Haag, K et al: The transjugular intrahepatic portosystemic stent-shunt procedure for refractory ascites. *NEJM.* **332**:1192-1197, 1995.

94. Rossle, M; Ochs, A; Gulberg, V et al: A comparison of paracentesis and Transjugular intrahepatic portosystemic shunting in patients with ascites. *NEJM.* **342**:**1701-1017**, 2000.

95. Gines, P; Uriz, J; Calahorra, B et al: Transjugular intrahepatic portosystemic shunting versus paracentesis plus albumin for refractory ascites in cirrhosis. *Gastroenterology.* **123**:1839-1847, 2002.

96. Sanyal, AJ; Genning, C; Reddy, KR et al: The North American study for the treatment of refractory ascites. *Gastroenterology.* **124**:634-641, 2003.

97. Moreau, R; Durand, F; Poynard, T et al: Terlipressin in patients with cirrhosis and type I hepatorenal syndrome: a retrospective multicentre study. *Gastroenterology.* **122**:923-930, 2002.

98. Ortega, R; Gines, P; Uriz, J: Terlipressin therapy with and without albumin for patients with hepatorenal syndrome: results of a prospective, non-randomised study. *Hepatology.* **36**:941-948, 2002.

99. Witzke, O; Bauman, M; Schand, P et al: Which patients benefit from haemodialysis therapy in Hepatorenal syndrome. *J. Gastroenterol. Hepatol.* **19**:1369-1373, 2004.

100. Fernandez, J; Navasa, M; Gomez, J et al: Bacterial infections in cirrhosis: epidemiological changes with invasive procedures and norfloxacin prophylaxis. *Hepatology.* **35**:140-148, 2002.

101. Singh, N; Gayowski, T; Yu, VL et al: Trimethoprim-Sulfamethoxazole for the prevention of spontaneous bacterial peritonitis in cirrhosis. *Arch. Int. Med.* **122**:595-598, 1995.

102. Artz SA, Paes IC, Faloon WW. Hypokalemia-induced Hepatic Coma in Cirrhosis.Gastroenterology.51:1046-1052 1966.

103. Kosko, JW; Kursh, ED; Resnick, MI: Metabolic complications of urological intestinal substitutes. *Urolog. Clinic. N. Amer.* **13**:193-199, 1986.

104. Cruz, DN; Hout, SJ: Metabolic complications of urinary diversions: an overview. *Amer. J. Med.* **102**:477-484, 1997.

105. McDougal, WS: Metabolic complications of urinary intestinal diversion. *J. Urology.* **147**:1199-1208, 1992.

106. Karveggia, FF; Thompson, JS, Schafer, EC et al: Hyperammonemic encephalopathy in urinary diversion with urea-splitting urinary tract infection. *Arch. Int. Med.* **150**:2389-2392.1990

107. McDougal, WS, Koch, MO: Effect of sulfate on calcium and magnesium homeostasis following urinary diversion. *Kidney Int.* **35**:105-115, 1989.

STARVATION, DIABETIC KETOACIDOSIS (DKA) and HYPERGLYCAEMIC HYPEROSMOLAR STATES (HHS)

KETONE FORMATION AND CONTROL OF GLUCOSE. [1-11]

Starvation.

Production of ketones in diabetic ketoacidosis (DKA) and fasting are similar. In fasting energy needs are provided by glycogenolysis (1-2 days); gluconeogenesis (up to 1 week); and ketosis, which starts after 2-3 days, is prolonged, and the main source of energy [12, 13]. Increase in ketones may be beneficial in minimising proteolysis by restraining alanine release from muscle. [14]

ßOH butyric acid is normally the main ketone body (ratio 3:1) but may increase to a ratio of 10:1 in severe acidosis. An increase in the ratio of NADH: NAD+ (REDOX state), from anaerobic metabolism or acidosis, increases conversion of acetoacetic acid to βOH butyric acid because H+ is taken up in its formation from acetoacetic acid. 1000-1500mmol ketone bodies produced daily are used as fuel by brain (600-1,500mmol/day), kidney (350-400mmol/day) and gut mucosa (~ 200mmol/day). [13]

The following are required for ketosis to occur (figure 1):

1) Fatty acid production must increase from lipolysis: a process inhibited by insulin and stimulated by glucagon and catecholamines.
2) Fatty acids pass into mitochondria, using carnitine as carrier, stimulated by glucagon.
3) Fatty acids must be converted to acetoacetic acid rather than be oxidised in Krebs cycle or converted into fat.

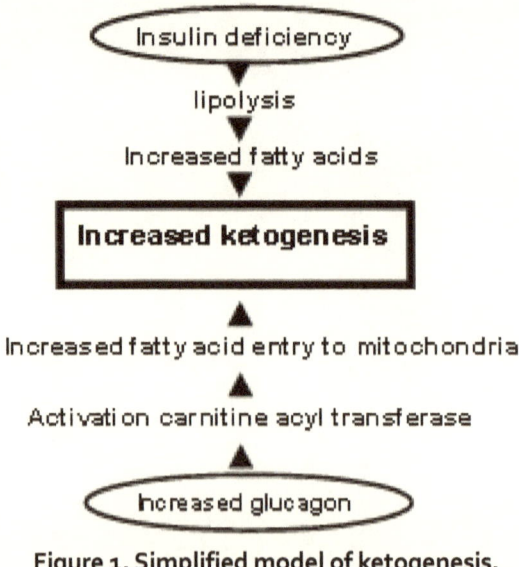

Figure 1. Simplified model of ketogenesis.

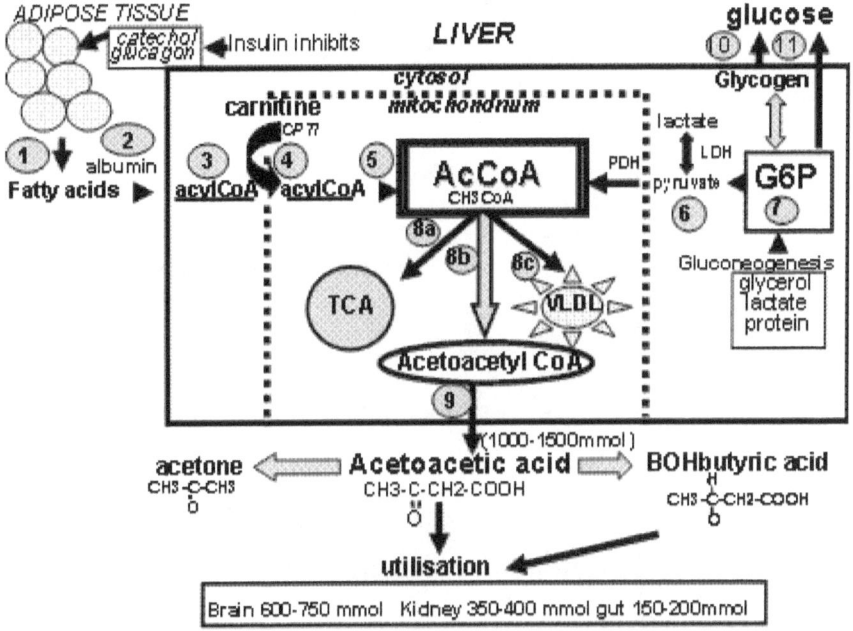

Figure 2: *Simplified model showing interrelationships of glucose, fatty acids, acetyl-CoA and production of ketones in liver. Actions occurring in mitochondria are shown in the centre between stipled lines. (Numbers in figure correspond to numbers in text.)*

In both starvation and diabetic ketoacidosis:

1. Fat breaks down to fatty acids by hormone sensitive lipase (not shown) which is inhibited by insulin and stimulated by catecholamines.

    Lipase

    Triglyceride ⟶ Glycerol and fatty acids

2. Fatty acids (and glycerol) are carried to liver bound to albumin.
3. Fatty acids are converted to acyL-CoA in liver cytosol by acyL-CoA synthetase. (not shown)

    Long chain acyL-CoA (or free fatty acids) cannot penetrate the inner mitochondria membrane. (shown as stippled line).
4. Acyl-Coa combines with carnitine forming acyl carnitine, catalysed by the enzyme carnitine palmitoly transferase-1 (CPT1). Acyl-Coa is reformed after passing through the inner mitochondrial membrane catalysed by CPT-II.

The above process is, in essence, the <u>shuttling of **acyL-Coa** through the inner mitochondrial membrane using carnitine (carnitine shuttle). This process is inhibited by insulin and stimulated by glucagon</u>.

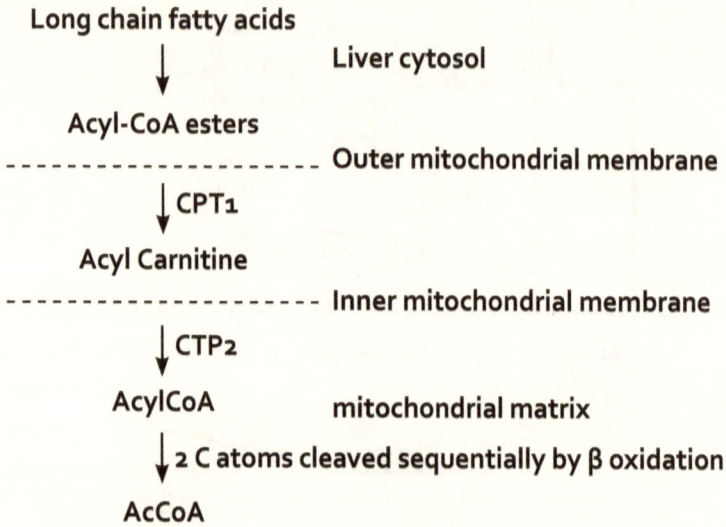

5. In mitochondria oxidation successively removes 2 carbon fragments from the carboxyl end of fatty acylCoA to form Acetyl CoA (AcCoA).
   <u>AcCoA is pivotal in fuel metabolism shown in Figure 2.</u>
6. AcCoA is also formed from pyruvate, stimulated by pyruvate dehydrogenase. Pyruvate is derived from lactate or G6P.
7. G6P is produced from either glycogenolysis or gluconeogenesis (6b) from amino-acids, glycerol and lactic acid.
8. <u>AcCoA</u> normally has 3 outcomes:
   * Oxidation in the TCA cycle (Krebs citric acid cycle) to form ATP.
   * <u>Condensation of 2 molecules to form Acetoacetyl COA.</u>
   * Reconversion into fatty acids for incorporation into triglycerides as VLDL particles.
   Energy from oxidation of AcCoA is obtained from hydrogen atoms (H), H^+ (proton without e^-) and electrons split off from fatty acids and glucose. This is discussed in the chapter on metabolic acidosis.
9. When ADP is unavailable for conversion to ATP two molecules of unutilised AcCoA condense to form one molecule of acetoacetic acid. Acetoacetic acid is reduced to βOH butyric acid and in the process changes NADH to NAD^+ and is also converted to acetone.

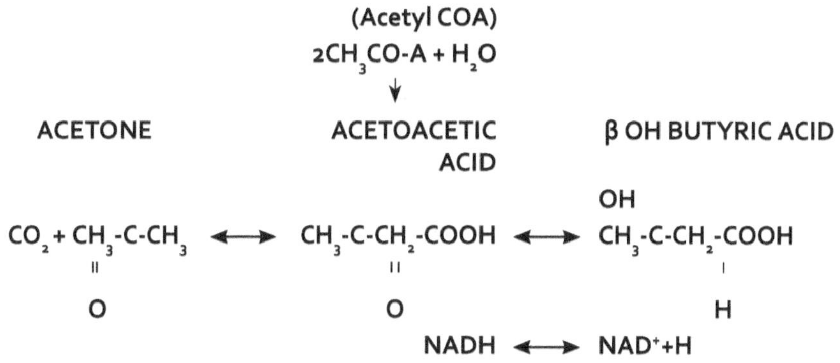

(Acetyl COA)

$2CH_3CO\text{-}A + H_2O$

↓

| ACETONE | ACETOACETIC ACID | β OH BUTYRIC ACID |

OH

$CO_2 + CH_3\text{-}C\text{-}CH_3$ ⟷ $CH_3\text{-}C\text{-}CH_2\text{-}COOH$ ⟷ $CH_3\text{-}C\text{-}CH_2\text{-}COOH$

‖   ‖ |

O   O   H

NADH ⟷ $NAD^+ + H$

GLUCOSE.

During fasting insulin secretion is inhibited and glucagon secretion stimulated. Glucose (G) is synthesised by liver from Glucose 6 phosphate (G-6-P) by the action of G-6-phosphatase.

G-6-phosphatase

G-6-P ⟶ G (glucose)

G-6-P(figure 2) is generated by:

Glycogenolysis (figure 2(7): breakdown of liver glycogen stimulated by glucagon. Muscle glycogen does not contribute because it lacks the enzyme G-6-phosphatase.

Gluconeogenesis– from lactic acid (via pyruvic acid), glycerol and amino-acids. Amino-acids for gluconeogenesis are derived from protein breakdown. Insulin secretion is necessary to inhibit proteolysis. [14]

Following food insulin levels increase and glucose is taken up by liver, muscle, adipose and other tissues. Glucose has three fates:

* Conversion to glycogen in liver and muscle. Insulin increases glucose uptake by tissues, including muscle, by shifting transporters, (GLUT4) from cytosol to cell membranes; stimulates synthesis of protein; and inhibits proteolysis.
* Oxidation to Acetyl-CoA for production of ATP from ADP.
* Conversion to fat in liver, as VLDL particles, and adipose tissue as stored triglyceride.

Muscle glycogen synthesis is the principal method of glucose disposal. [15, 16] Man's capacity to change carbohydrate into fat is limited. During starvation all stored fuels are mobilised: glycogen, aminoacids and fat. [12]

* Muscle decreases utilisation of glucose and increases use of fatty acids. [12]
* Brain increasingly uses ketoacids. [12, 13]
* Following depletion of glycogen stores glucose is synthesised by gluconeogenesis from glycerol, lactate and aminoacids derived from proteolysis. [12]

Pathogenesis of Diabetic Ketoacidosis and Hyperglycaemia. [1-11]

Diabetes is due to relative or absolute deficiency of insulin.

Diabetic ketoacidosis can be regarded as an exaggerated fasted state [2, 11, 17] in which a similar quantity of ketoacids are produced, compared to starvation, but ketones are utilised less well:[17] brain and other tissues fail to utilise ketones [12]; and a reduction of GFR, which decreases excretion of glucose and ketones, leads to rapid increase in ketoacidosis. [17] For diabetic ketoacidosis to develop there must be:

* Increase in lipolysis.
* Increase in fatty acid conversion to ketoacids in liver rather than for synthesis of fat or glucose.

Ketoacidosis is due to both deficiency of insulin and excess glucagon [18]—an increase in the glucagon insulin ratio. [18, 19]

Patients withdrawing from insulin, following pancreatectomy, [20] or those with insulin dependence treated with somatostatin, [21] have delayed development of and decrease in ketoacidosis than would otherwise occur. Insulin suppresses glucagon secretion and in its absence glucagon secretion increases. Insulin inhibits hormone sensitive lipase. Insulin deficiency therefore increases lipolysis and fatty acid delivery to liver.

Glucagon excess increases secretion of hepatic carnitine and decreases malonyl CoA, a crucial intermediate in synthesis of long chain fatty acids. Increase in the glucagon: insulin ratio increases conversion of fatty acids to ketones in liver as in starvation.

Glucose.

Insulin normally inhibits and glucagon stimulates glycogenolysis in liver. Insulin deficiency increases glucose produced by both glycogenolysis and gluconeogenesis and decreases peripheral utilisation of glucose by tissues which use glucose uptake transporters (GLUT) to transport glucose into cells. Insulin normally facilitates glucose entry into cells by mobilising GLUT from the cytosol to cell membranes. However, brain and kidney utilise glucose without insulin, and muscles can partially utilise glucose by non-insulin mediated glucose transport (NIMGU).

Glucagon, catecholamines, cortisol and growth hormone, which are markedly elevated in both diabetic ketoacidosis and Hyperglycaemic Hyperosmolar states, contribute to both ketoacidosis and hyperglycaemia. [2-8] Catecholamines increase both lipolysis and glycogenolysis. Cortisol deficiency attenuates both hyperglycaemia and ketoacidosis. [22,]

IN GENERAL UNSULIN PLAYS THE MAIN ROLE IN MOBILISATION OF FATTY ACIDS WHILE THE GLUCAGON-INSULIN RATIO CONTROLS OXIDATION OF FATTY ACIDS. [5]

DIABETIC KETOACIDOSIS (DKA) AND HYPERGLYCAEMIC HYPEROSMOLAR' NON-KETOCIDOTIC CRISES (HHS).

Acute diabetic crises are usually separated into Diabetic Ketoacidosis and (non-keto acidotic) Hyperglycaemic Hyperosmolar States (HHS).

The difference may be due to secretion of sufficient insulin in HHS to prevent ketoacidosis but insufficient to prevent hyperglycaemia: less insulin is required to inhibit ketoacidosis than to inhibit glycogenolysis and transport glucose into cells. [23, 24-31] De Fronzo et al [23] showed that only one unit of insulin administered per hour was sufficient to inhibit lipolysis but 8 units/ hour were required to inhibit hepatic glucose output. Others have shown that only one tenth as much insulin is required to suppress lipolysis compared to glucose utilisation. [27]

Moreover the amount of insulin secreted depends on severity of hyperglycaemia: the level of serum glucose influences insulin secretion so that residual functioning β cells can increase insulin secretion sufficiently to prevent ketoacidosis during severe hyperglycaemia. [26, 28, 32] Renal function is also important in influencing excretion of glucose and ketones.

Hyperglycaemia, resulting from low GFR, for example from hypovolaemia or pre-existing renal dysfunction, may enhance insulin secretion sufficiently to inhibit lipolysis and ketosis. [26]

Some studies have reported similar serum insulin levels in DKA and HHS on presentation. [33, 34] However portal vein insulin is much higher than in peripheral veins because insulin is degraded on passing through liver. [25, 30, 35] The differential effect of insulin resistance on tissues, such as muscle compared to liver, may also play a role, because insulin resistance is common in non-insulin dependent compared to insulin dependent diabetes. A small, but critical amount of insulin in liver, increases oxidation of fatty acids but is insufficient to inhibit gluconeogenesis and prevent peripheral uptake of glucose. [35]

Chupin et al [29] compared subjects with Diabetic Ketosis (DKA) with subjects with HHS. Although serum insulin was similar at presentation, C-Peptide levels, which escape liver degradation, were over five times higher in HHS. Following recovery both tolbutamide stimulated serum insulin and c-Peptide levels did not increase in subjects with DKA but both showed a clinically significant increase in subjects with the non-ketotic Hyperosmolar state.

This is in keeping with the more potent effect of adequate residual insulin secretion in preventing ketoacidosis and glucagon in causing hyperglycaemia. In one study serum glucose levels correlated with serum glucagon levels whereas ketoacid levels correlated best with serum insulin levels and body mass index. [34]

The correlation between serum glucose, serum insulin (or C-Peptide), fatty and ketoacids is poor in Diabetic ketoacidosis [33, 34]. Various hormones may have a differential effect in modulating glucose and ketoacid metabolism.

Some authors [36, 37] separate diabetic metabolic crises into DKA, HSS and DKA-HHS because of the considerable overlap between DKA and HHS.

DIABETIC KETOACIDOSIS:

Ketoacids.

βOH butyrate usually exceeds the concentration of acetoacetate. Urinary nitroprusside test for ketones reacts with acetoacetate but not with βOH butyrate. Occasionally acetoacetate is sufficiently low, compared to βOH butyrate, that the test is weakly positive or even negative and may lead to misdiagnosis. Plasma acetone is also elevated two or three times more than acetoacetate and remains elevated for longer than βOH butyrate and acetoacetic acid. [7, 38] This may cause persistence of the characteristic breath odour when Diabetic Ketoacidosis resolves.

Peripheral tissues have a limited capacity to metabolise ketoacids generated over a short duration and these progressively increase.

Each mmol of keto acid gives rise to 1mmol H^+. Keto acids are strong acids and are therefore buffered by $NaHCO_3$ in blood.

βOH butyric acid + $NaHCO_3$ ➝ Na butyrate + H_2CO_3 ➝ CO_2 + H_2O.

CO_2 is eliminated by ventilation and decreases the amount of H^+ ions that would otherwise occur but at the cost of lowering serum HCO_3^- and total body buffering capacity.

Keto anions are excreted in 3 ways: [1, 2, 13]

- Initially ketoanions are excreted with cations, predominantly Na^+ and K^+, because NH_4^+ synthesis takes time to develop. This causes hyperchloraemic acidosis because of loss of $NaHCO_3$, which initially buffered keto acids. An alternative explanation, according to the Stewart model, is that loss of Na^+ and K^+, which accompany excreted anions, decreases the strong ion difference (SID).[chapter 6]
- When renal synthesis of NH_4^+ increases in response to acidosis NH_4^+ combines with keto anions and takes the place of and decreases loss of cations. This has a neutral effect on [H^+] (pH).
- When GFR decreases further, to approximately 25-30mL/minute,ketoanions are retained and cause anion gap acidosis.[23] Retention of other unmeasured anions, $H_2Po_4^-$/HPo_4^{2-}, SO_4^{2-}, creatinate and organic acids may accumulate in prerenal failure and also decrease the SID or serum HCO_3^-.

There is, on average, an anion gap acidosis on presentation in which the reduction of serum HCO_3^- is matched by increase in anion gap ($\Delta AG:\Delta HCO_3^-$ = 1:1). [Δ=change] However there is considerable individual variation:

hyperchloraemic acidosis in some patients and anion gap acidosis with varying $\Delta AG \Delta HCO_3^-$ ratios in others. [39]

Hyperchloraemic acidosis often develops or increases on treatment because:

- Volume depletion, which decreases the bicarbonate space, is corrected. [2]
- Anions, which would otherwise be converted to bicarbonate, continue to be excreted with cations.
- Treatment with saline and/or KCL delivers a fluid devoid of HCO_3^- and containing Cl^- in greater amounts than the ratio in plasma- therefore decreasing the SID.
- The anion gap (AG) may also decrease from hypoalbuminemia or alkalosis from vomiting. On the other hand, hyperalbuminemia from haemoconcentration, secondary to hypovolaemia, may increase the anion gap on presentation (2.5mEq per g/L of albumin above normal). This normalises on treatment.
- Ketoanions may move into cells more readily than HCO_3^- in intracellular buffering of H^+. [40] Thus the distribution space of HCO_3^-, keto and lactate anions may vary. [1, 39]

The traditional concept of an anion gap acidosis in DKA, due to an increase in keto anions with an equivalent decrease in HCO_3^-, is not always correct:

There was no correlation between initial serum total CO_2 and plasma anion gap (AG) in DKA, whereas there was a good correlation with severity of prerenal failure. [39] Following treatment hyperchloraemic acidosis developed in the majority of patients because of retention of Cl^- from sodium chloride infusion; and continued excretion of keto anions. The HCO_3^- deficit equaled the increase in AG on average but there was considerable individual variation.

Lactic acid contributes to acidosis if volume depletion becomes sufficiently severe to compromise tissue perfusion.

Hyperglycaemia.

Lack of insulin decreases glucose entry into cells which utilise glucose transporters (GLUT). Muscle is the principal organ of glucose disposal in the formation of glycogen. [15, 16] Insulin is not required for glucose transport into brain, kidney tubules and intestinal mucosa. Increased plasma glucose levels also facilitate transfer of glucose into cells by non insulin mediated pathways and high extracellular glucose levels stimulate insulin secretion in those with residual β cell function.

Hyperglycaemia has two important effects: cellular dehydration [41] and osmotic diuresis causing loss of electrolytes and water. [41, 42]

When the renal threshold for glucose is exceeded glycosuria results. Glycosuria causes an increase in water, sodium and potassium losses in urine [41] depending on the rate of flow of fluid down tubules. [42] Each gram of glucose excreted adds a solute load of $\approx$ 55 mOsmol. Excretion of ketones contributes to osmotic diuresis which may amount to to ½ of the additional osmotic load in diabetic ketosis. [23]

Water exceeds solute losses. In one study urine contained approximately 40-50mmol sodium and 20-30mmol of potassium in each litre of urine containing 300mmol of glucose. In another study losses were approximately 60-75mmol of sodium and 12-35mmol of potassium per litre of urine. [42]

Potassium excretion increases because osmotic diuresis increases Na^+ delivery to distal tubules where it exchanges with K^+. When volume depletion increases glomerular filtration rate (GFR) falls. This decreases urinary glucose losses, increases hyperglycaemia, decreases H^+ and keto anion excretion. The concentration of plasma glucose depends on renal function.

Cellular dehydration.

Hyperglycaemia causes water transfer from cells to extracellular fluid causing cellular dehydration but at the same time increasing extracellular volume and supporting circulatory volume.

Estimated or measured serum osmolality on presentation may not accurately reflect (free) water balance or total body osmolality because extracellular water re-enters cells on resolution of hyperglycaemia following treatment. This has two important potential consequences:

* Rapid reduction of extracellular glucose, without adequate volume repletion, decreases vascular volume. For example an increase in serum glucose to 50mmol/L theoretically increases the extracellular fluid by 1.5L [1] and reduction of serum glucose of 50 mmol/L to normal decreases extracellular fluid by a similar amount. [1]

* More importantly cellular osmolality decreases as serum glucose levels decrease, because water held by glucose reenters cells. Water influx predisposes to swelling of brain cells, which have adapted to cellular hypertonicity, by losing osmoles. Rapid reduction of serum osmolality or extracellular glucose, from use of hypotonic fluids, may predispose to cerebral oedema.

Sodium Depletion.

Loss of sodium in urine not only results from osmotic diuresis but also from excretion of sodium with ketoanions.Sodium loss causes hypovolaemia, hypotension, tachycardia and decrease in GFR.

Osmolality (free water) Disturbances.

Estimated or measured plasma osmolality may be high, normal or rarely low on presentation. Although hyperglycaemia is a poor stimulus, volume depletion stimulates thirst. Thus, in those with access to water and without severe vomiting, clinically significant hypertonicity is rare at presentation, compared to HHS.

Serum sodium may also be normal, low or high on presentation regardless of tonicity. If serum sodium is used as an indication of serum tonicity (not free water status) half serum glucose above normal should be added and hyperlipidaemia taken into account.

Potassium:

Potassium depletion is due to an increase in potassium excretion from osmotic diuresis; K^+ accompanying ketoanion excretion in urine; K^+ lost in exchange for Na^+ in distal tubules, stimulated by hypovolaemia; K^+ loss from glycogenolysis and proteolysis. Potassium depletion may be mild, moderate or severe. Although potassium depletion is usually present the serum potassium is usually normal or even raised on presentation due to the following:

* Hyperchloraemic acidosis. Cells buffer acidosis by exchanging K^+ for H^+ because Cl^- does not readily enter cells. Ketoacidosis does not cause cellular potassium loss (in exchange for H^+) because ketoanions can enter cells with H^+ in buffering [39, 40].
* Insulin deficiency. Insulin keeps K^+ in cells.

* <u>Cellular dehydration</u>: when water is lost from cells, cellular potassium concentration increases. K^+ may accompany water to maintain normal intracellular: extracellular K^+ concentration gradient or accompany water in solvent drag.
* <u>Loss of K^+ from muscle breakdown</u> to provide for gluconeogenesis and from breakdown of glycogen to which K^+ is complexed.
* <u>Cell catabolism.</u>

Magnesium and phosphate deficiency result from increased losses in urine; cell catabolism, which releases both phosphate and magnesium; phosphate losses from glycogenolysis and in excretion of titratable acid. Hypophosphataemia and hypomagnesaemia are rare on presentation but may develop following treatment. The changes resulting from diabetic ketoacidosis, summarised in Figure 4, are as follows.

* <u>Sodium depletion</u>, resulting from osmotic diuresis and excretion of keto anions with sodium, causes interstitial fluid depletion, hypovolemia and renal failure.
* <u>Cellular Dehydration</u> from water transfer out of cells due to hyperglycaemia.
* <u>Plasma tonicity disturbances</u> (estimated or measured) may be high, normal or low. Severe (free) water depletion, however, is rare unless vomiting is present.
* <u>Plasma Na^+</u> however is usually low due to the osmotic effect of glucose in causing trans-cellular movement of water, which dilutes plasma Na^+; or from hypertriglyceridemia.
* <u>Severe metabolic acidosis</u> -anion gap due to ßhydroxybutyric and acetoacetic acid and hyperchloraemic acidosis from urine loss of Na^+ and K^+ with ketoanions.
* <u>Potassium depletion</u> of varying severity but with low, normal or high serum K^+ on presentation.
* <u>Increased urinary magnesium and phosphate losses</u>: hypophosphataemia and hypomagnesaemia usually only develop following treatment but are rarely sufficiently severe to require replacement.
* <u>Increase in serum Triglyceride (VLDL) from liver synthesis.</u> Fatty acids are converted to VLDL by liver. This may increase triglyceride sufficiently to cause lactescence and may cause abdominal pain, rarely pancreatitis, and pseudo-hyponatraemia.

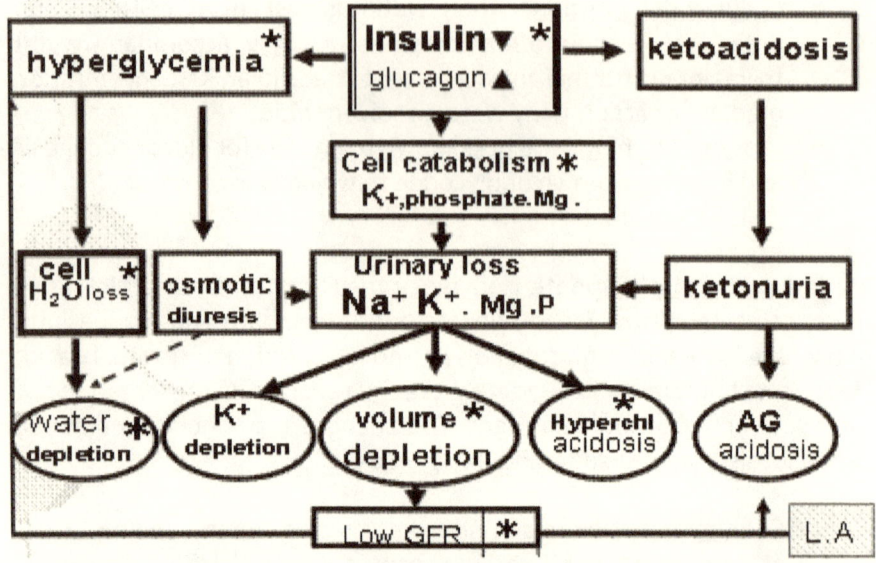

Figure 4: *Changes produced in diabetic ketoacidosis. Renal losses of potassium are offset by cellular efflux of K+ shown by asterisk (*) in the diagram: from insulinopenia, hyperglycaemia, hyperchloraemic acidosis, cellular water depletion, hypovolaemia and cell catabolism. L.A =Lactic acidosis. AG = anion gap. Hyperchl= hyperchloraemic*

QUANTITATIVE DATA.

This is based on few studies on small numbers of selected subjects, mainly carried out over 30 years ago, when patients presented at a later stage than occurs today.

Several texts give average values for electrolyte and water deficiencies in patients presenting with diabetic ketoacidosis. These report water losses of approximately 100mL/kg, [6, 23] Na+ losses of 5-10mmol/Kg, [11, 23] K+ losses of 3-10mmol/kg [1,6,9,11,23] and free water losses of 3L. [1] Some authors suggest that losses of 3L saline and 3L free water occur on average, [23]

Carefully conducted balance studies by Nabarro et al [43] showed a positive balance of 428mmol sodium, 339mmol potassium and 39mmol magnesium per 1.73m² following treatment. The mean deficit in extracellular fluid was 2.9L and free water 1.7 L corrected to 1.73m². De Fronzo reported overall losses of 5-7L water, 300-450mmol Na+ and 200-400mmol K+ based on six studies. [23]

Average values of electrolytes on presentation are more consistent. These are shown in the following table from five studies on DKA.

References	(44)	(37)	(29)	(45)	(9)	
Number	56	171	22	48	-	Average
Serum						
Glucose mmol/L	33.4	28	34.2	39	34	34
Osmolality mOsm/kg/H2o	-	313	323	316	323	319
Total CO_2	8.8	7.9	9.4	7.9	9.4	9.0
Arterial Blood pH	7.17	7.l1	7.12	7.14	7.12	7.10
Na^+ mmol/L	134	-	134	137	134	134
K^+ mmol/L	5.5	-	4.5	5.7	4.5	5.0
Creatine μmol/L	168	-	97.3	-	-	132
Anion Gap	32				29	

Table 1: Results of laboratory tests on presentation of diabetic ketoacidosis from 5 publications (n) = number of cases).

However data on water and electrolyte losses are highly variable and influenced by severity on presentation. Data on an "average" patient is of doubtful usefulness when applied to individual patients who presents with DKA. Moreover variable urinary losses during treatment, which are substantial, confound accurate prediction of fluid and electrolytes required for correction.

Treatment should therefore be guided by response of blood pressure, mental state, urine output, other physiological variables and changes in serum electrolyte levels.

PRINCIPLES ON WHICH MANAGEMENT IS BASED.

Management should be based on personal experience and physiological principles (biological plausibility) because of the absence of randomised trials and few high quality observational studies. The mortality should be close to zero in developed countries. Thus an enormous number of patients would have to be randomised to achieve significant results.

For example the mortality of DKA in Australian and New Zealand hospitals has recently varied between 1.9 and 4.9 %. [37] In one series of 160 consecutive cases only one patient died, of a metabolic cause, due to an error in management. [46] Thus randomised trials are unlikely to have the power to detect differences in outcome from variations in management.

Even expert recommendations show considerable differences on the type of fluid, speed of infusion, potassium, magnesium and phosphate administration. Biological plausibility and observational data suggest the following:

Sodium and Water Depletion.

A reasonable rule of thumb is that losses of saline and free water are approximately 3L each. [11, 23] In patients who are hypotensive or oliguric, however, 4-5L saline may have been lost in addition to free water. However additional losses of sodium occur on treatment from osmotic diuresis and excretion of ketoanions. Saline should be given rapidly in seriously ill patients with hypotension or oliguria until their resolution.

- Rapid correction of circulatory failure is important in prevention of irreversible shock, kidney damage, correction of infection and metabolic abnormalities (chapter 5, part 2).
- Development of irreversible renal failure depends on the duration of pre-renal failure especially in elderly diabetic patients.
- Hypotension predisposes to cardiac infarction, stroke and acute tubular necrosis in older diabetics with narrowed arteries.
- Volume repletion alone, without insulin, decreases serum glucose, arterial blood pH, counter regulatory hormone levels and osmolality appreciably. [23, 47] Overall serum glucose falls by 6-22mmol from the initial level and by over 1mmol/hour from saline infusion alone. [47] Thus priority should be given to volume replacement.
- Rapid correction of hyperglycaemia alone may worsen hypovolaemia by decreasing extracellular volume as water transfers back into cells.

2L saline should be infused rapidly, within 10-30 mins, in seriously ill patients and not for example 1L in one hour followed by 1L in four hours as some advocate. Rapid infusion of saline should continue until <u>hypotension</u> and <u>oliguria</u> resolve.

There is inadequate evidence that colloids are superior to crystalloids. Colloids do not correct interstitial fluid depletion and may worsen it. Hypotonic electrolyte fluids should be avoided in initial therapy because rapid change of osmolality may theoretically cause cerebral oedema, especially in conjunction with decrease in extracellular glucose, which holds water in the extracellular space.

Glucose should be decreased slowly, as it approaches normal levels, because:

* Volume depletion may worsen because glucose holds water in the extracellular space.
* Osmolality may fall too rapidly.
* Glucose receptors may have down regulated and hypoglycaemic symptoms develop at higher serum glucose levels than usual. [32]

Sodium Bicarbonate (Na HCO3) (chapter 6).

This is rarely, if ever, required. Some consultants still advocate its use in extreme acidosis because a further reduction will result in a disproportionate worsening of acidosis if very low bicarbonate is not increased. For example, reduction of serum HCO_3^- from 4.0 to 2.0mmol/L, theoretically doubles $[H^+]$.

$$[H^+] = 24 \, pCO_2 / HCO_3^-$$

However $NaHCO_3$ may : [48-51]

* Transiently increases plasma $[H^+]$.
  $NaHCO_3 + H^+$ keto- anion $\longrightarrow Na^+$ ketoanion $+ H_2CO_3 \longrightarrow CO_2 + H_2O$.
* More importantly CO_2 generated from H_2CO_3 rapidly passes into cells and increases intracellular $[H^+]$ including that in the brain.
* Metabolism of ketoacids is decreased by increase in pH. [48, 50]
* Increase in pH decreases oxygen offloading to tissues.
* $NaHCo_3$ promotes K^+ loss in urine. [13]

However $NaHCo_3$ administration has been advocated if there is a reduced capacity to excrete urinary NH_4^+ because of renal tubular acidosis, very low GFR or decreased capacity to oxidise ketones rapidly. [1] There are concerns that saline infusion increases hyperchloraemic acidosis due to its higher ratio of Cl^-: Na^+ than occurs in plasma [51]—thus increasing the strong ion difference (SID) or decreasing serum bicarbonate. There is no evidence that this is of practical importance. Alternative fluids have other problems, including hypotonicity, which is important if they are infused rapidly.

(Free) Water Depletion.

Some "experts" advocate mathematical calculation to correct serum sodium because osmolality on presentation does not reflect free water balance. There is dissociation between cellular and extracellular water which resolves when glucose normalises: water previously lost from cells to extracellular space moves back into cells, increases serum sodium concentration and restores cellular hydration.

Therefore it has been suggested that a correction factor should be applied to estimate what serum sodium should become following normalisation of elevated glucose—considered to reflect water balance more accurately when hyperglycaemia is present.

Katz [52] suggested that a correction factor of 1.6 mmol should be added to serum Na$^+$ for each 100mg/dL (5.6mmol) increase in serum glucose above normal. This was derived entirely theoretically and based on several unproven assumptions. The assumption that glucose was entirely confined to the extracellular space is flawed because glucose enters cells in brain, heart and 50% of skeletal muscle by non-insulin mediated glucose uptake (NIMGU) and osmotic shifts from hyperglycaemia do not occur in liver. [1]

A correction factor, derived experimentally in healthy volunteers depended on severity of hyperglycaemia [53] and varied between 1.6-2.4mol for each 5.6mmol increase in serum glucose. This may not be relevant in patients with diabetes or hyperglycaemia of longer duration and use of hypotonic saline in the experiment may have distorted results.

Correction factors probably vary considerably from:

- Variations in both severity and duration of hyperglycaemia.
- Variations in glucose transport into different tissues due to differences in non-insulin mediated glucose uptake.
- Estimates of total body water (TBW) and extracellular volume (ECV) based on body weight which is inaccurate, [54] especially when based on weight on presentation.
- Considerable variations of urinary solute output during treatment which changes serum Na$^+$ independently of the correction factor.
- The extent of adaption of brain to hypertonicity is difficult to predict and depends on serum sodium rather than severity of hyperglycaemia [55]. Brain is relatively permeable to both urea and

glucose [56].Gradual development of hyperglycaemia may allow brain to adapt to hyperosmolality by losing osmoles. Sudden deterioration or lack of water intake may then raise serum sodium further. Mental changes correlate with serum sodium but not serum glucose levels. On presentation normal or raised serum sodium rather than hyperglycaemia implies that severe cellular dehydration is present. [55]

- The extent of potassium depletion: total body osmolality is due to both potassium and sodium.
  Osmolality = 2(Na$_e^+$ + K$_e^+$) / TBW (e = exchangeable). [57]
  Thus variations in extent of potassium depletion and correction of potassium depletion, which increases sodium efflux from cells, influences water balance appreciably.

Regardless of the above, water deficiency should be corrected slowly, but should not influence the speed of correction of hypovolaemia with isotonic saline. The early use of hypotonic fluids or rapid correction of serum glucose is potentially harmful.

In conclusion using correction factors lacks reliability, is of questionable relevance and has not been shown to change management.

Potassium.

Hypokalaemia was a common cause of death in the past. [58, 59] Average potassium losses were reported to vary between 3-10 mmol/kg [1, 2, 6,11,] or 200-400mmol in total. [23] Two balance studies showed losses of 89-190mmol [58] and 339mmol. [43] However this does not take ongoing urinary losses on treatment, which may amount to 20-50% of administered potassium, into account. Although K$^+$ losses of 89-190 mmol occurred in the study by Soler et al [58] 225-343 mmol were required to correct serum K$^+$ levels. [58] Biegelman [60] infused up to 620mmol (Mean 170 mmol) to maintain a normal serum K$^+$ level.

Serum K$^+$ is normal or raised in the majority of patients with DKA on presentation despite presence of potassium depletion: In 340 consecutive episodes only 4% were hypokalaemic. [60] The severity of metabolic acidosis is the main determinant of the magnitude of hyperkalaemia on admission [61] despite the absence of an effect of ketoacids in transferring K$^+$ out of cells. [40] The severity of ketoacidosis may however be a marker for severe cellular catabolism. Potassium decreases to its lowest level within 1-2 hours of treatment. [60] This is due to:

- Insulin which transfers K$^+$ into cells.
- Correction of hypovolaemia which dilutes concentration of plasma electrolytes.
- Decrease in extracellular osmolality which moves K$^+$ into cells.
- Formation of glycogen which requires potassium and phosphate for phosphorylation of glucose intermediates.
- Correction of hyperchloraemic acidosis.
- Marked ongoing urinary losses of potassium—20-50% of K$^+$ administered when glomerular filtration rate improves. [58]

Apart from serum K$^+$ on presentation, the amount of insulin [23] and bicarbonate [60, 61] administered correlate with the decrease of serum potassium. Although insulin infusion of only 1-2u/hour is sufficient to inhibit hepatic glucose output serum potassium decreases further from increasing insulin infusion. [23]

Very large losses of potassium are present when serum is low on admission. [62-66] Intravenous administration of 300 to over 700mmol (Mean 466) of potassium, in addition to oral potassium, were required over 24 hours in patients with hypokalaemia on admission, some of whom remained hypokalaemic. [62-66]

Several deaths or respiratory paralysis occurred from DKA in the past when insufficient potassium was given, often exacerbated by bicarbonate administration and high dose insulin administration. [62-73]

Thus it is vital to give potassium early to patients with low serum K$^+$ on admission. However deficiencies of K$^+$ are probably less compared to the past because patients usually present at an earlier stage.

When serum K$^+$ is raised potassium should usually not be given until urine output is adequate. I have found the following rule of thumb useful for K$^+$correction—discussed further in chapter 7.

Serum K+ High: o-mild K$^+$depletion is present.
No potassium is infused initially until urine output is >30 mL/hour.

Serum K+ normal: Mild to moderate K$^+$depletion is present.
Anticipate early hypokalaemia and add K$^+$20mmol to normal saline or 40-60mmol

to half strength saline following the first 1-2 litres of normal saline.

Initial Serum K+ low.   Severe potassium depletion is present. Add 20-40mmol K$^+$ to initial saline depending on the rate of infusion. Subsequently 60-80mmol/L potassium should be added to each litre of ½ n.Saline or 5% dextrose water depending on estimation of sodium status.

There are two further important factors in potassium administration: K$^+$ chloride added to normal saline results in a hypertonic fluid.

For example 20mmol KCL + 150mmol NaCl = 340mosm/kg H$_2$o. Na$^+$ will leave cells in exchange for K$^+$. Giving potassium contributes to correction of sodium deficiency. Indeed until potassium is excreted potassium contributes to osmolality to the same extent as sodium. Thus adding 70mmol KCL to one litre 5% glucose water provides a near half isotonic fluid and added to half strength saline an isotonic fluid. Serum K$^+$ should be remeasured frequently because of marked variations in the factors listed above.

Phosphate and Magnesium:

Hyperphosphataemia is present in the majority of patients with diabetic ketoacidosis before treatment—in one study 3.0mmol/L, on average, but normalises within 12 hours of treatment [74]. Hyperphosphataemia correlates with severity of hyperglycaemia, osmolality and acidosis.

Hypophosphataemia may develop at a later stage of treatment [11, 75] from action of insulin in phosphorylating glucose intermediates; [75] reversal of acidosis (which caused phosphaturia) and cellular repair, which requires phosphate—the main intracellular anion. However the majority of trials have failed to show benefit from routine use of phosphate replacement. [6, 23, 75] A randomised study of phosphate therapy in Diabetic Ketoacidosis failed to show benefit. [76] However serum phosphate should be measured if deterioration occurs and very low serum phosphate levels(<0.3mmol/L) should be treated.[11]

Hypomagnesaemia may also occur in the later stages of treatment but severe hypomagnesaemia is uncommon and rarely requires treatment.

In conclusion phosphate and magnesium uncommonly require treatment. The clinical importance of phosphate depletion has not been established satisfactorily.

Insulin-Glucose.

Continuous "low dose" insulin at 5-10 IU/hour, [77] following a bolus of 0.1μ/kg, is now established for treatment of DKA, although some consider that a bolus is unnecessary. However "low dose" insulin is a misnomer, as pointed out by De Fronzo et al: [23] a bolus initially results in a serum insulin level of ~2000μU/ml [78], but has a very short half life. Continuous insulin, given at 5 units/hour, results in serum insulin levels of approximately 100 μU/mL. [79] The table below, modified from De Fronzo et al [79], shows the serum insulin levels at various rates of insulin administration and the glucose infused to keep serum glucose constant in an insulin clamp experiment.

Insulin U/ hour	Serum Insulin. μU/mL	Glucose g/hour	Inhibition of Lipolysis %
1	20	13	100
2	40	21	100
4	80	34	100
8	160	50	100
16	320	50	100
40	1000	50	100

Table 2: *Insulin administration, serum insulin levels and glucose needed to keep serum glucose constant during an insulin clamp study.* Modified from De Fronzo et al. [79]

Table (2) illustrates several important points:

- Increasing insulin infusion above 8 units/hour has no effect on glucose disposal: the dose of glucose administered remains the same.
- Insulin infusion, as low as 1U/hour, completely inhibits lipolysis.
- However increasing insulin progressively decreases serum potassium up to a level of 500μU/mL. Thus high dose insulin increases hypokalaemia. [79]

DKA has been effectively treated by hourly doses of intramuscular insulin. [80] Comparison of intravenous, subcutaneous and intramuscular insulin showed no difference in the rate of decline of plasma glucose or ketones after the first two hours. [81] In a randomised study Lispro insulin, given by subcutaneous injection, (0.3μ/kg) followed by 0.1μ/kg/hour, resulted in similar biochemical and clinical outcomes and length of stay compared to intravenous insulin given in an Intensive Care Unit. [82] However subcutaneous insulin may take 90-120 minutes to be fully effective [23] and is less effective if injected into fat, which commonly occurs, rather than muscle. [83, 84]

Duration of Insulin-Glucose Therapy.

It is essential that insulin is not discontinued when serum glucose levels, urine output and overall status improve. Plasma glucose decreases predictably by 4-8mmol/hour although this may be less during infection. [11, 23]

When serum glucose reaches 12-15mmol/L the rate of decline should be slowed by decreasing the rate of insulin or increasing the amount of glucose administered: 5% dextrose water can be changed to 10% dextrose water. [23] This is important because:

* Continuing ketone metabolism requires insulin and therefore glucose.
* Glycogen stores require repletion.
* Gluconeogenesis must be inhibited and reformation of protein promoted.
* Rapid decrease in serum glucose predisposes to cerebral oedema, secondary to a decrease in tonicity.
* Hypoglycaemic symptoms may occur at higher serum glucose levels—as high as 6.2mmol/L, probably because of down regulation of glucose receptors. [32]

Plasma glucose declines at an average of 5mmol/L (4-8mmol/L) per hour, regardless of the insulin dose and reaches 15-16mmol in 4-6 hours. [11, 23] When serum glucose reaches approximately 15-16mmol/L further rapid decrease should be prevented by giving 5-10% glucose. 1L of 10 % glucose given in 2 hours should prevent a further decrease in serum glucose because, 50gm glucose, on average, can be metabolised per hour. [23] (Table 3).

DIAGNOSIS

This is based on clinical manifestations and biochemical results.

Clinical manifestations:

- Signs of extracellular volume depletion, hypotension, tachycardia, thirst, decreased skin turgor.
- Hyperventilation due to acidosis—regular deep respirations (Kussmaul).
- Acetone odour.
- Visual blurring due to hyperglycaemia.
- Weight loss, depending on duration, extent of fluid and tissue loss.
- Nausea, vomiting and abdominal pain. Up to 25% of patients with vomiting show positive occult blood on testing. Rarely severe gastric dilatation due to gastroparesis occurs. The plasma lipase and amylase (usually salivary source) are commonly increased, but pancreatitis is uncommon.
- Hepatomegaly, due to fatty liver, may be present.
- Semicoma or confusion are rare but serious and correlate with serum sodium or tonicity rather than acidosis. [85]

Serum shows the following:

- Plasma glucose varies considerably from 12-50mmol/L.
- Total CO_2 varies from <5 to20 mmol/L. Arterial blood pH varies from 6.8-7.3; [H^+] 160-50 nmol/L.
- Anion gap is usually but not always present.
- Plasma Na^+ may be low, normal or high. Marked elevation of serum triglyceride may cause spuriously low plasma sodium.
- Serum K^+ may be high, normal or low.
- Effective plasma osmolality (tonicity) may be normal, low or high but does not accurately reflect cellular osmolality or water balance.
- Plasma β hydroxybutyrate exceeds acetoacetate levels and occasionally results in a negative test for ketones because ketostix or acetest react with acetoacetate, but not ßOHbutyrate. [86, 87]
- Urea-creatinine ratio is increased from volume depletion.
- Serum creatinine may be spuriously elevated because of interference in measurement by ketoacids. [88]
- Plasma triglyceride may be markedly elevated and can cause plasma lactescence. Serum transaminases (ALT, AST) may be elevated. [23]

The following are important:

- Some patients, especially pregnant women, have severe ketoacidosis but near normal plasma glucose—Euglycaemic ketoacidosis. [89]
- Urine may test negative for ketones if β OH butyrate, which does not react, is the only ketone present. This is especially common when the redox state (NADH>NAD⁺) increases acetoacetic acid conversion to βOH butyrate as in lactic acidosis from shock. Paradoxically ketonuria may increase following improvement: increasing urine ketone levels are not a sign of deterioration.
- Starving patients, or those with alcoholic ketoacidosis, may show ketonuria and hyperglycaemia following infusion of 5% Dextrose water and be misdiagnosed as Diabetic Ketoacidosis.
- The combination of euglycaemia and negative urine test for ketones may cause misdiagnosis.
- Hypoglycaemic coma is rarely a diagnostic problem but rebound hyperglycaemia may follow a syncopal event or confusion in a hypoglycaemic patient.
- Poisons, especially salicylate and isopropyl alcohol, cause anion gap metabolic acidosis and ketonuria.
- Severe mental dysfunction, in the absence of serum hypertonicity or hypernatraemia, should alert to a diagnosis other than Diabetic Ketoacidosis.
- Abdominal pain and elevation of serum amylase or lipase may be misdiagnosed as Acute Pancreatitis.
- Fever is often absent in infection and marked neutrophilia is an expected finding. Thus infection may be overlooked. High CRP is a useful alert to infection.

MANAGEMENT OF DIABETIC KETOACIDOSIS SHOULD BE ORGANISED IN 4 STAGES AND BE KEPT SIMPLE:

1. Immediate management and Assessment.
2. Rapid restoration of volume with saline and initiation of insulin.
3. Slower correction of glucose with insulin, correction of glycogen and potassium depletion. Once hypotension and oliguria resolve potassium, concentration 20-70mmol/L depending on plasma K^+, can be added to 5% dextrose water or 0.45% saline in dextrose water, if sodium depletion is present. A lower dose is added in earlier if hypokalaemia develops.
4. Introduction of rapid acting insulin, before or with meals, with continuous insulin for basal purposes.

   If improvement is sufficient and vomiting absent change to the insulin regime the patient normally uses. The majority of patients should be off intravenous fluid and insulin within 12-24 hours.

First stage: Immediate Management and assessment

- In seriously ill patients establish a large bore IV line, ensure the airway is adequate, and determine SO_2 (saturation oxygen) on room air. Give oxygen if desaturation is present and exclude gastric dilatation.
- Take blood for electrolytes, creatinine, and total CO_2 and in seriously ill patients' arterial blood gas and blood cultures. Arterial blood gas sampling is uncommonly indicated, contrary to some recommendations: In a recent study arterial blood gas determinations in an emergency department did not influence management. [90]
- Start saline or other isotonic electrolyte solution and give as rapidly as possible (1L in 10-15 minutes).
- Ensure gastric dilatation is absent. If present pass a nasogastric tube.

Assessment

- Assess volume status and electrolytes

Shock or supine hypotension:	3-6L saline deficit $\propto$ size and sex
Postural Tachycardia > 100	
BP < 100 systolic on standing:	3-5L deficit $\propto$ size and sex
No postural hypotension or	
Tachycardia:	1-3L saline deficit

There is on average a deficit of 2-5L of saline and 2-3L free water. It is essential to vary initial therapy on the basis of body size or ideal body weight and gender. Females and the elderly have on average less TBW and extracellular water than do young males.

It is important that sepsis may contribute to effective hypovolaemia.

- Correct plasma Na^+ to indicate plasma osmolality:
  Corrected plasma Na^+ = 2 x Na^+ + 10 + Glucose above 5mmol/L. If corrected plasma Na> 145mmol/L there is severe free water deficit.
- Assess K^+ Status on presentation:
  Plasma K   >5.5mmol minimal depletion is likely
                    3.5-5.0mmol mild to moderate depletion is likely
                    <3.5mmol severe depletion is likely. Severe hypokalaemia will occur on treatment with low K^+ containing fluids.

Generally potassium should not be given on presentation. The need to give K^+ early however is suggested by the initial plasma K^+. If serum potassium is low 20mmol KCL should be added to the first or second litre of saline infused.

Remember that KCL added to n.Saline is a hypertonic fluid: rapid infusion in 10 minutes to ½ hour may cause an excessive increase in serum osmolality.

Calculate the Anion Gap (normal anion gap = 12):

Na – (Cl + HCO_3 + 12) = Ketones ± Lactic Acid—approximately.

Making allowances for albumin, phosphate, K^+, Mg^{2+}, Ca^{2+} improves the usefulness of the anion gap—especially albumin. However calculation of the anion gap rarely, if ever, changes management.

- Blood gas measurement can often be avoided by using total CO_2 on venous blood and oximetry to assess saturation of oxygen.

Establish the cause of Deterioration of Diabetic Control

This may be due to:

- Failure to take insulin because of vomiting, illness, psychological problems or alcohol.
- Increased need for insulin because of infection, myocardial infarction, stroke, trauma, intoxication or other disease.
- New diabetic or deterioration of the capacity to secrete insulin in Type II, previously non insulin requiring diabetic.

Second stage of Management

- Correct hypovolaemia rapidly. Isotonic electrolyte fluid such as saline should be given rapidly—in an average adult male 2L within 1 hour or until urine output is $\geq$ 50mls/hour. Once this occurs volume replacement can be slowed.
- Give rapid acting insulin intravenously, 5-6 units/hour, via a side arm—preferably controlled by a pump. Administration of a bolus (7-10 units) is controversial.

Third Stage of Management

Once urine output is satisfactory and plasma glucose levels decrease to 15–17mmol/L slowly correct free water deficit if present; replete glycogen stores with glucose; promote metabolism of keto-acids; and replace potassium. Continuing therapy with glucose and insulin is essential to metabolise ketones and regenerate bicarbonate.

There are several important points:

Serum hypotonicity or hypertonicity should be corrected slowly to avoid risk of cerebral oedema and osmotic demyelination.

When plasma glucose reaches 15-17mmol/L further reduction should be slowed. 1L 10% glucose water given over 2-4 hours should prevent further reduction of serum glucose [23] but usually must contain K^+ at a minimum concentration of 40 mmol/L if hypokalaemia is present. Hyperglycaemia contributes to osmolality.

When potassium is given for hypokalaemia most of the amount administered initially exchanges with cellular Na^+ and thus contributes to sodium correction. Indeed if all K^+ given were retained it would increase osmolality and or volume to the same extent as the same amount of Na^+ because total Body Osmolality is approximately $Na_e^+ + K_e^+ / TBW$.

Potassium replacement. (see Potassium Section).

Remember <u>considerable urine K^+ losses (20-50% of that administered) occurs during treatment.</u>

KCL is given in proportion to serum K^+: usually 20-70mmol per litre in either 5% dextrose water (DW) or ½ strength normal saline depending on the need for sodium replacement. Occasionally larger amounts are needed but venous pain increases as the concentration rises above 60mmol/L. Additional K+ can be given orally if vomiting is absent. If serum K^+ is <3.0mmol/L the minimum concentration of potassium in 5% DW should be 60mmol/L (see chapter on potassium).

Glucose solutions containing potassium, with or without sodium, (1L every 6-8 hours) should continue until vomiting is absent, plasma bicarbonate improves and feeding resumed.

Consider measuring plasma phosphate and magnesium during the later stages of hydration and especially when plasma K^+ becomes normal.

Phosphate occasionally needs replacement. If the plasma level is <u><0.3-0.5mmol/L</u> 10.0mmol potassium phosphate can be given in 4-6 hours (chapter 9).

Magnesium depletion can be corrected by infusing 10-20mmol of $MgSO_4$ in 5% DW (compatible with KCL) or half normal saline in dextrose water and infused over 12-24 hours. A single bolus is ineffective in replacement (see chapter on Magnesium). However magnesium, phosphate and calcium can be given orally as milk or oral preparations (chapters 8,9).

Note: *Fluid composition given at this stage depends on assessment of the need for further sodium replacement; potassium replacement; whether the decline of serum glucose should be slowed; and the amount of saline given previously.*

Once urine output and blood pressure are satisfactory potassium can be infused in 5 or 10% dextrose water slowly to prevent a rapid decrease in serum osmolality. If significant sodium depletion is considered to be present half strength n.Saline should be given with added potassium. For example 1L of half strength saline with 60mmol KCL added will provide a near isotonic electrolyte solution of 135mmol/L (combined $Na^+ + K^+$). This will contribute to the correction of sodium depletion, potassium depletion and change serum osmolality slowly.

Initial goals in management are:

- Urine output >50mls/hour
- Improvement in plasma HCO_3^- (total CO_2) or SID reflecting elimination of keto-acids.
- Slow change of hyper-osmolality or hypo-osmolality—if present.
- Avoidance of oxygen desaturation and arrhythmias.

Plasma glucose decreases by 4-8mmol/L per hour. Urinary ketones may remain positive for a considerable time and urine nitroprusside test may become more positive because of conversion of βOH butyrate to acetoacetate as the redox state improves. Serum bicarbonate may take a long time to normalise, despite clinical and metabolic improvement, especially if saline and KCl are given in treatment (Excess Cl^- compared to cations $Na^+ + K^+$). There is delay in excretion of chloride compared to metabolism of ketones. Acetone may also take 48 hours to be metabolised and the characteristic fruity odour may persist. [38]

If deterioration or confusion occurs:

- Measure arterial blood pH, pCO_2, HCO_3^-, pO_2.
- Remeasure plasma glucose—exclude (relative) hypoglycaemia.
- Remeasure serum electrolytes and creatinine to exclude hyponatraemia, hypokalaemia and renal failure.
- Measure plasma phosphate, magnesium and calcium.
- Repeat ECG for ischaemia, infarct or arrhythmia.
- Check SO_2 to rule out pulmonary oedema, pneumonia or aspiration.
- Reconsider if infection is present or antibiotics used are appropriate. Measure serum CRP(C-reactive protein)
- Consider whether cerebral oedema or osmotic demyelination is present.

Note: An increase in the urine ketotest should not cause concern but serum bicarbonate should increase.

Cerebral oedema. [91-103]

Cerebral oedema is a rare but serious problem which has been recognised for over 40 years. The cause has not been established but may be due to rapid change in osmolality from use of hypotonic fluids or rapid reduction of plasma glucose to normal.

It more commonly occurs in children who are recovering from Diabetic Ketoacidosis [91, 92] may occur suddenly without warning, [93, 94] and is the most common cause of death. [91, 92] Subclinical brain swelling, based on sequential CT scans, occur in children recovering from Diabetic Ketoacidosis. [94] Osmotic disequilibrium due to rapid correction of hyperglycaemia or excessive administration of hypotonic fluids is an accepted cause. [95-97] In one study using computed tomography the progression of brain oedema correlated with the rapidity of decrease in effective osmolality. [98]

There are many other theoretical causes: excessive use of crystaloid fluid which may decrease oncotic pressure [99]; impaired brain autoregulation; [100] increase in activity of Na: K^+ pumps in cells- perhaps activated by insulin; [101] bicarbonate use; [7] or respiratory alkalosis. [102] Mannitol may be effective in treatment. [92, 97]

The best evidence, and most plausible cause, is rapid decrease of osmolality from rapid correction of hyperglycaemia or early use of hypotonic fluids. Brain cells in animal models normalise brain water within four hours of severe hyperglycaemia, [96] either by transferring osmoles out of cells or because brain cells are permeable to glucose. Sudden decrease in osmolality cause adapted brain cells to develop oedema. The implications are that hyperosmolality and hyperglycaemia should be corrected slowly (chapter 4).

Fourth Stage of Treatment—Refeeding

Feeding should be started when urine output is satisfactory, an overall improvement has occurred and vomiting is absent.

Give subcutaneous rapid acting insulin before each main meal—either before or during eating. This can be given immediately before or after meals, if vomiting is a risk, using a rapid acing insulin analogue such as Lispro insulin. Subcutaneous insulin takes 1-2 hours to be fully effective, although newer analogues act more rapidly. Therefore overlap intravenous insulin with the initiation of subcutaneous insulin. [23]

Continue intravenous glucose with insulin via a side arm with instructions to increase or decrease by 1 unit/hour to maintain plasma glucose between

8-12mmol/L. Continuous basal infusion also ensures adequate basal insulin levels overnight.

Once normal feeding is established the patient's usual insulin regime can be implemented.

Alternatively, or for new diabetics, order rapid acting insulin before each main meal and intermediate or long acting insulin before sleep at night and fine tune the insulin dose based on capillary glucose levels.

HYPERGLYCAEMIC HYPEROSMOLAR STATE (HHS) [7, 9, 37,104-112]

HHS is the opposite end of a spectrum from DKA, distinguished by absence of (or minimal) ketoacidosis, despite severe hyperglycaemia and hyperosmolality.

In reality a considerable overlap occurs [8, 9, 23, 37,104-109] with different degrees of ketoacidosis and osmolar disturbances to the point that some divide patients into DKA, HHS and mixed DKA-HSS. [9, 37]

The most likely reason for absence of ketoacidosis, despite severe hyperglycaemia, is secretion of sufficient insulin to prevent ketosis but insufficient to inhibit glycogenolysis and facilitate peripheral glucose uptake—especially in muscle. Severe hyperglycaemia causes the following:

- Loss of water from cells to extracellular fluid in response to increase in extracellular osmolality from glucose. This expands extracellular volume (EVC) at the expense of the intracellular volume and causes.
- Hyponatraemia without extracellular hypotonicity, cellular dehydration and hypertonicity.
- Osmotic diuresis occurs when glucose exceeds the renal threshold for reabsorption.
- This leads to loss of free water, sodium, approximately 30-50mmol/L, potassium, 20-30mmol/L, and lesser amounts of phosphate and magnesium. Urine potassium losses are due to K^+ exchange with Na^+ from an increase in sodium delivery to distal nephrons, and stimulation of aldosterone secretion secondary to hypovolaemia; glycogenolysis; and proteolysis which liberate potassium.
- Increasing sodium depletion causes hypovolaemia and decreases GFR.

- Decrease in GFR decreases glycosuria which increases serum glucose.
- Hypokalaemia is uncommon, despite potassium depletion from urinary loss, because of hyperosmolality and cell catabolism. However residual insulin secretion facilitates cellular potassium uptake.
- Hypertonicity increases as a result of hyperglycaemia, urinary loss of free water (greater than solute) and in some cases failure to drink fluids: hyperosmolality from hyperglycaemia is a poor stimulus to thirst.
- Brain cells adapt to hypertonicity by generating osmoles to prevent loss of cellular volume (shrinking).
- Despite this, increasing tonicity causes confusion and clouding of consciousness.
- Confusion and clouding of consciousness may decrease water intake.

There are two important implications for treatment from the events outlined:

* Sudden decrease in osmolality, either from a rapid reduction in hyperglycaemia or from rapid infusion of hypotonic fluids, predisposes to cerebral oedema, especially if brain cells have adapted to hypertonicity, by generating osmoles.
* Sudden decrease in hyperglycaemia results in transfer of extracellular water back into cells which may worsen hypovolaemia.

For example consider a 72kg man with total body water (TBW) of 43L (28L intracellular water, 15L ECW and plasma sodium of 140mol/L:

Estimated effective osmolality = approximately 290mOsm/kg H_2O (140 x 2 + 10).

Theoretically rapid infusion of 1000mmol glucose increases serum glucose from 5 to ~71mmol/L (1000÷15(ECV) = approximately 66mmol/L.

Total body osmoles increase from 12,500 to 13,500mOsm.

New osmolality =13,500÷43 (TBW).) = 314mOsm/kg/water

The total extracellular solute increases to (290x15) +1000 = 5350mOsm/ kgH_2O assuming 1000mmol glucose is initially confined to the extracellular volume (ECV):

Therefore ECV increases to $(5350 \div 314mOsm/kgH_2o) = 17L$; an increase of 2L.

If glucose normalises 2 L returns to intracellular fluid and decreases ECV by 2L.

CLINICAL MANIFESTATIONS. [4, 7-9, 37,104-106,108-112]

Patients are older [4, 37,104-111] than those with DKA; either have known maturity onset diabetes without previous ketosis [108] or are previously undiagnosed. [111]

Comorbidity is much higher. Onset is insidious and duration longer before presentation [4, 7-9,106,108-112] because of absence of severe ketosis. Patients present with unresponsiveness, abnormal behaviour, delirium, inability to cope, manifestations of the precipitating illness, or seizures.

Polyuria, polydipsia, severe fatigue, somnolence and symptoms of the provoking illness are followed by increasing confusion, clouding of consciousness, coma and seizures. Coma, however, occurs in a minority [9,106] and some have no cerebral symptoms on presentation. [113] Cerebral symptoms correlate with serum sodium rather than serum glucose levels or estimated osmolality. [105,113]

Patients may be asymptomatic, despite serum glucose levels between 45-92mmol/L, provided hyponatraemia is present. [7,113] Serum osmolality <340mOsm/kgH2o in the presence of coma should suggest another diagnosis.

Focal neurological signs such as hemiparesis may also occur. Thirst is sometimes surprisingly absent. [103] perhaps because glucose stimulates thirst less than sodium. A decrease in access to fluids may predispose to water depletion.

The majority have a precipitating illness: [1, 3, 7-9, 105, 108-110] Infection is the most common, [7,104,106,108-110] but myocardial infarction, stroke, use of diabetogenic drugs, renal failure and excessive carbohydrate consumption are responsible for some cases. HHS may rarely occur in patients with burns or sepsis, without diabetes, who are given large quantities of intravenous glucose or carbohydrate.

Risk factors for HHS are age, dementia, nursing home residence, absent history of diabetes, infection, [112] and decrease in intake of water from dementia. [105] Diabetogenic drugs, [105,106,109] associated with HHS, are corticosteroids, thiazide diuretics and phenytoin.

Physical Findings.

Volume depletion and manifestations of hypertonicity are more severe at presentation than occurs in DKA because of the longer duration of polyuria; more severe hyperglycaemia causing osmotic diuresis; and inadequate intake of fluids. Ketoacidosis is usually absent and mild if present.

Supine tachycardia and hypotension suggest that severe hypovolaemia is present because free water depletion alone is rarely sufficiently severe to cause these signs. However these signs may be due to a precipitating illness such as severe infection or myocardial infarction.

Skin inelasticity and enophthalmos are often present but have poor specificity and predictive value. Hyperventilation and acetone odour of the breath are usually absent. [8] Mental changes, and occasionally focal neurological signs are commonly present.

Laboratory Manifestations:

Biochemical manifestations are highly variable. [104,105] Serum osmolality, sodium, glucose, bicarbonate and the arterial blood pH are higher than occurs in DKA and serum potassium usually lower. (Table 2).Renal function is worse than occurs in DKA and the urea: creatinine ratio increased due to severe volume deletion. The table below shows the results from six studies and compares this to results from Table 1 on DKA.

Reference	37	112	105	29	106	104	HSS Mean	DKA Mean
Glucose mmol/L	54	41	65	52	54	61	54.5	34
Osmolality mOsm/kg/H_2O	370	380	384	380	373	353	373	319
Sodium mmol/L	-	153	144	149	142	141	146	134
TOTAL CO_2 mmol/L	24	-	17	-	22		21	9
Arterial blood pH units	7.39	7.4	7.26	7.30	7.39		7.33	7.10
Serum Potassium mmol/L	-	4.8	5.0	3.9	3.0		4.2	5.0
Serum Creatinine µmol/L			477	124			300	97

Table 3: Biochemical results from six series on HSS contrasted with five series of DKA from Table 1. [9, 29, 37, 44, 45]

Haematocrit and haemoglobin are raised. Serum free fatty acids (FFA) [105] and 3 ß hydroxybutyrate are both lower. In the review by Kitabchi et al [7] concentration of ßhydroxybutyrate was 1.0mmol/L compared to 9.1mmol/L in DKA. Insulin levels have been reported to be similar in some studies but lower in DKA in others. [105,106] C-Peptide levels are several fold higher in HHS compared to DKA. [29] Serum glucagon levels are increased in both DKA and HSS. Arterial blood lactate is sometimes elevated above 5.0mmol/L. There are few quantitative data on water, sodium and potassium losses. The average fluid deficit has been reported to be approximately 9L: 3.1L extracellular and 5.1L intracellular fluid. [109,110] Arieff and Carol [105] measured the loss of plasma volume on presentation in six cases: this was approximately 3L. Sodium losses in 33 cases were approximately 500 mmol, potassium 300-1000mmol and water 100-200mL per kg.

Mortality is much higher than for DKA; [7,36,104,106,] varies from 10-33%; but is often due to the underlying illness, [7,37,104,106,] especially infection. Mortality is also related to the severity of hypertonicity [37] and comorbidity.

Complications include rhabdomyolysis; [4,111,114] vascular thrombosis, probably due to volume depletion; coexistent infection; and increase in serum viscosity. [4,111] Adult respiratory distress syndrome is rare. [9] Surprisingly cerebral oedema has been reported rarely [110] but rapid change in osmolality should be avoided. [108] Osmotic demyelination rarely follows treatment.

TREATMENT.

There is controversy about the composition of fluid which should be used and other recommendations for treatment. However the majority of reports stress the need for initial isotonic saline if hypovolaemia is severe. Shock may follow use of hypotonic fluids. [108] Large volumes of fluid have often been administered, for example 11.9L and 8.2L in the acute phase.

I believe that treatment should be organised in four stages, as for DKA.

Stage 1: Immediate treatment—similar to DKA previously outlined.

Stage 2: Rapid correction of hypotension and oliguria with isotonic saline; and initiation of low dose insulin until urine output and blood pressure normalise.

Stage 3: Slow correction of both glucose and serum sodium to avoid rapid change in osmolality. Rapid increase in serum osmolality may cause osmotic demyelination. Once urine output increases potassium should be included. Serum glucose should be corrected slowly to avoid rapid decrease in ECV and cerebral oedema.

Stage 4: Commence feeding, ensuring that swallowing is adequate, and use oral drugs or insulin as appropriate.

If deterioration or failure to improve occurs:

- Measure or remeasure arterial blood pH, pCO_2, HCo_3^- and pO_2.
- Repeat glucose, electrolyte measurements (± osmolality).
- Measure serum phosphate, calcium and magnesium.
- Order an ECG.
- Ensure urine output and serum total CO_2 are satisfactory.
- Most importantly strongly consider whether infection is present, antibiotics are appropriate or other underlying illness is present.

REFERENCES

1. Ketoacidosis p89-99 in Fluid, Electrolyte and Acid-base physiology. A problem-based approach. Ed. Halperin, ML; Goldstein, MB.Third edition 1999

2. Shafiee MA, Kamel KS, Halperin ML. A conceptual Approach to the patient with Metabolic Acidosis. Application to a patient with Diabetic Ketoacidosis. *Nephron.* 2002, 92(Suppl 1):46-55.

3. Ruderman NNB; Myers MG; Chipkin SR; Tornheim K: Hormone-Fuel Interrelationships: Fed State, starvation and diabetes mellitus in Joslins diabetes mellitus. 14th Edition.2005. Eds. Kahn, CR; Weir, GC; King, GL; Jacobson, AM; Smith, RJ. Lippincott, Williams and Wilkins.

4. Krentz AJ, Nattrass M: Acute metabolic complications of diabetes, Hyperosmolar non-ketotic hyperglycaemia and Lactic acidosis. in Textbook of Diabetes. Eds. Pickup, JC and Williams, G. 3rd Edition.2003 Blackwell.

5. Foster DW, McGarry JD: The metabolic derangements and treatment of Diabetic Ketoacidosis. 1983, *NEJM.* 309:159-169.

6. Kitabchi, AE, Wall, BM: Diabetic Ketoacidosis. Endocrine Emergencies. *Med. Clin. N. Amer.* 1995, 79:9-37.

7. Kitabchi AE, Murphy MB: Diabetic Ketoacidosis and Hyperosmolar hyperglycaemic non-ketotic coma. *Med. Clinic. N. Amer.* 1988, 72:1545-1563.

8. Adrogue, HJ: Fluid-electrolyte and acid-base disorders complicating diabetes mellitus, p 2661-2686 in Disease of the Kidney and Urinary tract. 7 edition 2001.Schrier RW ed.Lippincott,Williams and Wilkins.

9. Kitabchi AE,Kreisberg LA; Umpierrez GE, et al:Management of hyperglycaemic crises in patients with diabetes. *Diabetes Care.* 2007, 24:131-153.

10. Lippincott's Illustrated Reviews: Biochemistry. 2nd Edition.2004 Eds. Champe, PC; Harvey, RA. JB Lippincott Company.

11. Kreisberg RA. Diabetic Ketoacidosis: New concepts and Trends in pathogenesis and Treatment. *Ann Intern Med.* 1978, 88:681-695.

12. Cahill GF: Starvation in Man. *Clin. Endocrin and Metab.* 1976, 5(2):397-415.

13. Kamel KS, Lin SH, Cheema-Dhadli S et al: Prolonged total fasting : A feast for the integrative Physiologist. *Kidney Int.* 1998, 53:531-539.

14. Castellino P, Luzi L, Simonson DC et al: Effects of insulin and plasma amino acid concentrations on leucine metabolism in man. *J. Clin. Invest.* 1987, 80:1784-1793.

15. Shulman GI, Rothman DL: Jue T et al: Quantitation of muscle glycogen synthesis in normal subjects and subjects with non-insulin dependent

diabetes by 13C nuclear magnetic resonance spectroscopy. *NEJM.* 1990, 322:223-228.

16.   Bjorntorp P, Sjostrom L: Carbohydrate storage in Man: Speculations and some quantitative considerations. *Metabolism.* 1978, 27(Suppl 2):1853-1864.

17.   Fery F, Balasse EO: Ketone body production and disposal in Diabetic Ketosis. A comparison with fasting ketosis. *Diabetes.* 1985, 34:326-332.

18.   Unger RH, Orci L: The essential role of glucagon in the pathogenesis of diabetes mellitus. *Lancet.* 1975, 1:14-16.

19.   Alberti KGMM, Christensen NJ, Iversen J, Orskov, H: Role of glucagon and other hormones in development of Diabetic Ketoacidosis. *Lancet.* 1975, 1307-1311.

20.   Barnes AJ, Bloom SR, Alberti KGMM et al: Ketoacidosis in pancreatectomised man. *New Eng J Med.* 1977, *296:1260*-1253.

21.   Gerich JE, Lorenzi M; Bier DM et al: Prevention of human Diabetic Ketoacidosis by somatostatin. *New Eng J Med.* 1975, 292:985-989.

22.   Barnes AJ, Kohner EM, Bloom SR et al: Importance of pituitary hormones in etiology and Diabetic Ketoacidosis. *Lancet.* 1978, 1:1171-1174.

23.   De Fronzo RA, Matsuda M, Barrett EJ: Diabetic Ketoacidosis.A combined metabolic-nephrologic approach to therapy.*Diabetes Reviews* 1994, 2:209-238.

24.   Rabinowitz D, Liljenquist JE: Glucose metabolism in intact man. The responsiveness of splanchnic and peripheral tissues to insulin. *Metabolism.* 1978, 27:1832-1866.

25.   Brown PM, Tomkins CV, Juul S, Sonksen PH: Mechanism of action of insulin in diabetic patients: a dose related effect on glucose production and utilization. *BMJ.* 1978, 5:1239-1242.

26.   Kingston ME, Skoog WC: Maintenance of basal insulin secretion in severe non-insulin dependent diabetes. *Diabetes Care.* 1986, 9:232-235.

27.   Zierler KI, Rabinowitz D: Effect of very small concentrations of insulin in forearm metabolism. Resistance of its action on potassium and free fatty acids without its effect on glucose. *J. Clin. Invest.* 1964, 43:8950.

28.   Madsbad S, Alberti KGMM, Binder C et al: Role of residual insulin secretion in protecting against Ketoacidosis in insulin-dependent diabetes. *BMJ.* 2:1257-1259.

29.   Chupin M, Charbonnel B, Chupin F: C-Peptide blood levels in Ketoacidosis and in Hyperosmolar non-ketotic coma. *Acta Diabet.* 18:123-128, 1981.

30.   Blackard WG, Nelson NC. Portal and peripheral vein immunoreactive insulin concentrations before and after glucose. *Diabetes.* 1970, 19:302.

31.   Turner, RC, Holman RK: Insulin rather than glucose homeostasis in the pathophysiology of diabetes. *Lancet.* 1976, 6:1272-1274.

32. Halter JB, Graf RJ, Porte D: Potentiation of insulin secretory responses by plasma glucose levels in man: Evidence that hyperglycaemia in diabetes compensates for impaired glucose potentiation. *J. Clin. Endocrin and Metab.* 1979, 48:946.

33. Watkins PJ, Hill DM, Fitzgerald MG, Malins JM: Ketonaemia in uncontrolled diabetes mellitus. *BMJ.* 1970, 4:522-525.

34. Malchoff CD, Pohl SL, Kaiser DL, Carey RM: Determinants of glucose and ketoacid concentrations in acutely hyperglycaemic diabetic patients. *Amer. J. Med.* 1984, 77:275-285.

35. Joffe BI, Goldberg RB, Krut LH, Seftel HC: Pathogenesis of non-ketotic Hyperosmolar diabetic coma. *Lancet.* 1975 1: 1069-1071.

36. Wachtel TJ, Tetu-Mouradjian LM, Goldman DL et al: Hyperosmolarity and acidosis in diabetes mellitus. *J. Gen. Intern Med.* 1991, 6: 495-502.

37. MacIsaac RJ, Lee LY, McNeil KJ et al: Influence of age on the presentation and outcome of acidotic and Hyperosmolar diabetic emergencies. *Intern. Med. J.* 2002, 32:379-385.

38. Sulway MJ, Malins JM. Acetone in diabetic ketoacidosis. *Lancet.* 1970, 2:736-740.

39. Androgue HJ, Wilson H, Boyd A et al: Plasma acid-base patterns in Diabetic Ketoacidosis. *New Eng J Med.* 1982, 307:1603-1610.

40. Fulop M: Serum potassium in lactic acidosis and Ketoacidosis. *New Eng J Med.* 1979. 300:1087-1089.

41. Gennari JF, Kassirer JP:Osmotic diuresis. *New Eng J Med.* 1974, 291:714-720.

42. Brodsky WA, Raprorts, West CD: the mechanism of glycosuric diuresis in diabetic man. *J Clin Invest* 1950, 29:1021-1032.

43. Nabarro JDN, Spencer AG, Stowers JM: Metabolic studies in severe diabetic ketosis. *Quart. J. Medicine.* 1952, 21:225-243.

44. Musey VC, Lee JK, Crawford R et al: Diabetes in urban African-Americans. Cessation of insulin therapy is the major precipitating cause of Diabetic Ketoacidosis. *Diabetes Care.* 1995,18:483-490.

45. Kitabchi AE; Young R; Sacks H; Morris L: Diabetic Ketoacidosis : Reappraisal of therapeutic approach. *Ann. Rev. Med.* 1979, 30:339-357.

46. Davoren PM, Bowen K: Ten years of Diabetic Ketoacidosis. *Med. J. Australia.* 1990, 152:327-328.

47. Waldhausl W, Kleinberger G, Korn A et al: Severe hyperglycaemia: Effects of rehydration on endocrine derangements and blood glucose concentration. *Diabetes.* 1979, 28:577-584.

48. Hale PJ, Crase J, Nattrass M: Metabolic effects of bicarbonate in the treatment of Diabetic Ketoacidosis. *BMJ.* 1984, 289:1035-1038.

49. Morris LR, Murphy MB, Kitabchi AE: Bicarbonate therapy in severe Diabetic Ketoacidosis. *Ann. Int. Med.* 1986, 105:836-840.

50. Hood VL, Tannen RL. Protection of acid-base balance by pH regulation of Acid Production. *New Eng J Med.* 1998, 339:819-25.

51. Adrogue HJ, Barrero J, Eknoyan G: Salutary effects of modest fluid replacement in the treatment of adults with Diabetic Ketoacidosis. *JAMA.* 1989, 262:2108-2113.

52. Katz Murray A: Hyperglycaemia-Induced Hyponatraemia—Calculation of Expected serum Sodium Depression. *New Eng. J. Med.* 1973, 289(16):843-844.

53. Hillier Teresa, Abbott Robert et al: Hyponatraemia: Evaluating the Correction Factor for Hyperglycaemia. *Amer. J. Med.* 1999, 106:400-402.

54. Kashyap AS: Hyperglycaemia-Induced Hyponatraemia: Is It Time to Correct the Correction Factor. *Arch Intern Med.* 1999, 159:2745-2746.

55. Daugirdas John T, Kronfol Nouhad O, et al: Hyperosmolar Coma: Cellular Dehydration and the Serum Sodium Concentration. *Ann Intern. Med.* 1989, 110(11):855-857.

56. Lund-Andersen H: Transport of glucose from blood to brain. *Physiol. Rev.* 1979, 59:305-352.

57. Edelman I, Leibman J, O'Meara MP: Interrelations between serum sodium concentration, serum osmolarity and total exchangeable potassium and total body water. *J. Clin. Invest.* 1958, 37:1236-1256.

58. Soler NG, Dixon K, Bennett MA, et al. Potassium balance during treatment of diabetic ketoacidosis. *Lancet.* 1972, 2:665-667.

59. Soler NG, Bennett MA, Fitzgerald MG, Malins JM: Intensive care in the management of Diabetic Ketoacidosis. *Lancet.* 1973, 1:951-953.

60. Beigelman PM: Potassium in severe Diabetic Ketoacidosis. *Amer. J. Med.* 1973, 54:419-420.

61. Androgue HJ, Ledderer ED, Suki WN, Eknoyang WN: Determinants of plasma potassium levels in Diabetic Ketoacidosis. *Medicine.* 1986, 65:163-172.

62. Stephens FI: Paralysis due to reduced serum potassium concentration during treatment of diabetic acidosis: Report of case treated with 33 grams of potassium chloride intravenously. Annals Intern Med 1948, 301272-1286.

63. Pullen H, Doig A, Lambie AT: Intensive intravenous potassium replacement therapy. *Lancet.* 1967, 2 809-811.

64. Clementsen HJ: Potassium therapy. A break with tradition. *Lancet.* 1962, 2 175-177.

65. Seftel HC, Kew MC: Early and intensive potassium replacement in diabetic acidosis. *Diabetes.* 15:694-696.

66. Abramson E, Arky R: Diabetic acidosis with initial hypokalaemia. *JAMA.* 1966, 196:115-117.

67. Dorin RI, Crapo LM: Hypokalaemic respiratory arrest in Diabetic Ketoacidosis. *JAMA.* 1987, 257:1517-1518.

68. Nicholson WM, Branning W: Potassium deficiency in diabetic acidosis. *J. Amer. Med. Ass.* 1947, 134:1292.

69. Frenkel M, Groen J, Willebrands AF: Reduction of serum potassium content and general muscular weakness during diabetic coma. *J Amer. Med. Ass.* 1947, 135:602.

70. Holler JW: Potassium deficiency occurring during the treatment of diabetic acidosis. *J. Amer. Med. Ass.* 1946, 131:1186.

71. Logsdon CS, McGavack TH: Death, probably due to potassium deficiency, following control of diabetic coma. J. Clin. Endocrin. 1948, 8:659.

72. Frenkel M, Groen J, Willebrands AF: Low serum potassium level during recovery from diabetic coma. Arch. Int. Med. 1947, 80:728.

73. Tuyman PE, Wilhem SK: Potassium deficiency associated with diabetic acidosis. Ann. Int. Med. 1948, 29:356.

74. Kebler R, McDonald FD; Cadnapaphornchai, P: Dynamic changes in serum phosphate levels in Diabetic Ketoacidosis. Amer. J. Med 1985. 79:571-576.

75. Stoff JS: Phosphate homeostasis and hypophosphataemia. Amer. J. Med. 1982 72:489-495.

76. Fisher JN, Kitabchi AE: A randomised study of phosphate therapy in the treatment of Diabetic Ketoacidosis. J. Clin. Endocrinol. Metab. 1983, 57:177-180.

77. Alberti GGMM: Low dose insulin in the treatment of Diabetic Ketoacidosis. Arch. Int. Med. 1977, 137:1367-1376.

78. Turner RC, Grayburn TA, Newman GB, Nabarro JDN: Measurement of insulin delivery rate in man. Clin, Endocrin. 1971, 33:279-286.

79. De Fronzo RA, Felig P, Ferranninie W, Wahren J Effect of graded doses of insulin on splanchnic and peripheral potassium metabolism in man. Amer. J. Physiol. 1980 238:E421-E427.

80. Alberti KGMM, Hockaday TDR, Turner RC: small doses of intramuscular insulin in the treatment of diabetic coma. Lancet. 1973, 2:512-522.

81. Fisher JN, Shahshahani MN, Kitabchi AE: Diabetic Ketoacidosis: Low dose insulin therapy by various routes. *New Eng J Med.* 1977, 297:238-241.

82. Umpierrez GE, Latif K, Stoever, J et al: Efficacy of subcutaneous insulin Lispro versus continuous intravenous regular insulin for the treatment of patients with Diabetic Ketoacidosis. Amer. J. Med. 2004, 117:291-296.

83. Thow J, Home P: Insulin injection technique. BMJ. 1990, 301:3-4.

84. Frid, A, Linden, B: where do lean diabetics inject their insulin? A study using computed tomography. BMJ. 1986, 292:1638.

85. Fulop M, Tannenbaum H, Dreyer N: Ketotic Hyperosmolar coma. Lancet. 1973, 2:635-639.

86.   Alberti KGMM, Hockaday TTR: Rapid ketone body estimation in the diagnosis of Diabetic Ketoacidosis. BMJ. 1972, 2:565-568.

87.   Schade DS, Eaton P: Differential diagnosis and therapy of hyperketonaemic state. JAMA. 1979, 241:2064-2065.

88.   Molitch ME, Rodman E, Hirsch CA, Dubinsky E: Spurious serum creatinine elevations in Ketoacidosis. Ann. Int. Med. 1980, 93:280-281.

89.   Munro J, Campbell IW, McCuish AC, Duncan LJP. Euglycaemic Diabetic Ketoacidosis. BMJ. 1973, 9:578-580.

90.   Rush MOJ, Godfrey MM, Geddis G: Arterial blood gas results rarely influence emergency physician management of patients with suspected Diabetic Ketoacidosis. Academic Emergency Medicine. 2003, 10:836-841.

91.   Fitzgerald MG, O'Sullivan DJ, Malins JM: Fatal diabetic ketosis. BMJ. 1961, 1:247-250.

92.   Winegrad AI, Kern EFO, Simmons DA: Cerebral oedema in Diabetic Ketoacidosis. *New Eng J Med*. 1985, 312:1184-1185.

93.   Carlotti APCP, Bohn D; Halperin ML: Importance of timing of risk factors for cerebral oedema during therapy for Diabetic Ketoacidosis. Arch. Dis. Child. 2003, 88:170-173.

94.   Krane EJ, Rockoff MA, Wallman JK, Wolfdorf JI: Subclinical brain swelling in children during treatment of Diabetic Ketoacidosis. *New Eng J Med*. 1985, 312:147-151.

95.   Silver SM, Clark, EC, Schroeder, BM, Sterns, RH: Pathogenesis of cerebral oedema after treatment of Diabetic Ketoacidosis. Kidney Int. 1997, 51:1237-1244.

96.   Arieff, AI, Kleeman DR, Keushkerian A, Bagdoyan H: Oedema in diabetic comas—effects of hyperglycaemia and rapid lowering of plasma glucose in normal rabbits. J. Clin. Invest. 1973, 52:571-5;

97.   Bello FA, Sotos JF: Cerebral oedema in Diabetic Ketoacidosis in children. Lancet. 1990, 336:64.

98.   Durr JA, Hoffman WH, Sklar AH et al: Correlates of brain oedema in uncontrolled IDDM. Diabetes. 1992, 41:627-632.

99.   Fein IA, Rackow EC, Sprung CL, Grodman R: Relation of colloid osmotic pressure to arterial hypoxaemia and cerebral oedema during crystalloid volume loading of patients with Diabetic Ketoacidosis. Ann. Int. Med. 1982, 96:570-575.

100. Roberts JS; Vavilala MS; Schenkman KA et al: Cerebral hyperaemia and impaired cerebral autoregulation associated with Diabetic Ketoacidosis in critically ill children. Crit. Care Med. 2006, 34:2217-2223.

101. Van Der Meulen JA; Klip A; Grinstan S: Possible Mechanism for Cerebral Oedema in Diabetic Ketoacidosis. Lancet. 1987, 2:306-308.

102. Glasier N, Barnett P, McCaslin I et al: Risk factors for cerebral oedema in children with Diabetic Ketoacidosis. *New Eng J Med*. 2001, 334:264-269.

103. Durr JA, Hoffman WH, Sklar AT et al: Causes of brain oedema in uncontrolled IDDM. Diabetes. 1992, 41:627-632.

104. McCurdy DK: Hyperosmolar hyperglycaemic non-ketotic diabetic coma. Med. Clin. N. Amer. 1970, 54:683-699.

105. Arieff AI, Carroll HJ: Non-ketotic Hyperosmolar coma with hyperglycaemia : Clinical features, pathophysiology, renal function, acid-base balance, plasma-cerebrospinal fluid equilibria and the effects of therapy in 37 cases. Medicine. 1972, 51:73-93.

106. Gerich JE, Martin MM, Recant L: Clinical and metabolic characteristics or Hyperosmolar non-ketotic coma. Diabetes. 1971, 20:228-238.

107. Westphal SA: The occurrence of Diabetic Ketoacidosis in non-insulin dependent diabetes and newly diagnosed diabetic adults. Amer. J. Med. 1996, 101:19-24.

108. Gordon EE, Kubadi UM. The hyperglycaemic Hyperosmolar syndrome. Amer. J. Med. Science. 1976, 271:252-268.

109. Ennis ED, Stahl EJVB, Kreisberg RA. The Hyperosmolar hyperglycaemic syndrome. Diabetic Reviews. 1994, 2:115-126.

110. Braaten JT. Hyperosmolar non-ketotic diabetic coma : diagnosis and management. Geriatrics. 1987, 42:83-92.

111. Lorber D: Non-ketotic hypertonicity in diabetes mellitus. Med. Clin. N. Amer. 1995, 79:39-51.

112. Pinies JA, Cairo G Gaztambide S, Vasquez JA: Course and prognosis of 132 patients with diabetic non-ketonic Hyperosmolar state. Diabetes and Metabolism. 1994, 20:43-48.

113. Popli S, Leehey DJ, Daugirdas JT et al: Asymptomatic non-ketotic severe hyperglycaemia with hyponatraemia. Arch. Int. Med. 1990, 150:1962-1964.

114. Singhal PC, Ambramovici M, Venkatesan J: Rhabdomyolysis in the hyperosmolar state. Amer. J. Med. 1990 88:9-12.

Diuretics and genetic disorders of tubular transport.

First you must define the problem. Confucius.

Despite filtration of 20,000-25,000mmol of sodium less than 1% is excreted (filtration fraction <1%). Reabsorption is achieved using the electrochemical gradient for sodium and negative potential generated by action of Na^+: K^+ pumps. Sodium reabsorption in different segments of the nephron, site of action of diuretics [1-6] and genetic disorders which mimic them are shown in the figure 1.

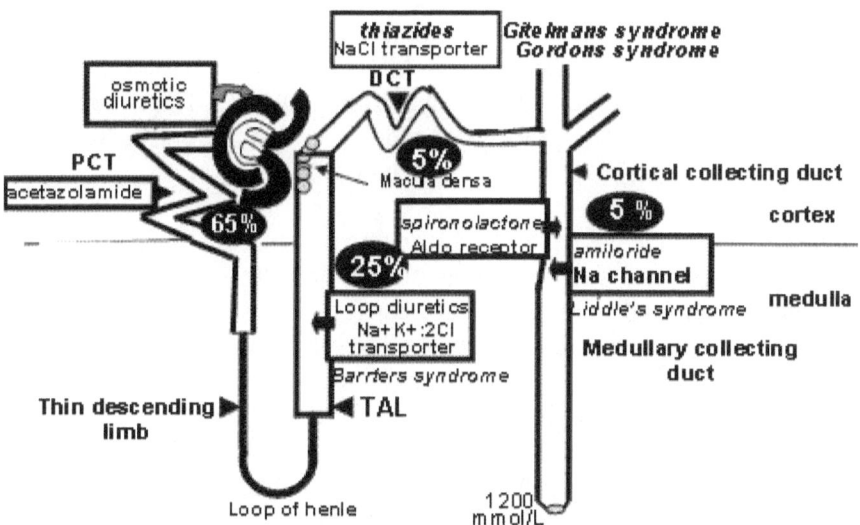

Figure: 1. Approximate percent of sodium reabsorption in different segments of the nephron are shown in black ovals. [1-6]

The site of action of diuretics (in italics) and mechanism of action are shown in boxes.PCT=proximal convoluted tubule; TAL= thick ascending loop.DCT=distal convoluted tubule. Aldo = aldosterone receptor; the site of action of genetic tubular defects is shown outside of boxes in italics.

OSMOTIC DIURETICS.

Mannitol is used to decrease cerebral oedema. Intravenous mannitol diffuses from blood stream to interstitial space and its osmotic action attracts water. It is filtered and excreted in urine unchanged [3].Increase in tubular osmotic pressure decreases passive reabsorption of water. Sodium reabsorption decreases secondary to its dilution in proximal tubular fluid. [3]

Mannitol therefore causes a relative water diuresis-water is lost more than solute. In addition renal blood flow, both within cortex and medulla, increases and may cause medullary washout. Expansion of extravascular volume may cause pulmonary oedema.

Glucose and urea act as endogenous osmotic diuretics by increasing renal loss of sodium, potassium and water.

NON-OSMOTIC DIURETICS.

Commonly used diuretics are carbonic anhydrase inhibitors, such as acetazolamide, which act on proximal tubules; loop diuretics, which act on thick ascending loops of Henle (TALH); thiazide diuretics (and indapamide), which act on distal convoluted tubules (DCT) and collecting ducts; and distal tubule diuretics, aldosterone antagonists and Na+ channel antagonists, which act on principal cells.

Diuretics are bound to plasma proteins, which trap diuretics in the vascular space, and decrease their glomerular filtration. [1,3] All except spironolactone (and eprelenone) are carried to the perivascular plexus surrounding proximal tubules and are secreted into the tubular lumen by either the organic acid pathway—loop diuretics, thiazides and carbonic anhydrase inhibitors; or organic base pathway—amiloride. [1,3,4] Impairment of renal function therefore limits transfer to the lumen and site of action. Spironolactone is carried by the circulation to its site of action on aldosterone receptors in distal tubules.

All diuretics initially cause net loss of sodium. The maximum loss occurs following administration of the first dose; but with continued use a steady state develops, provided dietary sodium intake remains the same. [5] Further net losses cease but total body sodium decreases from its initial level. Once a steady state is reached further volume depletion or electrolyte abnormalities usually only occur when dietary sodium changes, renal dysfunction or volume depletion develop from diarrhoea or vomiting. Diuretic potency depends on:

Dose.
Site of action.
Ability of more distal tubular sites to reabsorb sodium.

Carbonic Anhydrase Inhibitors. (3-5) (chapter 3)

Carbonic anhydrase inhibitors, such as acetazolamide, act in proximal tubules to inhibit carbonic anhydrase and thus bicarbonate reabsorption. Acetazolamide and other carbonic anhydrase inhibitors are weak diuretics. They increases bicarbonate excretion by approximately 25-30 %[3] but sodium is reabsorbed further down the nephron which limits their potency. Delivery of poorly reabsorbed anions such as HCO_3^- to collecting ducts increases luminal negativity and promotes secretion of K^+ in exchange for Na^+ which is reabsorbed. Acetazolamide therefore causes metabolic acidosis, hypokalaemia and mild sodium loss. [3, 6] Acetazolamide is well absorbed; 90% is protein bound; acts within 30 minutes; and for approximately two hours. It is predominantly used to counteract respiratory alkalosis of altitude sickness; for glaucoma; and rarely for metabolic alkalosis secondary to chronic respiratory failure.

LOOP DIURETICS. [1-6] (Figure 2)

Loop diuretics act on thick ascending limbs loops of Henle (TAL) by inhibiting $Na^+ K^+ 2Cl^-$ (NKCC2) transporters. Therefore Na^+, K^+ and chloride reabsorption decrease. K^+ secretion into the lumen, via K^+ channels, normally occurs to provide K^+ for operation of NKCC2 transporters because potassium concentration in tubular fluid is low. K^+ transfer provides a positive lumen gradient which promotes paracellular Ca^{2+} [8] and Mg^{2+} [9] reabsorption. Loop diuretics decrease calcium and magnesium reabsorption by interfering with K^+ recycling into the lumen.

Increased delivery of Na^+ and Cl^- to collecting ducts increases Na^+ reabsorption in exchange for K^+ by principal cells and leads to urinary loss of potassium. Inhibition of Cl^- reabsorption by $Na^+K^+2Cl^-$ transporters leads to metabolic alkalosis. Thus losses of urine Na^+, K^+ Cl^-, Mg^{2+}, and Ca^{2+} increase; and urine osmolality is low because of interference with generation of medullary hypertonicity by the large volume of tubular fluid passing down collecting ducts.

Loop diuretics are powerful because they act on the segment of the nephron where 25% of filtered sodium is reabsorbed. All currently used loop diuretics are rapidly absorbed in 1 to 2 hours:50% Furosemide, 10-50% Bumetanide and nearly all Torsemide. Furosemide is excreted in urine whereas Bumetanide and Torsemide are metabolised by liver. [7] Torsemide is more rapidly absorbed, has better bioavailability and longer half life. [7]

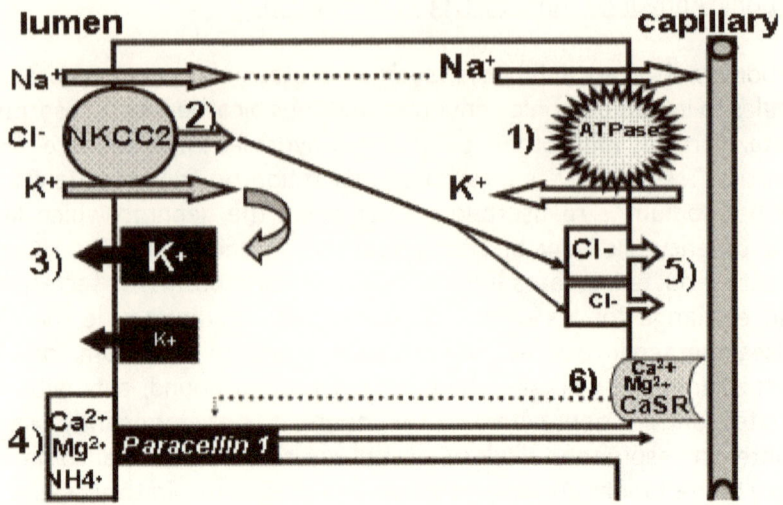

Figure 2: _Model of cell function in the cell of the thick ascending loop of Henle._

1. Na^+:K^+ pumps create low sodium concentration and negative intracellular potential.
2. This drives NKCC2 cotransporters to reabsorb Na^+, K^+ and Cl^-.
3. K^+, of low concentration in the tubular lumen, is recycled into the tubular lumen by K^+ channels to provide K^+ for NKCC2 cotransporters to function.
4. Recycling K^+ produces a positive lumen which promotes passive reabsorption of Ca^{2+} and Mg^{2+} by the paracellular route (between cells) facilitated by Paracellin 1.
5. Cl^- exits through Cl channels on basolateral membranes and Na^+ via Na^+:K^+ pumps
6. The CaSR (Ca^{2+} Mg^{2+} sensing receptor) controls paracellin related reabsorption of Ca^{2+} and Mg^{2+} by decreasing activity of K^+ channels which decrease lumen positivity.

Intravenous administration.

Intravenous loop diuretics act within 5-10 minutes and peak in 1-2 hours. In (diuretic naïve) healthy volunteers 40mg furosemide, 20mg Torsemide and 1mg Bumetanide, given intravenously, led to excretion of 200-250mmol sodium in 3-4 litres of urine, over 3-4 hours. [7] The response is blunted in heart failure: 45mmol Na^+, 24mmol K^+ and 0.78L urine were excreted in six hours in patients (New York heart Association Class III—IV) given 20mg of intravenous furosemide. [7] An oral dose of 40mg furosemide results in losses of hypotonic fluid containing approximately 60mmol of Na^+ /L over 3-4 hours in normal subjects. Electrolyte free water is excreted. Loop diuretics are therefore used when unsuppressed ADH secretion causes severe hyponatraemia, especially when fluid overload is also present.

Following infusion furosemide results in venodilation, possibly by causing release of prostaglandin E2 from the TALH, and stimulates renin release. Aspirin and NSAIDS block prostaglandin stimulated vascular dilatation. Secretion of renin is unopposed and may cause vasoconstriction secondary to Angiotensin 2, rather than vasodilatation. Hemodynamics may worsen in congestive cardiac failure. [7]

THIAZIDE DIURETICS AND INDAPAMIDE. [1-6,8,9] (Figure 3)

Thiazide diuretics act on NaCl cotransporters (NCC) of distal convoluted tubules (DCT) and collecting ducts to decrease Na^+ Cl^- reabsorption. Na^+ reabsorption, in exchange for K^+ by principal cells distally, results in hypokalaemia and less severe sodium loss than would otherwise occur. Urine osmolality is often high because this segment of the nephron normally reabsorbs NaCl without water, which further dilutes urine. Alkalosis results from increase in Na^+: H^+ exchange in distal nephrons or from loss of Cl^- greater than the ratio of $Na^:$ Cl^- in extracellular fluid.

Calcium reabsorption increases compared to loop diuretics.

Luminal Ca^{2+} (TRPV5) channels, which are voltage gated, increase luminal Ca^{2+} reabsorption. Secondly, continued transfer of Na^+ out of the cell by Na^+ K^+ pumps, while Na^+ influx from Na^+:Cl^- transporters is inhibited, results in low cellular Na^+. This activates basolateral Na^+:Ca^{2+} exchangers to increase sodium and thus Ca^{2+} entry into cells. [6] Thiazide induced volume depletion also increases proximal tubule Ca^{2+} reabsorption. [8] The cause of magnesuria is uncertain but rarely causes hypomagnesaemia. Thiazide diuretics are well absorbed and variably metabolised: bendrofluazide and indapamide by liver and chlorothiazide and hydrochlorothiazide by renal excretion [1] Therefore higher doses should be given in renal failure: for example 500-100mg/day hydrochlorothiazide in severe and 100-200mg/day in moderate renal failure Recently thiazide diuretics have been found to act on collecting ducts.(Eldari D,Hubner C.Current Opinion Nephrology Hypertension 2011.**20** 1120:506-511).

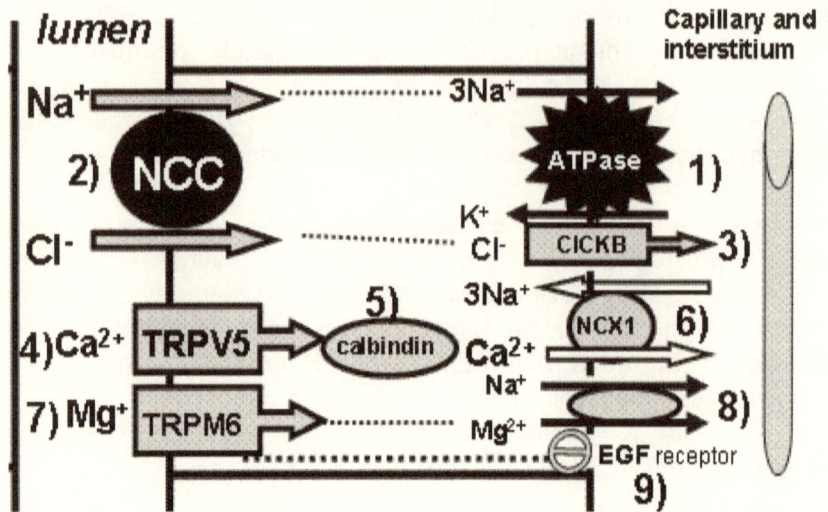

Figure 3 : Distal convoluted tubule cell showing Na+Cl luminal transporter (NCC), Ca2⁺channel (TRPV5),Mg2⁺channel (TRPM6) basolateral 3Na+:Ca²⁺exchanger(NCX1) and Cl⁻ channel (ClCKB).

1. *Na⁺:K⁺ ATPase pumps create low Na⁺ concentration and negative intracellular potential,*
2. *This promotes reabsorption of sodium and chloride by Na⁺ Cl⁻ transporters (NCC).*
3. *Cl⁻ exists by Cl⁻ channels (ClCKB) and Na⁺ via Na⁺ K⁺ pumps (1).*
4. *Ca²⁺ enters cell via calcium channels, TRPV5, (transient receptor protein vanilloid 5).*
5. *Ca²⁺ is transported across cell by calbindin, a Ca²⁺ binding protein.*
6. *Ca²⁺ exits the basolateral membrane on Ca²⁺: 3 Na⁺ exchangers (NCX1).*
7. *Mg²⁺ enters cell by TRPM6 (transient receptor protein melastin 6) channel.*
8. *Magnesium exits the basolateral membrane on Na⁺:Mg²⁺ exchangers.*
9. *Stimulation by epidermal growth factor (EGFR) receptor is important for optimum function of TRPM6.*

DIURETICS ACTING ON COLLECTING DUCT PRINCIPAL CELLS

Aldosterone antagonists, spironolactone and eprelenone, act on aldosterone receptors in principal cells to prevent transfer of the aldosterone—aldosterone receptor complex to the nucleus where it acts. Amiloride directly inhibits action of ENaC sodium channels. Both spironolactone and amiloride, called potassium sparing diuretics, decrease K⁺ loss because K⁺ exchanges for luminal Na⁺ reabsorption. Both spironolactone and amiloride are well absorbed (bioavailability ~ 90%) but cause only mild natriuresis because only 3% of filtered sodium is reabsorbed in collecting ducts. Their main role is to prevent potassium loss by inhibiting K⁺: Na⁺ exchange. Spironolactone causes mild metabolic acidosis due to decreased H⁺ secretion; and amiloride stimulates calcium reabsorption.

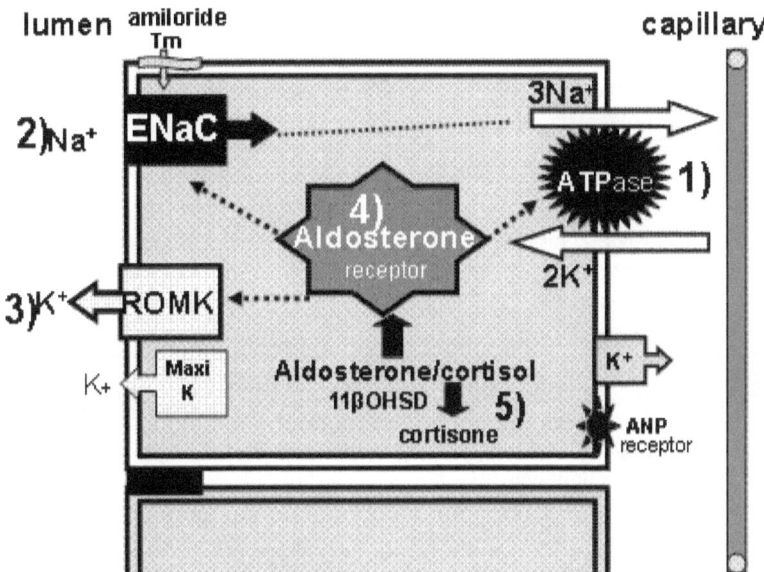

Figure: 4 **Actions of Principal cell.(excluding water reabsorption). Numbers correspond to text.**
ENaC = sodium channel. ROMK = K⁺ channel—high open probability. Maxi K = K⁺ channel = high flow conductance channel. Tm = trimethoprim- inhibits ENaC. ANP=Atrial natriuretic peptide.IIβOHSD= 11βhydroxysteroid dehydrogenase type 2.

1. *Na⁺: K⁺ pumps generate negative intracellular and lower Na gradient within cells.*
2. *Increases Na⁺ entry across the luminal membrane through sodium channels—EnaC and increases the negative potential in the lumen.*
3. *K⁺ moves into the tubular lumen through K⁺ channels in response to the negative lumen potential created by Na⁺ reabsorption. Na⁺ exits and K⁺ enters cells via Na⁺: K⁺ ATPase pumps as in 1.*
4. *The aldosterone receptor stimulates activity of ENaC channels, K⁺ channels and Na⁺: K⁺ pumps.*
5. *Cortisol, which acts with equal affinity to aldosterone on the receptor, is converted to inactive cortisone by 11 β hydroxysteroid dehydrogenase II before it can act.*

The differences between the diuretics are summarised in Table 1.

	LOOP (Furosemide) (Torsemide. Bumetanide)	THIAZIDES (Indapamide)	K+ SPARING (Amiloride, spironolactone)
Bioavailability	10-100%, average 50% decreased in heart failure.	Variable 50-90%	90%
Site of action	Lumen of TAL Na+K+2Cl- co-transporter	Lumen of DCT. Na+Cl- co-transporter	Principal cell Amiloride –Na+ channel Spironolactone, Eprelenone— aldosterone receptor
Transport to site of action	Secretion into proximal tubule by organic acid transporters.		Amiloride by proximal tubule organic base transporters Spironolactone— circulation to basolateral membrane.
Elimination	Furosemide—renal Bumetanide—liver 50% Torsemide—liver 80%	Renal except bendrofluazide and Indapamide by liver	Amiloride—renal
Duration	6-8 hours ↑ by renal failure. Bumetanide 4-6 hrs Torsemide 6-8 hrs	Long. Less effect in renal failure.	Amiloride 6-10 hours Spironolactone 24 hours
Potency	High. Effective to GFR of 3 mL/min.	Low. Less effect in renal failure.	Only 25-30 mmol/L excretion of Na+.
Urine losses	Na+K+Cl- Ca²+Mg²+ Low tonicity	Na+K+Cl- Mg²+ No Ca²+ loss High tonicity	Na+ HCO$_3$- excretion
Side effects	Hypovolaemia Hypokalaemia Hyponatraemia Hypocalcaemia Hypomagnesaemia Interstitial nephritis Gout Skin rash. Ototoxicity if IV	Volume depletion Hypokalaemia Hyponatraemia Hypercalcaemia Hypomagnesaemia Diabetes Interstitial nephritis Gout Skin rash. Impotence pancreatitis	Hyperkalaemia Acidosis Gynecomastia Loss of libido Anti-androgen due to spironolactone

Table 1: Properties and differences of commonly used diuretics [1-6] *(TAL=thick ascending limb (loop of Henle). (DCT= Distal Convoluted tubule).*

PROBLEMS WITH DIURETICS. [1, 5, 7, 10-13-29]

Provided intake of solute remains stable most complications occur within the first week of use. [5] Side effects are summarised in Table 1. The main problems are hypovolaemia, due to excessive sodium depletion, and electrolyte abnormalities.

When a steady state develops, after the first weeks of use, electrolyte disorders and change in volume status (or oedema) usually only occur when dietary intake of sodium changes, episodes of diarrhoea, deterioration of renal function or infection occur.

Decrease in cardiac output may cause hypotension, fatigue, depression, renal dysfunction [10, 11] and impotence. GFR decreases and may cause renal dysfunction in hospitalised patients. [12]

A sudden drop in diastolic filling and peripheral vasoconstriction, from low cardiac output, may worsen diastolic dysfunction.

Decrease in cardiac output or hypotension stimulates RAAS activation: [7, 10, 13, 14] an increase in renin, norepinephrine and AVP secretion occurs within 30 minutes following intravenous furosemide [7]. Vasoconstriction may impair cardiac output, whereas in the long term, RAAS activation increases ventricular remodelling. [10, 13]

Consider whether diuretics should be discontinued when volume excess has been corrected in chronic heart failure because of these risks; and the absence of evidence that diuretics decrease mortality or myocardial remodelling-except spironolactone.

Electrolyte Disorders.

These vary depending on diuretic used: loop and thiazide diuretics cause loss of Na^+, K^+, Cl^-, Mg^{2+} and alkalosis. Loop diuretics increase, whereas thiazide diuretics, decrease calcium loss.

Hyponatraemia. [15-19]

Thiazide diuretics predispose to hyponatraemia because they act on distal convoluted tubules which dilute urine and do not interfere with generation of medullary hypertonicity. They impair further tubular fluid dilution from Na^+:Cl^- reabsorption without water in the DCT. They may cause hyponatraemia, in the absence of clinically significant hypovolaemia, which may be sufficiently severe to cause death. [15-17] Women, especially post menopausal, are much more commonly affected than men. [16] Factors other than action of thiazides on distal convoluted tubules contribute to thiazide associated hyponatraemia. [15, 18, 19] 72% had one or more of increased ADH secretion, hypokalaemia or polydipsia in one review.

Friedman et al [17] tested those presenting with hyponatraemia with a single dose of thiazide-amiloride. Hyponatraemia developed again in these subjects, associated with weight gain and polydipsia, but not in young or old controls.

Loop diuretics usually only cause hyponatraemia secondary to severe hypovolaemia because they do not affect dilution in distal convoluting tubules; and they wash out medullary hypertonicity in the collecting duct which decreases maximal urinary concentration, and limits free water reabsorption.

Hypokalaemia and Hypomagnesaemia.

Both thiazide and loop diuretics cause hypokalaemia although severe hypokalaemia is uncommon. [20] The frequency and severity of hypokalaemia and other electrolyte disorders are related to the type of diuretic used, dose, underlying cause for which diuretics are given, dietary content of sodium and potassium and extent to which secondary hyperaldostereonism, a common problem in cirrhosis, is present.

The extent to which diuretics predispose to arrhythmias and sudden death is controversial. There are no randomised controlled trials using potassium supplements or potassium sparing diuretics and many observational studies, mainly done on those taking thiazide diuretics, are methodologically flawed. [20]

Thiazide diuretics are reported to cause an increase in arrhythmias [21,22-29] and sudden death. [21,23,25,27,29] Ventricular extrasystoles correlated with serum K^+ in a substudy of the MRC Mild Hypertension Trial but correlation with serum uric acid was similar suggesting that this was an association rather than cause. [30] Other studies have not shown an increase in arrhythmias [31-35] or sudden death. [24, 31-35] An increase in arrhythmias may only occur in those with severe hypokalaemia [36] or acute coronary syndromes. [37] Catecholamine secretion may lower serum potassium further in these cases. [38] However these studies were methodologically flawed [39] and normalisation of serum potassium with potassium-insulin infusion did not reduce arrhythmias or mortality. [40]

There are two strategies which potentially decrease risk of hypokalaemia and or arrhythmias: treatment with potassium supplements or cotreatment with potassium sparing diuretics. Use of potassium sparing diuretics has shown a decrease in sudden death in some studies but not in others.

There is no consensus on routine use of either potassium sparing diuretics or use of potassium supplements. An editorial, "Our National Obsession with potassium", contains a robust critique of the evidence on which potassium "pushing" is based. [39] Potassium sparing diuretics may increase the risk of hyperkalaemia and death. [39]

There is consensus, however, that low rather than high doses of thiazides should be used in treatment of hypertension because complications, including hypokalaemia, are reduced. [41] Metabolic alkalosis is an important complication associated with hypokalaemia and is discussed further in Acid-base disorders.

Hyperkalaemia and mild hyperchloraemic acidosis, due to inhibition of Na^+ reabsorption in distal nephrons, are uncommon complications of distal acting diuretics and decreases K^+ and H^+ exchange for Na^+.

Hypomagnesaemia and Magnesium Depletion.

Magnesium depletion is reported from use of loop or thiazide diuretics [42] but is uncommon, its significance uncertain, and severe hypomagnesaemia is rare. There are several publications claiming diuretics cause magnesium depletion, arrhythmias and other harmful effects, in the absence of hypomagnesaemia. [43] These studies are methodologically or conceptually flawed and are discussed further in the chapter on magnesium.

Hypocalcaemia and Hypercalcaemia.

An Increase in calcium loss from loop diuretics may cause secondary hyperparathyroidism [5] whereas hypercalcaemia may occur from thiazide diuretics, in association with immobilisation or primary hyperparathyroidism. The clinical importance is uncertain.

Metabolic Complications.

Thiazide diuretics increase insulin resistance and cause a slight increase in serum LDL cholesterol, [44] uric acid and slight decrease in HDL.[44] This is of minor degree and uncertain clinical importance provided low doses are used. [41] Serum cholesterol decreases to pre-treatment levels on more prolonged use. [44, 45] The incidence of diabetes is probably not increased when low rather than high doses are used. [35]

Sexual dysfunction.

Thiazide diuretics are associated with male sexual dysfunction but do not have a major effect on quality of life. [47]

Diuretic potency depends on Na^+ delivery to the site of action and magnitude of transport inhibition of Na^+. Loop diuretics are potent because they act on the TAL where 25-30% of Na^+ is reabsorbed. Increased delivery of Na^+ exceeds the capacity of more distal nephron segments for reabsorption. An initial 40 mg dose of furosemide in normal individuals results in maximum losses of 3-4L of hypotonic fluid containing approximately 60 mmol/L of Na^+ over 3-4 hours. This is probably less in ill patients and becomes less with additional doses.

Thiazides and potassium sparing diuretics are less potent because they act on the DCT and principal cells of collecting ducts respectively where 5-10% and ~ 3% of Na^+ are reabsorbed respectively. Thiazide are ineffective in renal failure whereas loop diuretics are effective, in higher doses, to a GFR of <15mls/min. The dose of thiazide diuretics should be increased in mild, but avoided in severe renal failure.

In severe renal failure (<15ml/min) only 1/5-1/10 of administered Furosemide is secreted into the tubule lumen resulting in the excretion of only 25mmol of sodium. The maximum effect in renal failure is achieved by an intravenous dose of 160-200mg or an oral dose of 250-400mg given three times a day.

Cardiac Failure.

Diuretics are recommended for treating volume overload in decompensated heart failure: [7] they relieve congestion, decrease intracardiac pressure and improve cardiac performance. However their efficacy is based on few trials of limited quality and contradictory findings. [7]

In acute decompensated heart failure a bolus of intravenous furosemide (10-100mg); Torsemide or 0.5-4mg Bumetanide are recommended. [7] A bolus peaks in 1-2 hours and lasts for 6 hours. [7]

Their action is decreased by renal failure (dependent on GFR) and by impaired gastrointestinal absorption, which is decreased in congestive cardiac failure: the response to Furosemide may be delayed for several hours.

More importantly loop diuretics such as furosemide act over 2-4 hours. [7] Therefore sodium loss is followed by avid sodium retention during the remainder of the day in those with heart failure. An increase in frequency, rather than a higher single dose, should be given, or salt restriction imposed, if sodium excess occurs. [1]

Renal dysfunction prolongs their action but decreases effectiveness [1]. Thiazide diuretics are relatively ineffective when renal failure develops. They are less effective when non-steroidal anti-inflammatory drugs, including aspirin and thiazolidenediones, are used.

Hypertension.

Thiazide diuretics are recommended, for initial therapy of hypertension, [46] but this is controversial. They are especially useful in 'salt sensitive' hypertension. The majority of complications are avoided if low dose thiazides are used.

Renal failure.

Diuretics are contraindicated in acute renal failure or oliguria of uncertain cause in the absence of hypovolaemia or heart failure.

Loop diuretics may be used to treat sodium excess in chronic renal failure. However many renal patients are prone to develop sodium depletion, especially in diseases affecting the renal medulla. Caution should be exercised in their use. Thiazides are ineffective in severe renal failure. The dose of Furosemide should be increased in renal failure: If the glomerular filtration ratio is 15mL/minutes only 1/5-1/10 of a loop diuretic will be secreted into tubular fluid. [1] The maximum intravenous dose of Furosemide is 160-200mg which results in excretion of approximately 20% of filtered sodium. [1] The maximum oral dose is double the intravenous dose.

NON CARDIOGENIC OEDEMA OR ASCITES.

Nephrotic syndrome.

Diuretics are bound by albumin which decreases their transport into proximal tubule cells. Binding with filtered albumin in the lumen decreases delivery to the transporters or channels which mediate sodium reabsorption. [6]

Liver cirrhosis.

Loop diuretics are relatively ineffective for treatment of ascites because hypovolaemia limits Na^+ delivery to distal tubules and secondary hyperaldostereonism increases Na^+ exchange with K^+. Furosemide may only result in a loss of 25-50mmol sodium and may causes severe hypokalaemia. Spironolactone is especially effective in counteracting secondary hyperaldostereonism, potassium loss and hypokalaemia.

Diuretic resistance.

Diuretic resistance reflects the intensity of stimulation of sodium retention secondary to 'effective' hypovolaemia, a low cardiac output or arterial under filling (arterial dilatation in cirrhosis). [1]Compensation for Na^+ loss begins as soon as the action of diuretics decrease. Compensation decreases GFR, increases Na^+ reabsorption in proximal tubules and in distal tubules in exchange for K^+. [1] Hypertrophy may also occur in distal nephron cells with long term use. Thiazides which block hypertrophy, at least in animals, may be synergistic. [1, 2]

Management of diuretic resistance.

- Consider whether effective hypovolaemia is sufficiently severe that increasing sodium loss may cause more harm than good: postural hypotension, tachycardia, dizziness, depression, rising serum creatinine and hyponatraemia suggest effective hypovolaemia is present.
- Exclude poor compliance.
- Reduce dietary sodium.

- Consider whether diminished drug bioavailability is present—eg congested liver and intestine from cardiac failure.
- Discontinue drugs which interfere with diuretic action or cause sodium retention—eg NSAIDs, thiazolidenediones; or interfere with organic acid transporters.
- Change from a thiazide to a loop diuretic.
- Increase dose in renal failure.
- Administer diuretics several times daily if high sodium diet is responsible in heart failure.
- Consider the intravenous route to overcome poor bioavailability.
- Consider diuretic combinations: add Thiazide to a loop diuretic. Add in distal tubule diuretics—amiloride, spironolactone, especially if hypokalaemia is a problem.
- Consider intravenous albumin if oncotic pressure is low—especially following paracentesis.
- Improve cardiac function.
- Consider a large intravenous bolus of Furosemide.
- Give a bolus of 40 mg furosemide followed by a continuous infusion of 10 mg/hour or 20-40 mg/hour if GFR <25ml/min.

Lithium induced Nephrogenic Diabetes Insipidus.

An unusual use of diuretics is the administration of amiloride in Nephrogenic Diabetes Insipidus caused by lithium therapy: Amiloride decreases lithium entry via sodium channels (EnaC) into principal cells where it decreases water reabsorption. [48]

GENETIC DISORDERS OF TUBULAR TRANSPORT.

Genetic disorders primarily involving magnesium, calcium and phosphate are described in the relevant chapters.

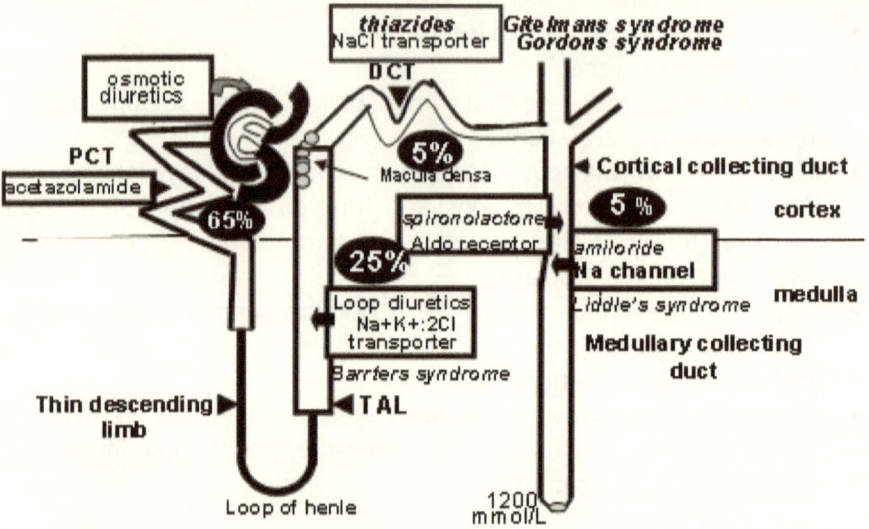

Figure: 5 *Genetic disorders causing sodium reabsorption disorders*.

Bartter's syndrome. [49, 50-55] (Figure 6)

This is due to several mutations which cause malfunction of Na$^+$ K$^+$ 2Cl$^-$ (NKCC2) transporters in thick ascending limbs of loops of Henle (TAL) (figure 7). [49-53]

The disorders which cause malfunction of NKCC2 channels are shown in the following figure 6. Adequate function of the NKCC2 transporter requires: [49-52]

- Normal function of NKCC2 transporters.
- Recycling of potassium into the tubular lumen.
- Normal function of the basolateral chloride channels and associated protein called Barrtin.
- Normal function of the calcium sensing receptor (CaSR).

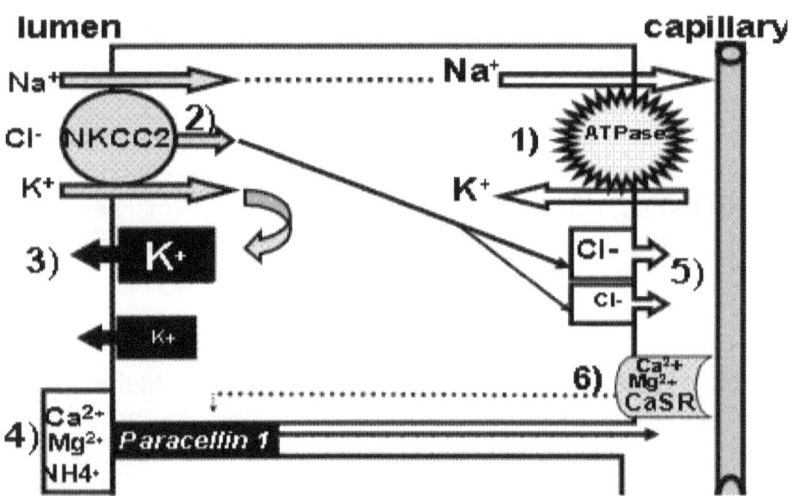

Figure: 6 *Ascending loop of Henle showing sites of disorders in Bartter's Syndrome.*

1. $Na^+:K^+$: pumps generate negative intracellular potential and low Na^+ gradient
2. Na^+, Cl^- and K^+ are transported from lumen into cell by $Na^+K^+2Cl^-$ cotransporters (NKCC2).
3. K^+, of low concentration in tubular fluid, is recycled into the lumen to enable NKCC2 transporters to work.
4. Ca^{2+} and Mg^{2+} are reabsorbed through the paracellular route because of the positive luminal voltage resulting from K^+ recycling into the lumen.
5. Cl^- is transported into the interstitial space by Cl^- channels.
6. CaSR stimulates paracellin to increase Mg^{2+} and Ca^{2+} reabsorption if hypocalcaemia or hypomagnesaemia occurs.

Recycling of K^+ into the tubular lumen by (ROMK) K^+ channels is necessary to provide sufficient potassium for Na^+ K^+ $2Cl^-$ transporters to function (3 in figure 6)because of the very low tubular concentration of K^+, compared to Na^+ and Cl^-, in tubular lumen.

Stimulation by hypercalcaemia decreases action of the CaSR (calcium sensing receptor). This decreases action of K^+ channels which decrease activity of NKCC2 due to low intratubular fluid K^+. A gain in function mutation of the CaSR decreases K^+ recycling and is a cause of Barrters syndrome. Adequate function of <u>basolateral</u> chloride channels (figure 6) are required to transfer reabsorbed Cl^- out of the cell in order to maintain a chloride gradient and positive cellular potential. Chloride channel dysfunction may involve ClCAKb; ClC-Kb plus ClCka [54, 55] or an abnormality of the protein Barrtin which is required to bind to chloride channels for transfer to the membrane. [53, 54]

Barrters syndrome is therefore due to any of the disorders described above: abnormal NKCC2, abnormal K$^+$ channel function, abnormal basolateral Cl channel function and associated protein Barrtin, and abnormal function of the CaSR.

Bartters Syndrome causes urinary loss of Na$^+$, K$^+$, Cl$^-$, Ca^{2+} and Mg^{2+}. Urinary loss of calcium and magnesium occur because their paracellular reabsorption depends on the tubular positive potential provided by K$^+$ recycling into the lumen. Bartter's Syndrome mimics the effect of loop diuretics which act on NKCC2 transporters. Potassium loss increases because of downstream exchange for sodium reabsorption in collecting ducts.

Bartter's Syndrome is therefore characterised by sodium depletion, hypovolaemia, hypokalaemia, metabolic alkalosis due to Cl$^-$ depletion, increased urinary calcium and magnesium losses. However hypocalcaemia and hypomagnesaemia are uncommon. Renin levels Increase secondary to sodium depletion. Bartter's Syndrome varies in severity depending on the transporters or channels involved. It may present in the antenatal period with polyhydramnios and premature labour; [51, 53] in neonates, children and rarely adults. Development is often stunted and deafness associated in some causes. [54, 55]

Gitelmans Syndrome. [49-53, 55-61]

Gitelman syndrome is usually a recessive disorder [49, 51, 53], due to mutation of the SLC12A gene, which codes the NCC (Na$^+$: Cl$^-$) transporters in distal convoluted tubules (DCT). This causes underactivity of the NCC. The function of the NCC transporters may be normal but routing to plasma membranes may be defective: retention of the NCC transporters in endoplasmic reticulum is followed by proteosomal digestion. This is important because of the potential for drug therapy to promote rerouting to plasma membranes. [50] (Figure 7)

A small minority of patients with the Gitelman phenotype have mutations of genes encoding chloride channels (ClC-kb). The basolateral K$^+$ channels (Kir 1 and 4) recycles K$^+$ for use by Na$^+$: K$^+$ ATPase pumps. Rare mutations, which decreases function of basolateral K^+ channels, decreases function of Na^+: K^+ pumps which in turn decreases the Na^+ and negative gradient required for normal function of NCC transporters. This is a cause of Gitelmans syndrome.

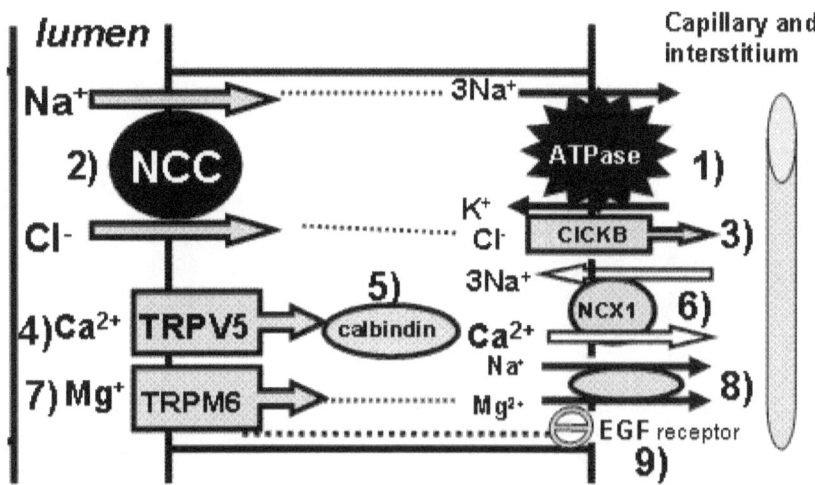

Figure 7. Function of the distal convoluted tubule.

1. *Na^+:K^+ ATPase pumps create low Na^+ concentration and negative intracellular potential.*
2. *This promotes reabsorption of sodium and chloride by Na^+ Cl^- transporters (NCC).*
3. *Cl^- exists by Cl^- channels (ClCKθ) and Na^+ via Na^+ K^+ pumps (1).*
4. *Ca^{2+} enters cell via calcium channels, TRPV5, (transient receptor protein vanilloid 5).*
5. *Ca^{2+} is transported across cell by calbindin, a Ca^{2+} binding protein.*
6. *Ca^{2+} exits basolateral membrane on Ca^{2+}: 3 Na^+ exchangers (NCX1).*
7. *Mg^{2+} enters cell by TRPM6 (transient receptor protein melastin 6) channel.*
8. *Magnesium exits the basolateral membrane on Na^+:Mg^{2+} exchangers.*
9. *Stimulation by epidermal growth factor (EGFR) receptor is important for optimum function of TRPM6.*

Both genetic [59] and phenotypic [51] heterogeneity are present. Malfunction of the Na^+ Cl^- (NCC) transporters in distal convoluted tubules (DCT) mimics the action of thiazide diuretics. However, severe hypomagnesaemia is characteristic of Gitelmans syndrome, but is much less common from thiazide diuretics. [49-53]

Reabsorption of Na^+ and Cl^- decreases. Electrogenic reabsorption of Na^+, in exchange for K^+, occurs down stream in collecting ducts causing potassium deficiency and hypokalaemia. This and chloride deficiency causes metabolic alkalosis. Hypocalciuria is characteristic compared to Bartter's Syndrome. Both Ca^{2+} and Mg^{2+} are reabsorbed by the transcellular route in DCT. There are three proposed mechanisms for hypocalciuria:

1. Hypovolaemia increases proximal tubule Ca^{2+} reabsorption.[8]
2. Continued transfer of Cl- out of cells via basolateral chloride channels, in the absence of luminal Cl^- entry, depolarises the cell (makes it more positive) [8, 51,52] Ca^{2+} reabsorption by the TRPV5 calcium channels, which are voltage gated, increases.
3. When Na^+ entry into cells decrease continued activity of Na^+: K^+ pumps, increases activity of Na^+:Ca^{2+} exchangers in basolateral membranes. [50, 51]

The cause of hypomagnesaemia and increased magnesium loss in urine is uncertain. The TRPM6 magnesium channels are down regulated.

Urine contains inappropriate increases in sodium, potassium, chloride and magnesium but low calcium. Only patients on thiazide diuretics or with Gitelmans Syndrome show this urinary profile. Patients usually have moderate hypovolaemia, hypokalaemia, alkalosis and hypomagnesaemia. Serum Ca^{2+} is usually normal but rarely decreases due to severe hypomagnesaemia. [56]

Muscle cramps (84%), paraesthesias (46%), especially of the face, dizziness, muscle weakness, fatigue (22%), palpitations and salt craving are common. [57, 58] Although less severe than Barrters syndrome, Emergency Room visits are increased and Quality of life decreased. [58] Chondrocalcinosis and sclerochoroidal calcifications are uncommon manifestations. Serious arrhythmias are surprisingly uncommon but can be life threatening. [58] Progressive renal failure is rare.

Large doses of potassium and magnesium supplements, a high salt diet, amiloride [60] 10-30 mg/day) and/or spironolactone, [61] 200-300mg/day, are used in treatment but are uncommonly fully effective in reversing hypovolaemia and electrolyte abnormalities. [60] This is shown in the shown by the following case:

A 25-year-old man presented with muscle weakness, cramps, dizziness, paraesthesias of the nose and hands and palpitations due to runs of paroxysmal supraventricular tachycardia. A niece had been diagnosed with Gitelmans Syndrome. Urine and stool tests for diuretics and cathartics were negative. Serum electrolytes were: K^+ 1.9 mmol/L, Na^+ 140mmol/L, HCo_3^- 27mmol/L, Mg^{2+} 0.49mmol/L, Ca^{2+} 2.5mmol/L, creatinine .06mmol/L.

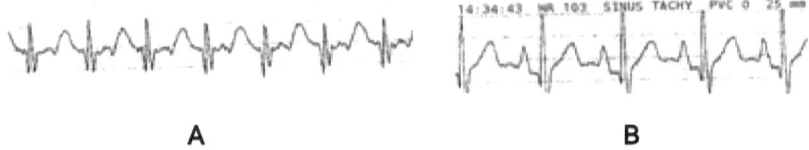

A	B

Figure 9. *(A) ECG on admission showing supraventricular tachycardia and hypokalaemia with giant U waves, and (B) Following normalisation of serum potassium: sinus rhythm and normal T waves.*

He was given over 1000 mmol potassium (intravenous 700mmol, oral supplements >300mmol) and normal diet. Despite this serum potassium rose to only 3.0mmol/L. Later urine results showed 24 hour excretion of sodium of 183mmol, potassium 160 mmol, despite serum K^+ of 2.9mmol/L, Mg^{2+}, 12.7mmol, despite serum Mg^{2+} of 0.6mmol/L, and urine calcium of only 0.8mmol.

During the next year of follow up the serum potassium varied between 3.0-3.5mmol/L, serum magnesium between 0.6-0.7mmol/L and moderate hypovolaemia persisted: marked postural tachycardia (figure 10), high serum renin 1070μU/L and aldosterone 2460 pmol/L.

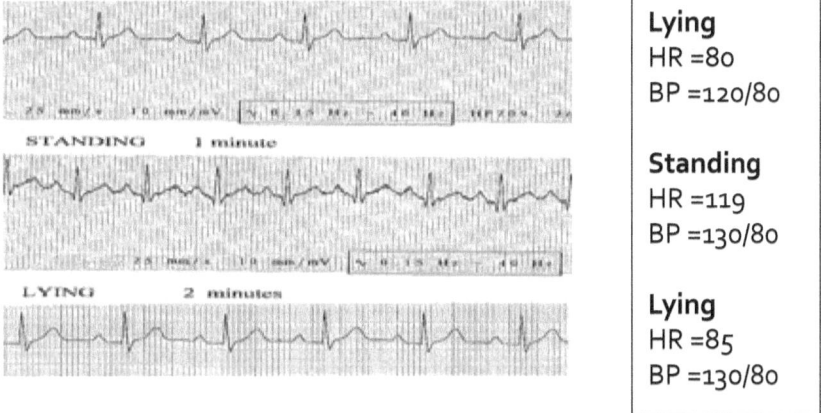

Figure 10. *Monitor showing orthostatic tachycardia without hypotension.*

This occurred despite a combination of a high sodium diet, potassium supplements, 60mmol/day, magnesium supplements, 20mmol day, amiloride 10mg twice daily and Eprelenone 50mg daily. Amiloride may be less effective than spironolactone. [59]Spironolactone should be avoided in male subjects because of its antitesterone side effects.Eprelenone can be used instead as in the case described.

Gordon's Syndrome. [49, 50, 52, 62-64]

This autosomal dominant disorder is due to overactivity of Na^+: Cl^- transporters of the DCT compared to underactivity in Gitelmans syndrome. This results in hyperkalaemia, but compared to other similar conditions, is associated with hypertension and a decrease in both renin and aldosterone secretion. This may be asymptomatic and present in adults. Increased NaCl reabsorption, proximal to the CCD, decreases Na^+ delivery to principal cells. Cl^- reabsorption is increased by the paracellular pathway. This decreases electrogenic sodium reabsorption, the negative lumen potential necessary for tubular K^+ secretion and results in excessive K^+ reabsorption. An increase in Na^+ and Cl^- reabsorption causes hypertension and hyperchloraemic acidosis respectively.Thiazide diuretics, which decrease action of the NCC transporters, are effective in treatment.

Gordon's syndrome is not due to mutations involving NCC transporters, but to mutations in WNK4 and WNK1 (with no lysine kinase). WNK4 normally modulates action of aldosterone by inhibiting NCC in the DCT thus increasing NaCl delivery to collecting ducts; inhibits K^+ secretion in the collecting duct principal cells by phosphorylating K^+ channels; and stimulates paracellular Cl^- reabsorption. This increases Na^+ reabsorption with Cl^-, rather than in exchange for K^+, and leads to hypertension, hyperkalaemia and metabolic acidosis. [45, 97, 185]

Liddle's Syndrome. [49, 52, 63]

This autosomal dominant disorder is due to gain in function of ENaC sodium channels in luminal membranes of Principal cells. This causes increased Na^+ reabsorption and K^+ secretion (in exchange for Na^+) into the tubular lumen. This causes hypertension, hypokalemia but low serum renin and aldosterone levels. Amiloride is effective for treatment.

Gain in function is due to mutations in beta or gamma subunits of EnaC channels which interact with Nedd 4, a cytoskeletal protein, which normally retrieves EnaC from apical membranes and degrades it. [64] Increased channel occupation on membranes results in increased Na^+ reabsorption and electrogenic K^+ secretion.

Gain in function of mineralocorticoid receptor. [63]

This autosomal dominant disorder resembles Liddles Syndrome but is less severe except in pregnancy. The hormone binding domain of the mineralocorticoid receptor may have an increased affinity for several steroids, including progesterone. This may explain the increase in severity in pregnancy.

Loss of ENaC and Aldosterone Receptor Function. [49, 52]

These rare conditions cause Pseudohypoaldostereonism (type 1) and clinically resemble hypoaldosteronism by causing sodium depletion, hyperkalaemia and hyperchloraemic acidosis but in association with raised aldosterone and renin levels.

Decrease in function of ENaC sodium channel or aldosterone receptor activity decreases reabsorption of Na^+, K^+ and H^+ secretion. Several recessive mutations, which decrease function of ENaC channels, and four different mutations affecting the mineralocorticoid receptor (Pseudohypoaldostereonism.Type II) have been described. Carbenoxolone which inhibits 17 β hydroxy steroid dehydrogenase Type II is partially effective in treatment [49].

The following disorders may also affect sodium reabsorption:

Decreased action of β ßhydroxysteroid dehydrogenase II. [52, 63]

(Apparent mineralocorticoid excess)

Cortisol acts with equal affinity to aldosterone on aldosterone receptors, but its concentration is approximately 1000 times higher (aldosterone picomol/L cortisol micromol/L). Cortisol is converted to cortisone, which is inactive, by II ßhydroxysteroid dehydrogenase Type II before it can occupy the receptor. Rare hereditary defects of II ßhydroxysteroid dehydrogenase and liquorice, which inactivates the enzyme, may cause hypokalaemia and hypertension.

Corticosteroid excess.

Very high serum cortisol or large doses of synthetic corticosteroids exceed the capacity of 11 β hydroxysteroid dehydrogenase type 2 enzymes to inactivate corticosteroids: this stimulates Na⁺ reabsorption by ENaC channels, K⁺ secretion by the (ROMK) potassium channels and causes hypertension, hypokalaemia and alkalosis.

Congenital Adrenal Hyperplasia. [63] (chapter 7)

Enzyme deficiencies in the cascade leading to cortisol synthesis result in increased stimulation by ACTH. This leads to formation of the mineral corticosteroid deoxycorticosterone which causes hypertension and hypokalaemia, suppression of renin and aldosterone secretion.

11 β hydroxylase deficiency: adrenal androgens are also increased resulting in ambiguous genitalia in female and pseudoprecocious puberty in male infants.

17 α hydroxylase deficiency decreases synthesis of gonadal hormones resulting in ambiguous genitalia in males and lack of secondary sexual characteristics in females.

Glucocorticoid remedial hypertension (Aldosterone-cortisol hybrids). [52, 64, 65]

Aldosterone is normally produced in the zona glomerulosa of adrenal glands following stimulation by both angiotensin II and hyperkalaemia; whereas cortisol is produced in the zona fasciculata following stimulation by ACTH. Defective genes results in production of a C18 cortisol—aldosterone hybrid in the zona fasciculata driven by ACTH rather than aldosterone. Thus ACTH rather than Angiotensin II stimulates aldosterone secretion. Increased aldosterone secretion, which results from stimulation by ACTH, causes hypertension and hypokalaemia. Aldosterone secretion is suppressed by a small dose, 0.5 mg, of dexamethasone, which suppresses ACTH and improves hypertension.

Familial Hyperaldosteronism type 2.

This autosomal dominant disorder is due to a lack of suppression of aldosterone synthesis and is associated with bilateral adrenocortical hyperplasia or adrenal adenomas. It is similar to sporadic Hyperaldosteronism.

Mutations in CaSR (see chapter on Calcium).

Familial Hypocalciuric Hypercalcaemia. Autosomal dominant mutation of genes controlling CaSR decreases sensitivity of calcium receptors in parathyroids, kidney and other organs. Higher levels of Ca^{2+} than normal are needed to suppress PTH secretion. Serum PTH is normal or increased despite hypercalcaemia and urine Ca^{2+} excretion is low because of abnormal function of calcium sensors (CaSR) in thick ascending loops of Henle.

Familial hypocalcaemia with hypercalciuria.

Mutations from gain of function of the CaSR cause hypocalcaemia and hypercalciuria. This resembles and should be distinguished from hypoparathyroidism because treatment with Vitamin D may increase hypercalciuria and cause nephrocalcinosis.

X-linked Hypophosphatemic Ricketts—(Chapter 9)

Mutations Affecting Voltage Gated Chloride Channels. [49]

Mutations of chloride channels cause several abnormalities of proximal tubule function of varying severity and phenotypic expression. These include proteinuria, hypercalciuria, Ricketts, nephrocalcinosis, sodium and chloride loss and are referred to under various names including Dents disease.

REFERENCES

1. Brater DC. Diuretic Therapy. *NEJM.* 1998, **339**:387-395.
2. Ellison DH. The Physiologic Basis of Diuretic Synergism: It's Role in Treating Diuretic Resistance. *Ann. Int. Med.* 1991, **114**:886-894.
3. Ellison DH, Okusa MD, Schrier RW. Mechanisms of Diuretic Action. p2423-244; in Diseases of the Kidney and Urinary Tract. 7th Edition 2001 Ed. Schrier RW, Lippincott, Williams and Wilkins.
4. The Kidney. Chapter 24, p368-380 in Rang and Dales Pharmacology. Ed. HP Rang, MM Dale, JM Ritter, RJ Flower. 6th Edition, 2006 Churchill, Livingstone and Elsevier.

5. Clinical use of Diuretics. P 447-472 in Clinical Physiology of Acid-Base and Electrolyte Disorders. Ed. Rose B, Post TW, 5th Edition, 2001 McGraw-Hill.

6. Morrison RT. Edema and Principles of Diuretic use. *Med. Clin. N. Amer.* 1997, **81**:689-704.

7. Cleland JG, Coletta A, Witte K. Practical Applications of Intravenous Diuretic Therapy in Decompensated Heart Failure. *Amer. J. Med.* 2006, **119**:S26-S36.

8. Mesenkamp AR, Hoenderop JGJ, Bindels RJM. Recent advances in Renal Tubular Calcium Reabsorption. *Current Opinion in Nephrology and Hypertension.* 2006, **15**:524-529.

9. Chubanov V, Guderman T, Schlingmann KP. Essential role for TRPM6 in Epithelial Magnesium Transport and Body Magnesium Homeostasis. *Eur. J. Physiol.* 2005, **451**:228-234.

10. Hill JA, Yancy CW, Abraham WT: Beyond Diuretics: Management of Volume Overload in Acute heart Failure Syndromes. *Amer. J. Med.* 2006, **119**:S37-S44.

11. Mehta RL, Pascual MT, Soroko S, Chertow GM. Diuretics, Mortality and Non-recovery of Renal Function in Acute Renal Failure. *JAMA.* 2002, **288**:2547-2553.

12. Butler J, Forman DE, Abraham WT, et al. Relationship between heart failure treatment and development of worsening renal function among hospitalised patients. *Am. Heart J.* 2004, **147**:331-338.

13. Francis GS, Siegel RM, Goldsmith SR, et al. Acute vasoconstrictor response to intravenous Furosemide in patients with chronic congestive heart failure. *Ann. Int. Med.* 1985, **103**:1-6.

14. Agostoni P, Marenzi G, Lauri G, et al. Sustained improvement in functional capacity after removal of body fluid with isolated ultra filtration in chronic cardiac insufficiency: Failure of Furosemide to provide the same results. *Amer J. Med.* 1994, **96**:191-199.

15. Sonnenblick M, Friedlander Y, Rosin A J. Diuretic-induced severe hyponatraemia—Review and Analysis of 129 reported patients. *Chest.* 1993, **103(2)**:601-606.

16. Ayus J. Carlos, Arieff Allen I. Chronic Hyponatraemic Encephalopathy in Postmenopausal Women. *JAMA.* 1999, **281(24)**:2299.

17. Friedman E, Shadel M, Halkin H, Farfel Z. Thiazide-induced Hyponatraemia. *Ann. Int. Med.* 1989, **110**:24-30.

18. Hamburger S, Koprivca B, Ellerbeck et al. Thiazide-induced Syndrome of inappropriate Secretion of Antidiuretic Hormone. *JAMA.* 1981, **246**:1235-1236.

19. Beresford HR. Polydipsia, Hydrochlorothiazide and Water Intoxication. *JAMA.* 1970, **214**:879-883.

20. Greenberg A. Diuretic Complications. *American J of Medical Sciences.* 2000, **319**. 10-24
21. Cooper HA, Dries DL, Davis CE et al. Diuretics and risk of arrhythmic death in patients with left ventricular dysfunction. *Circulation.* 1999, **100**:1311-1315.
22. Ryan MP, Diuretics and Potassium/Magnesium Depletion. *Amer. J. Medicine.* 1987, **82(suppl 3A)**:381-42.
23. Bigger JT. Diuretic therapy, Hypertension and Cardiac Arrest. *NEJM.* 1994, **330**:1899-1900.
24. Multiple Risk Factor Intervention Trial Research Group. Multiple Risk Factor intervention Trial: Risk Factor changes and mortality results. *JAMA* 1982, **248**:1465-77.
25. Greenberg G, Brennan PJ, Miall WE. Effects of Diuretic and Beta-Blocker Therapy in the Medical Research Council Trial. *Amer. J. Med.* 1984, **76**:45-51.
26. Shivkumar K. Do diuretics cause heart disease? *Ann. Int. Med.* 1995, **123**:891.
27. Siscovick DS, Raghunathan TE, Psaty BM et al. Diuretic Therapy for Hypertension and the Risk of Primary Cardiac Arrest. *NEJM.* 1994, **330**:1852-7.
28. Dyckner T, Wester PO. Potassium/Magnesium Depletion in patients with Cardiovascular Disease. Amer J med.**82**:11-17.1987
29. Hoes AW, Grobbee DE, Lubsen J. et al. Diuretics, Beta-Blockers and the Risk for Sudden Cardiac Death in Hypertensive patients. *Ann. Int. Med.* 1995, **123**:481-487.
30. Ventricular extrasystoles during thiazide treatment: sub study of MRC mild hypertension trial. Medical research Council working Party on Mild to Moderate Hypertension. *BMJ.* 1983, **287**:1249-1253.
31. Narayan P, Papademetriou V. Effect of Hydrochlorothiazide therapy on cardiac arrhythmias in African-American men with systemic hypertension and moderate to severe left ventricular hypertrophy. *Amer. J. Cardiol.* 1996, **78**:886-889.
32. Kostis JB, Lacy CR, Wilson AC, et al. Chlorthalidone does not increase ventricular ectopic activity in isolated systolic hypertension. *J. Amer. College Cardiol.* 1992, **19**:1910.
33. Papademetriou V, Notargiacomo A, Heine D, et al. Effects of diuretic therapy and exercise-related arrhythmias in systemic hypertension. *Amer. J. Cardiol.* 1989, **64**:1152-6.
34. Papademetriou V, Burris JF, Notargiacomo A. Thiazide therapy is not a cause of arrhythmias in patients with systemic hypertension. *Arch. Int. Med.* 1988, **145**:1272-8.

35. Freis ED. The efficacy and safety of diuretics in treating hypertension. *Ann. Int. Med.* 1995, **122**:223-226.

36. Siegel D, Hulley SB, Black DM, et al. Diuretics, Serum and intracellular electrolyte levels and ventricular arrhythmias in hypertensive men. *JAMA.* 1992, **267**:1683-8.

37. Duke M.Thiazide Induced Hypokalemia.Association with acute myocardial infarction and ventricular fibrillation.JAMA 239:43 1978

38. Struthers AD, Whitesmith R, Reid JL. Prior thiazide diuretic treatment increases adrenaline-induced hypokalaemia. *Lancet.* 1983, **1**:1358-60.

39. Harrington JT, Isner JM, Kassirer JP. Our National Obsession with Potassium. *Amer J. Med.* 1982, **73**:155-158.

40. Rogers WJ, Segal PH, McDaniel HG, et al. Prospective randomised trial of glucose-insulin potassium in acute myocardial infarction. Effects on myocardial haemodynamics, substrate and rhythm. *Amer. J. Cardiol.* 1979, **43**:801-9.

41. Carlsen JE, Kober L, Torp-Pedersen C, Johansen P. Relation between dose of bendrofluazide, antihypertensive effect and adverse biochemical effects. *BMJ.* 1990, **300**:975-978.

42. Sheehan J, White A. Diuretic-associated hypomagnesaemia. *BMJ.* 1982, **285**:1157-1159.

43. Hollifield JW. Magnesium Depletion Diuretics and Arrhythmias. *Amer. J. Med.* 1987, **82**(suppl 3A):30-36.

44. Lasser NL, Grandits G, Caggiula AW, et al. Effects of Antihypertensive Therapy on Plasma Lipids and Lipoproteins in the Multiple Risk Factor intervention Trial. *Amer. J. Med.* 1984, **76**:52-66.

45. Miettinen TA, Huttunen JK, Naukkarinen V, et al. Multifactorial primary prevention of cardiovascular disease in middle-aged men. Risk factor changes, incidence and mortality. *JAMA.* 1985, **254**:2097-102.

46. The Sixth Report of the Joint National Committee on Prevention, Detection, Evaluation and Treatment of High Blood Pressure. *Arch. Int. Med.* 1997, **157**:2413-2434.

47. Chang SW, Fine R, Siegel D, et al. The impact of diuretic therapy on reported sexual function. *Arch. Int. Med.* 1991, **151**:2402-2407.

48. Battle DC, Von Riotte AB, Gaviria M et al. Amelioration of Polyuria by Amiloride in patients receiving long term lithium therapy. *NEJM.1985* **312**:408-414.

49. Scheinman SJ, Guay-Woodford LM, Thakker RJ, Warnock DG. Mechanisms of Disease. Genetic Disorders of Renal Electrolyte Transport. *NEJM.* 1999, **340**:1177-1187.

50. Flatman PW. Cotransporters, WNKs and hypertension: an update. Current Opinion Nephrol hypert.17:186-192.2008

51. Nine Vam Knoers. Gitelman Syndrome. Advances in Chronic Kidney Disease. 2006, **13**:148-154.
52. Warnock DG. Hereditary disorders of potassium homeostasis. *Best Practice and Research Clinical Endocrinology and Metabolism.* 2003, **17**:505-527.
53. Bhandar S. The Pathophysiological and molecular basis of Bartter's and Gitelman's syndromes. *Postgrad Med. J.* 1999, **75**:391-396.
54. Bichet DG, Fumiwara TM. Reabsorption of Sodium Chloride—Lessons from the Chloride Channels. *NEJM.* 2004, **350**:1281-1283.
55. Schlingmann KP, Konrad M, Jeck N, et al. Salt wasting and Deafness resulting from Mutations in Two Chloride Channels. *NEJM.* 2004, **350**:1314-1319.
56. Pantanetti P, Arnaldi G, Balercia G, et al. Severe hypomagnesaemia-induced hypocalcaemia in a patient with Gitelman's Syndrome. *Clinical Endocrinology.* 2002, **56**:413-418.
57. Pachulski RT, Lopez F, Sharaf R. Gitelman's Not-So-Benign Syndrome. *NEJM.* 2005, **353**:850-851.
58. Cruz DN, Shaer AJ, Bia MG, Borella P et al. Gitelman's Syndrome revisited: An evaluation of symptoms and health-related quality of life. *Kidney Int.* 2001, **59**:710-717.
59. Bettinelli A, Bianchetti MG, Borella P, et al. Genetic heterogeneity in tubular hypomagnesaemia-hypokalaemia with hypocalciuria (Gitelman's Syndrome). *Kidney Int.* 1995, **47**:547-551.
60. Griffing GT, Komanicky P, Aurecchia SA, et al. Amiloride in Bartter's Syndrome. *Clin. Pharmacol Therapeutics.* 1982, **31**:713-718.
61. Colussi G, Rombola G, De Ferrari ME, et al. Correction of hypokalaemia with antialdosterone therapy in Gitelman's Syndrome. *Amer. J. Nephrology.* 1994, **14**:127-135.
62. Huang C-L, Kuo E, Toto RD. WNK kinases and essential hypertension. Current Opinion Nephrol Hypertens.17:133-137.2008
63. Mulatero P, Verhovez A, Morello F Veglio F. Diagnosis and treatment of low –renin hypertension. Clinical Endocrinology.67:324-334 2007.
64. Take C, Ikeda K, Kurasawa T, Kurokawa K. Increased chloride reabsorption as an inherited renal tubular defect in familial type II pseudohypoaldosteronism. New England Journal of Medicine, 1991. 324(7): 472-6
65. Rich, G.M, Ulick S, Cook S, et al., Glucocorticoid-remediable aldosteronism in a large kindred: clinical spectrum and diagnosis using a characteristic biochemical phenotype. Annals of Internal Medicine, 1992. 116(10): p. 813-20.

ELECTROLYTE, FLUID DISTURBANCES IN RENAL DISEASE.

- Obstructive uropathy.
- Tubulo-interstitial disease.
- Acute renal failure.
- Chronic renal failure.

OBSTRUCTIVE UROPATHY. (1-3)

The most Common Causes are shown in table 1.

Prostatic enlargement, bladder neck obstruction
Urethral stricture or phimosis
Extrinsic compression from mass lesion
Bilateral pelvi-ureteric calculi or uric acid crystal obstruction from chemotherapy
Retroperitoneal fibrosis, haemorrhage, mass lesion, inflammation
Bladder mass lesions
Neurological Disease: Cauda equina syndrome, diabetes, transverse myelitis.
Drugs: Anticholinergic action
Trauma: Pelvic fracture

Table 1 Common causes of obstructive uropathy.

Urine normally moves into the ureter from the renal pelvis stimulated by electrical impulses, generated by a calyceal pacemaker. Obstruction leads to ureteral dilatation, cessation of peristalsis, a rise in intratubular pressure and filtration fraction.GFR decreases because pressure increases in Bowmans space. Blood flow to the medulla progressively decreases. Glomerular capillary pressure increases from afferent arteriolar dilatation and maintains GFR but at a lower rate.

The effects of obstruction depend on its degree of completeness and duration. Tubular functions of distal nephrons are especially affected and results in the following:

- Decrease in maximal urinary concentration and polyuria, resistant to ADH, occurs in partial obstruction and following relief of complete obstruction. This is probably due to decreased concentrations of medullary urea and sodium.
- Defective urinary ammonium secretion and acidification occurs in partial obstruction or following relief of complete obstruction.
- Decreased potassium excretion occurs from either Hyporeninaemic hypoaldostereonism or defective H$^+$ secretion. [4, 5].
- Marked losses of sodium, potassium and magnesium may follow resolution of obstruction, especially following bilateral obstruction. [1, 5]
- Loss of renal function occurs early and may be marked and permanent following relief of obstruction.

Clinical manifestation: are shown in table 2.

Following relief of obstruction marked diuresis and losses of sodium, potassium and magnesium may lead to volume depletion, hypokalaemia, hypomagnesaemia and hypernatraemia.

Pain in both loins due to renal capsular distension or pain typical of ureteric stone.
Hypertension—from unilateral or bilateral obstruction.
Manifestations of urinary tract infection.
Hyperchloraemic acidosis and hyperkalaemia. [4]
Hypernatraemia and increase in thirst due to polyuria.
In partial obstruction functional abnormalities similar to those in interstitial kidney disease.

Table 2. Clinical manifestations of obstructive uropathy.

Complete urinary tract obstruction results in renal failure This is suggested by anuria or oliguria alternating with polyuria. Partial obstruction may cause chronic renal failure.

Investigations:

Renal ultrasound should be done urgently in all patients with intrinsic renal failure, symptoms suggesting obstruction or evidence of an acidification defect, sodium wasting, polyuria or hyperkalaemia without cause. <u>Dilatation of the urinary tract takes time to develop following obstruction and may cause misdiagnosis.</u> On the other hand Diabetes insipidus and pregnancy cause non-obstructive dilatation of the pelvi-calcyceal system and ureters.

TUBULO-INTERSTITIAL DISEASE. [6,7] (Table 3)

Disease of interstitiium of the kidney but with only secondary glomerular involvement: the glomeruli are relatively normal until late. Inflammation, scarring, tubular atrophy and papillary necrosis develop in severe cases.

Chronic Pyelonephritis.
Drugs.
Autoimmune disease: Sjogrens syndrome, Systemic lupus erythematosus, cryoglobulinaemia.
Reflux nephropathy.
Uric acid nephropathy, oxalate nephropathy.
Infection: tuberculosis, brucellosis, leptospirosis.
Sickle cell disease.
Obstructive uropathy.
AIDS. [8].
Medullary cystic disease.
Renal transplantation.

Table 3. Causes of Tubulo-interstitial disease.

<u>Drugs</u> are an important cause: proton pump inhibitors, allopurinol, penicillins, ß lactam antibiotics, non-steroidal anti-inflammatory drugs, colchicine, cyclosporine-tacrolimus and diuretics but all medications should be considered as possible causes. Fever, rash and eosinophilia are clues that drugs are responsible. Symptoms occur late and are usually due to the underlying cause. Early diagnosis is important. Tubulo-interstitial disease is distinguished from glomerular disease by the following:

	Glomerular disease	Interstitial disease
Proteinuria	>3g (albumin)	≤1.5g (α_2 β_2 globulin)
Na⁺ status	Normal until late	Sodium wasting
Hypertension	Common	Less common
Acidosis	Late	Early
Hyperkalaemia	Late	Early
Uric acid	Normal	Increased fever, rash, eosinophilia

Table 4. Comparison between glomerular and interstitial disease.

Tubular-interstitial disease may be acute or chronic. Acute disease presents with fever, loin pain and renal failure. Urinalysis shows proteinuria, haematuria and white cell casts.Tubulo-interstitial disease may be asymptomatic until a late stage or present with:

- Manifestations of the primary illness—e.g. infection, diabetes, gout, drug reactions etc.
- Proteinuria usually <3g/day, pyuria, white cell casts.
- Renal failure.
- Acute onset due to a drug reaction.

Proximal tubule involvement may cause aminoaciduria, proteinuria, phosphaturia, glycosuria, uricosuria and urinary bicarbonate loss.

Distal tubule involvement causes four main functional defects. (chapter 6 with references)

- Sodium wasting.
- Impaired urine concentration.
- Defective renal acidification :decreased capacity to secrete NH_4^+ and or H^+.
- Hyperkalaemia.[9,-10]

Papillary necrosis occurs in severe cases.

ACUTE RENAL FAILURE. [11-13]

The diagnosis of acute renal failure is considered in those with oliguria, urine output <400mls/day, an unexpectedly raised or a rising serum creatinine ('polyuric' renal failure).Acute renal failure may be due to:

- Pre-renal failure.
- Urinary tract obstruction.
- Intrinsic renal disease.

Differentiation is discussed in the chapter on Oliguria, Hyponatraemia, Hypotension and Cardiac failure.

Urinary tract obstruction is suggested by anuria, oliguria alternating with polyuria, or a history of a potential cause. Acute tubular necrosis, compared to prerenal failure, is suggested by the following:

	Acute Tubular Necrosis	Pre-renal failure
Urine Na$^+$	>40mmol/L	<20 mmol/L
Fractional excretion Na	>1	<1
Urea : creatinine ratio (both in micromol/L)	<60	>60
Response to treatment	Inadequate	Adequate
Urine sediment	Normal	Granular casts, tubular epithelial cells

Table 5. Acute tubular necrosis compared to prerenal failure.

Acute compared to chronic renal failure is suggested by:

- Symptoms <3 months,
- A marked increase from a previous serum creatinine.
- Absence of anaemia.
- Normal kidneys or ultrasound.

Causes of Acute Renal Failure are shown in table 6:

The main causes of pre-renal failure are low cardiac output from effective hypovolaemia or cardiac dysfunction, sepsis, less commonly anaphylaxis, the hepato-renal syndrome and drugs.

Acute tubular necrosis due to shock, sepsis or hypovolaemia
Sepsis
Glomerular- tubular disease
Vasculitis
Acute interstitial nephritis—drugs, infection
Nephrotoxic agents
Rhabdomyolysis, Incompatible blood transfusion
Acute uric acid or myeloma nephropathy
Haemolytic uraemic syndrome, Thrombotic Thrombocytopaenic purpura, HELLP syndrome
Malignant hypertension
Bilateral renal artery occlusion
Atheroembolic disease
Acquired Immune Deficiency Syndrome associated acute renal failure
Hepato-renal syndrome
Falciparum malaria Postoperative

Table 6. Causes of acute renal failure.

Drugs are an important cause—NSAIDs, Angiotensin inhibitors, Angiotensin receptor blockers, aminoglycosides and intravenous contrast.

Non-Steroidal Anti-inflammatory Drugs (NSAIDS): during low cardiac output GFR is maintained by decrease in pre-glomerular arterial resistance and increase in efferent arteriolar pressure. The increase in efferent arteriolar pressure is modulated) by prostaglandins PG12 and PPGE2 which attenuate the reduction in renal blood flow: This compensatory response is decreased by NSAID drugs and increases the risk of renal failure.

Aminoglycoside Toxicity : this may develop after aminoglycosides are stopped because of their long half life. Renal failure is usually non-oliguric and reversible. Volume depletion, older age, and co administration of other nephrotoxins predispose to toxicity.

Contrast Nephropathy: this is probably due to hypoxic tubular injury especially in the medulla. Risk factors are volume depletion, older age, diabetes, coincident use of nephrotoxic drugs and underlying renal disease. Saline infusion ± acetyl cysteine decreases its incidence.

ACE Inhibitors and Angiotensin Receptor Blockers: the risk of renal failure developing from their use is increased by volume depletion, renal artery stenosis, cirrhosis, diabetes and cardiac failure.

Atheroembolic disease: follows angiography or cardiovascular surgery and often manifests with eosinophilia, high ESR and decrease in complement levels.

Rhabdomyolysis: is suspected in those who fall and remain immobilized, trauma, compartment syndrome, multiple seizures, medications, illicit drugs, poisons and muscle disorders and who have elevated plasma creatinine phosphocreatinase (CPK).

Multiple causes are implicated in many cases: older age, sepsis, nephrotoxic drugs,-especially statins, hypovolaemia, comorbid conditions such as diabetes, and underlying kidney disease. Volume depletion is probably the most important reversible predisposing cause. [14] A trial of fluids should be undertaken unless there are contraindications. [14]

Complications due to Acute Renal Failure.

Electrolyte fluid disorders : hyperkalaemia, hyperphosphataemia, hypermagnesaemia, metabolic acidosis, hyponatraemia.

Hypertension, pulmonary oedema, hyperuricaemia, infection.

Uraemic manifestations: Nausea, vomiting, anorexia, inadequate nutrition, asterixis, confusion, seizures, pericarditis, pleuritis, arrhythmias.

Prevention of renal failure:

- Assess risk factors: chronic renal failure, age, Multiple myeloma, diabetes, drugs.
- Avoid contrast, aminoglycosides and other nephrotoxins.

- Ensure volume status is optimum in high risk patients: prior to intravenous contrast, rhabdomyolysis or renal dysfunction.
- Stop NSAID's and ACE inhibitors if hypovolaemia or cardiac failure is present.
- Give prophylaxis before contrast (discuss protocol with Radiologist).
- Give Allopurinol prior to cancer chemotherapy.
- Avoid using loop diuretics (frusemide) blindly to increase urine output when oliguria is present.

Immediate treatment for Acute Renal Failure:

- Stop ACE inhibitors, NSAIDs, aminoglycosides, other potential nephrotoxins and potential culprit drugs.
- Treat the cause, relieve obstruction, if present, and give effective antibiotics if infection is likely.
- Treat volume depletion/overload (heart failure and arrhythmias). Consider central line, fluid challenge ± inotropes.
- Correct acidosis and hyperkalaemia. (See relevant chapters).
- Prevent and treat infections promptly.
- Maintain good nutrition.

Maintenance fluids. Insensible water loss, approximately 500-1000mL, (less in humid environments, more in low humidity environments) approximately equals the combination of preformed water and water of oxidation in food. Therefore additional water required to maintain water balance is roughly equivalent to urine output. Measure or estimate losses of urine, vomitus and diarrhoea.

Indications for Dialysis:

Early referral to a Nephrologist is essential if renal failure progresses despite volume challenge.

CHRONIC RENAL FAILURE. [15-17]:

Common causes of chronic renal failure are diabetes, hypertension, glomerular disease, interstitial nephritis and hereditary renal disease. This is often asymptomatic until glomerular filtration rate falls below 25mL/minute. Early manifestations are proteinuria, hypertension and slight increase in uric acid. When the GFR falls below 25 mL/minute there is a variable disturbance of:

Electrolyte and acid base abnormalities
Impaired urinary dilution and concentration
Excessive natriuresis in interstitial renal disease
These are discussed in more detail in the chapters 4,6,7,10.

Sodium, Volume Status.

The kidneys regulate volume status remarkably well even when 90% of renal function is lost [18]. Decrease in sodium conservation is due to osmotic diuresis resulting from protein catabolism which imposes a solute load on surviving nephrons. Acidosis and tubular dysfunction contribute. The major abnormality is loss of rapid adaption to changes in volume, sodium intake or loss. Adaption to a gradual change is well preserved and a gradual, rather than rapid, decrease of sodium intake to less than 5-10mmol can be tolerated without adverse effects [18].

Water Balance.

Polyuria, polydipsia and nocturia commonly occur in chronic renal failure. Osmotic diuresis decreases medullary hypertonicity. The ability to concentrate is lost earlier than the ability to dilute urine [18]. Delivery of sodium to distal diluting tubules, to enable dilution, decreases and impairs urinary dilution. However hypernatraemia is uncommon because intact thirst usually leads to adequate water intake. Hyponatraemia is potentially more serious and especially prone to occur when hypovolaemia is superimposed on chronic renal failure. Postural hypotension and tachycardia are important clues to hypovolaemia resulting from diuretics, changes in salt intake, diarrhoea and vomiting.

Acidosis. [19, 21]

When GFR decreases below 25mL-30 mL /minute either an anion "gap" or hyperchloremic acidosis develops. The following factors are involved in varying degrees:

- Diminished NH_4^+ synthesis, from decrease in nephron mass, occurs when GFR falls below 30-40 mL/min. This causes decrease in Cl^- excretion. Hyperkalaemia also decreases NH_4^+ synthesis.
- Interference with medullary recycling of NH_4^+.
- Interference with distal tubular acidification—(chapter on Acid-base Disorders).

- Retention of anions: SO_4^{2-} phosphate, urate, hippurate and organic acids.H_2SO_4, from meat, is buffered by $NaHCO_3$

$$H_2SO_4 + NaHCO_3^- \leftrightarrow Na_2SO_4 + 2H_2CO_3 \rightarrow 2CO_2 + 2H_2O.$$

SO_4^{2-} is lost as Na_2SO_4 and decreases SID.
- Less commonly decreased reabsorption of bicarbonate and bicarbonaturia occur. [21]

Early renal failure usually causes hyperchloraemic acidosis. "Anion gap" acidosis increases as renal failure progresses. However the severity of each is also determined by the cause of renal failure: medullary disease causes earlier and more severe renal tubular acidosis. Metabolic acidosis occurs in the majority of patients when GFR decreases to 20% of normal. [20] Even in advanced renal disease serum HCO_3^- rarely falls below 12 mmol/L.[20]

Plasma HCO_3^- stabilizes at a low level because of buffering of acidosis, mainly by bone buffers. This causes hypercalciuria, contributes to hyperphosphataemia and causes bone disease.

Medullary disease, interstitial nephritis and lithium toxicity cause RTA by more than one mechanism: defective $NH4^+$ synthesis or recycling, distal tubule dysfunction or failure to generate a negative voltage.

Potassium [22-30]

Decreased capacity to excrete potassium is due to lower numbers of relatively normal functioning nephrons. However, the failing kidney has a remarkable capacity to excrete potassium loads despite a marked reduction in nephrons. [22-24] It does this by increasing K^+ excretion per nephron.

Collecting ducts in cortex and medulla increase K^+ secretion by increasing the number of $Na^+:K^+$ pumps on basolateral membranes and K^+ channels on luminal membranes. Both a raised extracellular K^+ concentration and aldosterone play a role. Increase in urea excretion per nephron increases flow rate in CCD and facilitates K^+ secretion [28]. This may be important because many foods with high K^+ also contain high potential urea content.

Aldosterone is important for adaption to potassium loads but not essential. [25, 25, 26]

Uptake of K^+ by non-renal cells increases. The colon increases K^+ excretion [29] 3-4 times above normal which comprises an appreciable percent of K^+ excretion in between dialyses.

The extent to which internal redistribution contributes to potassium disposal is controversial but probably does not play a major role. Insulin secretion increases in response to hyperkalaemia [25] but probably only when this is severe [27] and an increase within the physiological range may not be clinically important. [25]

However once the serum K^+ rises above normal the capacity to take up further potassium is limited and may be confined to extracellular space alone. [24] A small additional load of potassium of only 0.25mmol/kg may cause severe hyperkalaemia. [24]

Hyperkalaemia is uncommon provided GFR is above 10mls/minute. This may occur at higher GFR in the following circumstances:

- Ingestion of high potassium containing fluids, foods or salt substitutes.
- Severe acidosis.
- Effects of drugs: NSAID's, spironolactone, ACE inhibitors, β blockers.
- Hyporeninaemic hypoaldostereonism.
- Insulin requiring diabetics.
- This is discussed further in the section on Potassium.

Calcium, Phosphate and Bone disease in Chronic Renal Failure

This should be read at the end of the chapter on Calcium where it is discussed with references.

Magnesium. Hypermagnesaemia is rarely an important manifestation of chronic renal failure.

Other Manifestations:

Anaemia:

Due to decrease in erythropoietin synthesis by proximal tubules and decrease in red cell life span.

Bleeding susceptibility:

This is due to various factors including platelet dysfunction and abnormality of Factor VIII.

Serositis: Pericarditis and pleuritis occur in the late stages of renal failure.

Gastrointestinal manifestations: Nausea, vomiting, anorexia, stomatitis, enlargement of salivary glands and poor nutrition.

Neuromuscular: Fatigue, insomnia, decreased concentration, confusion, uraemic neuropathy.

Generalised Pruritis: uncertain cause.

Metabolic: Insulin resistance, hypertriglyceridaemia, decreased HDL.

MANAGEMENT:

- Diagnose cause and correct (if possible).
- Delay deterioration.
- Prevent and treat complications.
- Refer to a Nephrologist if the diagnosis is uncertain or when serum Cr >0.26 mmol/l.

DELAY DETERIORATION.

Avoid and treat the following early.(table 8)

Infection—systemic or urinary.

Hypertension ACE inhibitors slow deterioration if proteinuria is present. End stage renal failure may respond to volume reduction.

Intraglomerular Hypertension and proteinuria—ACE inhibitors decrease both.

Metabolic acidosis –Give $NaHCo_3^-$ 1 g $\equiv$ 12mmol 2-3 times daily.

Anaemia—Subcutaneous erythropoietin analogue. Ensure iron stores are adequate. BP may increase following treatment.

Calcium, phosphate and Bone –Implement low phosphorus diet but avoid causing protein malnutrition. $CaCo_3$ or calcium acetate 1-2g with meals to bind phosphate. chapter 10.

Hyperuricaemia—Administer allopurinol but at a decreased dose depending on GFR.

Metabolic—Maintain good insulin control in diabetics and optimum nutrition. Statins are controversial.

Pruritis and Dry Scaly Skin –Use moisturizing creams.

Avoid and treat.

* **Obstruction** from Prostatic enlargement, stones, sloughed papillae, prevent hyperuricaemia

* **Nephrotoxins**—NSAID, x-ray contrast, Aminoglycosides, Tetracycline.

Maintain optimum volume electrolyte status.

Table 8. Factors required to delay deterioration.

Maintain optimum volume-electrolyte state.

• Glomerular disease often leads to sodium retention; tubulo interstitial disease to sodium depletion.
• Volume overload and oedema—thiazides are ineffective when serum Cr > 0.20 mmol/l. Gradually increase frusemide to 250mg twice daily for volume overload or heart failure if present.

- Volume depletion—Administer high sodium diet, sodium bicarbonate or salt tabs; in severe cases IV saline.
- Avoid volume overload and optimise treatment of heart failure.

Electrolytes—Prevent and treat hyperkalaemia and hypocalcaemia or hypercalcaemia. Dietary restriction is not required in the majority.

Hypercholesterolemia—Administration of Statins are relatively ineffective and controversial.

Caution with drug use—<u>avoid</u> NSAIDs, Aminoglycosides, Tetracycline, and d<u>ose reduction:</u> Allopurinol, Digoxin, and Aminoglycosides.

Prevent malnutrition—give protein 1g/kg/d and an adequate calorie intake.

Prevent Hyperkalaemia—see chapter on Potassium. Avoid NSAID, β Blockers, K^+ sparing diuretics, Trimethoprim. Give high quality low protein diet. Resonium 15-30g 3 times daily or 50g per rectum

Emergency treatment.

- IV insulin 10 units, 35 gm glucose → continuous insulin/glucose + Salbutamol inhalation via spacer.
- Correct acidosis (NaCO3 100-150mmol/l IV (controversial) unless in heart failure.
- Dialysis.

Acidosis—treat with sodium bicarbonate tablets.

TARGETS.

- Consider nephrology referral when Cr ≥ 0.2 mmol/l.
- BP 130/80 ;< 120 systolic in diabetics
- Consider ACE Inhibition, statin? Stop smoking.
- Maintain haemoglobin at 110-120g/l.
- Maintain serum HCO_3 >22mmol/l; PO_4 <1.6 mmol/l ;PTH ~ 3 x normal.
- Maintain good nutrition and HbA1C <7%.

REFERENCES

1. Klahr, S: Obstructive Nephropathy: Pathophysiology and Management. p 498-538 in *Renal and Electrolyte Disorders 6th Edition.2003* Ed Schrier, RW; Lippincott, Williams and Wilkins.

2. Klahr, S: Obstructive Nephropathy, 986-1003 in *Textbook of Nephrology*. Ed Massry, SG; Glassock RJ, 4 edition 2001; Lippincott, Williams and Wilkins.

3. Curhan, GC; Leidel, ML. Urinary Tract Obstruction. p1936-1958 in *The Kidney 5th Edition*.1996 Editor Brenner, BM. WB Saunders.

4. Battle, DC; Arruda, JAL; Kurtzman, NA: Hyperkalaemic distal renal tubular acidosis associated with obstructive uropathy. *New Engl J Med*. 304:973, 1981.

5. Sabatini, S; Kurtzman, NA: Enzyme activity in obstructive uropathy and basis for salt wastage and the acidification defect. *Kidney International*. 37:79, 1990.

6. Kelly, CJ; Neilson, EG: Tubulo-interstitial Disease.p1655-1679 in *The Kidney*. Ed. Brenner, BM.5 edition 1996. WB Saunders.

7. Eknoyan, G: Tubulo-interstitial Nephropathies. P 746-758 in *Textbook of Nephrology*. 4 edition 2001 Eds Massry, SG; Glassock, RJ. Lippincott,Williams and Wilkins.

8. Glassock, RJ; Cohen, AH et al: Human Immunodeficiency Virus (HIV) infection and the kidney. *Ann. Intern. Med.* 112:35, 1990.

9. Caramelo, C; Bello, E et al: Hyperkalaemia in patient's infected with the Human immunodeficiency Virus: Involvement in systemic mechanism. *Kidney International.* 56:198, 1999.

10. Lee, FO; Quismorio, FP; Troum, OM: Mechanisms of hyperkalaemia in systemic lupus erythematosus. *Arch, Intern. Med.* 148:397, 1988.

11. Edelstein, CL; Schrier, RW: Acute Renal Failure: Pathogenesis Diagnosis and Management p401-455 in *Renal and Electrolyte Disorders, 6th Edition*. Ed. RW Schrier. Lippincott, Williams and Wilkins.

12. Brady, HR; Brenner, BM, Lieberthel, W: Acute Renal Failure, p1200-1252 in *The Kidney 5th Ed.1996. Ed* Brenner, BM, WB Saunders.

13. Kleinknecht, Dieter: Management of Acute Renal Failure, p1015-1026 in *Oxford Textbook of Clinical Nephrology*. Eds. Cameron, S; Davison, AM; Grunfeld, JP; Kerr, D; Ritz, E. 1992. Oxford Medical Publications.

14. Sladen, RN; Oliguria in the ICU. *Anaesiology Clinics of North America.* 18(4), 739-52.2000.

15. Disturbances in Fluid, Electrolyte and Acid-Base Balance. Chronic Renal Failure. Bourgoigne, JJ; p 1381-1386 in *Textbook of Nephrology.4 edition 2001* Eds. Massry, SG; Glassock, RJ. Lippincott, Williams and Wilkins.

16. Wang, W; Chan, LL: Chronic Renal Failure: Manifestations and Pathogenesis. p 456-497 in Renal and Electrolyte Disorders, 6th Edition.2003 Ed. RW Schrier, Lippincott Williams and Wilkins.

17. Mitch, WE; Wilcox, CS: Disorders of Body Fluids, Sodium and Potassium in Chronic Renal Failure. *Amer. J. Med.* 72:536-550, 1982.

18. Warnock, DG: Uremic Acidosis. *Kidney International.* 34:278-287, 1988.

19. Acid-Base Metabolism p 380-443 in *Massry & Glassock's Textbook of Nephrology.*Eds. Massry, Shaul, G; Glassock, Richard J: 4 edition 2001

20. Kraut, JA; Kurtz, I: Metabolic Acidoses of CKD: Diagnosis Clinical Characteristics and Treatment. *Amer. J. Kidney Diseases.* 45:978-993, 2000.

21. Warnock, DG: Uremic Acidosis. *Kidney International.* 34:278-287, 1988.

22. Silva, P; RS Brown and FH Epstein: Adaptation to Potassium. *Kidney International.* 11(6):466-75, 1977.

23. Alexander, EA and Levinski, EA: An Extrarenal Mechanism of Potassium Adaptation. *Journal of Clinical Investigation.* 47(4):740-748, 1968.

24. Sterns, RH, et al: Disposition of Intravenous Potassium in Anuric Man: A Kinetic Analysis. *Kidney International.* 15(6):651-660, 1979.

25. Cox, M; Sterns, RH and Singer, I: The Defence Against Hyperkalaemia: the roles of insulin and aldosterone. *New England Journal of Medicine.* 299(10):525-532, 1978.

26. Sugarman, A and Brown, RS: The Role of Aldosterone in Potassium Tolerance: studies in anephric humans. *Kidney International.* 34(3):397-403, 1988.

27. Van Ypersele de Strihou, C: Potassium Homeostasis in Renal Failure. *Kidney International.* 11(6):491-504, 1977.

28. Halperin, ML, et al: Urea Recycling: an aid to the secretion of potassium during antiduiresis. *Nephron.* 72(4):507-511, 1996.

29. Basti, C; Hayslett, JP and Binder, HJ: Increased large intestinal secretion of potassium in renal insufficiency. *Kidney International.* 12(1):9-16, 1977.

30. Rabelink, TJ, et al: Early and late adjustment to potassium loading in humans. *Kidney International.* 38(5):942-947, 1990.

URINE ELECTROLYTES.

The pisse-prophet or, Certaine pisse-pot lectures.

Wherein are newly discovered the old fallacies, deceit and juggling of the pisse pot science, used by all those (whether quacks and empiricks or other methodicall physicians) who pretend knowledge of diseases, by the urine, in giving judgement of the same.   Thomas Brian.1637

The art of the "Pisse Prophet", who relied on the smell, colour and taste of urine, has given way to biochemical analysis. This is useful in diagnosis of low cardiac output, acid-base disorders, potassium disorders, osmolar disorders and in diagnosis of poisoning.

URINE SODIUM, CHLORIDE.

Low Cardiac Output (CO).

Urinary sodium and/or chloride decrease within a short time of reduction in CO from effective hypovolaemia or cardiac failure. Indeed low urinary sodium predicted the cause of hyponatraemia better than clinical signs. [1] Whether the predominant decrease occurs in sodium or chloride depends on acid-base balance: In alkalosis, due to vomiting for example, bicarbonate excretion obligates sodium excretion because HCO_3^- is poorly absorbed (poorly absorbed anion) in distal tubules. Thus urine sodium may initially exceed 30mmol/L despite the presence of hypovolaemia. However urinary chloride is extremely low (<10mmol/L). If metabolic acidosis accompanies hypovolaemia, as occurs in diarrhoea, chloride excretion increases and results in high urine Cl^- accompanying NH_4^+ during acidosis, but urinary sodium is usually < 10-20 mmol/L. Both sodium and chloride should be measured in assessment of hypovolaemia. [2, 3]

Low urinary sodium (<20 mmol/L) usually requires and implies:
- Need to conserve Na^+: evidence for low CO, arterial underfilling, losses of sodium greater than intake or cardiac failure.
- Normal renal function—in most cases.
- Adequate aldosterone secretion.
- Absence of osmotic diuresis or marked ketonuria.
- Absence of current diuretic use.
- Absence of poorly reabsorbable anions.

Low urinary sodium concentration occurs in some cases of renal failure, for example: in acute glomerular tubular nephritis, myoglobinuria and contrast nephropathy. Accuracy is increased by calculating the fractional excretion of sodium (Fe Na) on spot urine. [2, 4]

Fe Na$^+$ = urine Na$^+$ / plasma Na$^+$ X plasma creatinine/urine creatinine X 100(%).

Units should be the same for sodium and creatinine; mmol/L or mg/dL.

Fe Na should be less than 0.5% In sodium depletion [4]. Low fractional excretion of sodium plus fractional excretion urea better predicts hypovolaemia than sodium alone. [2, 4]

Spot urine sodium is useful in the differential diagnosis of hyponatraemia: it is low in sodium depletion or effective hypovolaemia, increased in severe renal failure, diuretic use and in the syndrome of inappropriate ADH secretion (SIADH).

Urine sodium should be high in the SIADH because hypovolaemia is characteristically absent. In practice there is considerable overlap between SIADH and sodium depletion. [4, 5] During low sodium intake, or low urine output, (reflected in high urine creatinine/plasma ratio), even FeNa may be low (<0.5%) in the SIADH. [5] The combination of FeNa<0.5% and fractional excretion urea (Fe urea) improves prediction of the response to saline. [4, 5]

However, during low urine output (antidiuresis) from sodium depletion, the FeNa is even lower, <0.15 %, and the Fe urea <45 % [5].

If the differential diagnosis between SIADH and sodium depletion is uncertain a trial of saline infusion can be carried out safely provided serum Na$^+$ is monitored. Infusion of 2 L of n.Saline over 24 hours increase plasma sodium by at least 5 mmol/L, and combined with low FeNa, identified sodium depletion.[6,7] Decrease in plasma sodium of up to 4 mmol/L occurred in a minority with the SIADH who had a urinary concentration of Na$^+$ + K$^+$ of 300 mmol/L or over suggesting that this strategy is safe. [7]

Urine Potassium.

Urine potassium indicates whether hypokalaemia is due to renal or gastrointestinal causes.

Urine potassium should be < 20mmol/L during diarrhoea, for example from laxative abuse. Apart from diarrhoeal disorders external potassium losses nearly always occur from the kidney. Nearly all K^+ is reabsorbed proximal to collecting ducts so that urinary K^+ is mainly due to secretion by Principal cells in collecting ducts. Common renal causes of potassium depletion are vomiting, diuretics, hereditary tubular disorders, diabetic ketoacidosis, excessive action of mineralocorticoids and rarely sweating. Hypokalaemia from vomiting is due to high urinary losses of potassium: hypovolaemia increases Na^+ reabsorption in exchange for K^+ in cortical collecting ducts (CCD). Figure (1) shows an approach for the analysis of hypokalaemia.

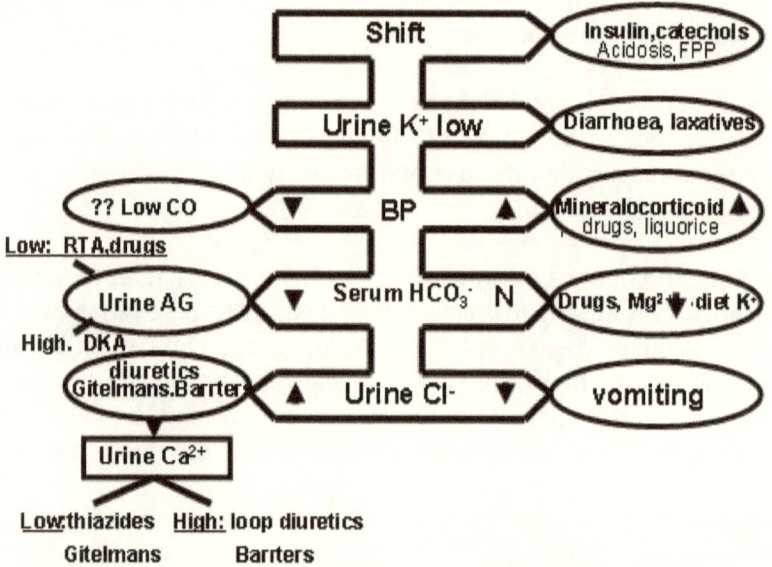

Figure 1: Approach to the Diagnosis of Hypokalaemia. catechols = catecholamines.

- Urinary Cl- is low from vomiting and sweating but increased from diuretic use and mineralocorticoid action.
- Raised blood pressure helps distinguish hypokalaemia due to raised mineralocorticoid secretion, in which blood pressure is raised, from surreptitious diuretic use.
- Loop diuretics and Barrter's syndrome can be differentiated from thiazide diuretic (or indapamide) use and Gitelman syndrome by urinary calcium concentration: this is raised from loop diuretics and lower than normal from thiazide use and Gitelman syndrome. A high Fe K^+ (>20%) is useful in predicting diuretic intake.[4]

Severe Hypomagnesaemia is a clue to the diagnosis of Gitelman syndrome because it is uncommon from use of thiazide diuretics.

Hyperkalaemia. Urine potassium is raised in patients with hyperkalaemia with rare exceptions, such as Familial Hyperkalaemic Periodic Paralysis Relatively low urine potassium suggests a defect in K^+ secretion in the CCD. Spot urine potassium concentration may be misleading, however, because it also depends on water reabsorption, which concentrates K^+ as tubular fluid passes down medullary collecting ducts. [2, 7] The transtubular potassium gradient (TTKG) gives a more sensitive indication of the efficiency of the CCD in both excreting and conserving potassium. [2, 8, 9]

$$TTKG = \frac{(K^+ \text{ urine})}{K^+ \text{ serum}} \times \frac{\text{Serum osmolality}}{\text{Urine osmolality}}$$

The rationale is as follows: tubular fluid in the CCD is in equilibrium with interstitium of renal cortex - ~300 $mOsmol/kgH_2O$, providing ADH is not suppressed. For example, If urine osmolality is $1200 mOsmol/kgH_2O$ and osmolality of tubular fluid assumed to be $300 mOsml/kgH_2o$, the concentration of tubular fluid K^+ in the CCD can be estimated as one quarter of the urinary K^+ concentration—Urine K x 300/1200. The estimate of K^+ concentration in the CCD is then related to serum K^+.

TTKG = urine K^+ concentration X (300 / actual urine osmolality) ÷ serum K^+.

For example if serum K^+ is 6.0mmol/L, urine K^+ 60mmol/L and urine osmolality 600 $mOsmol/kgH_2O$, tubular fluid concentration in the cortical collecting duct assumed to be 300 $mOsmol/kg/H_2O$:

TTKG = 60 ÷ 2 (= 30) divided by 6.0mmol/L = 5.0.

The TTKG, in the example above, indicates that function of the CCD is deficient despite a urinary K^+ concentration of 60mmol/L.

During hyperkalaemia TTKG should be >10.0. During hypokalaemia TTKG should be <2.0. [6]

However the assumptions above may not be correct: reabsorption of urea and recycling to the collecting duct may result in a higher osmolality than 300mOsmol/kg; and potassium may also be reabsorbed in the distal collecting ducts.

The usefulness of the TTKG has not been validated apart from case series. [8] It is most useful in the diagnosis of defective action of mineralocorticoids because improvement follows fludrocortisone administration [8]. The TTKG has also been shown to differentiate renal causes of hypokalaemia from Familial Periodic Paralysis: the TTKG was ≤2.0 in episodes of Familial Periodic Paralysis [10] because K^+ conservation by the kidney is normal.

Urine Magnesium.

Urine magnesium separates the two most common causes of hypomagnesaemia: urinary magnesium <0.5mmol/L occurs in gastrointestinal causes; a high level suggests renal losses of magnesium. There is a catch however: urinary magnesium may be low during severe hypomagnesaemia in Hereditary Hypomagnesaemia with secondary hypocalcaemia, due to a loss of function mutation of magnesium channels (TRPM6). Despite a decrease in transcellular reabsorption in both kidney and small intestine paracellular magnesium reabsorption can compensate for defective action of the TRPM6 and result in low urine magnesium when hypomagnesaemia is severe. To differentiate renal from gastrointestinal causes urine magnesium should ideally be measured when serum Mg^{2+} is above 0.45 mmol/L.

Urine Calcium.

This is important in separating disorders of thick ascending limbs loops of Henle, TALH, from distal convoluted tubules (DCT). Urine calcium is abnormally low (<5mmol/L) in patients with Gitelman syndrome or those taking thiazide diuretics. Urine calcium is increased in Barrters syndrome and in those taking loop diuretics. Memory is facilitated by recall that hypercalcaemia is treated with loop diuretics whereas thiazide diuretics, which decreases urinary calcium loss, is sometimes used in patients with osteoporosis or renal stones,

The diagnosis of Gitelmans syndrome and differentiation from Barrter's syndrome is supported by measuring urine electrolytes following administration of 50mg hydrochlorothiazide but is rarely required: patients with Gitelman's but not Barrter's syndrome have a blunted diuretic effect especially in fractional excretion of Cl^- (Fe Cl^-). [10]

Cause of Metabolic Acidosis. [11-14]: (Chapter 6)

Urinary pH measures free H^+ excretion but may mislead if used in assessment because this is a small part of total acid excretion.

Urine NH_4^+ excretion is the main component of acid excretion: the normal excretion of 30-40mmol/day can increase to >200mmol/day during severe metabolic acidosis. Thus low ammonium excretion during metabolic acidosis indicates that acid excretion is defective. However urinary ammonium measurement is rarely available outside of research laboratories. Urinary anion gap (net charge) gives an estimate of urinary ammonium concentration or excretion. This is derived as follows.

To satisfy electroneutrality urine cations must equal anions:

$$Na^+ + K^+ + 2Ca^{2+} + 2Mg^{2+} + NH_4^+ = Cl^- + H_2Po_4^- + 2HPO_4^{2-} + 2So_4^{2-} + HCo_3^- + \text{organic acids.}$$

Phosphate, sulfate, organic acids, calcium and magnesium do not change appreciably during metabolic acidosis and HCo_3^- is not excreted in acid urine. The average difference between the unmeasured anions and cations is 80mmol/L.

$$\underline{Na^+ + K^+ + NH_4^+ = Cl^- + 80.}$$

Therefore when urine AG is zero ammonium excretion is approximately 80mmol/L. An estimate of 24-hour excretion can be obtained using a spot urine creatinine which is normally 20mg/kg/day or approximately 1.4g/day.

During acidosis there should be a high net negative charge:

$Cl^- > (Na^+ + K^+)$ indicates a NH_4^+ excretion > 80mmol/L.

During acidosis net positive charge: $(NH_4^+ \leq 80mmol/L)$ is abnormal.

This concept was tested in normal subjects given oral NH_4Cl ; patients with diarrhoea; and those with distal renal tubular acidosis [13]. Urine pH of 5.64 units in subjects with diarrhoea was misleading as an index of acid secretion in suggesting less than maximum H^+ secretion was achieved. This occurs because maximum H^+ secretion is dependent on exchange of H^+ for Na^+ in distal tubules which is limited by decreased delivery of

Na$^+$ in patients with a low cardiac output from sodium depletion or heart failure. [11]

	Urine AG	Estimated NH4 excretion	Urine pH
Normal subjects given NH$_4$$^+$Cl	-27	107	4.9
Diarrhoea	-20	100	5.64
Distal Renal tubular acidosis Type I	+23	57	
Hyperkalaemia DTRA	+30	50	
Selective aldosterone ↓	+39	41	

Table 1: *Urine anion Gap (AG), arterial blood pH and ammonium excretion in normal subjects given NH$_4$Cl, subjects with Renal Tubular Acidosis and subjects with diarrhea.(modified from reference.* [13]

Administration of frusemide to increase Na$^+$ delivery to distal tubules in three of the above subjects with diarrhoea led to lower pH levels of 4.9, 4.3 and 5.1. [12]

In addition correction of sodium depletion led to a change in urine anion gap from -20 to -115mmol/L suggesting that decrease in free H$^+$ secretion, secondary to sodium depletion, also limited NH$_4$$^+$ excretion.

Thus maximum urine pH and NH$_4$$^+$ excretion during acidosis require adequate Na$^+$ delivery to distal tubules. The following table shows that urinary pH, anion gap and plasma K$^+$ is useful in the differential diagnosis of the causes of distal renal tubular acidosis.

	Urine AG	Urine pH	Plasma K$^+$
Normal	Negative	<5.5	N
Selective aldosterone deficiency	Positive	<5.5	↑
Hyperkalaemic DRTA	Positive	>5.5	↑
Type I DRTA	Positive	>5.5	N or ↓
Bicarbonate loss	Positive	>5.5	N or ↓

Table 2: *Urine pH, Anion Gap (AG) and plasma potassium in Distal Renal Tubular Acidosis (DRTA).*

Several factors may confound interpretation of urinary anion gap:

* Infection with urea splitting organisms may cause an increase in NH_4^+ and pH.
* Presence of unmeasured cations such as Lithium.
* Decreased Na^+ delivery to principal cells in collecting ducts, which limits $Na^+:H^+$ exchange reduces tubular fluid H^+ concentration, decreases trapping of NH_3 as NH_4^+ and decreases NH_4^+Cl excretion.
* The presence of unmeasured anions—which take the place of Cl^- lowers the difference between urinary Cl^- and measured cations ($Na^+ + K^+$) and thus decreases estimated urinary AG and NH_4^+ concentration. Unmeasured anions include HCo_3^- in alkaline urine, ketoanions; anions associated with Na^+ or K^+ in drugs such as penicillins acetyl salicylic acid, D lactate and SO_4^{2-}.

Decreased Na^+ delivery can be excluded as a cause of RTA by administering frusemide or infusing n.Saline.

The presence and effect of unmeasured anions can be estimated by measurement of urine osmolar gap.

Tests to Establish the Diagnosis of Renal Tubular Acidosis.

Urine anion gap is only useful if acidosis is present. Acidosis can be induced by NH_4^+Cl.

Oral NH4+Cl administration.: NH_4^+Cl o.1g per kg is administered. The urine pH and anion gap is measured for five hours. This has been superseded by the following.

Urine pH is measured following administration of both Furosemide and fludrocortisone. Urinary pH decreased to less than 5.3 in all controls compared to none of those with renal tubular acidosis. Furosemide increases sodium delivery to distal tubules and fludrocortisone stimulates Na^+ reabsorption in exchange for K^+ and H^+. [13].

Urine Osmolar Gap. (OG) [2, 15]

Estimation of NH_4^+ excretion using urine AG depends on the assumption that Cl^- is the main urinary anion. However if another anion is present in appreciable amounts, such as βOH butyrate, the AG will give a misleading estimate of NH_4^+ excretion because βhydroxybutyrate, which is not measured, is excreted with NH_4^+. The urine osmolar gap (OG) is independent of the type of anion. It is the difference between estimated and measured urine osmolality. A large difference is usually due to an unmeasured anion.

<u>Estimated Urine Osmolality = $2(Na^+ + K^+)$ + urea (mmol/L) + glucose (mmol/L)</u>

The Na^+ and K^+ are doubled to include accompanying anions whereas glucose and urea, which are non-ionic, have no accompanying anions and are not doubled.

<u>Urine OG = Measured—estimated urine osmolality.</u>

The difference should be $<15mOsm/kgH_2O$.

A large OG suggests that an unmeasured anion is present in abnormal amounts. Examples are βOH butyrate from starvation or diabetic ketoacidosis, aspirin poisoning, penicillinate anions from high dose penicillin therapy, sulfur containing compounds, which give rise to SO_4^{2-} and D.lactate. For example urine β hydroxybutyrate gives a negative test for ketones.Thus an abnormally low urine anion gap due to β hydroxybutyrate might suggest that ammonium excretion and acidification are defective but an abnormally high osmolar gap indicates that an unmeasured anion is present in urine. [15]

Urine pCO2. [16]

This measurement is used in the differential diagnosis of the cause of Renal Tubular Acidosis. The rationale of the test is that bicarbonate reaching distal tubule is converted to $H_2CO_3^-$ by H^+ secreted by Proton (H^+ ATPase) pumps.

$$HCO_3^- + H^+ \longrightarrow H_2CO_3^- \longrightarrow CO_2 + H_2O$$

Carbonic anhydrase is absent in the lumen of distal tubules so that $H_2CO_3^-$ is only slowly converted to CO_2. Permeability to CO_2 is low in the distal tubule so that CO_2 liberated from H_2CO_3 remains in tubular fluid. Therefore, in the presence of metabolic alkalosis, in which bicarbonate reaches distal tubules, <u>urine blood: PCO_2 ratio</u> increases.

When H^+ secretion is defective HCO_3^- is not converted to CO_2 and urinary PCO_2 is approximately the same as blood pCO_2. The test is carried out by giving intravenous $NaHCO_3^-$ 0.5-2.0mmol/kg so that the urine pH exceeds arterial blood pH. PCO_2 is measured on freshly voided urine. Collection under oil is unnecessary provided urine is not allowed to stand for more than 5 minutes.

This test distinguishes inadequate H^+ secretion from primary proton pump disorders due to voltage defects due to inadequate Na^+ delivery to distal tubules because increased $NaHCO_3^-$ is reabsorbed proximally in sodium depletion. In patients with Type I distal tubular acidosis, due to dysfunction of H^+ secretion, the urine blood difference in pCO_2 was 2.0mmHg($\pm$ 2.2) compared to 32.7mmHg($\pm$ 3.1) in controls.

Urine Osmolality.

Urine osmolality is mainly determined by urea and electrolytes (non-urea solutes). Urea excretion, usually ~ 500-600 mOsmol/day, depends on dietary protein intake and (endogenous) catabolism of tissue. Urine osmolality is useful in diagnosis of polyuria and hypernatraemia but adds little to measurement of urine sodium in the diagnosis of hypovolaemia and "inappropriate ADH secretion".

Water abstraction from tubular fluid in cortical collecting ducts should be maximal during hypernatraemia. Maximum osmolality depends on:

- Medullary tonicity. This decreases from malnutrition or a low protein diet and decreases maximal urine osmolality under conditions of water deprivation.
- The ratio between urea: non-urea solutes. (chapter 4). Urea obligates water excretion when urine electrolytes are low but does not obligate excretion of water when urine electrolytes are high: this depends on the ratio of urea: non-urea solutes. Maximum urine osmolality may vary between 600-1200mOsmol/kgH$_2$O because of this and the factors described above.

Urine osmolality is useful in assessment of hypernatraemia because this should be maximum when hypernatraemia is present. Thus urine osmolality estimates the adequacy of urine concentration. Urine osmolality is also useful in the differential diagnosis of Polyuria.

Polyuria may be due to a water diuresis from inadequate ADH secretion or solute diuresis as occurs in diabetes:

Urine osmolality is usually <150mOsmkg H$_2$o. In water diuresis.

Urine osmolality >300 mOsmol/kg H$_2$O. In solute diuresis.

Water diuresis may be due to inadequate ADH secretion; resistance to action of ADH (Nephrogenic diabetes insipidus); or Compulsive Polydipsia. (Details in chapter 4)

The best diagnostic test is to restrict water for 16-18 hours with careful monitoring of plasma sodium (or osmolality), urine osmolality (hourly), thirst, weight and access to water. If adequate urine osmolality is achieved (>600-800mOsm/L) diagnosis of compulsive water drinking is probable. Continued low urine osmolality, while serum osmolality rises, is usually diagnostic of central diabetes insipidus (inadequate ADH secretion) or less commonly nephrogenic diabetes insipidus.

If urine osmolality remains low, ADH is given which further increases urine concentration in Central Diabetes Insipidus but not in Nephrogenic Diabetes Insipidus. Following ADH or dDAVP urine osmolality is measured every 30 minutes for three hours. ADH should not increase osmolality in nephrogenic diabetes insipidus.

Nephrogenic Diabetes Insipidus may be hereditary or acquired from drugs, Lithium, hypercalcaemia, hypokalaemia or renal disease. Solute diuresis is usually due to glucose, or other solutes such as mannitol.

Inappropriate ADH Secretion.(Chapter 4)

Urine osmolality may be misleading in suggesting the diagnosis of inappropriate ADH secretion: a high urinary osmolality may be mainly due to urea which is an ineffective osmole.

Combined urinary Na^+ + K^+ gives a less misleading indication of excretion of solute free water. Alternatively urine Na^+ concentration alone indicates whether hypovolaemia is present and that unsuppressed ADH secretion is appropriate.

The sum of urinary concentration of Na^+ + K^+ is also better than urine osmolality in signaling return of normal tubular dilution when hyponatraemia due to unsuppressed ADH secretion is managed. [16]

Severe Sodium Depletion.

Urine osmolality has traditionally been considered to be raised in severe sodium depletion. However urine osmolality may be low, normal or high in severe sodium depletion depending on the concentration of K^+, urea and intake of free water. The urine sodium concentration is low and is useful in diagnosis; urine osmolality is not.

For example in breast feeding infants with diarrhoea[18] and in beer potomania[19] urinary osmolality is usually low because of low solute excretion and continued intake of milk or beer, both of low sodium and potassium concentration, despite severe sodium depletion. In infants with severe sodium depletion from diarrhoea urine refraction which correlates with urine osmolality was very low. [18]

Urinary Uric Acid. [20]

The fractional excretion of uric acid is useful in the diagnostic separation of diuretic related causes of hyponatraemia and inappropriate ADH secretion where it is lower.

The following summarizes the serum and urinary changes in disorders of vomiting, diarrhoea, diuretic use, urinary tubular disorders and Diabetic Ketoacidosis.

	SERUM					URINE					OTHER
	Na^+	K^+	HCO_3^-	AG	Other	Na^+	K^+	Cl^-	pH	AG	
Vomiting early	N	↓	↑+	N		↑	↑	↓	N↑	-	
Intermediate	N	↓	↓+	N		↓	↑	↓	↑N		
Late	N↓	↓++	↑++	N		↓	↓	↓	↓	-	
Diarrhoea (laxatives)	N↓	↓	↓	N		↓	↓	↑	↓	↑	↑urine NH_4^+
Diuretics -											
Current	N↓	↓	N↑	N		↑	↑	↑	-		Thiazides Urine Ca low Serum Na^+ may ↓
Remote	N	↓	↑	N		↓	↓	↓	-		Loop: urine Ca ↑
Barrters			Similar to loop diuretics								
Gitelman's			Similar To Thiazide Diuretics serum Mg↓ urine Ca low								
RTA I	N↓	↓	↓	↓		↑	↑	↓	<5.8	+ve	
RTA II	N	↓	↓	N		↑	↑	-		N	
RTA IV	N↓	↑	↓	N		↑	↓	↑	>5.8	N	
Keto Acid.	↑↓N	↓N	↓	↑		↑	↑	↑	<5.8	N+	

Table 3. Typical serum and urinary electrolytes in various conditions.
Remote refers to 2-4 days previous diuretic use. RTA=renal tubular acidosis. N=normal; Keto acid = ketoacidosis.

REFERENCES

1. Chung AM, Kluge R, Schrier RW, Anderson RJ: Clinical assessment of extracellular fluid volume in hyponatraemia. *Amer J. Med.* **83**:905-8, 1987.

2. Kamel KS, Ethier JH, Richardson RMA, et al: Urine Electrolytes and osmolality. When and How to use them. *Amer J. Nephrol.* **10**:89-102, 1990.

3. Kamel, KS. Magner,PO ElthierJH.Halperin ML. Urine electrolytes in the assessment of extracellular fluid volume contraction. American J Nephrology.**9**:344-347 1989.

4. Musch W, Thimpont J, Vandervede D, et al: Combined Fractional Excretion of sodium and urea. Better Predicts Response to Saline in Hyponatraemia. *Amer J. Med.* **99**:348-356, 1995.

5. Musch W, Hedeshi A, Decaux G: Low sodium excretion in SIADH.Patients with low Diuresis. Nephron Physiology **96** 11-18 2004.

6. Musch W, Hedeshi A, Decaux G: Treating the syndrome of inappropriate ADH secretion with isotonic saline.QJM **91** 749-753 1998

7. Musch W,Decaux G:Utility and limitations of biochemical parameters in the evaluation of hyponatraemia in the elderly.Int Urology & Nephrol **32** 475-493 2001

8. Choi MJ, Ziyadeh F: The Utility of the Transtubular Potassium Gradient in the Evaluation of Hyperkalaemia. *J. Am. Soc. Nephrol.* **19**:424-426, 2008.

9. Shua-Hua Lin, Yah-Feng L, Dung-Tsa C, et al: Laboratory tests to determine the cause of Hypokalaemia and Paralysis. *Arch. Int. Med.* **164**:1561-1566, 2004.

10. Colussi G, Bettinelli A, Tedeschi S, et al: A Thiazide Test for the Diagnosis of Renal Tubular Hypokalaemia Disorders. *Clin. J. Amer. Soc. Nephrol.* **2**:454-460, 2007.

11. Goldstein MB, B ear R, Richardson RMA, et al: The urine anion gap: a clinically useful index of ammonium excretion. *Amer J. Med Science.* **292**:198-202, 1986.

12. Battle DC, Riotte A, Schlueter W: Urinary sodium in the Evaluation of Hyperchloraemic Metabolic Acidosis. *New Engl J Med.* **316**:140-143, 1987.

13. Battle DC, Hizon M, et al: The use of the urinary anion gap in the diagnosis of Hyperchloraemic Metabolic Acidosis. *New Engl J med.* **318**:594-9, 1988.

14. Walsh SB, Shirley DG, Wrong OM, Unwin RJ: Urinary acidification assessed by simultaneous furosemide and fludrocortisone treatment: an

alternative to ammonium chloride. *Kidney International.* **71**:1310-1316, 2007.

15. Halperin ML, et al: The urine Osmolal Gap: A clue to estimating urinary ammonium in "Hybrid" types of Metabolic Acidosis. *Clinical & Investigative Medicine.* **11**:198-202, 1988.

16. Halperin ML, Goldstein MB, Haig A, et al: Studies on the pathogenesis of Type I (Distal) Renal Tubular Acidosis as revealed by the urinary PCO_2 tensions. *J. Clin. Invest.* **53**:669-677, 1974.

17. Kamel K S, Bear RA Treatment of Hyponatraemia: A Quantitative Analysis. Amer.J.Kid Dis.**21** 439-443 1993

18. Kingston ME: Electrolyte Disturbances in Breast-Fed Infants with Gastroenteritis and Dehydration. *J. Pediatr.* **83**:1073, 1973.

19. Sanghvi SR, Kellerman PS, Nanovic L: Beer Potomania: An unusual cause of hyponatraemia at high risk of complications from rapid correction. *Amer. J. Kid. Dis.* **50**; 673-680, 2007.

20. Wiebke F, Stork S, Koschker AC, et al: Value of fractional uric acid excretion in differential diagnosis of hyponatraemic patients on diuretics. *The Journal Clinical Endocrinol &Metabolism.* 2008, doi: 10.1210/jc.